# Handbook of Measurement Error Models

**Chapman & Hall/CRC**
**Handbooks of Modern Statistical Methods**

**Series Editor**
Garrett Fitzmaurice, *Department of Biostatistics, Harvard School of Public Health, Boston, MA, U.S.A.*

The objective of the series is to provide high-quality volumes covering the state-of-the-art in the theory and applications of statistical methodology. The books in the series are thoroughly edited and present comprehensive, coherent, and unified summaries of specific methodological topics from statistics. The chapters are written by the leading researchers in the field and present a good balance of theory and application through a synthesis of the key methodological developments and examples and case studies using real data.

**Published Titles**

**Handbook of Spatial Epidemiology**
*Andrew B. Lawson, Sudipto Banerjee, Robert P. Haining, and María Dolores Ugarte*

**Handbook of Neuroimaging Data Analysis**
*Hernando Ombao, Martin Lindquist, Wesley Thompson, and John Aston*

**Handbook of Statistical Methods and Analyses in Sports**
*Jim Albert, Mark E. Glickman, Tim B. Swartz, and Ruud H. Koning*

**Handbook of Methods for Designing, Monitoring, and Analyzing Dose-Finding Trials**
*John O'Quigley, Alexia Iasonos, and Björn Bornkamp*

**Handbook of Quantile Regression**
*Roger Koenker, Victor Chernozhukov, Xuming He, and Limin Peng*

**Handbook of Statistical Methods for Case-Control Studies**
*Ørnulf Borgan, Norman Breslow, Nilanjan Chatterjee, Mitchell H. Gail, Alastair Scott, and Chris J. Wild*

**Handbook of Environmental and Ecological Statistics**
*Alan E. Gelfand, Montserrat Fuentes, Jennifer A. Hoeting, and Richard L. Smith*

**Handbook of Approximate Bayesian Computation**
*Scott A. Sisson, Yanan Fan, and Mark Beaumont*

**Handbook of Graphical Models**
*Marloes Maathuis, Mathias Drton, Steffen Lauritzen, and Martin Wainwright*

**Handbook of Mixture Analysis**
*Sylvia Frühwirth-Schnatter, Gilles Celeux, and Christian P. Robert*

**Handbook of Infectious Disease Data Analysis**
*Leonhard Held, Niel Hens, Philip O'Neill, and Jacco Walllinga*

**Handbook of Meta-Analysis**
*Christopher H. Schmid, Theo Stijnen, and Ian White*

**Handbook of Forensic Statistics**
*David L. Banks, Karen Kafadar, David H. Kaye, and Maria Tackett*

**Handbook of Statistical Methods for Randomized Controlled Trials**
*KyungMann Kim, Frank Bretz, Ying Kuen K. Cheung, and Lisa Hampson*

**Handbook of Measurement Error Models**
*Grace Y. Yi, Aurore Delaigle, and Paul Gustafson*

**Handbook of Survival Analysis**
*John P. Klein, Hans C. van Houwelingen, Joseph G. Ibrahim, Thomas H. Scheike*

For more information about this series, please visit: https://www.crcpress.com/Chapman--Hall-CRC-Handbooks-of-Modern-Statistical-Methods/book-series/CHHANMODSTA

# Handbook of Measurement Error Models

Edited by

Grace Y. Yi, Aurore Delaigle, and Paul Gustafson

CRC Press
Taylor & Francis Group
Boca Raton London New York

CRC Press is an imprint of the
Taylor & Francis Group, an **informa** business
A CHAPMAN & HALL BOOK

First edition published 2021
by CRC Press
6000 Broken Sound Parkway NW, Suite 300, Boca Raton, FL 33487-2742

and by CRC Press
2 Park Square, Milton Park, Abingdon, Oxon, OX14 4RN



ISBN: 978-1-138-10640-6 (hbk)
ISBN: 978-1-032-07008-7 (pbk)
ISBN: 978-1-315-10127-9 (ebk)

DOI: 10.1201/9781315101279

Typeset in CMR10
by KnowledgeWorks Global Ltd.

Visit the companion website/eResources: https://www.routledge.com/Handbook-of-Measurement-Error-Models/Yi-Delaigle-Gustafson/p/book/9781138106406

MIX
Paper from responsible sources
FSC™ C013985
FSC www.fsc.org

Printed in the United Kingdom
by Henry Ling Limited

# Contents

# Preface

Valid inference results rely not only on sensible modeling and analysis methods, but also on good quality data. Error-contaminated data, however, are ubiquitous in applications. Measurement error has been a longstanding concern in various fields including clinical trials, cancer research, epidemiological studies, environmental studies, economics, survey sampling, and so on. Investigators often confront error-prone data with the urgent need to address measurement error impacts in their data analysis. Even though intensive research has been directed to measurement error problems, measurement error methods have not been used frequently in situations that merit their use. Lack of adequate understanding of measurement error effects and necessary analytical skills for handling them are perhaps the primary reasons.

While a large body of literature and several research monographs on measurement error models are available, research in this area has continued to attract growing attention. By carefully editing 24 chapters contributed from active scholars in the area, we hope this handbook will offer a good starting point for the readers who wish to start research and gain insight into measurement error models. This volume is also designed to serve as a quick reference to statistical methods and applications pertinent to measurement error models for researchers and analysts. The handbook is comprised of 7 parts which provide an overview of issues and challenges, measurement error impacts, modeling strategies, inference methods, and applications. It aims to strike a nice balance among different topics on methodology and application areas.

This handbook would not have been possible without the excellent contributions from the authors of the chapters. We are grateful for their outstanding commitment and immense patience during the course of assembling the volume. We are thankful for many colleagues for their discussions, enthusiasm, and support for this handbook. We are particularly indebted to Donna Spiegelman who helped plan the volume, contacted chapter contributors, and offered expertise. Special thanks go to Raymond Carroll, Leonard Stefanski, and Laurence Freedman. Finally, we express our sincere gratitude to John Kimmel of Chapman & Hall/CRC. His strong beliefs in this project, professional advice, and timely assistance have kept this project on track until reaching its final destination.

Grace Y. Yi, Aurore Delaigle, and Paul Gustafson
June 8, 2021

# *Editors*

**Grace Y. Yi** is a Professor in the Department Statistical and Actuarial Sciences and the Department of Computer Science at the University of Western Ontario where she holds a Tier I Canada Research Chair in Data Science. She is a Fellow of the Institute of Mathematical Statistics, Fellow of the American Statistical Association, the 2010 recipient of the CRM-SSC Prize in Statistics, and an Elected Member of the International Statistical Institute. Her research interests focus on developing methodology to address challenges concerning measurement error, causal inference, imaging data, missing data, high dimensional data, survival data, and longitudinal data. She authored the monograph "*Statistical Analysis with and Measurement Error or Misclassification: Strategy, Method and Application*" (2017, Springer). She has served the professions in various capacities. She was the Editor-in-Chief of *The Canadian Journal of Statistics* (2016–2018), is currently the Editor of Statistical Methodology Section for *The New England Journal of Statistics in Data Science*, and will be a co-Editor-in-Chief of *The Electronic Journal of Statistics* (2022–2024). She was the President of the Biostatistics Section of the Statistical Society of Canada in 2016 and the Founder of the first chapter (Canada Chapter, established in 2012) of International Chinese Statistical Association. Currently, she takes on the Presidency of the Statistical Society of Canada for the period of 2020–2022.

**Aurore Delaigle** is a Professor at the School of Mathematics and Statistics at the University of Melbourne. She is a Fellow of the Australian Academy of Science, a Fellow of the Institute of Mathematical Statistics, a Fellow of the American Statistical Association, and an Elected Member of the International Statistical Institute. She is a past recipient of the George W. Snedecor Award from the Committee of Presidents of Statistical Societies (COPSS), and of the Moran Medal from the Australian Academy of Science. Her research interests focus mainly on nonparametric methods, measurement error, group testing data, functional data and other types of indirect data. She is currently co Editor-in-Chief of *the Journal of the Royal Statistical Society, Series B*, and was the Executive Secretary of the Institute of Mathematical Statistics (2011–2017) and of the International Society for Nonparametric Statistics (2013–2018).

**Paul Gustafson** is a Professor in the Department of Statistics at the University of British Columbia. He is a Fellow of the American Statistical Association, the 2008 recipient of the CRM-SSC Prize in Statistics, and the 2020 Gold

Medallist of the Statistical Society of Canada. His research interests include Bayesian methods, causal inference, evidence synthesis, measurement error, and partial identification. He has authored two books: *Measurement Error and Misclassification in Statistics and Epidemiology: Impact and Bayesian Adjustments* (2004, Chapman and Hall / CRC Press), and *Bayesian Inference for Partially Identified Models* (2015, Chapman and Hall / CRC Press). He was the Editor-in-Chief of the Canadian Journal of Statistics (2007–2009) and is currently the Special Editor for Statistical Methods for the journal *Epidemiology.* Paul served as a founding Co-director of the Master of Data Science program at UBC, and currently serves as Head of the Department of Statistics.

# Contributors

**Tatiyana Apanasovich**
Department of Statistics
George Washington University
USA

**Jonathan W. Bartlett**
Department of Mathematical Sciences
University of Bath
United Kingdom

**John P. Buonaccorsi**
Department of Mathematics and Statistics
University of Massachusetts
USA

**Jeffrey S. Buzas**
Department of Mathematics and Statistics
University of Vermont
USA

**Howard H. Chang**
Department of Biostatistics and Bioinformatics
Emory University
USA

**Aurore Delaigle**
School of Mathematics and Statistics
University of Melbourne
Australia

**Annamaria Guolo**
Department of Statistical Science
University of Padova
Italy

**Paul Gustafson**
Department of Statistics
University of British Columbia
Canada

**Yicheng Kang**
Department of Mathematical Sciences
Bentley University
USA

**Joshua P. Keller**
Department of Statistics
Colorado State University
USA

**Ingrid Van Keilegom**
Faculty of Economics and Business
KU Leuven
Belgium

**Ruth H. Keogh**
Department of Medical Statistics
London School of Hygiene and Tropical Medicine
United Kingdom

DOI: 10.1201/9781315101279-0

**Arthur Lewbel**
Department of Economics
Boston College
USA

**Hua Liang**
Department of Statistics
George Washington University
USA

**Wei Liu**
Department of Mathematics and Statistics
York University
Canada

**Yanyuan Ma**
Department of Statistics
Pennsylvania State University
USA

**Peihua Qiu**
Department of Biostatistics
University of Florida
USA

**John W. Seaman, Jr.**
Department of Statistical Science
Baylor University
USA

**Pamela A. Shaw**
Department of Biostatistics, Epidemiology and Informatics
University of Pennsylvania
USA

**Samiran Sinha**
Department of Statistics
Texas A& M University
USA

**Weixing Song**
Department of Statistics
Kansas State University
USA

**James D. Stamey**
Department of Statistical Science
Baylor University
USA

**Linda Valeri**
Department of Biostatistics
Columbia University
USA

**Liqun Wang**
Department of Statistics
University of Manitoba
Canada

**Lang Wu**
Department of Statistics
University of British Columbia
Canada

**Grace Y. Yi**
Department Statistical and Actuarial Sciences
Department of Computer Science
University of Western Ontario
Canada

**Hongbin Zhang**
Department of Epidemiology and Biostatistics
City University of New York
USA

**David M. Zucker**
Department of Statistics
Hebrew University of Jerusalem
Israel

# Part I

# Introduction

# 1

# *Measurement Error Models - A Brief Account of Past Developments and Modern Advancements*

**Grace Y. Yi and Jeffrey S. Buzas**

## CONTENTS



## 1.1 Introduction

Measurement error arises in applications across many different fields and has been a longstanding concern in various disciplines including epidemiological studies, environmental studies, economics, survey sampling, etc.

While we may attempt to collect good quality data by careful design, measurement error is inevitable. Measurement error arises with different reasons and from different sources. Measurement error may refer to random noise, sampling error, or uncertainty and variation involved with the measuring process. An absence of clear and understandable rules, guidelines, and standards for

DOI: 10.1201/9781315101279-1

data collection and reporting processes can result in imprecise measurements. Due to the sensitivity of certain questions, reporting errors commonly arise so that the corresponding variables cannot be accurately measured. Sometimes, variables are impossible to measure precisely due to the nature of the variables themselves. For example, some variables represent averages of certain quantities over time, and any measurements at a particular time point would fluctuate around the long-term averages. In practice, we may artificially manipulate the measurements for security and confidentiality reasons. In other situations, it may be too expensive or time consuming to obtain a precise measurement of a variable, resulting in use of less expensive and/or convenient procedures to obtain surrogate measurements.

In this chapter, we take a brief tour of the development of measurement error strategies so as to appreciate the challenges facing analysts hoping to address measurement error in applications. To conduct sensible analyses for real world data which are commonly error-corrupted, it is critical to understand the impact of measurement error effects and develop correction adjustments for measurement error effects accordingly. Additionally, readers with an interest in the field of measurement error as a scientific discipline may gain an appreciation of the significant depth and breadth of results in the field of measurement error research.

In the literature, research on measurement error models may be categorized into three areas: (1) measurement error in covariates, (2) measurement error in the response variable, and (3) measurement error in both covariate and response variables. Our discussion here is directed to the first category with the highlight on how research in measurement error evolves over time.

## 1.2 Linear Measurement Error Model

In this section, we define a simple linear regression measurement error model and describe the effect of ignoring measurement error on estimation of the slope parameter.

Let $\{(Y_i, X_i) : i = 1, \ldots, n\}$ be a sequence of independent and identically distributed random variables, where $n$ is the sample size, $Y_i$ is a response variable, and $X_i$ is a covariate for $i = 1, \ldots, n$. In the presence of covariate measurement error, $X_i$ is often not observed, but a surrogate measurement $X_i^*$ is available for $i = 1, \ldots, n$. In the following discussion, we may drop the index $i$ and use the symbols $\{Y, X, X^*\}$ from time to time for ease of exposition.

Research on measurement error problems began with the simple linear regression measurement error model:

$$Y_i = \beta_0 + \beta_x X_i + \epsilon_i \tag{1.1}$$

with

$$X_i^* = X_i + e_i \tag{1.2}$$

for $i = 1, \ldots, n$, where $\beta_0$ and $\beta_x$ are regression parameters, $\epsilon_i$ is independent of $X_i$ with mean zero and a constant variance $\sigma^2$, and $e_i$ has zero mean and a constant variance $\sigma_e^2$. Usually, $e_i$ is assumed to be independent of $\{X_i, \epsilon_i\}$, which implies that *nondifferential* measurement error is considered, i.e., $f(y|x, x^*) = f(y|x)$, so that $X_i^*$ provides no additional information about the outcome $Y_i$ when $X_i$ is observed. Here and in the sequel, $f(\cdot|\cdot)$ represents the conditional probability density or mass function of the variables corresponding to the arguments.

Without a full distributional assumption for $\epsilon_i$, the least squares regression method is a natural option for estimation of the regression parameter $\beta = (\beta_0, \beta_x)^{\mathrm{T}}$. In the absence of measurements of the $X_i$, it is tempting to directly replace the $X_i$ with the available surrogate measurements $X_i^*$ in estimation procedures.

Let $\widehat{\beta}_x^*$ denote the resulting estimator of the slope $\beta_x$, given by

$$\widehat{\beta}_x^* = \frac{\sum_{i=1}^n (X_i^* - \overline{X}^*)(Y_i - \overline{Y})}{\sum_{i=1}^n (X_i^* - \overline{X}^*)^2},$$

where $\overline{X}^* = n^{-1}\sum_{i=1}^n X_i^*$ and $\overline{Y} = n^{-1}\sum_{i=1}^n Y_i$; this estimator is called a *naive* estimator of $\beta_x$.

The naive estimator $\widehat{\beta}_x^*$ is generally not a consistent estimator for the slope $\beta_x$ (Fuller, 1987). In fact,

$$\widehat{\beta}_x^* \xrightarrow{p} \beta_x^* \quad \text{as } n \to \infty \tag{1.3}$$

where $\beta_x^* = \lambda\beta_x$ with $\lambda = \sigma_x^2/(\sigma_x^2 + \sigma_e^2)$, and $\sigma_x^2$ is the variance of $X_i$. The factor $\lambda$, called the *reliability ratio*, is the ratio of the variability of $X_i$ to that of $X_i^*$:

$$\lambda = \frac{\mathrm{var}(X_i)}{\mathrm{var}(X_i^*)}.$$

Since $\lambda$ is no greater than 1, covariate measurement error in this case has an *attenuating* effect on estimation of the covariate effect $\beta_x$. The effects of measurement error on parameter estimation are much more complicated when multiple covariates are measured with error or there are additional covariates measured without error that are correlated with the mis-measured variable(s). For further details, see Carroll et al. (2006) and Gustafson (2021a).

## 1.3 Induced Regression and Regression Calibration

In contrast to the response model (1.1), we now examine the relationship between $Y$ and $X^*$ via the conditional expectation $E(Y|X^*)$. Assuming the nondifferential measurement error mechanism (the error model does not have to be (1.2)), iterating expectations gives that

$$\begin{aligned} E(Y|X^*) &= E\{E(Y|X^*)|X^*, X\} \\ &= E\{E(Y|X^*, X)|X^*\} \\ &= E\{E(Y|X)|X^*\}. \end{aligned}$$

The above identities hold for general linear or nonlinear regression models. Recognizing expectation as a smoothing operation, we conclude that the measurement error induced regression results in smoothing (or obscuring) the regression relationship between the outcome $Y$ and the predictor $X$.

For model (1.1),

$$\begin{aligned} E(Y|X^*) &= E\{E(Y|X)|X^*\} \\ &= \beta_0 + \beta_x E(X|X^*) \\ &= E\{Y|X = E(X|X^*)\}. \end{aligned}$$

This motivates the *regression calibration* method (Prentice, 1982), which estimates $\beta_x$ by regressing $Y$ on the conditional expectation $E(X|X^*)$. The implementation of the regression calibration method relies on the determination of $E(X|X^*)$, which requires the ability to estimate the density function of the latent variable $X$. This represents a difficult deconvolution problem, and typically approximations are used to avoid it. Assuming model (1.2), the best linear approximation to the regression of $X$ on $X^*$ is

$$E(X|X^*) \approx \mu_x + \sigma_{x|x^*}\sigma_{x^*}^{-2}(X^* - \mu_x),$$

where $\mu_x$ is the mean of $X$, $\sigma_{x|x^*} = \mathrm{Cov}(X, X^*) = \sigma_x^2$, and $\sigma_{x^*}^2 = \sigma_x^2 + \sigma_e^2$. The approximation suggests that additional data are needed for estimation and inference in the expanded model that includes $E(X|X^*)$. The need for additional informatoin is common to many estimation and inference approaches when there is covariate measurement error.

## 1.4 Identifiability

When the true covariate is not observed, it is natural to ask whether the model parameters can be consistently estimated, or even identifiable. In (1.1) and (1.2), if we impose a normal distribution on $\epsilon_i$ and $e_i$ as well as $X_i$, i.e.,

$$\epsilon_i \sim N(0, \sigma^2), \; e_i \sim N(0, \sigma_e^2), \text{ and } X_i \sim N(\mu_x, \sigma_x^2), \tag{1.4}$$

where $\sigma^2, \sigma_e^2, \mu_x$, and $\sigma_x^2$ are unknown parameters, then the joint distribution of $Y_i$ and $X_i^*$ is

$$N\left(\begin{pmatrix} \mu_y \\ \mu_x \end{pmatrix}, \begin{pmatrix} \sigma_y^2 & \sigma_{yx^*} \\ \sigma_{yx^*} & \sigma_{x^*}^2 \end{pmatrix}\right), \tag{1.5}$$

where $\sigma_y^2 = \beta_x^2\sigma_x^2 + \sigma^2$, $\sigma_{x^*}^2 = \sigma_x^2 + \sigma_e^2$, $\sigma_{yx^*} = \beta_x\sigma_x^2$, and $\mu_y = \beta_0 + \beta_x\mu_x$.

The initial models (1.1) and (1.2), together with (1.4), have six parameters, but the distribution (1.5) of $Y_i$ and $X_i^*$ involves only five parameters, expressed as functions of the original model parameters. This suggests that the original model parameters cannot be consistently estimated using the observed data $\{(Y_i, X_i^*) : i = 1, \ldots, n\}$, because they are not even identifiable from the model for the observed data.

To consistently estimate all the parameters, side conditions (or auxiliary data) are needed for estimation. Adcock (1877, 1878) considered estimation when the ratio $\sigma_x^2/\sigma_e^2$ is assumed to be known, resulting in orthogonal least squares estimation for $\beta_x$. Alternatively, other common identifiability choices are used in applications by adding a constraint on the parameters, including fixing the reliability ratio $\lambda = \sigma_x^2/(\sigma_x^2 + \sigma_e^2)$, $\sigma^2$, or $\sigma_e^2$ to be a given value or estimated with auxiliary data.

The linear model received much attention in the 1940s and 1950s, with many results focused on identifiability published in the econometrics literature. Neyman and Scott (1948) provided an interesting example of the failure of maximum likelihood when the number of parameters grows with the sample size, even when the model is identified.

Interestingly, if $X_i$ is not normal, the model is identified (Geary, 1942, 1943), and instrumental variable approaches (to be discussed below) can be used to construct consistent estimators. Geary developed instrumental variable estimators assuming higher central moments of $X_i$ are not zero. Wald (1940) developed an estimator based on grouping observations that seemed not to require additional identification information. However, his estimator requires an instrumental variable to define the groupings, and the existence of the instrumental variable requires certain knowledge of the measurement error distribution. Durbin (1954) provided another early example of an instrumental variable estimator in the context of Berkson measurement error. Some early references on identifiability issues include Reiersøl(1950), Robinson (1974), and Geraci (1976).

In a Bayesian context, Gustafson (2005) showed that there can be *indirect* learning about unidentified parameters that results from learning about identified parameters. Recently, Schennach and Hu (2013) showed that a very large class of regression models with covariate measurement error are identified without the need for auxiliary data. They proposed sieve regression for estimation. Bertrand, Van Keilegom and Legrand (2019) provided a novel method for estimating the measurement error variance that does not rely on auxiliary data, but assumes compact support for the distribution of the unobserved covariate $X$. Delaigle and Van Keilegom (2021) discussed estimation of the error distribution with or without extra data.

The recent identifiability results are impressive and in principle allow estimation without the need for auxiliary data (e.g., Gustafson, 2021b). However, while measurement error models may be identified without auxiliary data, Carroll et al. (2006) strongly recommended designing studies to obtain internal validation data whenever possible, because "... *it can be used with all known techniques, permits direct examination of the error structure, and typically leads to much greater precision of estimation and inference."* Most methods used in practice utilize auxiliary data; Wang (2021a) provided an overview of this topic.

## 1.5 Nonlinear Models

A substantial literature comprising impressive results was developed for linear measurement error models prior to 1980. Research for nonlinear models was sparse prior to 1980, but then exploded, beginning with the seminal papers by Prentice (1982) and Carroll et al. (1984). Prentice (1982) studied measurement error in survival models and suggested regression calibration as an approach to ameliorating the effects of measurement error. Carroll et al. (1984) proposed maximum likelihood estimators for Probit and other models for a binary outcome, with application to the Framingham data, and also suggested the use of regression calibration. Regression calibration was developed for logistic regression by Rosner, Willet and Spiegelman (1989) and Rosner, Spiegelman and Willet (1990). All those approaches require additional information for parameter estimation.

Using the same argument as in Section1.3 and again assuming nondifferential measurement error, with a nonlinear regression model with parameter $\beta_x$, we have that

$$\begin{aligned} E(Y|X^*) &= E\{E(Y|X)|X^*\} \\ &\neq E\{Y|X = E(X|X^*)\}. \end{aligned}$$

The non-equality results from the non-linearity of $E[Y|X]$ as a function of $X$. Therefore, regressing $Y$ on $E(X|X^*)$ may not produce consistent estimation of $\beta_x$ due to the nonlinear structure in the regression model. Using the regression calibration method may only lead to an *approximately* consistent estimator in nonlinear regression models.

For example, consider the logistic regression model for the binary response $Y$ and the covariate vector $X$,

$$P(Y = 1|X) = F(\beta_0 + \beta_x^{\mathrm{T}} X),$$

where $F(v) = (1+e^{-v})^{-1}$, and $\beta_0$ and $\beta_x$ are regression parameters. Under the nondifferential error assumption, Carroll et al. (1984) examined the induced regression model linking $Y$ and the surrogate $X^*$:

$$\begin{aligned} P(Y=1|X^*) &= \int P(Y=1|X=x, X^*=x^*) f(x|x^*) dx \\ &= \int P(Y=1|X=x) f(x|x^*) dx \\ &= \int F(\beta_0 + \beta_x^{\mathrm{T}} x) f(x|x^*) dx, \end{aligned}$$

where the integral is replaced by the summation if $X$ is discrete.

The final integral in the series of identities is typically analytically intractable, necessitating the approximation in the last line. When $\beta_x^2\sigma^2$ is not too large, $P(Y = 1|X^*)$ can be reasonably approximated by $F\{\beta_0 + \beta_x E(X|X^*)\}$ (Carroll et al. 1984). Therefore, in contrast to the linear model, replacing $X$ with $E(X|X^*)$ and running standard logistic analyses will only yield an approximately consistent estimator for the regression parameter $\beta_x$. An analogous statement holds for nonlinear models generally.

## 1.6 Development Timeline

While many important results on linear regression models with covariate measurement error were established in the mid-20th century, research on estimation and testing in nonlinear regression models with covariate measurement error increased rapidly beginning in the 1980s and continues to the present.

In this section we briefly discuss the development of several approaches to ameliorating the effects of covariate measurement error in a variety of inferential settings. We attempt a coarse-grained grouping of the methods according to the time (decade) when they emerged or were first most intensely studied, and mention a small sample of research articles that were important in the development of the methods. Not all papers cited fall within the designated decade.

### 1.6.1 1980-1989

In the period of 1980-1989, the following are major approaches and areas explored.

#### Likelihood Methods

Not surprisingly, likelihood methods were considered in some of the earliest papers to explore measurement error in nonlinear models, including the aforementioned Prentice (1982) and Carroll et al. (1984). Major challenges with likelihood approaches are modeling the unobserved distribution for $X$

and the potential sensitivity to mis-specification of this distribution, integrating over that distribution to obtain the likelihood of the observable data, and maximizing the resultant likelihood. These challenges, at least in part, spurred the development and use of regression calibration and other methods that do not require a model for the distribution of $X$.

Schafer (1987) is an early paper on the use of likelihood methods in covariate measurement error problems. He cast the measurement error problem as a missing data problem and proposed use of the EM algorithm to obtain approximate likelihood estimators. Fuller (1987) and Carroll et al. (1984) obtained the likelihood analytically for the linear regression and Probit models, respectively. Likelihood methods continued to be explored in the 1990s and beyond, with significant effort directed toward flexible parametric and semi-parametric approaches to modeling the latent distribution for $X$, see, for example, Roeder, Carroll and Lindsay (1996). Additional advancements were made in computation and maximization of likelihoods, see, for example, Schafer (2001, 2002). The Bayesian approach to measurement error adds priors to the likelihood and circumvents integration challenges with, typically, Markov chain Monte Carlo sampling (MCMC), discussed below. Research on likelihood methods continues to the present day, and discussions on this topic can be found in Yi (2021). Ma (2021) presented an account of semiparameteric methods rooted in the likelihood formation.

#### Regression Calibration

As noted in Section 1.3, regression calibration was proposed for proportional hazards models by Prentice (1982), and mention of the approach was made for linear models by Fuller (1987). Carroll and Stefanski (1990) developed regression calibration for a large class of models and expanded the model to provide better approximations in highly nonlinear models.

In its simplest guise, regression calibration imputes the unobserved $X$ with the best linear approximation to $E(X|X^*)$. The analyst then proceeds with the usual analysis (noting that standard errors will usually need revision). As noted above, regression calibration serves as an approximation to the induced regression of $Y$ on $X^*$, and can also be considered as an approximation to the likelihood for the observed data.

Although the regression calibration method only partially removes the bias induced from covariate measurement error in nonlinear models, its generality and straightforward implementation make this strategy popular in applications. A refined variant of regression calibration was developed by Freedman et al. (2004) using the moment reconstruction idea. Regression calibration has been implemented in Stata (Hardin, Schmiediche and Carroll, 2003). An account of this topic was provided by Shaw (2021).

### Conditional Scores

Stefanski and Carroll (1987) developed the conditional score approach to generalized linear models with covariate measurement error. Conditional scores are attractive because they essentially retain optimality properties enjoyed by likelihood estimators. The idea is to find a sufficient statistic for the unobserved covariate $X$ assuming other model parameters are known. Analysis is then conditional on this sufficient statistic, thereby removing dependence of the conditional likelihood score on the unobserved $X$, see also Lindsay (1982).

The conditional score for logistic regression with normally distributed additive measurement error is straightforward to construct, and in our experience is difficult to improve upon when the measurement error distribution is misspecified. The method was extended to the instrumental variable setting by Buzas and Stefanski (1996a), and to proportional hazards models with longitudinal covariates by Tsiatis and Davidian (2001). Conditional scores were developed for a large class of models by Tsiatis and Ma (2004). Research on conditional score methods is ongoing, with Stoklosa, Lee and Hwang (2019) as a recent example. See Zucker (2021) for the discussion on the methods.

### Hypothesis Testing

Tosteson and Tsiatis (1988) provided an early and important paper in the area of hypothesis testing for the association between $Y$ and $X$. They showed that, for generalized linear models, the optimal score test for no effects is obtained by replacing $X^*$ with $E(X|X^*)$, i.e., regression calibration results in the optimal score test when $X^*$ is observed. It follows that when $E(X|X^*)$ is linear in $X^*$, ignoring measurement error and proceeding with the usual score test results in the optimal test of no effects. Nevertheless, covariate measurement error can result in a significant loss of power, and tests of no effects due to the accurately observed $X$ may not be valid. Stefanski and Carroll (1990a) developed an estimator of $E(X|X^*)$ that results in approximately efficient score tests, and they also explored the Wald test.

A useful approximation for the sample size required to maintain power in the presence of covariate measurement error is $n_{X^*} = n_X/\rho^2_{XX^*}$, where $n_X$ is the sample size needed in the absence of measurement error and $\rho_{XX^*}$ is the correlation coefficient between $X$ and $X^*$. See McKeown-Eyssen and Tibshirani (1994) for the detail.

### Deconvolution/Nonparametric Inference

Under the classical error model (1.2), the observed covariate $X^*$ is a convolution of $X$ and the measurement error $e$. The distribution of $X$ is often of interest, either for scientific reasons or, for example, to estimate $E(X|X^*)$ (recall that $E(X|X^*)$ is used in both regression calibration estimation and construction of the optimal score test discussed by Tosteson and Tsiatis (1988)).

Estimation of the distribution of $X$ is termed *deconvolution*. Deconvolution estimators were studied intensely in the late 1980s and early 1990s, and research on the deconvolution problem continues to the present day. The first deconvolution kernel density estimators were proposed and studied by Carroll and Hall (1988) and Stefanski and Carroll (1990b). These authors showed that deconvolution kernel density estimators have very slow rates of convergence; see also Fan (1991). For example, if the measurement error $e$ is normally distributed, the deconvolution density estimator converges at a rate no faster than $(\log n)^{-2}$. This slow convergence rate would seem to rule out the use of deconvolution estimators. However, Stefanski and Carroll (1991) showed that estimation of the calibration function $E(X|X^*)$ using deconvolved density estimates enjoys rates of convergence reaching $n^{-4/5}$. Later studies of deconvolution estimators employed 'small sigma' asymptotics, i.e., deconvolution estimators were studied as $n \to \infty$ and $\sigma_e^2 \to 0$. This asymptotic scenario is relevant to the situation where $\text{Var}(X)$ is large relative to $\text{Var}(e)$. Estimators of the density of $X$ were obtained with standard nonparametric convergence rates without having to fully specify the distribution of the measurement error. Detailed discussion on this is given by Delaigle and Van Keilegom (2021).

Interest in this topic continues to grow, as is evident from, for example, Carroll and Hall (2004), Delaigle (2007, 2014), Delaigle, Hall and Qiu (2006), Carroll, Delaigle and Hall (2007), Delaigle and Meister (2011), and Delaigle and Hall (2014). See Delaigle (2016) and Carroll et al. (2006) for excellent summaries of results for deconvolution estimators. Detailed overiews of this topic can also be found in Apanasovich and Liang (2021), Delaigle (2021), Kang and Qiu (2021), and Song (2021).

### Misclassification

Research into the effects of misclassified categorical or discrete covariates/exposures has been spread over several decades, making it difficult to identify a decade where the area was studied most intensely.

An early example demonstrating the attenuating effects of misclassified binary exposures on the odds ratio was studied by Bross (1954). He concluded that, similar to the effects of measurement error on hypothesis testing mentioned above, misclassification may not affect the validity of a hypothesis test of no effects, but can affect power. See also Greenland (1980), Greenland and Robins (1985), and Greenland (1988).

Misclassified discrete covariates/responses are governed by the missclassification matrix consisting of entries, say $\pi_{jk}$, representing the probability that the covariate/response is classified as category $j$ when the true category is $k$. Successful analysis of misclassified data often requires validation data for estimation of the missclassification matrix (Spiegelman, Rosner and Logan 2000). Missclassified binary and ordinal responses have also been studied by Copas (1988) and Neuhaus (1999). Helmut et al. (2006) developed the simulation-extrapolation (SIMEX) method for misclassified covariates and/or missclassified responses. An R package implementing their methods is available through the **simex** function. A discussion on misclassification was given by Gustafson and Greenland (2014).

Breslow and Cain (1988) and Carroll, Gail and Lubin (1993) studied misclassification in logistic regression models for case-control data. Matched case-control studies with misclassification were studied by Gustafson, Le and Saskin (2001), Prescott and Garthwaite (2005), and Hogg et al. (2019). Mak, Best and Rushton (2015) studied the sensitivity of case-control studies to misclassification.

### 1.6.2 1990-1999

In the period of 1990-1999, the following are major approaches and areas explored.

#### Instrumental Variable Methods

Instrumental variables are additional measurements of $X$, denoted $V$, such that (i) $V$ is nondifferential, i.e., $f(y|x,v) = f(y|x)$; (ii) $V$ is correlated with $X$; and (iii) $V$ is independent of $X^* - X$. Replicate observations of $X$ are instrumental variables, but instrumental variables need not be replicates.

As mentioned above, instrumental variable estimators were proposed early in the study of covriate measurement error in linear models.

In the statistical literature, instrumental variable estimation in non-linear models began in earnest in the early 1990s. Stefanski and Buzas (1995) developed a measurement error correction method using instrumental variables for binary regression models. Buzas and Stefanski (1996a) discussed parameter estimation under Probit measurement error models using instrumental variables. Buzas and Stefanski (1996b) extended the conditional score method to instrumental variables in a class of generalized linear models, and Buzas (1997) developed an instrumental variable estimation approach for nonlinear models that provide consistent estimators without having to specify the measurement error distribution.

Carroll and Stefanski (1994) discussed using instrumental variables to handle problems that arise in regression meta-analysis when the predictor of interest is measured with error. They demonstrated that a single correction for attenuation is not possible when the measurement error variances differ across studies, and they suggested that study specific corrections are generally necessary.

Gustafson (2007) considered a strategy of measurement error modeling using an approximate instrumental variable. Hu and and Schennach (2008) discussed the use of instrumental variables for nonclassical measurement error models and established very general identifiability results. Under generalized linear mixed models, Wang (2021b) described semiparametric estimation using instrumental variables. For additional discussion of instrumental variable methods, see Lewbel (2021).

### Simulation Extrapolation

The simulation extrapolation (SIMEX) method, proposed by Cook and Stefanski (1994) and Stefanski and Cook (1995), is an attractive simple approach for reducing bias due to measurement error in a wide variety of models, and it has been widely used in practice. This approach is well suited to the settings with classical additive measurement error models with the error following a normal distribution, though the method is not limited to this model. Theoretical justification to this approach and the asymptotic distribution of the simulation extrapolation estimators were investigated by Carroll et al. (1996).

The idea is intuitive. To understand how the magnitude of covariate measurement error affects bias in parameter estimation, the analyst sequentially simulates increasing amounts of measurement error in the covariate, computes the naive estimate using a standard method developed for error-free settings, and then examines the naive estimates (averaged over simulated samples) against the amount of measurement error by fitting a regression model. The final step is to extrapolate the relationship between bias and magnitude of measurement error back to the case of no measurement error. Carroll et al. (2006) provided a detailed discussion of both the theoretical and practical aspects of the SIMEX method.

A commercial implementation of SIMEX is available in STATA, and SIMEX has also been implemented in R.

### Bayesian Approaches

Bayesian approaches to covariate measurement error problems are straightforward conceptually. As with general Bayesian approaches, Bayesian covariate measurement error models start with the likelihood and add priors to all unknown quantities. In the covariate measurement error setting, this requires specification of a distribution for the latent $X$, priors for parameters of this distribution, and priors for regression parameters in the model relating outcome to predictors. Finally, priors for parameters in the measurement error model also require specification. The resulting posterior is typically intractable analytically, and consequently there was limited research in Bayesian measurement error methods prior to around 1990.

The rapid development in the late 1980s and 1990s of computational approaches to approximating posterior distributions spurred research into Bayesian approaches for covariate measurement error problems. The result is that in the measurement error setting, MCMC sampling is typically used to obtain a sample from the (approximate) posterior distribution for all unknown quantities. A strength of this approach is that numerical evaluation of intractable integrals is avoided. Another advantage, at least in principle, is that no special techniques need to be developed for different types of regression models and measurement error models – simply apply the Bayesian machinery to the proposed models. However, the additional modeling required by covariate measurement error necessitates care in choosing priors and checking for sensitivity to mis-specification. More complex models may require specialized adaptations of MCMC algorithms, and/or careful selection of tuning parameters, starting values and scaling of covariates for use in existing algorithms.

Early research into application of Bayesian methods in the presence of covariate measurement error includes Stephens and Dellaportas (1992), Richardson and Gilks (1993), and Mallick and Gelfand (1996). Some recent work of Bayesian methods concerning error-prone data can be found in Gustafson, Le and Vallee (2002), Gustafson and Greenland (2006), Hossain and Gustafson (2009), and Xia and Gustafson (2018), among many others.

The book by Gustafson (2004) provides an excellent introduction to Bayesian models for covariate measurement error, and Carroll et al. (2006) contains a chapter devoted to Bayesian measurement error models. A recent account of this topic can be found in Sinha (2021) and Stamey and Seaman Jr. (2021).

**Survival Analysis**

Survival data pose new challenges for error-prone data, including censoring, skewed data, and semi-parametric hazard functions. Research on error-prone survival data dated back to the 1980s, marked by the seminal work of Prentice (1982) who considered the proportional hazards model with covariate measurement error. Since then, examining the measurement error effects on survival analysis has attracted attention. Available work in the period from 1990 - 1999 includes Pepe, Self and Prentice (1989), Hughes (1993), Gong, Whittemore and Grosser (1990), Nakamura (1992), Wang et al. (1997), Hu, Tsiatis and Davidian (1998), and Buzas (1998).

Since 2000, there has been extensive interest in accommodating measurement error effects into inferential procedures about survival data. A variety of inference methods have been developed from different perspectives. To name a few, Xie, Wang and Prentice (2001), Liao et al. (2011), and Shaw and Prentice (2012) developed variants of the usual regression calibration method by incorporating the risk set information, a feature which is typical for survival data. Hu, Tsiatis and Davidian (1998) developed a likelihood based method that requires the specification of the distribution of the true covariates. Huang and Wang (2000) proposed a nonparametric approach which requires repeated measurements for mismeasured covariates to be available for each subject. Gorfine, Hsu and Prentice (2003) examined estimation approaches for correlated failure times in the presence of covariate measurement error. Under stratified Cox models, Gorfine, Hsu, and Prentice (2004) explored nonparametric correction for covariate measurement error. With semiparametric survival regression, Zucker (2005) presented a pseudo-partial likelihood method to address the effects due to covariate measurement error. Yan and Yi (2016) developed several functional correction methods for measurement error effects under the additive hazards model.

Buzas (2021) offered an overview of covariate measurement error in survival data models.

### Analysis of Longitudinal/Correlated Data

Since the 1990s, attention on measurement error effects emerged from studies on correlated data, such as clustered data, multivariate data, longitudinal data, and times series. For example, with multivariate responses and error-contaminated covariates, Chesher (1991) derived approximations to distributions and then examined the resultant measurement error effects. With clustered data concerning covariate measurement error, Wang and Davidian (1996) examined measurement error effects under nonlinear mixed effects models. For longitudinal studies, Wang et al. (1998) and Tosteson, Buonaccorsi and Demidenko (1998) explored covariate measurement error effects, respectively under generalized linear mixed models and linear mixed models. With error in responses, Neuhaus (2002) investigated effects of misclassified binary response variables on analysis of longitudinal or clustered data. Regarding error-prone times series data, Koons and Foutz (1990) discussed estimation of moving average parameters. An overview of measurement error models in settings of time series was given by Buonaccorsi (2021), and discussion of time-varying covariates subject to measurement error was provided by Wu, Liu and Zhang (2021).

Methods of accommodating measurement error effects have spawned in late 1990s and continue to grow since 2000. To name a few, Higgins, Davidian and Giltinan (1997) proposed a two-stage estimation method for nonlinear mixed measurement error models. Zidek et al. (1998) discussed a nonlinear regression analysis method for clustered data. Wang, Wang and Wang (2000) proposed the expected estimating equations method, and Buonaccorsi, Demidenko and Tosteson (2000) developed likelihood-based methods for linear mixed models with measurement error. Chen, Yi and Wu (2011) proposed estimating equation methods to handle clustered binary responses subject to misclassification.

Attention on error-prone longitudinal data has been further paid to investigations of joint effects with other features. Some early work on joint modeling of survival data and error-contaminated longitudinal covariates was given by Tsiatis, Degruttola and Wulfsohn (1995), and later studied by Tsiatis and Davidian (2001), where the survival process was described by the Cox porportional hazards model. In contrast, with the accelerated failure time model employed to characterize the survival process, Tseng, Hsieh and Wang (2005) explored a joint modeling approach to handle error-contaminated covariates which are described by the linear mixed effects model.

When both measurement error and missing observations are present, Liang, Wang and Carroll (2007) derived estimation procedures under partially linear models. Wang et al. (2008), Yi (2005, 2008), and Yi, Ma and

Carroll (2012) developed marginal methods to incorporate measurement error and missingness effects. Liu and Wu (2007) and Yi, Liu and Wu (2011) took a mixed model framework for the response process and described likelihood-based methods. Detailed discussions on this topic were given by Carroll et al. (2006, Ch. 11), Buonaccorsi (2010, Ch.11, Ch.12), Wu (2009, Ch.3, Ch.8), and Yi (2017, Ch.5). A discussion of measurement error and missing data can be found in Keogh and Bartlett (2021).

### 1.6.3 After 2000

After 2000, the following are major approaches and areas explored.

#### Variable Selection

Variable selection methods for low dimensional data in the absence of covariate measurement error have been studied for decades. High dimensional variable selection methods in the absence of covariate measurement error began in earnest in the early 2000s. Variable selection methods in the presence of measurement error began around 2010, with Liang and Li (2009) and Ma and Li (2010) as early examples. These authors developed variable selection approaches using penalized regression methods. Yi, Tan and Li (2015) proposed variable selection methods in the longitudinal data setting when there is covariate measurement error and possibly missing observations. They developed a variation of SIMEX in their approach.

Several approaches for variable selection in the presence of covariate measurement error have been proposed that are applicable to the situation where the number of predictors is large relative to the sample size. Sørensen, Frigessi and Thoresen (2013) defined a corrected Lasso that results in consistent covariate selection in the presence of measurement error. Datta and Zou (2017) also developed a Lasso based method, dubbed CoCoLasso for convex conditioned Lasso, for variable selection in high dimensional settings with covariate measurement error.

Some of the aforementioned methods apply primarily to linear models. Recently, Brown, Weaver and Wolfson (2019) developed a variable selection procedure for high dimensional data where covariate measurement error is present. Their method, dubbed MEBoost, is extendable to a very large class of regression models where estimating equations that correct for the measurement error effects have already been proposed. In a somewhat reverse scenario, Stefanski, Wu and White (2014) developed an approach to variable selection for error-free settings utilizing ideas from measurement error modeling.

### Causal Inference

Interest in causal inference about error-prone data began with studying measurement error effects. Zidek et al. (1996) illustrated that measurement error may conspire with multicollinearity among confounders to mask the effects of causal variables. Hernán and Cole (2009) employed causal diagrams to represent various types of measurement error. Babanezhad, Vansteelandt and Goetghebeur (2010) studied the asymptotic bias of misclassified exposure on various causal effect estimators, and VanderWeele, Valeri and Ogburn (2012) examined measurement error effects on mediation analysis. Regier, Moodie and Platt (2014) conducted simulation studies to assess the effects of mismeasured confounders on the estimation of the causal effects.

Identifying conditions for conducting causal inference with measurement error is another topic of interest. For example, Lewbel (2007) discussed identification and estimation of the average treatment effect in nonparametric and semiparametric regression with misclassified treatment or exposure. Imai and Yamamoto (2010) investigated identification issues in the presence of a misclassified binary treatment variable. Díaz and van der Laan (2013) explored a sensitivity analysis to circumvent the cases with unidentifiable or not estimable model parameters.

Regarding estimation of the causal effects with error-corrupted confounders, McCaffrey, Lockwood and Setodji (2013) and Shu and Yi (2019ab) explored inverse-probability-weighted estimation approaches, and Shu and Yi (2019c) developed an R package for implementing the method of Shu and Yi (2019a). Further, Shu and Yi (2019d, 2020) studied the biases due to a misclassified binary outcome together with missingness or covariate measurement error, and developed estimation methods to accommodate those effects. A more detailed discussion on this topic is available in Valeri (2021).

## 1.7 Some Applications in Epidemiology

There are many applications of measurement error methodology in epidemiology. In one of the early papers on the topic of exposure error in studies of air pollution, Shy, Kleinbaum and Morgenstern (1978) described the measurement error problem and addressed its consequences in an epidemiologic framework. Willett (1989) provided an overview of issues related to the correction of nondifferential exposure measurement error in epidemiological studies. Rosner, Willett and Spiegelman (1989) considered the correction of logistic regression relative risk estimates and confidence intervals for systematic within person measurement error. They gave methodology (including regression calibration) and applied it to dietary fat intake and risk of breast cancer. MacMahon et al. (1990) was one of the first important practical applications, correcting for the regression dilution bias resulting from measurement error in diastolic blood pressure.

Gail (1991) included a bibliography and comments on the use of statistical models in epidemiology in the 1980s. Chen (1989) reviewed the methods for misclassified categorical data in epidemiological studies. Thomas, Stram and Dwyer (1993) presented an overview of the exposure error or misdassification problem from the general epidemiologic perspective. Spiegelman, McDermott and Rossner (1997) investigated the regression calibration scheme for correcting the bias due to measurement error in nutritional epidemiology. The central issues of measurement error modeling to progress in nutritional epidemiology were recognized and emphasized by many authors such as Prentice et al. (2002), Prentice and Huang (2011), and Buzas, Stefanski and Tosteson (2014), among others.

Recently there have been several systematic reviews of the use of corrections for measurement error in applied settings. The results are somewhat discouraging. Brakenhoff et al. (2018) found that almost half (247/565) of research studies published in 2016 in top 12 general medicine and epidemiological journals mention measurement error, but only 7% of the 247 (18) did something about it (investigated the effect or did a measurement error analysis). Brakenhoff et al. (2018) gave some recommendations for increasing the use of measurement error methods.

In a review article, Bennett et al. (2017) examined measurement error in a continuous exposure in nutritional epidemiology. They identified 126 studies that addressed measurement error. Among them, 43 were methodological and 83 applied existing methods. They found that regression calibration is by far the most widely used method in nutritional epidemiology. However, the underlying assumptions are not always met, and hence, they recommended that sensitivity analyses should be used to assess departures from model assumptions.

The review by Shaw et al. (2018) had findings consistent with those of the two aforementioned studies. Recently, Keogh et al. (2020) and Shaw et al. (2020) provided excellent and comprehensive overviews of measurement error and misclassification in epidemiological studies.

## 1.8 Monographs on Measurement Error Models

The effect of mismeasured variables in statistical and econometric analysis is one of the oldest known problems, dating from the 1870s in Adcock (1878). Long (1976) reviewed some methods of estimation and hypothesis testing in linear measurement error models. Research results based on a workshop on errors-in-variables were summarized in a volume of *Statistics in Medicine* (Byar and Gail, 1989). The volume, edited by Davidian et al. (2014), contains Raymond J. Carroll's research on measurement error models and commentary on its impact, together with history and anecdotes. The book provides a review and discussion on a range of topics including semiparametric and nonparametric regression, measurement error modeling, and quantitative methods for nutritional epidemiology. Chang and Keller (2021) provided an overview of methods to account for measurement error effects in the context of environmental epidemiology.

The problem of measurement errors in predictor variables in regression analysis has been carefully studied in the statistics and epidemiologic literature for several decades. Fuller (1987) summarized early research on linear regression with so-called "errors-in-x" variables. Carroll, Ruppert and Stefanski (1995) extended this literature to generalized linear models including Poisson, logistic, and survival regression analyses. Carroll et al. (2006) further documented up-to-date methods with a comprehensive discussion of various topics on nonlinear measurement error models, including Bayesian analysis methods. With an emphasis on the use of relatively simple methods, Buonaccorsi (2010) described methods to correct for measurement error and misclassification effects for regression models. Under the Bayesian paradigm, Gustafson (2004) provided a dual treatment of mismeasurement in both continuous and categorical variables. Other relevant books on this topic include Biemer et al. (1991), Cheng and Van Ness (1999), Wansbeek and Meijer (2000), and Dunn (2004).

A recent monograph by Yi (2017) emphasized unique features in modeling and analyzing measurement error and misclassification problems arising from medical research and epidemiological studies. The emphasis is on gaining insights into problems coming from a wide range of fields, including event history data (such as survival data and recurrent event data), correlated data (such as longitudinal data and clustered data), multi-state event data, and data arising from case-control studies.

## 1.9 Concluding Remarks

As the ease in collecting data increases, there is the growing use of data (e.g., EHR/EMR data, large scale administrative data) from sources not originally intended for answering scientific questions. Therefore, developing methods for handling faulty data becomes increasingly important. As pointed out by Brakenhoff et al. (2018), more guidance and tutorials are necessary to assist applied researchers with the assessment of the type and amount of measurement error as well as the steps that can subsequently be taken to minimize its impact on the studied relationships.

Even though there is intensive research into the development of methodology to handle measurement error, measurement error methods are not used frequently in the situations that merit their use. There are a couple of reasons which hinder the use of measurement error methodology. Lack of adequate understanding of measurement error impacts is perhaps the primary reason. Developing proper methods to address measurement error effects requires analytical skills and knowledge of the measurement error models. This presents a significant hurdle for introducing suitable corrections in the analysis. Furthermore, general-purposed software packages are lacking for analysts to implement the available correction methods developed in the literature, though some software packages have been available (e.g., Yi, 2017, Ch. 9; Guolo, 2021). Most importantly, the difficulty of obtaining auxiliary data often discourages the researchers to accommodate the feature of measurement error in their data analyses.

It seems difficult to offer universal guidelines. Study design, measurement error models, and analytic approaches can depend on many factors, including the form of the response and measurement error/misclassification models, the association structures among the covariates, the magnitude of mismeasurement in variables, and the availability of computing facilities, as noted by Carroll et al. (2006) and Yi (2017), among others.

The STRATOS initiative is a collaborative effort to "*to provide accessible and accurate guidance in the design and analysis of observational studies*" (STRATOS initiative website: https://www.stratos-initiative.org/). The group recently published a two part guidance document describing types of measurement error, the effect of measurement error on parameter estimation, and methods for amelioration (see Keogh et al., 2020 and Shaw et al., 2020). We are optimistic that continued efforts to interface with scientists through these types of publications, including this handbook, will result in an increased use of methods to correct for the effects of measurement error.

## Acknowledgments

Yi's reseach was supported by the Natural Sciences and Engineering Research Council of Canada (NSERC). Yi is Canada Research Chair in Data Science (Tier 1). Her research was undertaken, in part, thanks to funding from the Canada Research Chairs Program.

## References

Adcock, R. J. (1877). Note on the method of least squares. *Analyst*, 4, 183-184.

Adcock, R. J. (1878). A problem in least squares. *Analyst*, 5, 53-54.

Apanasovich, T. and Liang, H. (2021). Nonparametric measurement errors models for regression. In *Handbook of Measurement Error Models*, Yi, G. Y., Delaigle, A., and Gustafson, P. (Eds.), Chapman & Hall/CRC, Boca Raton, Florida, Chapter 14.

Babanezhad, M., Vansteelandt, S., and Goetghebeur, E. (2010). Comparison of causal effect estimators under exposure misclassification. *Journal of Statistical Planning and Inference*, 140, 1306-1319.

Bennett, D. A., Landry, D., Little, J., and Minelli, C. (2017). Systematic review of statistical approaches to quantify, or correct for, measurement error in a continuous exposure in nutritional epidemiology. *BMC Medical Research Methodology*, 17, 146.

Bertrand, A., Van Keilegom, I., and Legrand, C. (2019). Flexible parametric approach to classical measurement error variance estimation without auxiliary data. *Biometrics*, 75, 297-307.

Biemer, P. P., Groves, R. M., Lyberg, L. E., Mathiowetz, N. A., and Sudman, S. (1991). *Measurement Error in Surveys*. John Wiley & Sons, Inc., Hoboken, New Jersey.

Bross, I. (1954). Misclassification in $2 \times 2$ tables. *Biometrics*, 10, 478-486.

Brakenhoff, T. B., Mitroiu, M., Keogh, R. H., Moons, K. G. M., Groenwold, R. H. H., and van Smeden, M. (2018). Measurement error is often neglected in medical literature: A systematic review. *Journal of Clinical Epidemiology*, 98, 89-97.

Brown, B., Weaver, T., and Wolfson, J. (2019). MEBoost: Variable selection in the presence of measurement error. *Statistics in Medicine*, 38, 2705-2718.

Buonaccorsi, J. P., Demidenko, E., and Tosteson, T. (2000). Estimation in longitudinal random effects models with measurement error. *Statistica Sinica*, 10, 885-903.

Buonaccorsi, J. P. (2010). *Measurement Error: Models, Methods, and Applications*. Chapman & Hall/CRC, Boca Raton, Florida.

Buonaccorsi, J. P. (2021). Measurement error in dynamic models. In *Handbook of Measurement Error Models*, Yi, G. Y., Delaigle, A., and Gustafson, P. (Eds.), Chapman & Hall/CRC, Boca Raton, Florida, Chapter 18.

Buzas, J. S. and Stefanski, L. A. (1996a). Instrumental variable estimation in probit measurement error models. *Journal of Statistical Planning and Inference*, 55, 47-62.

Buzas, J. S. and Stefanski, L. A. (1996b). Instrumental variable estimation in generalized linear measurement error models. *Journal of the American Statistical Association*, 91, 999-1006.

Buzas, J. S. (1997). Instrumental variable estimation in nonlinear measurement error models. *Communications in Statistics - Theory and Methods*, 26, 2861-2877.

Buzas, J. S. (1998). Unbiased scores in proportional hazards regression with covariate measurement error. *Journal of Statistical Planning and Inference*, 67, 247-257.

Buzas, J. S. (2021). Covariate measurement error in survival data. In *Handbook of Measurement Error Models*, Yi, G. Y., Delaigle, A., and Gustafson, P. (Eds.), Chapman & Hall/CRC, Boca Raton, Florida, Chapter 15.

Buzas, J. S., Stefanski, L. A., and Tosteson, T. D. (2014). Measurement error. In Ahrens, W. and Pigeot, I. (Eds.), *Handbook of Epidemiology*, Vol. 3. Springer.

Byar, D. and Gail, M. (1989). Workshop on errors-in-variables. *Statistics in Medicine*, 8, 1027-1179.

Carroll, R. J., Delaigle, A., and Hall, P. (2007). Nonparametric regression estimation from data contaminated by a mixture of Berkson and classical errors. *Journal of the Royal Statistical Society, Series B*, 69, 859-878.

Carroll, R. J. and Hall, P. (1988). Optimal rates of convergence for deconvolving a density. *Journal of the American Statistical Association*, 83, 1184-1186.

Carroll, R. J., Ruppert, D., and Stefanski, L. A. (1995). *Measurement Error in Nonlinear Models*. Chapman and Hall, London.

Carroll, R. J., Ruppert, D., Stefanski, L. A., and Crainiceanu, C. M. (2006). *Measurement Error in Nonlinear Models*, 2nd ed., Chapman & Hall/CRC, Boca Raton, Florida.

Carroll, R. and Stefanski, L. (1990). Approximate quasi-likelihood estimation in models with surrogate predictors. *Journal of the American Statistical Association*, 85, 652-663.

Carroll, R. J. and Stefanski, L. A. (1994). Measurement error, instrumental variables and corrections for attentuation with applications to meta-analyses. *Statistics in Medicine*, 13, 1265-1282.

Carroll, R. J., Küchenhoff, H., Lombard, F., and Stefanski, L. A. (1996). Asymptotics for the SIMEX estimator in structural measurement error models. *Journal of the American Statistical Association*, 91, 242-250.

Carroll, R. J. and Hall, P. (2004). Low order approximations in deconvolution and regression with errors in variables. *Journal of the Royal Statistical Society, Series B*, 66, 31-46.

Carroll, R. J., Gail, M. H., and Lubin, J. H. (1993). Casecontrol studies with errors in covariates. *Journal of the American Statistical Association*, 88, 185-199.

Carroll, R. J., Spiegelman, C. H., Lan, K. K. G., Bailey, K. T., and Abbott, R. D. (1984). On errors-in-variables for binary regression models. *Biometrika*, 71, 19-25.

Chang, H. H. and Keller, J. P. (2021). Spatial exposure measurement error in environmental epidemiology. In *Handbook of Measurement Error Models*, Yi, G. Y., Delaigle, A., and Gustafson, P. (Eds.), Chapman & Hall/CRC, Boca Raton, Florida, Chapter 19.

Chen, T. T. (1989). A review of methods for misclassified categorical data in epidemiology, *Statistics in Medicine*, 8, 1095-1106.

Chen, Z., Yi, G. Y., and Wu, C. (2011). Marginal methods for correlated binary data with misclassified responses. *Biometrika*, 98, 647-662.

Cheng, C.-L. and Van Ness, J. W. (1999). *Statistical Regression with Measurement Error.* Edward Arnold Publishers Ltd., London and Baltimore.

Chesher, A. (1991). The effect of measurement error. *Biometrika*, 78, 451-462.

Cook, J. and Stefanski, L. A. (1994). A simulation extrapolation method for parametric measurement error models. *Journal of the American Statistical Association*, 89, 464-467.

Copas, J. B. (1988). Binary regression models for contaminated data (with discussion). *Journal of the Royal Statistical Society, Series B*, 50, 225-265.

Datta, A., and Zou, H. (2017). Cocolasso for high-dimensional error-in-variables regression. *Annals of Statistics*, 45, 2400-2426.

Davidian, M., Lin, X., Morris, J., and Stefanski, L. (2014). *The Work of Raymond J. Carroll: The Impact and Influence of a Statistician*, Springer, New York.

Delaigle, A. (2007). Nonparametric density estimation from data with a mixture of Berkson and classical errors. *The Canadian Journal of Statistics*, 35, 89-104.

Delaigle, A., Hall, P., and Qiu, P. (2006). Nonparametric methods for solving the Berkson errors-in-variables problem. *Journal of the Royal Statistical Society, Series B*, 68, 201-220.

Delaigle, A. and Meister, A. (2011). Nonparametric function estimation under Fourier-oscillating noise. *Statistica Sinica*, 21, 1065-1092.

Delaigle, A. (2014). Nonparametric kernel methods with errors-in-variables: Constructing estimators, computing them, and avoiding common mistakes. *Australian & New Zealand Journal of Statistics*, 56, 105-124.

Delaigle, A. and Hall, P. (2014). Parametrically assisted nonparametric estimation of a density in the deconvolution problem. *Journal of the American Statistical Association*, 109, 717-729.

Delaigle, A. (2016). Peter Hall's main contributions to deconvolution. *The Annals of Statistics*, 44, 1854-1866.

Delaigle, A. and Van Keilegom, I. (2021). Deconvolution with unknown error distribution. In *Handbook of Measurement Error Models*, Yi, G. Y., Delaigle, A., and Gustafson, P. (Eds.), Chapman & Hall/CRC, Boca Raton, Florida, Chapter 12.

Díaz, I. and van der Laan, M. J. (2013). Sensitivity analysis for causal inference under unmeasured confounding and measurement error problems. *The International Journal of Biostatistics*, 9, 149-160.

Dunn, G. (2004). *Statistical Evaluation of Measurement Errors: Design and Analysis of Reliability Studies.* 2nd ed., Oxford University Press Inc., New York.

Durbin, J. (1954). Errors in variables. *Review of the International Statistical Institute*, 22, 23-32.

Fan, J. (1991). On the optimal rates of convergence for nonparametric deconvolution problems. *Annals of Statistics*, 19, 1257-1272.

Freedman, L. S., Fainberg, V., Kipnis, V., Midthune, D., and Carroll, R. J. (2004). A new method for dealing with measurement error in explanatory variables of regression models. *Biometrics*, 60, 172-181.

Fuller, W. A. (1987). *Measurement Error Models.* John Wiley & Sons, New York.

Gail, M. H. (1991). A bibliography and comments on the use of statistical models in epidemiology in the 1980s. *Statistics in Medicine*, 10, 1819-1885.

Geary, R. C. (1942). Inherent relations between random variables. *Proceedings of the Royal Irish Academy, Section A*, 47, 63-76.

Geary, R. C. (1943). Relations between statistics: The general and the sampling problem when the samples are large. *Proceedings of the Royal Irish Academy, Section A*, 49, 177-196.

Geraci, V. J. (1976). Identification of simultaneous equation models with measurement error. *Journal of Econometrics*, 4, 263-283.

Gong, G., Whittemore, A. S., and Grosser, S. (1990). Censored survival data with misclassified covariates: A case study of breast-cancer mortality. *Journal of the American Statistical Association*, 85, 20-28.

Gorfine, M., Hsu, L., and Prentice, R. L. (2003). Estimation of dependence between paired correlated failure times in the presence of covariate measurement error. *Journal of the Royal Statistical Society, Series B*, 65, 643-661.

Gorfine, M., Hsu, L., and Prentice, R. L. (2004). Nonparametric correction for covariate measurement error in a stratified Cox model. *Biostatistics*, 5, 75-87.

Greenland, S. (1980). The effect of misclassification in the presence of covariates. *American Journal of Epidemiology*, 112, 564-569.

Greenland, S. and Robins, J. M. (1985). Confounding and misclassification. *American Journal of Epidemiology*, 122, 495-506.

Greenland, S. (1988). Variance estimation for epidemiologic effect estimates under misclassification. *Statistics in Medicine*, 7, 745-757.

Guolo, A. (2021). Measurement error and misclassification in meta-analysis. In *Handbook of Measurement Error Models*, Yi, G. Y., Delaigle, A., and Gustafson, P. (Eds.), Chapman & Hall/CRC, Boca Raton, Florida, Chapter 22.

Gustafson, P. (2004). *Measurement Error and Misclassification in Statistics and Epidemiology*. Chapman & Hall/CRC, Boca Raton, Florida.

Gustafson, P. (2005). On model expansion, model contraction, identifiability and prior information: Two illustrative scenarios involving mismeasured variables. *Statistical Science*, 20, 111-140.

Gustafson, P. (2021a). The impact of unacknowledged measurement error. In *Handbook of Measurement Error Models*, Yi, G. Y., Delaigle, A., and Gustafson, P. (Eds.), Chapman & Hall/CRC, Boca Raton, Florida, Chapter 2.

Gustafson, P. (2021b). Partial learning of misclassification parameters. In *Handbook of Measurement Error Models*, Yi, G. Y., Delaigle, A., and Gustafson, P. (Eds.), Chapman & Hall/CRC, Boca Raton, Florida, Chapter 4.

Gustafson. P., Le, N. D., and Saskin, R. (2001). Case-control analysis with partial knowledge of exposure misclassification probabilities. *Biometrics*, 57, 598-609.

Gustafson, P, Le, N. D., and Vallee, M. (2002). A Bayesian approach to case-control studies with errors in covariables. *Biostatistics*, 3, 229-243.

Gustafson, P. and Greenland, S. (2006). Curious phenomena in Bayesian adjustment for exposure misclassification. *Statistics in Medicine*, 25, 87-103.

Gustafson, P. (2007). Measurement error modeling with an approximate instrumental variable. *Journal of the Royal Statistical Society, Series B*, 69, 797-815.

Gustafson, P. and Greenland, S. (2014). Misclassification. In *Handbook of Epidemiology*, 2nd ed., Ahrens, W. and Pigeot, I. (Eds.), Springer, 639-658.

Hardin, J. W., Schmiediche, H., and Carroll, R. J. (2003). The regression-calibration method for fitting generalized linear models with additive measurement error. *The Stata Journal*, 3, 361-372.

Hernán, M. A. and Cole, S. R. (2009). Invited commentary: Causal diagrams and measurement bias. *American Journal of Epidemiology*, 170, 959-962.

Higgins, K. M., Davidian, M., and Giltinan, D. M. (1997). A two-step approach to measurement error in time-dependent covariates in nonlinear mixed-effects models, with application to IGF-I pharmacokinetics. *Journal of the American Statistical Association*, 92, 436-448.

Hogg, T., Zhao. Y., Gustafson, P., Petkau, J., Fisk, J., Marrie, R. A., and Tremlett, H. (2019). Adjusting for differential misclassification in matched case-control studies utilizing health administrative data. *Statistics in Medicine*, 38, 3669-3681.

Hossain, S. and Gustafson, P. (2009). Bayesian adjustment for covariate measurement errors: A flexible parametric approach. *Statistics in Medicine*, 28, 1580-1600.

Hu, Y. Y. and Schennach, S. M. (2008). Instrumental variable of nonclassical measurement error models. *Econometrica*, 76, 195-216.

Hu, P., Tsiatis, A. A., and Davidian, M. (1998). Estimating the parameters in the Cox model when covariate variables are measured with error. *Biometrics*, 54, 1407-1419.

Huang, Y. and Wang, C. Y. (2000). Cox regression with accurate covariates unascertainable: A nonparametric-correction approach. *Journal of the American Statistical Association*, 95, 1209-1219.

Hughes, M. D. (1993). Regression dilution in the proportional hazards model. *Biometrics*, 49, 1056-1066.

Imai, K. and Yamamoto, T. (2010). Causal inference with differential measurement error: Nonparametric identification and sensitivity analysis. *American Journal of Political Science*, 54, 543-560.

Kang, Y. and Qiu, P. (2021). Nonparametric deconvolution by Fourier transformation and other related approaches. In *Handbook of Measurement Error Models*, Yi, G. Y., Delaigle, A., and Gustafson, P. (Eds.), Chapman & Hall/CRC, Boca Raton, Florida, Chapter 11.

Keogh, R. H. and Bartlett, J. W. (2021). Measurement error as a missing data problem. In *Handbook of Measurement Error Models*, Yi, G. Y., Delaigle, A., and Gustafson, P. (Eds.), Chapman & Hall/CRC, Boca Raton, Florida, Chapter 20.

Keogh, R., Shaw, P., Gustafson, P., Carroll, R., Deffner, V., Dodd, K., Küchenhoff, H., Tooze, J., Wallace, M., Kipnis, V., and Freedman L. (2020). STRATOS guidance document on measurement error and misclassification of variables in observational epidemiology: Part I Basic theory, validation studies and simple methods of adjustment. *Statistics in Medicine*, 39, 2197-2231.

Koons, B. K. and Foutz, R. V. 1990. Estimating moving average parameters in the presence of measurement error. *Communications in Statistics*, 19, 3179-3187.

Kúchenhoff, H., Mwalili, S., and Lesaffre, E. (2006). A general method for dealing with misclassification in regression: The misclassification SIMEX. *Biometrics*, 62, 85-96.

Lewbel, A. (2007). Estimation of average treatment effects with misclassification. *Econometrica*, 75, 537-551.

Lewbel, A. (2021). Using instrumental variables to estimate models With mismeasured regressors. In *Handbook of Measurement Error Models*, Yi, G. Y., Delaigle, A., and Gustafson, P. (Eds.), Chapman & Hall/CRC, Boca Raton, Florida, Chapter 5.

Liang, H. and Li, R. (2009). Variable selection for partially linear models with measurement errors. *Journal of the American Statistical Association*, 104, 234-248.

Liang, H., Wang, S., and Carroll, R. J. (2007). Partially linear models with missing response variables and error-prone covariates. *Biometrika*, 94, 185-198.

Liao, X., Zucker, D. M., Li, Y., and Spiegelman, D. (2011). Survival analysis with error-prone time-varying covariates: A risk set calibartion approach. *Biometrics*, 67, 50-58.

Lindsay, B. (1982). Conditional score functions: Some optimality results. *Biometrika*, 69, 503-512.

Liu, W. and Wu, L. (2007). Simultaneous inference for semiparametric nonlinear mixedeffects models with covariate measurement errors and missing responses. *Biometrics*, 63, 342-350.

Long, J. S. (1976). Estimation and hypothesis testing in linear models containing measurement error: A review of Joreskog's model for the analysis of covariance structures. *Sociological Methods & Research*, 5, 157-206.

Ma, Y. (2021). Semiparametric methods for measurement error and misclassification. In *Handbook of Measurement Error Models*, Yi, G. Y., Delaigle, A., and Gustafson, P. (Eds.), Chapman & Hall/CRC, Boca Raton, Florida, Chapter 20.

Ma, Y. and Li, R. (2010). Variable selection in measurement error models. *Bernoulli*, 16, 274-300.

MacMahon, S., Peto, R., Cutler, J., Collins, R., Sorlie, P., Neaton, J., Abbott, R., Godwin, J., Dyer, A., and Stamler, J. (1990). Blood pressure, stroke, and coronary heart disease. Part 1, Prolonged differences in blood pressure: Prospective observational studies corrected for the regression dilution bias. *Lancet*, 335, 765-774.

Mak, T. S., Best, N., and Rushton L. (2015). Robust bayesian sensitivity analysis for case-control studies with uncertain exposure misclassification probabilities. *The International Journal of Biostatistics*, 11, 135-149.

Mallick, B. K. and Gelfand, A. E. (1996). Semiparametic errors in variables models: a Bayesian approach. *Journal of Statistical Planning and Inference*, 52, 307-321.

McCaffrey, D. F., Lockwood, J. R., and Setodji, C. M. (2013). Inverse probability weighting with error-prone covariates. *Biometrika*, 100, 671-680.

McKeown-Eyssen, G. E. and Tibshirani, R. (1994). Implications of measurement error in exposure for the sample sizes of case-control studies. *American Journal of Epidemiology*, 139, 415-421.

Nakamura, T. (1992). Proportional hazards model with covariates subject to measurement error. *Biometrics*, 48, 829-838.

Neuhaus, J. (1999). Bias and efficiency loss due to misclassified responses in binary regression. *Biometrika*, 86, 843-855.

Neuhaus, J. M. (2002). Analysis of clustered and longitudinal binary data subject to response misclassification. *Biometrics*, 58, 675-683.

Neyman, J. and Scott, E. L. (1948). Consistent estimates based on partial consistent observations. *Econometrica*, 16, 1-32.

Pepe, M. S., Self, S. G., and Prentice, R. L. (1989). Further results on covariate measurement errors in cohort studies with time to response data. *Statistics in Medicine*, 8, 1167-1178.

Prentice, R. L. (1982). Covariate measurement errors and parameter estimation in a failure time regression model. *Biometrika*, 69, 331-342.

Prentice, R. L. and Huang, Y. (2011). Measurement error modeling and nutritional epidemiology association analyses. *The Canadian Journal of Statistics*, 39, 498-509.

Prentice, R. L., Sugar, E., Wang, C. Y., Neuhouser, M., and Patterson, R. (2002). Research strategies and the use of nutrient biomarkers in studies of diet and chronic disease. *Public Health Nutrition*, 5, 977-984.

Prescott, G. J. and Garthwaite, P. H. (2005). Bayesian analysis of misclassified binary data from a matched case-control study with a validation substudy. *Statistics in Medicine*, 24, 379-401.

Richardson, S. and Gilks, W. R. (1993). A Bayesian approach to measurement error problems in epidemiology using conditional independence models. *American Journal of Epidemiology*, 138, 430-442.

Reiersøl, O. (1950). Identifiability of a linear relation between variables which are subject to errors. *Econometrica*, 18, 375-389.

Regier, M. D., Moodie, E. E., and Platt, R. W. (2014). The effect of error-in-confounders on the estimation of the causal parameter when using marginal structural models and inverse probability-of-treatment weights: A simulation study. *The International Journal of Biostatistics*, 10, 1-15.

Robinson, P. M. (1974). Identification, estimation and large-sample theory for regressions containing unobservable variables. *International Economic Review*, 15, 680-692.

Roeder, K., Carroll, R. J., and Lindsay, B. G. (1996). A nonparametric mixture approach to case-control studies with errors in covariables. *Journal of the American Statistical Association*, 91, 722-732.

Rosner, B., Willett, W. C., and Spiegelman, D. (1989). Correction of logistic regression relative risk estimates and confidence intervals for systematic within-person measurement error. *Statistics in Medicine*, 8, 1051-1070.

Rosner, B., Spiegelman, D., and Willett, W. C. (1990). Correction of logistic regression relative risk estimates and confidence intervals for measurement error: The case of multiple covariates measured with error. *American Journal of Epidemiology*, 132, 734-745.

Schafer, D. W. (1987). Covariate measurement error in generalized linear models. *Biometrika*, 74, 385-391.

Schafer, D. W. (2001). Semiparametric maximum likelihood for measurement error model regression. *Biometrics*, 57, 53-61.

Schafer, D. W. (2002). Likelihood analysis and flexible structural modeling for measurement error model regression. *Journal of Computational Statistics and Data Analysis*, 72, 33-45.

Schennach, S. M. and Hu, Y. (2013). Nonparametric Identification and Semiparametric Estimation of Classical Measurement Error Models Without Side Information. *Journal of the American Statistical Association*, 108, 177-186.

Shaw, P. (2021). Regression calibration for covariate measurement error. In *Handbook of Measurement Error Models*, Yi, G. Y., Delaigle, A., and Gustafson, P. (Eds.), Chapman & Hall/CRC, Boca Raton, Florida, Chapter 7.

Shaw, P., Gustafson, P., Carroll, R., Deffner, V., Dodd, K., Keogh, R., Kipnis, V., Tooze, J., Wallace, M., Kuchenoff, H., and Freedman L. (2020). STRATOS guidance document on measurement error and misclassification of variables in observational epidemiology: Part 2 - More complex methods of adjustment and advanced topics. *Statistics in Medicine*, 39, 2232-2263.

Shaw, P. A. and Prentice, R. L. (2012). Hazard ratio estimation for biomarker-calibrated dietary exposures. *Biometrics*, 68, 397-407.

Shaw, P. A., Deffner, V., Keogh, R. H., Tooze, J. A., Dodd, K. W., Küchenhoff, H., Kipnis, V., and Freedman, L. S. (2018). Epidemiologic analyses with error-prone exposures: Review of current practice and recommendations. *Annals of Epidemiology*, 28, 821-828.

Shu, D. and Yi, G. Y. (2019a). Causal inference with measurement error in outcomes: Bias analysis and estimation methods. *Statistical Methods in Medical Research*, 28, 2049-2068.

Shu, D. and Yi, G. Y. (2019b). Inverse-probability-of-treatment weighted estimation of causal parameters in the presence of error-contaminated and time-dependent confounders. *The Biometrical Journal*, 61, 1507-1525.

Shu, D. and Yi, G. Y. (2019c). ipwErrorY: An R Package for estimating average treatment effects with misclassified binary outcome. *The R Journal*, 11: 1, 337-351.

Shu, D. and Yi, G. Y. (2019d). Weighted causal inference methods with mismeasured covariates and misclassified outcomes. *Statistics in Medicine*, 38, 1835-1854.

Shu, D. and Yi, G. Y. (2020). Causal inference with noisy data: Bias analysis and estimation approaches to simultaneously addressing missingness and misclassification in binary outcomes. *Statistics in Medicine*, 39, 456-468.

Shy, C. M., Kleinbaum, D. G., and Morgenstern, H. (1978). The effect of misclassification of exposure status in epidemiological studies of air pollution health effects. *The Bulletin of the New York Academy of Medicine*, 54, 1155-1165.

Sinha, S. (2021). Bayesian approaches for handling covariate measurement error In *Handbook of Measurement Error Models*, Yi, G. Y., Delaigle, A., and Gustafson, P. (Eds.), Chapman & Hall/CRC, Boca Raton, Florida, Chapter 24.

Song, W. (2021). Nonparametric inference methods for Berkson errors. In *Handbook of Measurement Error Models*, Yi, G. Y., Delaigle, A., and Gustafson, P. (Eds.), Chapman & Hall/CRC, Boca Raton, Florida, Chapter 13.

Sørensen, ø., Frigessi, A., and Thoresen, M. (2013). Measurement error in LASSO: Impact and likelihood bias correction. *Statistica Sinica*, 25, 809-829.

Spiegelman, D., McDermott, A., and Rossner, B. (1997). Regression calibration method for correcting measurement-error bias in nutritional epidemiology. *The American Journal of Clinical Nutrition*, 65, 1179-1186.

Spiegelman, D., Rosner, B., and Logan, R. (2000). Estimation and inference for logistic regression with covariate misclassification and measurement error in main study/validation study designs. *Journal of the American Statistical Association*, 95, 51–61.

Stamey, J. D. and Seaman Jr., J. W. (2021). Bayesian adjustment for misclassification. In *Handbook of Measurement Error Models*, Yi, G. Y., Delaigle, A., and Gustafson, P. (Eds.), Chapman & Hall/CRC, Boca Raton, Florida, Chapter 23.

Stefanski, L. A. and Buzas, J. S. (1995). Instrumental variable estimation in binary regression measurement error models. *Journal of the American Statistical Association*, 90, 541-550.

Stefanski L. A. and Carroll, R. J. (1987). Conditional scores and optimal scores in generalized linear measurement error models. *Biometrika*, 74, 703-716.

Stefanski, L. and Carroll, R. (1990a). Score tests in generalized linear measurement error models. *Journal of the Royal Statistical Society, Series B*, 52, 345-359.

Stefanski, L. A. and Carroll, R. J. (1990b). Deconvoluting kernal density estimators. *Statistics*, 21, 165-184.

Stefanski, L. A. and Carroll, R. J. (1991). Deconvolution-based score tests in measurement error models. *The Annals of Statistics*, 19, 249-259.

Stefanski, L. A. and Cook, J. R. (1995). Simulation-extrapolation: The measurement error Jackknife. *Journal of the American Statistical Association*, 90, 1247-1256.

Stefanski, L.A., Wu, Y., and White, K. (2014). Variable selection in nonparametric classification via measurement error model selection likelihoods. *Journal of the American Statistical Association*, 109, 574-589.

Stephens, D. A. and Dellaportas, P. (1992). Bayesian analysis of generalised linear models with covariate measurement error. In *Bayesian Statistics 4*. Oxford University Press, Oxford.

Stoklosa, J., Lee, S. M., and Hwang, W. H. (2019). Closed-population capture - recapture models with measurement error and missing observations in covariates. *Statistica Sinica*, 29, 589-610.

Thomas, D., Stram, D., and Dwyer, J. (1993). Exposure measurement error: Influence on exposure-disease relationships and methods of correction. *Annu Rev Public Health*, 14, 69-93.

Tosteson, T. D., Buonaccorsi, J. P., and Demidenko, E. (1998). Covariate measurement error and the estimation of random effect parameters in a mixed model for longitudinal data. *Statistics in Medicine*, 17, 1959-1971.

Tosteson, T. D. and Tsiatis, A. A. (1988). The asymptotic relative efficiency of score tests in the generalized linear model with surrogate covariates. *Biometrika*, 75, 507-514.

Tseng, Y.-K., Hsieh, F., and Wang, J.-L. (2005). Joint modelling of accelerated failure time and longitudinal data. *Biometrika*, 92, 587-603.

Tsiatis, A. A. and Davidian, M. (2001). A semiparametric estimator for the proportional hazards model with longitudinal covariates measured with error. *Biometrika*, 88, 447-458.

Tsiatis, A. A., Degruttola, V., and Wulfsohn, M. S. (1995). Modeling the relationship of survival to longitudinal data measured with error. Applications to survival and CD4 counts in patients with AIDS. *Journal of the American Statistical Association*, 90, 27-37.

Tsiatis, A. A. and Ma, Y. (2004). Locally efficient semiparametric estimators for functional measurement error models. *Biometrika*, 91, 835-848.

Valeri, L. (2021). Measurement error in causal inference. In *Handbook of Measurement Error Models*, Yi, G. Y., Delaigle, A., and Gustafson, P. (Eds.), Chapman & Hall/CRC, Boca Raton, Florida, Chapter 21.

VanderWeele, T. J., Valeri, L., and Ogburn, E. L. (2012). The role of measurement error and misclassification in mediation analysis. *Epidemiology*, 23, 561-564.

Wald, A. (1940). The fitting of straight lines if both variables are subject to error. *Annals of Mathematical Statistics*, 11, 284-300.

Wang, C. Y., Hsu, L., Feng, Z. D., and Prentice, R. L. (1997). Regression calibration in failure time regression. *Biometrics*, 53, 131-145.

Wang, C. Y., Huang, Y., Chao, E. C., and Jeffcoat, M. K. (2008). Expected estimating equations for missing data, measurement error, and misclassification, with application to longitudinal nonignorable missing data. *Biometrics*, 64, 85-95.

Wang, C. Y., Wang, N., and Wang, S. (2000). Regression analysis when covariates are regression parameters of a random effects model for observed longitudinal measurements. *Biometrics*, 56, 487-495.

Wang, L. (2021a). Identifiability in measurement error models. In *Handbook of Measurement Error Models*, Yi, G. Y., Delaigle, A., and Gustafson, P. (Eds.), Chapman & Hall/CRC, Boca Raton, Florida, Chapter 3.

Wang, L. (2021b). Estimation in mixed-effects models with measurement error. In *Handbook of Measurement Error Models*, Yi, G. Y., Delaigle, A., and Gustafson, P. (Eds.), Chapman & Hall/CRC, Boca Raton, Florida, Chapter 17.

Wang, N. and Davidian, M. (1996). A note on covariate measurement error in nonlinear mixed effects models. *Biometrika*, 83, 801-812.

Wang, N., Lin, X., Gutierrez, R. G., and Carroll, R. J. (1998). Bias analysis and SIMEX approach in generalized linear mixed measurement error models. *Journal of the American Statistical Association*, 93, 249-261.

Wansbeek, T. and Meijer, E. (2000). *Measurement Error and Latent Variables in Econometrics*, North-Holland.

Willett, W. (1989). An overview of issues related to the correction of non-differential exposure measurement error in epidemiologic studies. *Statistics in Medicine*, 8, 1031-1040.

Wu, L. (2009). *Mixed Effects Models for Complex Data.* Chapman and Hall/CRC, Boca Raton, Florida.

Wu, L., Liu, W., and Zhang, H. (2021). Mixed effects models with measurement errors in time-dependent covariates. In *Handbook of Measurement Error Models*, Yi, G. Y., Delaigle, A., and Gustafson, P. (Eds.), Chapman & Hall/CRC, Boca Raton, Florida, Chapter 16.

Xia, M. and Gustafson, P. (2018). Bayesian inference for unidirectional misclassification of a binary response trait. *Statistics in Medicine*, 37, 933-947.

Xie, S. X., Wang, C. Y., and Prentice, R. L. (2001). A risk set calibration method for failure time regression by using a covariate reliability sample. *Journal of the Royal Statistical Society: Series B*, 63, 855-870.

Yan, Y. and Yi, G. Y. (2016). A class of functional methods for error-contaminated survival data under additive hazards models with replicate measurements. *Journal of the American Statistical Association*, 111, 684-695.

Yi, G. Y. (2005). Robust methods for incomplete longitudinal data with mismeasured covariates. *The Far East Journal of Theoretical Statistics*, 16, 205-234.

Yi, G. Y. (2008). A simulation-based marginal method for longitudinal data with dropout and mismeasured covariates. *Biostatistics*, 9, 501-512.

Yi, G.Y. (2017). *Statistical Analysis with Measurement Error or Misclassification: Strategy, Method and Application.* Springer Science+Business Media LLC, New York.

Yi, G. Y. (2021). Likelihood methods for measurement error and misclassification. In *Handbook of Measurement Error Models*, Yi, G. Y., Delaigle, A., and Gustafson, P. (Eds.), Chapman & Hall/CRC, Boca Raton, Florida, Chapter 6.

Yi, G. Y., Liu, W., and Wu, L. (2011). Simultaneous inference and bias analysis for longitudinal data with covariate measurement error and missing responses. *Biometrics*, 67, 67-75.

Yi, G. Y., Ma, Y., and Carroll, R. J. (2012). A functional generalized method of moments approach for longitudinal studies with missing responses and covariate measurement error. *Biometrika*, 99, 151-165.

Yi, G. Y., Tan, X., and Li, R. (2015), Variable selection and inference procedures for marginal analysis of longitudinal data with missing observations and covariate measurement error. *The Canadian Journal of Statistics*, 43, 498-518.

Zidek, J. V., Le, N. D., Wong, H., and Burnett, R. T. (1998). Including structural measurement errors in the nonlinear regression analysis of clustered data. *The Canadian Journal of Statistics*, 26, 537-548.

Zidek, J. V., Wong, H., Le, N. D., and Burnett, R. (1996). Causality, measurement error and multicollinearity in epidemiology. *Environmetrics*, 7, 441-451.

Zidek, J. V., Le, N. D., Wong, H., and Burnett, R. T. (1998). Including structural measurement errors in the nonlinear regression analysis of clustered data. *The Canadian Journal of Statistics*, 26, 537-548.

Zucker, D. M. (2005). A pseudo-partial likelihood method for semiparametric survival regression with covariate errors. *Journal of the American Statistical Association*, 100, 1264-1277.

Zucker, D. M. (2021). Conditional and corrected score methods. In *Handbook of Measurement Error Models*, Yi, G. Y., Delaigle, A., and Gustafson, P. (Eds.), Chapman & Hall/CRC, Boca Raton, Florida, Chapter 8.

# 2

# *The Impact of Unacknowledged Measurement Error*

**Paul Gustafson**

## CONTENTS



## 2.1 The Problem at Hand

Statistical investigations of relationships between two or more variables are ubiquitous in science. However, the ability to accurately measure variables of interest is often limited. To frame our discussion, say we are interested in how one or more *explanatory* variables or *predictors*, denoted $X$, impact an *outcome* or *response* variable, denoted $Y$. This is a regression task, and we can build a regression model for which some parameters, or *coefficients*, describe

DOI: 10.1201/9781315101279-2 

the population-level association between $X$ and $Y$. If we can collect data in the form of true (and independent) realizations of $(X, Y)$ for $n$ study units, then we can use these data to estimate the regression coefficients. Nice properties then ensue, particularly that the estimated coefficients will converge to the corresponding true values as the number of study units approaches infinity.

When measurement is challenging, however, the situation becomes much thornier. Say we can only record a surrogate $X^*$ in lieu of $X$. Plugging $(X^*, Y)$ data into our estimation procedure does not, in general, consistently estimate the coefficients describing the $(X, Y)$ data. Moreover, this arises even if the form of the surrogate seems amenable. For instance, even if $X^*$ has the form of $X$ plus some noise that is symmetrically distributed around zero, the regression relationship between $X^*$ and $Y$ will differ from that between $X$ and $Y$.

This phenomenon is often referred to as 'errors-in-variables' or 'errors-in-covariates' when $X$ is continuous, and 'misclassification' when $X$ is discrete. Generically we can refer to 'mismeasurement' of explanatory variables to encompass both cases. The following chapters in this volume cover a wide array of techniques for dealing with mismeasurement. That is, they describe ways of still validly learning the $(X, Y)$ relationship even though the available data are instances of $(X^*, Y)$. Such techniques can be applied given awareness that one has a surrogate $X^*$ rather than the $X$ of interest, and given a route to information about the nature and magnitude of the mismeasurement. First, however, this chapter peruses the impact of unacknowledged mismeasurement. How badly do we do if, wittingly or unwittingly, we use $(X^*, Y)$ data as if they were $(X, Y)$ data?

## 2.2 A Nondifferentially Mismeasured Predictor in a Linear Regression

Say we are interested in the regression relationship

$$E(Y|X, Z) = \beta_0 + \beta_1 X + \beta_2^T Z,$$

where $Y$ is a continuous, scalar outcome variable, $X$ is a scalar explanatory variable, and $Z$ is a vector of $p_z$ further explanatory variables. Here we view $X$ as the explanatory variable of most interest, while the elements of $Z$ are additional explanatory variables (or 'covariates') included out of scientific necessity. In a biostatistics context, for instance, $Y$ could be a health outcome, $X$ could be the exposure of interest, and $Z$ could consist of potential confounding variables (for instance, 'common causes' of $X$ and $Y$). In this setting, inference about $\beta_1$ would be key, since this parameter describes the conditional exposure-disease association given the confounding variables.

We presume that the elements of $Z$ can be measured accurately, whereas $X$ is prone to measurement error. That is, a surrogate $X^*$ is recorded in lieu of

$X$. In a biostatistics context, many exposure variables are indeed difficult to measure well, with prime examples being how much of a particular substance one eats, or drinks, or inhales.

A simple form of measurement error would be *nondifferential* with respect to both $Y$ and $Z$, whereby $X^*$ is conditionally independent of $(Y, Z)$ given $X$. In scientific terms, this corresponds to the poor measurement of $X$ being intrinsic to the measuring instrument, without any influence of a subject's health outcome or covariate values. Sometimes one might also encounter the weaker notion of measurement error that is nondifferential with respect to $Y$ only, whereby $X^*$ is conditionally independent of $Y$ given $(X, Z)$. This leaves open the possibility that $Z$ influences the measurement process. It is easy to verify that nondifferential measurement error with respect to $(Y, Z)$ is automatically nondifferential with respect to $Y$.

A consequence of either the weaker or stronger form of nondifferential error is that

$$\begin{aligned} E(Y|X^*, Z) &= E\{E(Y|X, Z)|X^*, Z\} \\ &= \beta_0 + \beta_1 E(X|X^*, Z) + \beta_2^T Z. \end{aligned} \quad (2.1)$$

Should it further happen to be that $E(X|X^*, Z)$ is linear in $X^*$ and $Z$, then $E(Y|X^*, Z)$ will have this property also, i.e., we can write:

$$E(Y|X^*, Z) = \beta_0^* + \beta_1^* X^* + \beta_2^{*T} Z. \quad (2.2)$$

Then the extent to which $\beta_1^*$ differs from $\beta_1$ is of primary concern. The discrepancy between these two coefficients directly informs how misled one will be upon analyzing $(Y, X^*, Z)$ data as if there were no measurement error, i.e., pretending that the (observed) $X^*$ values are identical to the (unobserved) $X$ values.

A prototype case arises if the stronger form of nondifferentiality holds, with both $(X^*|X)$ and $(X|Z)$ having simple normal structure. Say the nondifferential measurement error is described by $(X^*|X) \sim N(X, \tau^2)$. So our surrogate is unbiased for $X$, but noisy, with this noise being homoscedastic. Also, say that $(X|Z)$ is normally distributed with a mean that is a linear function of $Z$ and constant variance $\lambda^2$. Under these conditions, it is easy to verify that $E(X|X^*, Z)$ is linear in $X^*$, with coefficient $(1 + \tau^2/\lambda^2)^{-1}$. Consequently,

$$\beta_1^* = \frac{1}{1 + \tau^2/\lambda^2}\beta_1, \quad (2.3)$$

where we refer to $(1+\tau^2/\lambda^2)^{-1}$, which is between zero and one, as the *attenuation factor*. If we regress $Y$ on $X^*$ and $Z$ with the hope of actually estimating the association of $Y$ and $X$ given $Z$, we have a biased procedure. Our estimated coefficient for $X^*$ is consistent for $\beta_1^*$, which is attenuated by the factor $(1 + \tau^2/\lambda^2)^{-1}$ compared to the desired target $\beta_1$. For completeness we point out that (2.3) also applies to the simpler situation when there aren't covariates at play, i.e., when there is no $Z$. In this case, we simply have $\lambda^2 = \text{Var}(X)$.

As one expects, (2.3) shows the bias incurred worsens as more measurement error is present, since the attenuation factor $(1 + \tau^2/\lambda^2)^{-1}$ decreases as $\tau^2$ increases. We also see that association between the covariate of interest $X$ and the other covariates $Z$ worsens the situation. That is, more attenuation results as $Z$ becomes more predictive of $X$, i.e., as $\lambda^2$ decreases.

In fact, (2.3) is quite a general expression that holds in circumstances beyond those stated above. For instance, see Sections 2.2 and 2.9 of Gustafson (2004) for a motivation of (2.3) in terms of large-sample estimator limits irrespective of whether the presumed regression model for $(Y|X, Z)$ is correctly specified or not. Generally (2.3) is the basis for the oft-quoted maxim that typical measurement error structure induces *bias toward the null*, in the sense of a regression coefficient that is systematically shrunk toward zero.

### 2.2.1 What About a Mismeasured Confounder?

The attenuation described above arises when we try to infer the impact of $X$ on $Y$ adjusted for $Z$, but $X$ itself is poorly measured. In biomedical applications, this corresponds to inferring the impact of an exposure on a health outcome adjusted for confounders, with the challenge that the exposure is not well measured. Situations also arise, however, when it is a confounder, not the exposure, that is subject to measurement error.

To briefly investigate confounder measurement error without adding a further notational burden, we stick with the framework of (2.2) and presume $Z$ to be scalar. Then we temporarily regard $Z$ as the exposure and $X$ as the confounder which is subject to measurement error. Thus $\beta_2$ becomes the target parameter of most interest, but we incur a bias of $\beta_2^* - \beta_2$ when we simply take the $Z$ coefficient from the $Y$ on $(X^*, Z)$ regression as our estimator.

Under normal and linear structure, with $X|Z \sim N(\alpha_0 + \alpha_1 Z, \lambda^2)$ and $X^*|X \sim N(X, \tau^2)$, it is easy to work out that

$$\beta_2^* - \beta_2 = \alpha_1\beta_1 \left\{ \frac{\tau^2}{\lambda^2 + \tau^2} \right\}.$$

Intuitively, this bias grows in magnitude as the measurement error magnitude $\tau^2$ increases. It is also more pernicious when $\alpha_1$ and $\beta_1$ are larger in magnitude, i.e., when $X$ is more strongly associated with $Z$ and $X$ is more strongly associated with $Y$ given $Z$.

Interestingly, under the same conditions we have the marginal relationship between $Z$ and $Y$ governed by:

$$\begin{aligned} E(Y|Z) &= \beta_0 + \beta_1 E(X|Z) + \beta_2 Z \\ &= (\beta_0 + \alpha_0\beta_1) + (\beta_2 + \alpha_1\beta_1)Z. \end{aligned}$$

Note then that we can write $\beta_2^*$ as a weighted combination of the target parameter ($\beta_2$, the fully adjusted effect of $Z$ on $Y$) and the unadjusted target ($\beta_2 + \alpha_1\beta_1$, the $Z$ coefficient in $E(Y|Z)$). In this combination, the fraction of the weight on the unadjusted target is simply $\tau^2/(\tau^2 + \lambda^2)$, the proportion of the variance of $X^*$ due to measurement error. Thus a direct interpretation comes forth: Conditioning on a poorly measured surrogate for a confounding variable is intermediate between conditioning on the actual confounder and not conditioning at all. Sometimes then, using a poorly measured confounder is referred to as yielding 'partial control' of confounding. Some work that delves into this topic more closely includes Brenner (1993); Greenland (1980); Ogburn and VanderWeele (2012); Ogburn and Vanderweele (2013).

### 2.2.2 The Shape of the Regression Relationship

Next we briefly consider the impact of measurement error on the *shape* of an $(X, Y)$ relationship. We do so in the uncluttered circumstance of simply having the two variables in play, i.e., without any additional precisely measured explanatory variables. Say the true regression relationship is quadratic, with

$$E(Y|X) \quad = \quad \beta_0 + \beta_1 X + \beta_2 X^2.$$

If $X \sim N(\mu, \lambda^2)$ and $(X^*|X, Y) \sim N(X, \tau^2)$, then it is easy to establish that $Y$ will also relate to $X^*$ in a quadratic fashion. Thus we can write

$$E(Y|X^*) \quad = \quad \beta_0^* + \beta_1^* X^* + \beta_2^* X^{*2}.$$

While the expression for $\beta_0^*$ is cumbersome, the linear and quadratic coefficients are easily expressed. Specifically,

$$\begin{pmatrix} \beta_1^* \\ \beta_2^* \end{pmatrix} \quad = \quad \begin{pmatrix} (1 + \tau^2/\lambda^2)^{-1}\beta_1 + 2(1 + \tau^2/\lambda^2)^{-2}\mu\beta_2 \\ (1 + \tau^2/\lambda^2)^{-2}\beta_2 \end{pmatrix}. \qquad (2.4)$$

Whereas $(1+\tau^2/\lambda^2)^{-1}$ is the usual attenuation factor, we see this term plays a role in the linear term, but its square governs the attenuation for the quadratic coefficient. So there is a sense of extra attenuation being involved when the target parameter described the curvature of the regression function.

To give some flavor of this measurement error impact, Figure 2.1 superimposes $E(Y|X^*)$ and $E(Y|X)$, for some specific choices of $(\beta_0, \beta_1, \beta_2)$. Of course, in line with (2.4), $E(Y|X^*)$ has less curvature than $E(Y|X)$. This provides an example of what is referred to in Carroll, Ruppert, Stefanski, and Crainiceanu (2006, Sec. 1.1) as the third of the "triple whammy" of measurement error implications, namely that measurement error "masks the features of the data, making graphical model analysis difficult." For an in-depth discussion of how measurement error impacts the shape of a statistical relationship between an explanatory variable and an outcome variable, see Keogh, Strawbridge and White (2012).

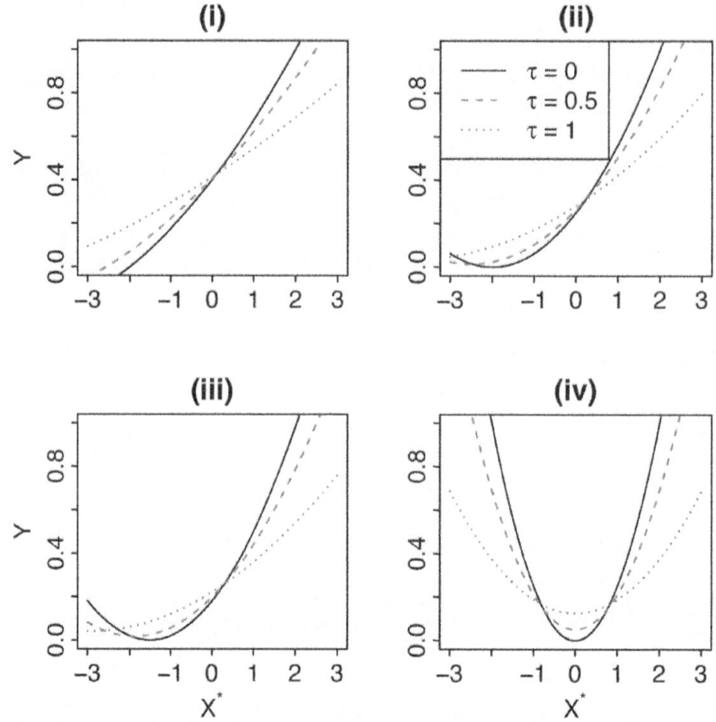


**FIGURE 2.1**
The impact of measurement error on a curved relationship. Each panel gives $E(Y|X^*)$ arising from $E(Y|X)$ under $\tau = 0$ (no measurement error), $\tau = 0.5$, and $\tau = 1$. In panels (i) through (iv), the underlying regression coefficients $(\beta_0, \beta_1, \beta_2)$ are $(0.4, 0.25, 0.025)$, $(0.25, 0.25, 0.0625)$, $(0.18, 0.24, 0.08)$, and $(0.25, 0.25, 0.0625)$, respectively. Throughout, $X \sim N(\mu, \lambda^2)$, with $\mu = 0$ and $\lambda = 1$.

## 2.3 A Nondifferentially Misclassified Predictor in a Linear Regression

When the error-prone explanatory variable $X$ is binary rather than continuous, the narrative concerning the attenuation factor is slightly more nuanced. A first reason for this is that now two parameters are needed to describe the measurement error. Upon defining $\theta_i = Pr(X^* = X|X = i)$, the *specificity* $Sp = \theta_0$ and *sensitivity* $Sn = \theta_1$ characterize how poorly or well $X^*$ performs as a surrogate for $X$. A second contributor to the nuance is that even nondifferential misclassification can spawn additional terms in $E(Y|X^*)$ that do not have counterparts in $E(Y|X)$, as explained below.

In the previous section, we saw with continuous $X$ subject to the simplest form of measurement error (nondifferential, unbiased, homoscedastic, normal), the impact of this error can be characterized by the map from $(\beta_0, \beta_1, \beta_2)$ describing $E(Y|X, Z)$ to $(\beta_0^*, \beta_1^*, \beta_2^*)$ describing $E(Y|X^*, Z)$. Implicit here is that an absence of interaction between $X$ and $Z$ in $E(Y|X, Z)$ transmutes to an absence of interaction between $X^*$ and $Z$ in $E(Y|X^*, Z)$. Such regularity is lost, however, in the case of a misclassified binary $X$. Presuming nondifferentiality of $X^*$ with respect to $(Y, Z)$, the structure of (2.1) still applies, but $E(X|X^*, Z)$ is generally not linear in $(X^*, Z)$, a point stressed by Buonaccorsi (2010, Sec. 6.7). This can be checked after using Bayes theorem to characterize $(X|X^*, Z)$ via

$$\text{Odds}(X = 1|X^*, Z) \quad = \quad \text{Odds}(X = 1|Z)\frac{(1-\theta_1)^{(1-X^*)}\theta_1^{X^*}}{\theta_0^{(1-X^*)}(1-\theta_0)^{X^*}},$$

where the odds of any event $A$ is defined, as usual, as $Odds(A) = Pr(A)/\{1 - Pr(A)\}$.

Given this complexity, one way to describe the situation is with an attenuation factor for each level of $Z$. Let

$$AF_z \quad = \quad \frac{E(Y|X^* = 1, Z = z) - E(Y|X^* = 0, Z = z)}{E(Y|X = 1, Z = z) - E(Y|X = 0, Z = z)}$$

characterize the attenuation within the $Z = z$ stratum. (Since we are characterizing an infinite population, we can think about this stratum whether $Z$ is continuous or categorical.) Then some algebraic manipulations give a somewhat intuitive form:

$$AF_z \quad = \quad \frac{(\theta_0 + \theta_1 - 1)}{1 + \theta_1\{c_z(1-\theta_1) - (1-\theta_0)\} + \theta_0\{c_z^{-1}(1-\theta_0) - (1-\theta_1)\}}, \tag{2.5}$$

where $c_z = \text{Odds}(X = 1|Z = z)$. To interpret (2.5), we can regard $c_z = 1$ (for all $z$) and $\theta_0 = \theta_1$ as a 'base case' corresponding to a 50% prevalence of $X$ given $Z = z$ (hence no association between $X$ and $Z$), with specificity and sensitivity being equal. In the base case we have $AF_z = \theta_0 + \theta_1 - 1$ (for all $z$), which very directly shows the attenuation worsening as the specificity $\theta_0$ and sensitivity $\theta_1$ decrease from one. The base case also matches the attenuation factor determined from a different perspective in Gustafson (2004, Sec. 3.2). (Specifically, the view taken there compares limiting coefficients from regression of $Y$ on $(1, X^*, Z)$ to those for regression of $Y$ on $(1, X, Z)$, so that the nonlinearity of $E(Y, X^*, Z)$ in $(X^*, Z)$ is not acknowledged.)

To explore the attenuation (2.5) beyond the base case, consider the situation of a binary $Z$. Table 2.1 reports $\beta^*$ values in

$$E(Y|X^*, Z) \quad = \quad \beta_0^* + \beta_1^* X^* + \beta_2^* Z + \beta_3^* X^* Z$$

arising from

$$E(Y|X,Z) = \beta_0 + \beta_1 X + \beta_2 Z,$$

when $(\beta_0, \beta_1, \beta_2) = (0, 1, 0.5)$. Two different settings for $(Sp, Sn)$ are considered, in tandem with four settings for the distribution of $(X|Z)$.

Some principal observations from Table 2.1 are that the attenuation in terms of $\beta_1^*/\beta_1$ can be far worse than the base case when the exposure is less common, i.e., when $Pr(X = 1|Z)$ is lower. And, as alluded to above, when $X$ and $Z$ are associated, an interaction is spawned.

To explore this theme further, the same calculations can be used to determine $\beta^*$ from $\beta$ when the $E(Y|X,Z)$ relationship does in fact involve an interaction term between $X$ and $Z$. Some examples of this arising when $(\beta_0, \beta_1, \beta_2, \beta_3) = (0, 1, 0.5, -2)$ appear in Table 4.1. Rather curiously, the $AF_0$ and $AF_1$ values seen are identical to those in Table 2.1. In fact, numerical experimentation reveals that the two attenuation factors do not vary as $\beta_3$ changes, though the algebra is sufficiently complicated to obscure why this happens.

## 2.4 Differential Misclassification of a Predictor

Next we extend the results of the previous section to the situation where the misclassification of $X$ has the more subtle structure of being differential. This narrative is most clearly expressed when the outcome $Y$ is binary. So we presume each of $Z$, $X$, $X^*$, $Y$ is binary, and the only conditional independence we assert is that between $X^*$ and $Z$ given $(X, Y)$. Hence we presume

**TABLE 2.1**
Regression coefficients $\beta^*$ describing $Y$ in terms of $(1, X^*, Z, X^*Z)$. The underlying coefficients for $Y$ in terms of $(1, X, Z)$ are $(\beta_0, \beta_1, \beta_2) = (0, 1, 0.5)$. The attenuation factors $AF_0$ and $AF_1$ are also reported. Different values of $Sn$, $Sp$, and $\gamma_z = Pr(X = 1|Z = z)$ are considered.

| $Sn$ | $Sp$ | $\gamma_0$ | $\gamma_1$ | $\beta_0^*$ | $\beta_1^*$ | $\beta_2^*$ | $\beta_3^*$ | $AF_0$ | $AF_1$ |
|---|---|---|---|---|---|---|---|---|---|
| 0.75 | 0.75 | 0.50 | 0.50 | 0.25 | 0.50 | 0.50 | 0.00 | 0.50 | 0.50 |
| 0.75 | 0.75 | 0.20 | 0.20 | 0.08 | 0.35 | 0.50 | 0.00 | 0.35 | 0.35 |
| 0.75 | 0.75 | 0.20 | 0.50 | 0.08 | 0.35 | 0.67 | 0.15 | 0.35 | 0.50 |
| 0.75 | 0.75 | 0.50 | 0.20 | 0.25 | 0.50 | 0.33 | -0.15 | 0.50 | 0.35 |
| 0.65 | 0.85 | 0.50 | 0.50 | 0.29 | 0.52 | 0.50 | -0.00 | 0.52 | 0.52 |
| 0.65 | 0.85 | 0.20 | 0.20 | 0.09 | 0.43 | 0.50 | 0.00 | 0.43 | 0.43 |
| 0.65 | 0.85 | 0.20 | 0.50 | 0.09 | 0.43 | 0.70 | 0.09 | 0.43 | 0.52 |
| 0.65 | 0.85 | 0.50 | 0.20 | 0.29 | 0.52 | 0.30 | -0.09 | 0.52 | 0.43 |

it is the outcome $Y$, not the covariate $Z$, that is having some influence on the exposure classification. Thus outcome-specific specificity and sensitivity, $Sp_y = Pr(X^* = 0|X = 0, Y = y)$ and $Sn_y = Pr(X^* = 1|X = 1, Y = y)$, completely describe the misclassification.

For a given distribution of $(X, Y|Z)$, and given $(Sp_0, Sp_1)$ and $(Sn_0, Sn_1)$ values, it is a straightforward exercise to compute the distribution of $(X^*, Y|Z)$. Specifically,

$$\begin{aligned}
Pr(X^* = x^*, Y = y|Z = z) &= \sum_{x=0}^{1} Pr(X^* = x^*, X = x, Y = y|Z = z) \\
&= \sum_{x=0}^{1} Pr(X^* = x^*|X = x, Y = y) \\
&\qquad \times Pr(X = x, Y = y|Z = z).
\end{aligned}$$

These calculations, however, do not spawn a general and easy-to comprehend relationship between the impact of $X^*$ on $Y$ relative to the impact of $X$ on $Y$. (In fact this is not surprising, since we already saw considerable 'messiness' in the special case of nondifferential misclassification in the previous section.) Thus we must resort to showing results of the calculation for specific inputs.

Often there is a plausible narrative for differential misclassification when $Y = 1$ and $Y = 0$ are diseased (case) and healthy (control) states respectively, and when the misclassification of $X$ arises from $X^*$ being based on questionnaire self-report. This can come into play in a cross-sectional study, with $Y$ and $X^*$ being ascertained simultaneously. And it is of particular concern in case-control studies where the questionnaire is administered at the time that $Y$ is ascertained, but participants are being asked to think back about an $X$ defined at a past time.

**TABLE 2.2**
Regression coefficients $\beta^*$ describing $Y$ in terms of $(1, X^*, Z, X^*Z)$. The underlying coefficients for $Y$ in terms of $(1, X, Z)$ are $(\beta_0, \beta_1, \beta_2, \beta_3) = (0, 1, 0.5, -2)$. The attenuation factors $AF_0$ and $AF_1$are also reported. Different values of $Sn$, $Sp$, and $\gamma_z = Pr(X = 1|Z = z)$ are considered.

| $Sn$ | $Sp$ | $\gamma_0$ | $\gamma_1$ | $\beta_0^*$ | $\beta_1^*$ | $\beta_2^*$ | $\beta_3^*$ | $AF_0$ | $AF_1$ |
|---|---|---|---|---|---|---|---|---|---|
| 0.75 | 0.75 | 0.50 | 0.50 | 0.25 | 0.50 | 0.00 | -1.00 | 0.50 | 0.50 |
| 0.75 | 0.75 | 0.20 | 0.20 | 0.08 | 0.35 | 0.35 | -0.70 | 0.35 | 0.35 |
| 0.75 | 0.75 | 0.20 | 0.50 | 0.08 | 0.35 | 0.17 | -0.85 | 0.35 | 0.50 |
| 0.75 | 0.75 | 0.50 | 0.20 | 0.25 | 0.50 | 0.17 | -0.85 | 0.50 | 0.35 |
| 0.65 | 0.85 | 0.50 | 0.50 | 0.29 | 0.52 | -0.08 | -1.04 | 0.52 | 0.52 |
| 0.65 | 0.85 | 0.20 | 0.20 | 0.09 | 0.43 | 0.31 | -0.85 | 0.43 | 0.43 |
| 0.65 | 0.85 | 0.20 | 0.50 | 0.09 | 0.43 | 0.12 | -0.95 | 0.43 | 0.52 |
| 0.65 | 0.85 | 0.50 | 0.20 | 0.29 | 0.52 | 0.11 | -0.95 | 0.52 | 0.43 |

If $X = 1$ corresponds to a behavioral choice that might be stigmatized, then those who fall ill might be particularly reticent to own up to a behavioral choice that might have contributed to their illness. In this situation, $Sn_1 < Sn_0$ is plausible. (Whereas, there might be no reason to question $Sp_0 = Sp_1$.) On the other hand, say $X = 1$ corresponds to an environmental factor. Those who fall ill might be quicker to think of an environmental externality as contributing to their ill health. In this situation, $Sp_1 < Sp_0$ is plausible, i.e., amongst those not actually exposed to the environmental agent, those who fall sick might be more likely to mistakenly report such exposure. (Whereas, $Sn_0 = Sn_1$ could still be plausible.)

To see the impact of differential misclassification in these two scenarios, Table 2.3 gives the distribution of $(Y|X^*, Z)$ arising when $Pr(Y = 1|X, Z) = 0.15 + 0.3X + 0.15Z$ and $X \perp Z$, with $Pr(X = 1) = 0.5$. For reference, the first row (the baseline scenario) of results is for nondifferential misclassification, with $Sp = 0.85$ and $Sn = 0.65$ (consequently, this row matches the appropriate row in Table 2.1). Then the two denial scenarios leave $Sp_0$, $Sp_1$, $Sn_0$ unchanged, but $Sn_1$ drops to either 0.55 or 0.45. Similarly, the two blame scenarios leave $Sn_0$, $Sn_1$, $Sp_0$ as per the baseline scenario, while dropping $Sp_1$ to either 0.55 or 0.45. Note that the two denial scenarios are particularly damaging, with virtually all of the impact of $X$ 'lost' due to the misclassification.

**TABLE 2.3**
Regression coefficients for $Y$ in terms of $(1, X^*, Z, X^*Z)$ when misclassification is differential. The underlying coefficients for $Y$ in terms of $(1, X, Z)$ are $(\beta_0, \beta_1, \beta_2) = (0.15, 0.3, 0.15)$. The distribution of $(X|Z)$ is given by $\gamma = (0.5, 0.5)$. The baseline scenario is nondifferential misclassification, with $Sn = 0.65$ and $Sp = 0.85$. In the denial scenarios, the sensitivity amongst cases is reduced to either 0.55 (i) or 0.45 (ii). In the blame scenarios, the specificity amongst cases is reduced to either 0.75 (i) or 0.65 (ii).

| Scenario | $\beta_0^*$ | $\beta_1^*$ | $\beta_2^*$ | $\beta_3^*$ | $AF_0$ | $AF_1$ |
|---|---|---|---|---|---|---|
| Baseline | 0.24 | 0.16 | 0.15 | -0.00 | 0.52 | 0.52 |
| Denial (i) | 0.27 | 0.09 | 0.15 | -0.00 | 0.31 | 0.30 |
| Denial (ii) | 0.29 | 0.03 | 0.15 | -0.01 | 0.09 | 0.07 |
| Blame (i) | 0.23 | 0.18 | 0.14 | 0.01 | 0.59 | 0.63 |
| Blame (ii) | 0.22 | 0.20 | 0.14 | 0.02 | 0.66 | 0.73 |

## 2.5 Other Topics

### 2.5.1 Generalized Linear Models

A key statistical concept is that properties and intuitions for linear models with continuous outcome variables tend to be preserved when we move to generalized linear models for other types of outcome variables. This certainly holds in the realm of the impact of measurement error, though the relevant mathematics becomes less amenable.

For instance, Gustafson (2004, Sec. 2.6) takes a close look at the parallel to the attenuation described by (2.2) and (2.3) when logistic models for binary $Y$ variables are considered. The starting point is

$$\text{logit}Pr(Y = 1|X, Z) \quad = \quad \beta_0 + \beta_1 X + \beta_2^T Z.$$

However, even under the nicest of circumstances, the logistic link function is not preserved. That is, $(Y|X^*, Z)$ does not exactly follow a logistic model. Nonetheless, we can compare the limiting coefficients from *fitting* such a model, and ask to what extent the $X^*$ coefficient (say in the large-sample limit) is attenuated relative to $\beta_1$. These calculations need to be done numerically, but Gustafson (2004, Sec. 2.6) gives a numerical demonstration that the attenuation factor (2.3) from the linear regression context still roughly applies in the logistic regression setting.

### 2.5.2 Survival Analysis and other Complex Data Settings

As we progress beyond linear models and generalized linear models, it becomes much more difficult to glean simple insights into the impact of unchecked measurement error. In the survival analysis context, for instance, it seems Prentice (1982) was the first to consider the impact via the hazard rate for a survival-time outcome in terms of predictors $(X, Z)$ inducing a different hazard rate for the outcome in terms of $(X^*, Z)$. While there is some scope to infer approximate relationships between the forms and parameters for the original and induced hazard functions, the mathematics is far less clean and general than that encountered with linear models. Recently, Yi (2017, Sec. 3.2.1) summarized the literature on hazard functions induced by measurement error, providing a number of relevant references.

In a similar spirit to her investigation of the survival time situation, Yi (2017, Sec. 4.2) also examines the biasing effects of measurement error when a Poisson process is used to model recurrent events over time. Here the mean function for $N(t)$, the number of events arising by time $t$, is the starting point. The situation is complicated, however, since a Poisson process for $(N(t)|X, Z)$ does not generally induce a Poisson process for $(N(t)|X^*, Z)$. Rather, the induced process is generally overdispersed relative to Poisson variation. While some special cases are amenable to a simple characterization of the bias due to misclassification, general expressions like those arising in linear models are not available.

In longitudinal data models it is similarly challenging to provide simple characterizations of measurement error bias, though Yi (2017, Sec. 5.2.1) is able to obtain an interesting closed-form expression for attenuation in a special case that the predictor measured with error is uncorrelated with other precisely measured predictors.

### 2.5.3 Polychotomous Predictors

In the setting of a categorical predictor with more than two categories, even 'nicely behaving' mismeasurement of this predictor will not necessarily induce bias toward the null. For instance, say $X$ and $X^*$ are ordinal and trichotomous, taking values in $\{0, 1, 2\}$. A number of authors have investigated how misclassification of $X$ into $X^*$, even if well-behaved, does not guarantee attenuation in this setting. See, for instance, Dosemeci, Wacholder and Lubin (1990), Birkett (1992), Weinberg, Umbach and Greenland (1994), and Gustafson (2004, Sec. 3.6).

Specifically, we can presume nondifferentiality in the sense that $X^*$ is conditionally independent of $Y$ given $X$, so that the mismeasurement is described by a $3 \times 3$ matrix of classification probabilities, with the $(i, j)$-th entry being $Pr(X^* = j|X = i)$. This matrix can be well-behaved in the sense that the probabilities decline as we move away from the diagonal, both within each row and within each column. (For rows, this decline is naturally interpreted as a worse classification being less likely, for each level of $X$. Ogburn and Vanderweele (2013) describe the classification probabilities as *tapered* when the condition holds for both rows and columns.) Yet it can be that a contrast for the outcome across adjacent levels involves *reverse attenuation*. For instance, we can find tapered classification probabilities such that $\{E(Y|X^* = k+1) - E(Y|X^* = k)\} > \{E(Y|X = k+1) - E(Y|X = k)\} > 0$. Progressing from two to even three levels of the categorical predictor suffices to remove much of the intuition and regularity around the bias due to misclassification.

### 2.5.4 Multiple Covariates Measured with Error

In practice it can easily arise that more than one explanatory variable is prone to mismeasurement. For instance, we might be interested in the $(Y|X_1, X_2)$ regression, but can only observe $(Y, X_1^*, X_2^*)$ data. Both Gustafson (2004, Sec. 2.4) and Carroll et al. (2006, Sec. 3.3.2) scrutinize this situation. Even with nondifferentiality and simple measurement error structure such as $(X_i^*|X_i) \sim N(X_i, \tau_i^2)$ for $i = 1, 2$, the situation is rather complex. This is particularly true if $X_1^*$ and $X_2^*$ are correlated given $(X_1, X_2)$, and one can imagine that such correlated measurement errors could easily arise in applications.

To give some flavor for what can happen, regard $(\beta_0, \beta_1, \beta_2)$ as the coefficients defining a linear form for $E(Y|X_1, X_2)$. With sufficient assumptions $E(Y|X_1^*, X_2^*)$ will also be linear, with coefficients $(\beta_0^*, \beta_1^*, \beta_2^*)$ induced. It is possible that reverse attenuation arises, e.g., $\beta_1^* > \beta_1 > 0$ is possible. Also, *transferal* can arise, in the following sense: Even if $\text{Var}(X_1) = \text{Var}(X_2)$, we can see $\beta_1^* > \beta_2^* > 0$ when in fact $\beta_2 > \beta_1 > 0$. This raises the spectre of identifying the 'wrong culprit' amongst two predictor variables, when in reality one is a strong predictor of the outcome while the other is weak. Again, much intuition and regularity is lost in the face of two or more predictors being simultaneously mismeasured.

### 2.5.5 Berkson Error

Throughout this chapter we have discussed situations where the observable $X^*$ arises as a corrupted version of the latent $X$, and inference procedures are applied to $(X^*, Y)$ data as if they were $(X, Y)$ data. Sometimes, however, the scientific context is really such that $X$ arises as a corrupted version of $X^*$, and this is referred to as *Berkson error* (Berkson, 1950). The prototype situation for this is when $X$ is a factor in a controlled experiment, such as the temperature at which a given experimental run is conducted. The experimenter may set the thermostat to a desired level $X^*$, but in reality the actual temperature achieved, $X$, may be slightly lower or higher than the thermostat setting. Hence it is natural to write $X|X^* \sim N(X^*, \tau^2)$ rather than $X^*|X \sim N(X, \tau^2)$. This may not seem like such a big deal, in that either way $\tau$ describes the measurement error magnitude. However, the difference between the two cases is rather profound.

Say that $(Y|X, X^*) \sim N(\beta_0 + \beta_1 X, \sigma^2)$, so that measurement error is nondifferential, and say that $(X, X^*)$ has a bivariate normal distribution. On the one hand, if $(X^*|X) \sim N(X, \tau^2)$ then we are immediately in the context of (2.3), and the $X^*$ coefficient in $E(Y|X^*)$ is biased toward the null, relative to $\beta_1$. On the other hand, if $(X^*|X) \sim N(X, \tau^2)$ then $E(Y|X^*) = \beta_0 + \beta_1 X^*$, hence no bias arises in estimating $\beta_1$ directly from the regression of $Y$ on $X^*$. As emphasized by Buonaccorsi (2010, Sec. 4.2) however, the fact that $\text{Var}(Y|X^*)$ exceeds $\text{Var}(Y|X)$ has implications. For instance, the naive regression of $Y$ on $X^*$ does not yield valid prediction intervals for predicting $Y$ from $X$. And in fact there are many further nuances concerning when Berkson error arises, and what it implies. For instance, see Küchenhoff, Bender and Langner (2007) and Hoffmann et al. (2018) in the context of modeling failure-time outcomes.

### 2.5.6 Mismeasured Outcome

This chapter, and indeed this volume, emphasizes mismeasurement of an explanatory variable. Of course scientific contexts can easily arise where it is the outcome variable $Y$ that is mismeasured. This situation generally raises less concern and has spawned less literature, for the following reason. In the simplest case of normal linear regression structure, we have seen that $(Y|X) \sim N(\beta_0 + \beta_1 X, \sigma^2)$ and $(X^*|X,Y) \sim N(0, \tau^2)$ causes problems: The $X^*$ coefficient in $E(Y|X^*)$ is not the same as the $X$ coefficient in $E(Y|X)$. But if $(Y^*|Y,X) \sim N(Y, \tau^2)$ then immediately $E(Y^*|X) = E(Y|X)$, i.e., we are working with the same regression function whether it is $Y$ or $Y^*$ that is observable. In the simplest of settings then, measurement error in the outcome is merely absorbed into the residual variance, via $\text{Var}(Y^*|X) = \text{Var}(Y|X) + \tau^2$.

As we move from a continuous outcome variable $Y$ described by a linear model to other outcome variable types, issues around mismeasurement of $Y$ become more prominent. For instance, if $Y$ and $X$ are binary and their odds-ratio is of interest, the symmetry inherent in this situation dictates that misclassification of $Y$ would be as damaging as misclassification of $X$.

### 2.5.7 Statistical Power

This chapter has centered on estimation, with a focus on how biased estimation procedures can be if they are used in a naive manner, i.e., if we pretend that we have higher-quality data than is actually the case. However, measurement error also has implications for hypothesis testing. Insofar as the first principle of statistical hypothesis testing is to control Type I error rate, some forms of measurement error do permit naivety. For instance, say the null hypothesis that $X$ and $Y$ are conditionally independent given $Z$ is of interest, versus a nondirectional alternative. With very well-behaved measurement error, such as $(X^*|X,Y,Z) \sim N(X, \tau^2)$, it is true (and intuitive) that $X \perp Y|Z$ if and only if $X^* \perp Y|Z$. Hence one has a 'hall pass' to simply test for a zero coefficient for $X^*$ in the $(Y|X^*, Z)$ regression, and the Type I error rate will be controlled as usual. In this sense, it is not invalid to apply the same procedure to $(X^*, Y, Z)$ data that one would apply to $(X, Y, Z)$ data, were it available.

There is a penalty in terms of power, however. Necessarily, the $(X^*, Y|Z)$ association is weaker than the $(X, Y|Z)$ association, with the extent of weakening governed by $\tau$. Thus for a given sample size, significance level, and strength of $(X, Y|Z)$ association, $(X^*, Y|Z)$ data possess less power to detect the alternative hypothesis than do $(X, Y, Z)$ data. This power loss is readily quantified. As emphasized by Buzas, Stefanski and Tosteson (2014, Sec. 33.3.1), to match the power inherent in $n$ independent instances of $(X, Y, Z)$, one needs approximately $(1 + \tau^2/\lambda^2)n$ independent instances of $(X^*, Y, Z)$. The same attenuation factor that describes the extent of multiplicative bias in estimating the $X$ coefficient also describes the reduction in effective sample size for hypothesis testing purposes.

As a final thought on power, we have seen in this chapter that unacknowledged mismeasurement of explanatory variables tends to produce bias in estimating relationships between the actual variables of interest. As is amply covered in this volume, with enough knowledge about the mismeasurement process, methods which acknowledge the problem can take the bias away. In contrast, the power loss is permanent. Knowledge of the $(X^*|X, Y)$ distribution plus observation of the $(X^*, Y)$ data does not let us reconstruct the actual $X$ data, hence the power based on $(X, Y)$ data is unattainable. A noisy observation (of $(X^*, Y)$) inherently has lower information content than a good observation (of $(X, Y)$). The 'no free lunch' principle that pervades so much of statistical work is very much at play here.

## 2.6 Conclusion

We have seen that error can propagate in nefarious ways. In simple situations, error in measuring explanatory variable $X$ may be 'fair,' say in the sense that the observable surrogate $X^*$ is distributed symmetrically around $X$. Yet this can produce a systemic bias, should we interpret the regression of $Y$ on $X^*$ as if it were the regression of $Y$ on $X$. The slope estimator has a sampling distribution which is pushed toward the null. And when me move beyond simple situations, we no longer have a simple relationship for how ignoring mismeasurement biases the estimation process. Though we generally have the means to evaluate this relationship under given circumstances, even if it is complex.

So we have some understanding of the biases at play, and we view such understanding as a first step in trying to remove these biases. But what are the next steps? To find out, read on. The following chapters in this volume describe a wide array of strategies, in a wide array of contexts, for appropriate statistical analysis in the face of mismeasured data.

## References

Berkson, J. (1950). Are there two regressions? *Journal of the American Statistical Association*, 45(250), 164-180.

Birkett, N. (1992). Effect of nondifferential misclassification on estimates of odds ratios with multiple levels of exposure. *American Journal of Epidemiology*, 136(3), 356-362.

Brenner, H. (1993). Bias due to non-differential misclassification of polytomous confounders. *Journal of Clinical Epidemiology*, 46(1), 57-63.

Buonaccorsi, J. P. (2010). *Measurement Error: Models, Methods, and Applications.* Chapman and Hall, CRC Press.

Buzas, J. S., Stefanski, L. A. and Tosteson, T. D. (2014). Measurement error. In W. Ahrens and I. Pigeot (Eds.), *Handbook of Epidemiology,* Volume 3. Springer.

Carroll, R. J., Ruppert, D., Stefanski, L. A., and Crainiceanu, C. M. (2006). *Measurement Error in Nonlinear Models: A Modern Perspective*, 2nd ed. Chapman & Hall, CRC Press.

Dosemeci, M., Wacholder, S., and Lubin, J. H. (1990). Does nondifferential misclassification of exposure always bias a true effect toward the null value? *American Journal of Epidemiology*, 19, 746-748.

Greenland, S. (1980). The effect of misclassification in the presence of covariates. *American Journal of Epidemiology*, 112(4), 564-569.

Gustafson, P. (2004). *Measurement Error and Misclassification in Statistics and Epidemiology: Impact and Bayesian Adjustments.* Chapman & Hall, CRC Press.

Hoffmann, S., Laurier, D., Rage, E., Guihenneuc, C., and Ancelet, S. (2018). Shared and unshared exposure measurement error in occupational cohort studies and their effects on statistical inference in proportional hazards models. *PLoS One*, 13(2), e0190792.

Keogh, R. H., Strawbridge, A. D., and White, I. R. (2012). Effects of classical exposure measurement error on the shape of exposure-disease associations. *Epidemiologic Methods*, 1(1), 13-32.

Küchenhoff, H., Bender, R., and Langner, I. (2007). Effect of Berkson measurement error on parameter estimates in cox regression models. *Lifetime Data Analysis*, 13(2), 261-272.

Ogburn, E. L and VanderWeele, T. J. (2012). On the nondifferential misclassification of a binary confounder. *Epidemiology*, 23(3), 433-439.

Ogburn, E. L and Vanderweele, T. J. (2013). Bias attenuation results for nondifferentially mismeasured ordinal and coarsened confounders. *Biometrika*, 100(1), 241-248.

Prentice, R. (1982). Covariate measurement errors and parameter estimation in a failure time regression model. *Biometrika*, 69(2), 331-342.

Weinberg, C. R., Umbach, D. M., and Greenland, S. (1994). When will nondifferential misclassification of an exposure preserve the direction of a trend? (with discussion). *American Journal of Epidemiology*, 140, 565-571.

Yi, G. Y. (2017). *Statistical Analysis with Measurement Error or Misclassification.* Springer.

# Part II

# Identifiability and Estimation

# 3

# *Identifiability in Measurement Error Models*

**Liqun Wang**

## CONTENTS



## 3.1 Introduction

Identifiability is a fundamental issue in the statistical estimation and inference in measurement error (ME) models. The problem is caused by the fact that measurement error in covariates introduces so much uncertainty that the main sample data, no matter how large the sample size, cannot provide sufficient amount of information to identify all unknown parameters.

Generally speaking, a parameter in a given model is identifiable, if it is uniquely determined by the sampling distribution of the observed random variables in the model. Specifically, suppose we observe a random vector $Z$ and the sampling distribution $F(z;\theta)$, $z \in \mathbb{R}^k$, is known up to an unknown parameter vector $\theta \in \Theta$, where $\Theta \subseteq \mathbb{R}^p$ is the parameter space. Then $\theta$ is said to be identifiable, if for any possible values $\theta_1, \theta_2 \in \Theta$, $F(z;\theta_1) \equiv F(z;\theta_2)$ implies $\theta_1 = \theta_2$ (Fuller, 1987; Hsiao, 1983). The model is said to be identifiable, if all unknown parameters in it are identifiable. In other words, $\theta$ is identifiable if it is uniquely determined by the sampling distribution $F(z;\theta)$. Therefore $\theta$ cannot be consistently estimated if it is not identifiable.

While the problem of identifiability in linear ME models has been well studied, e.g., Hsiao (1983) and Fuller (1987), it has been a long-standing and

DOI: 10.1201/9781315101279-3

challenging problem in nonlinear models. Usually direct and explicit answers are difficult to obtain because the analytic forms of the moments of the observed variables are not available. In such cases the problem has to be studied through the existence of consistent estimators for some or all of the unknown parameters in the model. In general, there are two different types of measurement error. One is the classical error, also called errors-in-variables, which is independent of the unobserved true covariates. The other is the Berkson error which is independent of the observed surrogate covariates. Examples of variables typically observed with classical ME include long-term average blood pressure or cholesterol level of a person measured during a clinic visit, or the viral load and CD4+ T cell counts measured in laboratories in an HIV trial. Examples of variables typically observed with Berkson ME include an individual's exposure to certain air pollutants that are measured at some monitoring stations in a city, or the actual absorption of a medical substance in a patient's blood stream measured by the predetermined doses.

To deal with classical ME models, some researchers used an instrumental variable (IV) approach. For example, Hausman et al. (1991) showed that the univariate polynomial model is identifiable, while Wang and Hsiao (1995, 1996, 2011) showed that identifiability holds for general nonlinear models. In addition, Wang and Hsiao (2007) developed consistent estimators for censored linear models, and Guan et al. (2019) used a similar approach for the ordinal probit models. A recent survey of the instrumental variable methods for the estimation in ME models is given by Lewbel (2021), while in longitudinal model is given by Wang (2021). Some other researchers assumed that the ME variance is known or can be estimated by replicate measurements of the surrogate covariates. For example, Wang (1994, 1998) studied the censored linear (Tobit) model, Hausman et al. (1995) showed that the polynomial model is identifiable, whereas Li (2002), Li and Hsiao (2004), and Schennach (2004) proposed consistent estimators in generalized linear or nonlinear models. However, Huang and Huwang (2001) showed that a polynomial model of order greater than two where all unobserved variables and errors have normal distribution is identifiable without extra information.

Interestingly, nonlinear models with Berkson ME are generally identifiable without extra information or data besides the main sample. This was shown for logistic models by Rudemo et al. (1989), and for polynomial models by Huwang and Huang (2000). Later, Wang (2003, 2004) showed that a nonlinear model is generally identifiable using the first two conditional moments of the response variable given the observed surrogate covariates.

In this chapter, we provide an account of identifiability results for general nonlinear regression models with either Berkson or classical ME in the covariates. In particular, we show that the Berkson ME models are generally identifiable without extra data. We study the IV approach to identifiability in the classical ME models, where a semiparametric approach is also presented. The rest of this chapter is organized as follows. In Section 3.2, we demonstrate the problem of identifiability in a simple linear model. In Section 3.3, we study the identifiability in nonlinear models with Berkson measurement error. In Section 3.4, we use the instrumental variable method to study the identifiability in nonlinear models with classical measurement error. Finally, conclusions an discussion are given in Section 3.5.

## 3.2 Linear Measurement Error Model

In this section we demonstrate how measurement error causes the problem of identifiability using a simple linear model with classical ME. Specifically, consider

$$Y = \beta_0 + \beta_x X + \varepsilon, \tag{3.2.1}$$

where $\varepsilon \sim N(0, \sigma_\varepsilon^2)$ and is uncorrelated with $X$. Suppose $X$ is unobservable and instead the observed covariate is

$$X^* = X + U, \tag{3.2.2}$$

where $U$ is the random ME independent of $X$ and $\varepsilon$. Further, suppose $X \sim N(\mu_x, \sigma_x^2)$ and $U \sim N(0, \sigma_u^2)$. Then the sampling distribution of the observed variables $(Y, X^*)$ is jointly normal which is completely characterized by its first two moments. Further, these two moments are related to the unknown parameters in model (3.2.1)–(3.2.2) as

$$\begin{aligned}
\mu_y &= \beta_0 + \beta_x \mu_x; &(3.2.3)\\
\mu_{x^*} &= \mu_x; &(3.2.4)\\
\sigma_y^2 &= \beta_x \sigma_{yx^*} + \sigma_\varepsilon^2; &(3.2.5)\\
\sigma_{yx^*} &= \beta_x \sigma_x^2; &(3.2.6)\\
\sigma_{x^*}^2 &= \sigma_x^2 + \sigma_u^2. &(3.2.7)
\end{aligned}$$

It is easy to see that the above five moment equations contain six unknown parameters $(\beta_0, \beta_x, \mu_x, \sigma_x^2, \sigma_u^2, \sigma_\varepsilon^2)$ on the right-hand sides. Therefore, except for $\mu_x$, all other parameters cannot be uniquely determined by the observed moments on the left-hand sides. Hence the model is not identifiable.

In fact, by simple algebra we can find the range constraints of the unknown parameters imposed by (3.2.3)–(3.2.7). Suppose $\beta_x \neq 0$, then the constraints are

$$\frac{\sigma_{yx^*}}{\sigma_{x^*}^2} \leq \beta_x \leq \frac{\sigma_y^2}{\sigma_{yx^*}};$$

$$\mu_y - \frac{\mu_{x^*}\sigma_y^2}{\sigma_{yx^*}} \leq \beta_0 \leq \mu_y - \frac{\mu_{x^*}\sigma_{yx^*}}{\sigma_{x^*}^2};$$

$$\frac{\sigma_{yx^*}^2}{\sigma_y^2} \le \sigma_x^2 \le \sigma_{x^*}^2;$$

$$0 \le \sigma_u^2 \le \sigma_{x^*}^2 - \frac{\sigma_{yx^*}^2}{\sigma_y^2};$$

$$0 \le \sigma_\varepsilon^2 \le \sigma_y^2 - \frac{\sigma_{yx^*}^2}{\sigma_{x^*}^2},$$

if $\sigma_{yx^*} > 0$, and the inequalities for $\beta_x, \beta_0$ are reversed if $\sigma_{yx^*} < 0$. In other words, any set of parameter values falling in these intervals is compatible with the sampling distribution of $(Y, X^*)$.

The lack of identifiability of the normal linear model remains true in the censored linear models. Wang (1994, 1998) studied the so-called Tobit model (3.2.1)–(3.2.2) where the response variable $Y$ is censored so that one observes $Y^* = \max\{Y, 0\}$. Due to the censoring, now the parameters $\mu_y, \sigma_{yx^*}, \sigma_y^2$ on the left-hand sides of (3.2.3)–(3.2.7) are not directly observable. However, these parameters can be identified through the following observed (conditional) moments

$$\mu_{y^*} = \Phi(\eta)\mu_{y^*}^+; \tag{3.2.8}$$
$$\mu_{y^*}^+ = \mu_y + \sigma_y\phi(\eta)/\Phi(\eta); \tag{3.2.9}$$
$$\mu_{y^*x^*}^+ = \sigma_{yx*} + \mu_{x^*}\mu_{y^*}^+; \tag{3.2.10}$$

where $\mu_{y^*}^+ = E(Y^* \mid Y^* > 0)$, $\eta = \mu_y/\sigma_y$, and $\Phi(\cdot)$ and $\phi(\cdot)$ are the standard normal distribution and density functions, respectively. Therefore, as in the case of the linear model, prior restrictions on the parameters $(\beta_0, \beta_x, \sigma_x^2, \sigma_\varepsilon^2, \sigma_u^2)$ are needed to achieve model identifiability.

The situation in Berkson ME models is slightly different than in classical ME models. To illustrate, instead of (3.2.2) we assume that we observe $X^*$, where $X = X^* + U$ with $U$ independent of $X^*$ and $\varepsilon$. Then by substituting $X^* + U$ for $X$ in equation (3.2.1), we obtain

$$Y = \beta_0 + \beta_x X^* + \delta,$$

where $\delta = \varepsilon + \beta_x U$ is uncorrelated with $X^*$. Hence $\beta_0, \beta_x$ and $\sigma_\delta^2 = \sigma_\varepsilon^2 + \beta_x^2\sigma_u^2$ can be identified by the least squares regression of $Y$ on $X^*$. However, without any extra information, only the regression parameters $\beta_0, \beta_x$ are identifiable and the variance parameters $\sigma_\varepsilon^2, \sigma_u^2$ are not identifiable.

In practice, usually certain restrictions on unknown parameters are imposed in order to ensure identifiability. The commonly used restrictions are (1) ME variance $\sigma_u^2$ is known; (2) error variance ratio $\sigma_u^2/\sigma_\varepsilon^2$ is known; or (3) signal-to-noise (reliability, heritability) ratio $\sigma_x^2/\sigma_{x^*}^2$ is known. If there is no strong theoretical justification for these assumptions, these quantities can be estimated if additional data besides the main sample $(Y, X^*)$ is available. For example, (1) validation data, i.e., an observed subsample on $(Y, X)$; (2)

replicate data, i.e., two or more independent and unbiased measurements $X^*$ for the same $X$; (3) instrumental variables that are correlated with $X$ but uncorrelated with errors $U$ and $\varepsilon$. For more discussion see, e.g., Fuller (1987) and Carroll et al. (2006).

## 3.3 Nonlinear Model with Berkson Error

In this section we study the identifiability in nonlinear models with Berkson ME. Specifically, consider the model

$$Y = g(X, \beta) + \varepsilon, \tag{3.3.1}$$

where $Y \in I\!R$ is the response variable, $X \in I\!R^{p_x}$ is the vector of covariates, $\varepsilon$ is the random error, and $\beta \in I\!R^p$ is the vector of unknown parameters. In general, $g(x; \beta)$ is nonlinear in $x$. The unobserved true covariate $X$ is related to its observed surrogate $X^*$ as

$$X = X^* + U, \tag{3.3.2}$$

where $U$ is the measurement error that has a density $f_u(u; \theta)$ with unknown parameters $\theta$. Throughout this section we make the following assumptions.

**Assumption 1** *(1) $U$ is independent of $X^*$ and $E(U) = 0$; (2) $\varepsilon$ satisfies $E(\varepsilon \mid X, X^*) = 0$ and $E(\varepsilon^2 \mid X, X^*) = \sigma_\varepsilon^2$.*

Under these model assumptions the first two conditional moments of the response $Y$ given the observed surrogate $X^*$ are given by

$$\begin{aligned} E\left(Y \mid X^*\right) &= E[g(X, \beta) \mid X^*] + E(\varepsilon \mid X^*) \\ &= \int g\left(X^* + u, \beta\right) f_u(u; \theta)\, du \end{aligned} \tag{3.3.3}$$

and, similarly

$$\begin{aligned} E\left(Y^2 \mid X^*\right) &= E[g^2(X, \beta) \mid X^*] + 2E[\varepsilon g(X, \beta) \mid X^*] + E(\varepsilon^2 \mid X^*) \\ &= \int g^2\left(X^* + u, \beta\right) f_u(u; \theta)\, du + \sigma_\varepsilon^2. \end{aligned} \tag{3.3.4}$$

It is apparent that, when the conditional moments in (3.3.3) and (3.3.4) admit closed forms, the parameters $\beta, \theta, \sigma_\varepsilon^2$ can be identified by the nonlinear least squares method because both $Y$ and $X^*$ are observable. This is illustrated by the following examples.

**Example 3.3.1** First, consider the quadratic model

$$Y = \beta_0 + \beta_1 X + \beta_2 X^2 + \varepsilon,$$

where $\beta_2 \neq 0$ and $Var(U) = \theta$. For this model the first conditional moment of $Y$ given $X^*$ is given by:

$$\begin{aligned} E(Y|X^*) &= \beta_0 + \beta_1 E[(X^* + U)|X^*] + \beta_2 E[(X^* + U)^2|X^*] \\ &= \beta_0 + \beta_1 X^* + \beta_2 X^{*2} + \beta_2\theta \\ &= \varphi_1 + \varphi_2 X^* + \varphi_3 X^{*2}, \end{aligned} \tag{3.3.5}$$

where $\varphi_1 = \beta_0 + \beta_2\theta$, $\varphi_2 = \beta_1$ and $\varphi_3 = \beta_2$. Similarly, the second conditional moment of $Y$ is

$$\begin{aligned} E(Y^2|X^*) &= E[(\beta_0 + \beta_1 X + \beta_2 X^2)^2|X^*] + E(\varepsilon^2|X^*) \\ &= \varphi_4 + \varphi_5 X^* + \varphi_6 X^{*2} + 2\varphi_2\varphi_3 X^{*3} + \varphi_3^2 X^{*4}, \end{aligned} \tag{3.3.6}$$

where

$$\begin{aligned} \varphi_4 &= \beta_0^2 + (2\beta_0\beta_2 + \beta_1^2)\theta + 3\beta_2^2\theta^2 + \sigma_\varepsilon^2, \\ \varphi_5 &= 2\beta_1(\beta_0 + 3\beta_2\theta), \\ \varphi_6 &= 2\beta_0\beta_2 + \beta_1^2 + 6\beta_2^2\theta. \end{aligned}$$

It is easy to see that $(\varphi_i)$ are identified by the nonlinear least squares regression using (3.3.5) and (3.3.6). Further, we can show that the mapping $(\beta_i, \theta, \sigma_\varepsilon^2) \mapsto (\varphi_i)$ is bijective. In fact, by using simple algebra we can find the inverse mapping

$$\begin{aligned} \beta_0 &= \varphi_1 - \varphi_3\theta; \\ \beta_1 &= \varphi_2; \\ \beta_2 &= \varphi_3; \\ \theta &= (\varphi_6 - 2\varphi_1\varphi_3 - \varphi_2^2)/(4\varphi_3^2); \\ \sigma_\varepsilon^2 &= \varphi_4 - \varphi_1^2 - \varphi_2^2\theta - 2\varphi_3^2\theta^2. \end{aligned}$$

Therefore, the original parameters $(\beta_i, \theta, \sigma_\varepsilon^2)$ are identifiable.

**Example 3.3.2** Next, consider model $g(X;\beta) = \beta_1 X_1 + \beta_3 \exp(\beta_2 X_2)$, where $\beta_2\beta_3 \neq 0$. In addition, we assume that $U = (U_1, U_2)^\top \sim N(0, \theta I_2)$, where $\theta > 0$ and $I_2$ is the 2-dimensional identity matrix. Then using the expression of the normal moment generating function, we obtain the conditional moment of $Y$ given $X^*$ as

$$\begin{aligned} E(Y|X^*) &= \beta_1 X_1^* + \beta_1 E(U_1) + \beta_3 \exp(\beta_2 X_2^*) E\left(\exp(\beta_2 U_2)\right) \\ &= \varphi_1 X_1^* + \varphi_3 \exp(\varphi_2 X_2^*), \end{aligned} \tag{3.3.7}$$

where $\varphi_1 = \beta_1$, $\varphi_2 = \beta_2$ and $\varphi_3 = \beta_3 \exp(\beta_2^2\theta/2)$. Similarly, the second conditional moment of $Y$ given $X^*$ is

$$\begin{aligned}
E(Y^2|X^*) &= \beta_1^2 E[(X_1^* + U_1)^2|X^*] + \beta_3^2 E[\exp(2\beta_2(X_2^* + U_2))|X^*] \\
&\quad +2\beta_1\beta_3 E[(X_1^* + U_1)\exp(\beta_2(X_2^* + U_2))|X^*] + E(\varepsilon^2|X^*) \\
&= \beta_1^2(X_1^{*2} + \theta) + \beta_3^2 \exp(2\beta_2 X_2^*) E\left[\exp(2\beta_2 U_2)\right] \\
&\quad +2\beta_1\beta_3 X_1^* \exp(\beta_2 X_2^*) E[\exp(\beta_2 U_2)] + \sigma_\varepsilon^2 \\
&= \varphi_4 + \varphi_1^2 X_1^{*2} + \varphi_5 \exp(2\varphi_2 X_2^*) \\
&\quad +2\varphi_1\varphi_3 X_1^* \exp(\varphi_2 X_2^*), \qquad (3.3.8)
\end{aligned}$$

where $\varphi_4 = \beta_1^2\theta + \sigma_\varepsilon^2$ and $\varphi_5 = \beta_3^2 \exp(2\beta_2^2\theta)$. Again, $(\varphi_i)$ are clearly identified by (3.3.7) and (3.3.8) and the nonlinear least squares method. Furthermore, it is straightforward to obtain the inverse relationship

$$\begin{aligned}
\beta_1 &= \varphi_1; \\
\beta_2 &= \varphi_2; \\
\beta_3 &= \varphi_3^2/\sqrt{\varphi_5}; \\
\theta &= \log(\varphi_5/\varphi_3^2)/\varphi_2^2; \\
\sigma_\varepsilon^2 &= \varphi_4 - \varphi_1^2 \log(\varphi_5/\varphi_3^2)/\varphi_2^2.
\end{aligned}$$

Therefore the mapping $(\beta_i, \theta, \sigma_\varepsilon^2) \mapsto (\varphi_i)$ is bijective and hence the original parameters $(\beta_i, \theta, \sigma_\varepsilon^2)$ are identifiable.

The above examples suggest that in many situations, the parameters in nonlinear models can be identified using the first two conditional moments of $Y$ given $X^*$ and the least squares method. This fact is shown for polynomial models by Huwang and Huang (2000), and for general nonlinear models by Wang (2003, 2004). When the closed forms of the conditional moments in (3.3.3) and (3.3.4) are not available, a simulation-based method can be used to identify and consistently estimate parameters $\beta, \theta, \sigma_\varepsilon^2$ (Wang, 2004).

## 3.4 Nonlinear Model with Classical Error

In this section, we consider the general nonlinear model (3.3.1) with classical ME, where the the unobserved true covariate $X$ is related to its observed surrogate $X^*$ as

$$X^* = X + U, \qquad (3.4.1)$$

and the ME $U$ is independent of $X$. Unlike in the Berkson ME model (3.3.1)–(3.3.2), model (3.3.1) and (3.4.1) is generally unidentifiable without extra information. In this section, we show how the model can be identified by using the instrumental variable approach. In general, an IV is an observed variable that is correlated with the unobserved true covariate $X$ but independent of measurement and model errors $U$ and $\varepsilon$. Here, we assume that a vector of instrumental variables $W \in \mathbb{R}^{p_w}$ is available and is related to $X$ through

$$X = \Gamma W + \delta, \tag{3.4.2}$$

where $\Gamma$ is a $p_x \times p_w$ matrix of unknown parameters and $\delta$ is the random error. In addition, we assume that the random errors in (3.3.1), (3.4.1) and (3.4.2) satisfy the following conditions.

**Assumption 2** *(1) $U$ satisfies $E(U \mid X, W) = 0$ and $E(UU^\top \mid X, W) = \Sigma_u$; (2) $\varepsilon$ satisfies $E(\varepsilon \mid X, X^*, W) = 0$ and $E(\varepsilon^2 \mid X, X^*, W) = \sigma_\varepsilon^2$; (3) $\delta$ is independent of $W$ and has $E(\delta) = 0$; (4) $\Gamma$ has full row rank $p_x \le p_w$.*

Note that the assumptions of zero conditional mean for the measurement and model errors in Assumption 2 (1) and (2) are weaker than the usual requirement for the IV that it is independent of the errors. Moreover, the independence assumption between $W$ and $\delta$ in Assumption 2 (3) is made to simplify notation in the following derivations, where the conditional distribution of $\delta$ given $W$ can be used instead of the marginal distribution of $\delta$. Further, the full rank condition of $\Gamma$ ensures that (3.4.2) does not contain redundant IVs. It also implies that at least as many IVs as the number of mismeasured covariates are needed in order to ensure model identification.

There is no distributional assumptions for $X, U$ and $\varepsilon$, so model (3.3.1), (3.4.1) and (3.4.2) represent a semiparametric model. In the following, we show that the model is identifiable based on the observed data $(Y, X^*, W)$. Our approach is based on the first two conditional moments of $(Y, X^*)$ given the instrumental variables $W$.

First, substituting (3.4.2) in (3.4.1) results in a usual regression equation

$$E(X^* \mid W) = \Gamma W. \tag{3.4.3}$$

Therefore $\Gamma$ can be identified by the least squares regression of $X^*$ on $W$. Hence, subsequently we assume that $\Gamma$ is identified. Further, the second moment of $X^*$ given $W$ is:

$$\begin{aligned} E(X^* X^{*\top} \mid W) &= E(XX^\top \mid W) + E(UU^\top \mid W) \\ &= \Gamma W W^\top \Gamma^\top + E(\delta\delta^\top \mid W) + E(UU^\top \mid W) \\ &= \Gamma W W^\top \Gamma^\top + \Sigma_\delta + \Sigma_u. \end{aligned} \tag{3.4.4}$$

Therefore $\Sigma_u$ can be identified by the above equation if $\Sigma_\delta$ is identified. In order to identify the other parameters, we need the conditional moments of the response variable $Y$ given $W$. Under the model assumptions the conditional moment of $Y$ given $W$ is given by:

$$\begin{aligned} E(Y \mid W) &= E[g(X, \beta) \mid W] + E(\varepsilon \mid W) \\ &= E[g(\Gamma W + \delta, \beta) \mid W] \\ &= \int g(x + \Gamma_w W, \beta)\, dF_\delta(x). \end{aligned} \tag{3.4.5}$$

Similarly, the second order conditional moments are

$$\begin{aligned}
E(YX^* \mid W) &= E[Xg(X,\beta) \mid W] + E[Ug(X,\beta) \mid W] + E(X\varepsilon \mid W) \\
&\quad + E(U\varepsilon \mid W) \\
&= E[(\Gamma W + \delta)g(\Gamma W + \delta, \beta) \mid W] \\
&= \int (x + \Gamma W) g(x + \Gamma W, \beta)\, dF_\delta(x) \qquad (3.4.6)
\end{aligned}$$

and

$$\begin{aligned}
E(Y^2 \mid W) &= E[g^2(X,\beta) \mid W] + E(\varepsilon^2 \mid W) \\
&= \int g^2(x + \Gamma W, \beta)\, dF_\delta(x) + \sigma_\varepsilon^2. \qquad (3.4.7)
\end{aligned}$$

From the above moment equations we can see that, if $\beta$ and the distribution $F_\delta$ (hence $\Sigma_\delta$) can be identified by (3.4.5) and (3.4.6), then $\sigma_\varepsilon^2$ will be identified by (3.4.7). The following examples demonstrate how $\beta$ and $F_\delta$ are identified by (3.4.5) and (3.4.6).

**Example 3.4.1** Consider a polynomial model $g(x;\beta) = \beta_1 + \beta_2 x^2$, where $p_x = 1$, $\Gamma = 1$ and $Var(\delta) = \theta$. Then moments (3.4.5) and (3.4.6) are respectively

$$\begin{aligned}
E(Y \mid W) &= (\beta_1 + \beta_2\theta) + \beta_2 W^2; \\
E(YX^* \mid W) &= (\beta_1 + 3\beta_2\theta)W + \beta_2 W^3.
\end{aligned}$$

We can see that $\beta_1 + \beta_2\theta$ and $\beta_2$ can be identified by the least squares method from the first equation, while $\beta_1 + 3\beta_2\theta$ is identified by the second equation. It follows that $\beta_1, \beta_2$ and $\theta$ are identifiable.

**Example 3.4.2** Another example is an exponential model $g(x;\beta) = \beta_1 \exp(\beta_2 x)$, where $\beta_1\beta_2 \neq 0$ and $\delta \sim N(0,\theta)$. In this model moments (3.4.5) and (3.4.6) are respectively

$$\begin{aligned}
E(Y \mid W) &= \beta_1 \exp\left(\beta_2 W + \beta_2^2\theta/2\right); \\
E(YX^* \mid W) &= \beta_1(\beta_2\theta + W)\exp\left(\beta_2 W + \beta_2^2\theta/2\right).
\end{aligned}$$

Again, $\beta_2$, $\beta_1 \exp\left(\beta_2^2\theta/2\right)$ and $\beta_1\beta_2\theta \exp\left(\beta_2^2\theta/2\right)$ can be identified by nonlinear least squares method, implying that $\beta_1, \beta_2$ and $\theta$ are identifiable.

In the rest of this section we derive sufficient conditions for $\beta$ and $F_\delta$ to be identifiable based on moment equations (3.4.5)–(3.4.6). The basic idea is to apply Fourier deconvolution to these equations to separate $\beta$ and $F_\delta$. This approach is based on the following assumptions.

**Assumption 3** *The distribution of $W$ is absolutely continuous with respect to Lebesgue measure and has support $I\!R^{p_w}$.*

**Assumption 4** *$g(x;\beta)(\|x\|+1) \in L^1(I\!R^{p_x})$, the space of absolutely integrable functions on $I\!R^{p_x}$. Further, the set $\mathcal{T} = \{t \in I\!R^{p_x} : \varphi_g(t;\beta) \neq 0\}$ is dense in $I\!R^{p_x}$, where $\varphi_g(t;\beta) = \int \exp(it^\top x) g(x;\beta)\,dx$ is the Fourier transform of $g(x;\beta)$ and $i = \sqrt{-1}$.*

The integrability of $g(x;\beta)$ in Assumption 4 implies the existence of the Fourier transform $\varphi_g(t;\beta)$ (Lukacs 1970). The second part of the assumption means that the zeros of $\varphi_g(t;\beta)$ are isolated points in $I\!R^{p_x}$. The examples given at the end of this section show that this assumption is fairly general. Define the functions

$$h_1(\beta) = \int g(x;\beta)\,dx; \tag{3.4.8}$$

$$h_2(\beta) = \int x g(x;\beta)\,dx. \tag{3.4.9}$$

Then we have the following result.

**Theorem 3.1** *Under Assumptions 2–4, suppose $h_1(\beta)$ and $h_2(\beta)$ are differentiable in an open neighborhood of the true parameter value, and the Jacobian*

$$J(\beta) = \left( \frac{\partial h_1(\beta)}{\partial \beta}, \frac{\partial h_2^\top(\beta)}{\partial \beta} \right) \tag{3.4.10}$$

*has full rank $p = \dim(\beta)$. Then $\beta$ and $F_\delta$ are identifiable.*

**Proof.** For every $v \in I\!R^{p_x}$, define

$$m_1(v) = \int g(x+v;\beta) dF_\delta(x). \tag{3.4.11}$$

Then by (3.4.5) $m_1(\Gamma W) = E(Y \mid W)$ which is fully observable on $I\!R^{p_x}$ because of Assumption 3 and that $\Gamma$ has full rank. Moreover, by Assumption 4 we have $m_1(v) \in L^1(I\!R^{p_x})$ and, further, taking Fourier transformation on both sides of (3.4.11) yields

$$\begin{aligned}
\varphi_{m_1}(t) &= \int \exp(it^\top v) m_1(v)\,dv \\
&= \int \exp(it^\top x) g(x;\beta)\,dx \cdot \int \exp(-it^\top v)\,dF_\delta(v) \\
&= \varphi_g(t;\beta)\varphi_\delta(-t),
\end{aligned} \tag{3.4.12}$$

where $\varphi_\delta(t)$ is the characteristic function of $\delta$. It follows from (3.4.12) that, for any $t \in \mathcal{T}$, $\varphi_\delta(t)$ is uniquely determined by

$$\varphi_\delta(t) = \frac{\varphi_{m_1}(-t)}{\varphi_g(-t;\beta)}. \tag{3.4.13}$$

Moreover, by Assumption 4 the value of $\varphi_\delta(t)$ at any zero of $\varphi_g(-t,\beta)$ is also uniquely determined, because any characteristic function is uniformly continuous in $I\!R^{p_x}$ (Lukacs, 1970). Therefore $F_\delta$ is identifiable as long as $\beta$ is.

In order to obtain the identifiability condition for $\beta$, we define, for every $v \in I\!R^{p_x}$,

$$m_2(v) = \int (x+v)g(x+v;\beta)\,dF_\delta(x). \tag{3.4.14}$$

Then by (3.4.6) $m_2(\Gamma W) = E(YZ \mid W)$ which is observable. Further, by Assumption 4 $m_2(v) \in L^1(I\!R^{p_x})$ and, therefore, by integrating both sides of (3.4.11) and (3.4.14) and applying Fubini's Theorem we obtain

$$\int m_1(v)dv = \int g(x;\beta)\,dx = h_1(\beta); \tag{3.4.15}$$

$$\int m_2(v)dv = \int xg(x;\beta)\,dx = h_2(\beta). \tag{3.4.16}$$

Since the Jacobian $J(\beta)$ of the above equations has full rank $p$, by the Rank Theorem (Zeidler, 1986, p.178), $\beta$ is the unique solution of (3.4.15) and (3.4.16) in its neighborhood. It follows that $\beta$ is identified by (3.4.5)–(3.4.6). □

Note that since $J(\beta)$ has dimensions $p \times (p_x + 1)$, for $J(\beta)$ to have full rank it is necessary that $p \leq p_x + 1$. In addition, if $\varphi_\delta(t) \in L^1\,(I\!R^{p_x})$, then the density of $\delta$ exists and is given by

$$f_\delta(x) = \frac{1}{(2\pi)^{p_x}} \int \exp(it^\top x)\frac{\varphi_{m_1}(t)}{\varphi_g(t;\beta)}\,dt.$$

From a practical point of view, the integrability of $g(x;\beta)$ in Assumption 4 is not as restrictive as it appears, if $X$ is bounded with probability one. In the case where $X$ is unbounded, the truncated Fourier transform $\varphi_g^c(t;\beta) = \int_{-c}^{c}\exp(it'x)g(x;\beta)\,dx, c \to \infty$, can be used so that this assumption may be weaken to the condition that $E[|g(X;\beta)|(\|X\|+1)] < \infty$ (Wang and Hsiao, 2011).

In the rest of this section, we use some examples to illustrate how to apply Theorem 3.1 to check model identifiability. To simplify notation, we consider cases where all variables are scalars and $\Gamma = 1$.

**Example 3.4.3** Consider an exponential model $g(x;\beta) = \exp(-\beta x^2)$ where $\beta > 0$ and hence $g(x;\beta)$ is integrable. Further, the Fourier transform of $g(x;\beta)$ is

$$\begin{aligned}\varphi_g(t;\beta) &= \int \exp(itx)\exp(-\beta x^2)\,dx \\ &= \sqrt{\frac{\pi}{\beta}}\exp\left(-\frac{t^2}{4\beta}\right),\end{aligned}$$

which clearly satisfies Assumption 4. To check the rank condition, we calculate

$$h_1(\beta) = \int \exp(-\beta x^2)\, dx = \sqrt{\frac{\pi}{\beta}}$$

and

$$h_2(\beta) = \int x \exp(-\beta x^2)\, dx = 0.$$

It follows that $J(\beta) = \left(-\sqrt{\pi}/(2\beta\sqrt{\beta}), 0\right)$ which has rank one. Therefore, by Theorem 3.1 the model is identifiable.

**Example 3.4.4** Now consider the quadratic model $g(x;\beta) = \beta_1 x + \beta_2 x^2$ where $E\|X\|^3 < \infty$. It is clear that condition $E[|g(X;\beta)|(\|X\| + 1)] < \infty$ holds. Further, for any $c > 0$, the truncated Fourier transform is

$$\begin{aligned} \varphi_g^c(t;\beta) &= \int_{-c}^{c} \exp(itx)(\beta_1 x + \beta_2 x^2)\, dx \\ &= 2c\cos(ct)\left(\frac{\beta_2}{t^2} - \frac{i\beta_1}{t}\right) + 2\sin(ct)\left(\frac{\beta_2 c^2}{t} + \frac{i\beta_1}{t^2} - \frac{2\beta_2}{t^3}\right), \end{aligned}$$

which satisfies Assumption 4. To check the rank condition, we calculate $h_1(\beta) = 2\beta_2 c^3/3$ and $h_2(\beta) = 2\beta_1 c^3/3$. Hence the Jacobian is

$$J(\beta) = \frac{2c^3}{3}\begin{pmatrix} 0 & 1 \\ 1 & 0 \end{pmatrix},$$

which has rank two. Therefore, by Theorem 3.1 the model is identifiable.

**Example 3.4.5** Finally consider another exponential $g(x;\beta) = \exp(\beta x)$, $\beta \neq 0$ and $X$ has a normal distribution. In this case condition $E[|g(X;\beta)|(\|X\| + 1)] < \infty$ is satisfied. Further, for any $c > 0$ and $t \neq i\beta$, the truncated Fourier transform is

$$\varphi_g^c(t;\beta) = \frac{\exp[c(\beta + it)] - \exp[-c(\theta + it)]}{\beta + it},$$

which satisfies Assumption 4. Moreover, since $h_1(\beta) = [\exp(c\beta) - \exp(-c\beta)]/\beta$, and

$$h_2(\beta) = \frac{c(\exp(c\beta) + \exp(-c\beta))}{\beta} - \frac{\exp(c\beta) - \exp(-c\beta)}{\beta^2},$$

the Jacobian $J(\beta)$ is of rank one, implying that the model is identifiable.

## 3.5 Conclusions and Discussion

We have studied the problem of identifiability in regression models with covariate measurement error. We have shown that in general a nonlinear model with

Berkson measurement error can be identified by using the first two conditional moments of the response variable given the surrogate predictors. However, for a nonlinear model with classical measurement error, or a linear model with either classical or Berkson error, to be identifiable, certain restrictions or extra data are required. We have shown how instrumental variables can help to achieve model identifiability. We derived a sufficient rank condition for the identifiability of the regression coefficients, which is easy to check in practice. As in most theoretical works on nonlinear systems, we only obtained the results for local identifiability. More restrictive assumptions and theoretical techniques would be needed to achieve global identifiability, if it is possible at all.

In practice, any variables that are correlated with the error-prone covariates but independent of the measurement and model errors can serve as instrumental variables, such as a second independent measurement taken with a different method, or repeated measurements at different time points in longitudinal studies. For example, a second measurement of the systolic blood pressure can be taken by a different physician at a different time, or the cholesterol level, which is measured by laboratory blood test, can be measured again by using the home test kit. A further example is the CD4+ T cell counts in a HIV patient tested by two different laboratories using two different methods. It is worthwhile to note that the assumption of instrumental variables is weaker than that of replicate data because they can be biased measurements of the unobserved true covariates (Carroll and Stefanski, 1994; Carroll et al., 2006). The instrumental variable approach is also used in the literature of causal inference to deal with the problem of unobserved confounders, where usually additional conditions are imposed to achieve model identification (Angrist et al., 1996; Baiocchi et al., 2014).

In this Chapter, we are mainly concerned with the case where the error-prone covariates and measurement errors are continuous random variables. For the misclassification problem and Bayesian approach, see Gustafson (2003, 2021) and Yi (2017). A survey of semiparametric methods for both measurement error and misclassification problems is given in Ma (2021). Moreover, we focused on the parametric identifiability in regression models. There is a large literature on nonparametric identification, which is usually called deconvolution problems, e.g., Schennach (2007), Zinde-Walsh (2014), and Delaigle and Van Keilegom (2021). For an overview of nonparametric methods of estimation with classical measurement errors, see Delaigle (2021), and Apanasovich and Liang (2021), who introduce kernel deconvolution methods of density and regression, respectively, or Kang and Qiu (2021) who survey Fourier transformation and other related approaches. For a survey of nonparametric methods for Berkson measurement error models, see Song (2021). See also Delaigle (2007) for nonparametric density estimation with a mixture of Berkson and classical errors.

## Acknowledgments

The author is grateful to co-editor Aurore Delaigle for the kind invitation to write this chapter and for her helpful comments and suggestions on the previous version. This research is supported by the Natural Sciences and Engineering Research Council of Canada (NSERC).

## Bibliography

Angrist, J. D., Imbens, G. W., and Rubin, D. B. (1996). Identification of causal effects using instrumental variables. *Journal of the American Statistical Association*, 91(434), 444-455.

Apanasovich, T. and Liang, H. (2021). Nonparametric measurement errors models for regression. In Yi, G. Y., Delaigle, A., and Gustafson, P. (Eds.), *Handbook of Measurement Error Models*, CRC, Chapter 14.

Baiocchi, M., Cheng, J., and Small, D. S. (2014). Instrumental variable methods for causal inference. *Statistics in Medicine*, 33(13), 2297–2340.

Carroll, R. J., Ruppert, D., Stefanski, L. A., and Crainiceanu, C. M. (2006). *Measurement Error in Nonlinear Models: A Modern Perspective.* CRC Press.

Carroll, R. J. and Stefanski, L. A. (1994). Measurement error, instrumental variables and corrections for attenuation with applications to meta-analyses. *Statistics in Medicine*, 13(12), 1265–1282.

Delaigle, A. (2007). Nonparametric density estimation from data with a mixture of Berkson and classical errors. *Canadian Journal of Statistics*, 35(1), 89–104.

Delaigle, A. (2021). Deconvolution kernel density estimator. In Yi, Y. G., Delaigle, A., and Gustafson, P. (Eds.), *Handbook of Measurement Error Models*, CRC, Chapter 10.

Delaigle, A. and Van Keilegom, I. (2021). Deconvolution with unknown error distribution. In Yi, G. Y., Delaigle, A., and Gustafson, P. (Eds.), *Handbook of Measurement Error Models*, CRC, Chapter 12.

Fuller, W. A. (1987). *Measurement Error Models*, Volume 305. John Wiley & Sons.

Guan, J., Cheng, H., Bollen, K. A., Thomas, D. R., and Wang, L. (2019). Instrumental variable estimation in ordinal probit models with mismeasured predictors. *Canadian Journal of Statistics*, 47(4), 653–667.

Gustafson, P. (2003). *Measurement Error and Misclassification in Statistics and Epidemiology: Impacts and Bayesian Adjustments.* CRC Press.

Gustafson, P. (2021). Partial learning of misclassification parameters. In Yi, G. Y., Delaigle, A., and Gustafson, P. (Eds.), *Handbook of Measurement Error Models*, CRC, Chapter 4.

Hausman, J. A., Newey, W. K., Ichimura, H., and Powell, J. L. (1991). Identification and estimation of polynomial errors-in-variables models. *Journal of Econometrics*, 50(3), 273–295.

Hausman, J. A., Newey, W. K., and Powell, J. L. (1995). Nonlinear errors in variables estimation of some engel curves. *Journal of Econometrics*, 65(1), 205–233.

Hsiao, C. (1983). Identification. In Griliches, Z. and Intriligator, M. D. (Eds.), *Handbook of Econometrics*, Volume 1, North-Holland, pp. 223–283.

Huang, Y. S. and Huwang, L. (2001). On the polynomial structural relationship. *Canadian Journal of Statistics*, 29(3), 495–512.

Huwang, L. and Huang, Y. S. (2000). On errors-in-variables in polynomial regression-Berkson case. *Statistica Sinica*, 10, 923–936.

Kang, Y. and Qiu, P. (2021). Nonparametric deconvolution by Fourier transformation and other related approaches. In Yi, G. Y., Delaigle, A., and Gustafson, P. (Eds.), *Handbook of Measurement Error Models*, CRC, Chapter 11.

Lewbel, A. (2021). Using instrumental variables to estimate models with mismeasured regressors. In Yi, G. Y., Delaigle, A., and Gustafson, P. (Eds.), *Handbook of Measurement Error Models*, CRC, Chapter 5.

Li, T. (2002). Robust and consistent estimation of nonlinear errors-in-variables models. *Journal of Econometrics*, 110(1), 1–26.

Li, T. and Hsiao, C. (2004). Robust estimation of generalized linear models with measurement errors. *Journal of Econometrics*, 118(1-2), 51–65.

Lukacs, E. (1970). *Characteristic Functions.* Griffin.

Ma, Y. (2021). Semiparametric methods for measurement error and misclassification. In Yi, G. Y., Delaigle, A., and Gustafson, P. (Eds.), *Handbook of Measurement Error Models*, CRC, Chapter 9.

Rudemo, M., Ruppert, D., and Streibig, J. (1989). Random-effect models in nonlinear regression with applications to bioassay. *Biometrics*, 45, 349–362.

Schennach, S. M. (2004). Estimation of nonlinear models with measurement error. *Econometrica*, 72(1), 33–75.

Schennach, S. M. (2007). Instrumental variable estimation of nonlinear errors-in-variables models. *Econometrica*, 75(1), 201–239.

Song, W. (2021). Nonparametric inference methods for Berkson errors. In Yi, G. Y., Delaigle, A., and Gustafson, P. (Eds.), *Handbook of Measurement Error Models*, CRC, Chapter 13.

Wang, L. (1994). Identifiability and estimation of censored errors-in-variables models. In *ASA Proceedings of the Business and Economic Statistics Section*, 351–354. American Statistical Association (Alexandria, VA).

Wang, L. (1998). Estimation of censored linear errors-in-variables models. *Journal of Econometrics*, 84(2), 383–400.

Wang, L. (2003). Estimation of nonlinear Berkson-type measurement error models. *Statistica Sinica*, 13, 1201–1210.

Wang, L. (2004). Estimation of nonlinear models with Berkson measurement errors. *Annals of Statistics*, 32(6), 2559–2579.

Wang L. (2021). Estimation in mixed-efects models with measurement error. In Yi, G.Y., Delaigle A., and Gustafson P., (Eds.), *Handbook of Measurement Error Models*, CRC, Chapter 17.

Wang, L. and Hsiao, C. (1995). Simulation-based semiparametric estimation of nonlinear errors-in-variables models. *Working Paper, University of Southern California.*

Wang, L. and Hsiao, C. (1996). A semiparametric estimation of nonlinear errors-in-variables models. In *ASA Proceedings of the Business and Economic Statistics Section*, American Statistical Association (Alexandria, VA). 231–236.

Wang, L. and Hsiao, C. (2007). Two-stage estimation of limited dependent variable models with errors-in-variables. *The Econometrics Journal*, 10(2), 426–438.

Wang, L. and Hsiao, C. (2011). Method of moments estimation and identifiability of semiparametric nonlinear errors-in-variables models. *Journal of Econometrics*, 165(1), 30–44.

Yi, G. Y. (2017). *Statistical Analysis with Measurement Error or Misclassification.* Springer.

Zeidler, E. (1986). *Nonlinear Functional Analysis and Its Applications I.* Springer.

Zinde-Walsh, V. (2014). Measurement error and deconvolution in spaces of generalized functions. *Econometric Theory*, 30, 1207–1246.

# 4

# *Partial Learning of Misclassification Parameters*

**Paul Gustafson**

## CONTENTS



## 4.1 Motivation

We generally see imprecision in a continuous variable referred to as measurement error, while imprecision in a discrete variable is referred to as misclassification. Much of the literature deals with one case or the other, though several recent books in the area cover both (Buonaccorsi, 2010; Yi, 2017). Gustafson (2004) also covers both, albeit from a Bayesian perspective. Later in the present volume, Sinha (2021) concentrates on the Bayesian approach to measurement error, while Stamey and Seaman (2021) take a broad look at using Bayesian inference to adjust inferences for misclassification of one or more variables. In particular, the latter chapter surveys situations where direct validation data are available, situations where multiple imperfect measurements are available, and situations where prior information about the misclassification is the only help at hand.

The present chapter foreshadows the methodological narrative taken up by Stamey and Seaman (2021), particularly when the only available information about the extent of misclassification comes in the form of prior information. Said foreshadowing arises by focusing on an underlying theoretical issue concerning *parameter identification* in the face of misclassified data. We pose, and address, the following question. Theoretically, how good can posterior knowl-

DOI: 10.1201/9781315101279-4

edge about the extent of misclassification be, relative to prior knowledge? The answer to this question has implications for the value of doing a fully Bayesian analysis, compared to 'plugging in' *a priori* best guesses of misclassification parameters as if they were known truth.

To frame our problem, say that $X \in \{0, \ldots, p-1\}$ is ordinal with $p$ categories, $X^* \in \{0, \ldots, q-1\}$ is ordinal with $q$ categories, and $Y \in \{0, 1\}$ is binary. Generally the scientific goal is to learn about the $(X, Y)$ association, but with the handicap that we observe only $(X^*, Y)$ data on a number of study subjects.

We take it as read that $X^*$ is a surrogate for $X$, i.e., $X^*$ is positively associated with $X$, regardless of whether these two ordinal variables have the same number of levels ($q = p$) or not. We also take it as read that $X^*$ is *non-differential*, i.e., $(X^* \perp Y \mid X)$. This is a precise mathematical encapsulation of the notion that the mismeasurement process offering up $X^*$ in lieu of $X$ is 'blinded' to a study subject's outcome status.

While the ultimate scientific goal is learning about the $(X, Y)$ association, this chapter focusses on an intermediate step. In the absence of any validation data, what can the observed data contribute to advance knowledge about the mismeasurement process? In essence, we investigate the extent to which posterior knowledge about the distribution of $(X^*|X)$ is better than the prior knowledge.

## 4.2 The Case That $p = q = 2$

Generally misclassification of $X$ into $X^*$ is governed by a $p \times q$ misclassification matrix, with each row describing a probability mass function. However, in the simplest case of binary variables ($p = q = 2$), this can be reduced to parameters $\gamma = (\gamma_0, \gamma_1)$, where $\gamma_x = Pr(X^* = X|X = x)$. In common parlance then, $\gamma_0$ and $\gamma_1$ are respectively the *specificity* and *sensitivity* of $X^*$ as a surrogate for $X$.

Let $\theta$ parameterize $(X|Y)$, say via $\theta_y = Pr(X = 1|Y = y)$. With this parameterization, it is convenient to imagine data arising via case-control sampling, in which the marginal distribution of $Y$ is fixed by the study investigator. Hence only the $(X|Y)$ distribution contributes to the likelihood function. What follows, however, is equally applicable to cross-sectional data collection, in which case the marginal distribution of $Y$ is unknown and commensurately estimated.

We can combine a joint prior distribution for the unknown parameters $(\theta, \gamma)$ with data in the form of two independent Binomial observations: respectively the number of the $n_0$ *controls* (subjects with $Y = 0$) for whom $X^* = 1$, and the number of the $n_1$ *cases* (subjects with $Y = 1$) for whom $X^* = 1$. Note that the 'success' probabilities for these binomial datapoints are functions of $(\theta, \gamma)$. Using $\phi = (\phi_0, \phi_1)$ to denote these probabilities, we immediately have

$$\begin{aligned} \phi_y &\doteq Pr(X^* = 1|Y = y) \\ &= \theta_y\gamma_1 + (1 - \theta_y)(1 - \gamma_0). \end{aligned}$$

As an illustration of a practical choice of prior distribution for $(\theta, \gamma)$, we first assume that $\gamma$ is *a priori* independent of $\theta$. This seems quite reasonable, as generally there should be no overt link between background information about the mismeasurement process on the one hand, and background information about the exposure-disease relationship on the other. For illustration, we also take a simple and neutral prior specification for $\theta$, namely a uniform distribution on $(0, 1)^2$. Thus it remains only to specify the prior distribution for $\gamma$.

A very weak prior assertion about the quality of $X^*$ as a surrogate for $X$ would be that the association is positive, i.e., $(1 - \gamma_0) < \gamma_1$. A more stringent specification would be that there are known lower bounds, $\underline{\gamma}_0$ and $\underline{\gamma}_1$, respectively for the specificity $\gamma_0$ and sensitivity $\gamma_1$ (and it is convenient to presume both lower bounds exceed 0.5). That is, the study investigator is willing to commit to worst-case scenarios for the performance of $X^*$ as a surrogate for $X$. For illustration, we simply presume a uniform prior distribution for $(\gamma_0, \gamma_1)$ over $(\underline{\gamma}_0, 1) \times (\underline{\gamma}_1, 1)$. Thus the joint prior density over all unknown parameters takes the form:

$$\pi(\theta, \gamma) \quad \propto \quad I_{(0,1)}(\theta_0)I_{(0,1)}(\theta_1)I_{(\underline{\gamma}_0,1)}(\gamma_0)I_{(\underline{\gamma}_1,1)}(\gamma_1), \tag{4.1}$$

where here, and throughout, $I_A(\cdot)$ is the indicator function of set $A$.

To see what happens when this prior distribution is combined with data, it is illuminating to reparameterize from $(\theta, \gamma)$ to $(\phi, \gamma)$, with the implication that only $\phi$, and not $\gamma$, will appear in the likelihood function. Expressed in the new parameterization, our prior distribution is, upon change of variables applied to (4.1), expressed as:

$$\begin{aligned} \pi(\phi, \gamma) \quad \propto \quad & (\phi_0 + \phi_1 - 1)^{-2}\, I_{(0,1)}(\phi_0)\, I_{(0,1)}(\phi_1) \;\times \\ & I_{(g_0(\phi),1)}(\gamma_0)I_{(g_1(\phi),1)}(\gamma_1), \end{aligned} \tag{4.2}$$

where $g_0(\phi) = \max\{\underline{\gamma}_0, 1 - \phi_0, 1 - \phi_1\}$ and $g_1(\phi) = \max\{\underline{\gamma}_1, \phi_0, \phi_1\}$. (For ease of exposition in what follows, we leave implicit the dependence of $g_i()$ on $\underline{\gamma}_i$, for $i = 0, 1$.) For a longer narrative on the route from (4.1) to (4.2), see Gustafson, Le and Saskin (2001).

Upon combining the joint prior distribution (4.2) with the binomial-based likelihood for the observed data, and then considering the sample size going to infinity, we have a simple characterization for the limiting posterior distribution of $(\phi, \gamma)$. It is composed of a point mass distribution for $\phi$ at the true value $\phi^\dagger$, along with the conditional prior distribution of $(\gamma|\phi = \phi^\dagger)$ implied by (4.2). This has density proportional to (4.2), as a function of $\gamma$ with

$\gamma = \gamma^\dagger$ fixed. (Here, and throughout, we use a 'dagger' notation to indicate true parameter values giving rise to observed data.)

The form of the limiting posterior distribution makes clear that two things are happening to our knowledge of the classification parameters, as more data are collected. First, whereas the prior only restricts $\gamma$ via the lower bounds $\underline{\gamma}_0$ and $\underline{\gamma}_1$, we learn more stringent lower bounds, $g_0(\phi^\dagger)$ and $g_1(\phi^\dagger)$ as we collect more data (since, in the limit, we learn that $\phi = \phi^\dagger$). In common parlance for partial identification settings, whether approached in a Bayesian or non-Bayesian fashion, the rectangle $(g_0(\phi), 1) \times (g_1(\phi), 1)$ would be referred to as the *identification region* for $\gamma$, i.e., the set of all possible values of the classification parameters which are consistent with the law of the observable data.

A second finding is that whereas the prior on $\gamma$ is uniform above the lower bounds, the limiting posterior has a 'tilt.' The term $(\gamma_0 + \gamma_1 - 1)^{-2}$ in (4.2) shows that the (limiting) posterior involves a favoritism for smaller values of $\gamma_0$ and $\gamma_1$.

In terms of point estimation in a finite sample, the posterior mean of $\gamma$ is a natural estimator (particularly if a squared-error loss function is considered). From our characterization of the limiting posterior, this estimator will converge to $E(\gamma|\phi = \phi^\dagger)$ as the sample size increases. The form of (4.2) admits a closed form for this (bivariate) conditional mean, namely having components

$$E(\gamma_i|\phi) = \frac{\{1 - g_{1-i}(\phi)\}[\log g_{1-i}(\phi) - \log\{g_0(\phi) + g_1(\phi) - 1\}]}{\log g_0(\phi) + \log g_1(\phi) - \log\{g_0(\phi) + g_1(\phi) - 1\}},$$

for $i = 0, 1$.

For some illustrative values of $\theta^\dagger$ and $\gamma^\dagger$, Figure 4.1 displays features of the limiting posterior distribution of $\gamma$, namely the identification region and the limiting posterior mean. These show that, depending on the underlying parameter values, the data will sharpen either one or both of the lower bounds for the classification probabilities. The tilt mentioned above is also evident, with the limiting posterior mean of $\gamma$ always lying southwest of the identification region midpoint. As a further observation from Figure 4.1, for given underlying parameter values the learning of the classification parameters is not guaranteed to be in the correct direction. In some figure panels, the limiting posterior mean is further from the true classification parameters than is the prior mean. It turns out, however, that improvement is guaranteed in an aggregate sense.

To quantify the aggregate amount of learning about the classification parameters, note that the large-$n$ limit of *any* estimator of $\gamma$ can only depend on $(\theta^\dagger, \gamma^\dagger)$ via $\phi^\dagger$. Let $h(\phi^\dagger)$ be this (bivariate) limit for a given estimator. The large-sample limit of the estimator mean-squared-error (MSE) is therefore $\text{MSE}(\theta^\dagger, \gamma^\dagger) = \|h(\phi^\dagger) - \gamma^\dagger\|^2$. Subsequently averaging the MSE across the parameter space, and particularly taking this average with respect to the prior distribution, gives an aggregate measure of (large-sample) estimator performance across the parameter space. For clarity, we will refer to this

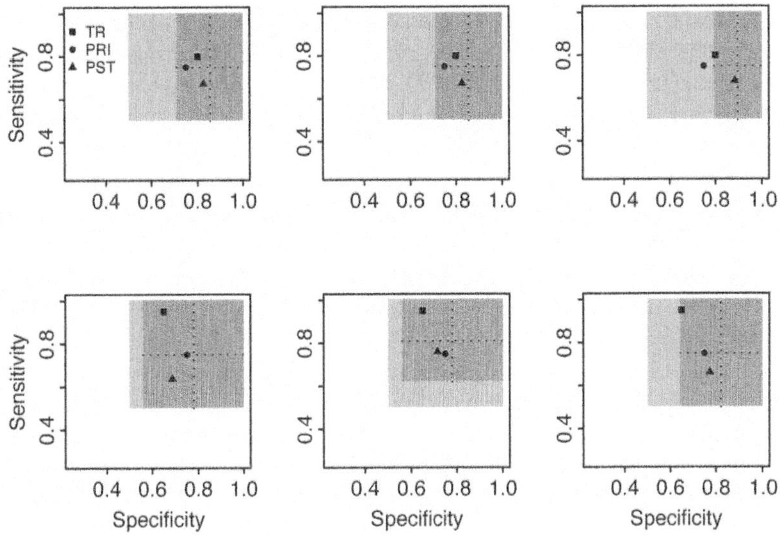


**FIGURE 4.1**
Visualization of learning about misclassification parameters when $p = q = 2$. In each panel, the darker rectangle is the identification region, while the lighter shading indicates values which are supported by the prior but discredited upon learning the law of the observable data. The true value, prior mean, and limiting posterior mean of specificity ($\gamma_0$) and specificity ($\gamma_1$) are also plotted. For reference, the dotted line segments bisect the identification region. The underlying values for $\gamma^\dagger$ are $(0.8, 0.8)$ in the top panels and $(0.65, 0.95)$ in the lower panels. The underlying values for $\theta^\dagger$ are $(0.15, 0.15)$, $(0.15, 0.45)$, and $(0.01, 0.03)$, in the left, middle, and right panels, respectively.

as *average mean-squared error* (AMSE). Of course amongst *all* functions $h()$, $E\left(\|h(\phi) - \gamma\|^2\right)$ is minimized by $h(\phi) = E(\gamma|\phi)$ (where again we emphasize that expectation here is under the specified prior distribution). Hence, according to this aggregate measure of performance, the posterior mean of the classification probabilities is the optimal estimator. In fact, this narrative is nothing more than the usual decision-theoretic argument that Bayes risk is minimized by the Bayes estimator. However, it has a slightly different 'look and feel' in the present context, due to the lack of full identification, and consequent positive large-sample limits of MSE.

We can now characterize the value of the information in the data concerning the classification parameters. Specifically, we can compare the aggregate performance of the optimal pre-data estimator to that of the optimal infinite-data estimator. That is, we can see how much the $AMSE$ for the limiting posterior mean of the classification parameters (hereafter $AMSE_{lpst}$) is reduced compared to the $AMSE$ of the prior mean (hereafter $AMSE_{pri}$). As detailed in Table 4.1, for the prior distribution as specified above, a 42.2% reduction is achieved. (This is perhaps more relevantly interpreted as a 24% reduction in the square-root of $AMSE$—hereafter $RAMSE$— which speaks to estimation error on the absolute scale.) The magnitude of the reduction speaks strongly against simply 'plugging in' best-guess values of the classification parameters as if they were known, since this would nullify the evident benefit of prior-to-posterior updating for these parameters.

In fact, the prior-to-posterior reduction in $RAMSE$ can be regarded as having two components. Table 4.1 also reports $RAMSE$ achieved by an estimator whose large-sample limit is the midpoint of the identification region. (This could be a relevant limit for a non-Bayesian procedure which involves estimating the identification region but has no sense of the tilt mentioned above.) This estimator yields a reduction of only 10.8% relative to $RAMSE_{pri}$. And in turn it is beaten by a further 14.8% reduction achieved by the limiting posterior. Thus we see the full benefit of the prior-to-posterior updating requires both learning the identification region and applying the tilt across the region. This idea of decomposing the benefit into these two components is pursued in much more generality and depth by Gustafson (2014).

As a final remark about Table 4.1, note that the average squared distance from the prior mean to the limiting posterior mean (hereafter $AMSD$) is also reported, as a summary of how much the Bayesian updating moves opinion about the misclassification parameters. In fact, it is easy to verify that necessarily $AMSD = AMSE_{pri} - AMSE_{lpst}$, i.e., the aggregate amount by which opinion is moved equals the aggregate improvement in estimating $\gamma$ by its (limiting) posterior mean rather than its prior mean. Similar decompositions are considered in Gustafson (2006), in a broader context of study design.

**TABLE 4.1**

Root-average-mean-squared error (RAMSE) when estimating $\gamma$ using (i), the prior mean, (ii), the identification interval midpoint, and (iii), the limiting posterior mean. The root-average-mean-squared distance (RAMSD) from the prior mean to the limiting posterior mean is also reported. Whereas $RAMSE_{pri}$ is computed exactly, the remaining table entries are computed using Monte Carlo averages of 40000 draws from the joint prior distribution.

| $RAMSE_{pri}$ | $RAMSE_{mid}$ | $RAMSE_{lpst}$ | $RAMSD$ |
|---|---|---|---|
| 0.204 | 0.182 | 0.155 | 0.133 |

## 4.3 The Case That $p = q = 3$

Now say that both $X$ and $X^*$ are ordinal with three levels, each taking values in $\{0, 1, 2\}$. Nondifferential misclassification can be parameterized by $\gamma_{ij} = Pr(X^* = j|X = i)$, i.e., $\gamma$ is a $3 \times 3$ classification matrix, with nonnegative entries and rows summing to one. One characterization of well-behaved misclassification is that for $k \geq 0$ both $\gamma_{i,i+k}$ and $\gamma_{i,i-k}$ are decreasing, i.e., rows of $\gamma$ are unimodal with mode at the entry corresponding to correct classification. We restrict consideration to such $\gamma$, describing this as *monotone* misclassification.

An interesting algebraic feature of monotone classification matrices is that the three pairs of the form $(\gamma_{i2}, \gamma_{i0})$, for $i = 0, 1, 2$, live in three disjoint regions of the unit square. Thus, as depicted in the left panel of Figure 4.2, we can visualize a particular monotone classification matrix as two connected line segments. For instance, both the rather poor classification corresponding to

$$\gamma = \begin{pmatrix} 0.65 & 0.24 & 0.11 \\ 0.28 & 0.41 & 0.31 \\ 0.18 & 0.23 & 0.59 \end{pmatrix}, \tag{4.3}$$

and the much better classification corresponding to

$$\gamma = \begin{pmatrix} 0.91 & 0.06 & 0.03 \\ 0.08 & 0.85 & 0.07 \\ 0.04 & 0.11 & 0.85 \end{pmatrix}, \tag{4.4}$$

are visualized in the right panel of this figure. Both are visualized as intermediate between perfect classification and complete futility. (In the case of perfection, $X^* \equiv X$, and the two connected line segments would comprise the 'L' of the coordinate axes. In the case of complete futility, $X^*$ is independent of $X$, and (to satisfy monotonicity) $X^*$ is uniformly distributed over the three levels. Hence the two connected line segments would collapse to a single point at $(1/3, 1/3)$.)

As in the previous section, we envision the end purpose as inference about the relationship between $X$ and a binary $Y$, based on observations from the distribution of $(X^*|Y)$. We start with $\theta$ (a $3 \times 2$ matrix) parameterizing the distribution of $(X|Y)$, according to $\theta_{ij} \doteq Pr(X = i|Y = j)$. The consequent distribution of $(X^*|Y)$ can be expressed via $\phi_{ij} \doteq Pr(X^* = i|Y = j)$, with the columns (indicated by a 'dot' notation) of $\phi$ determined from the columns of $\theta$ according to

$$\phi_{\cdot j} = \gamma^T \theta_{\cdot j}, \tag{4.5}$$

for $j = 0, 1$.

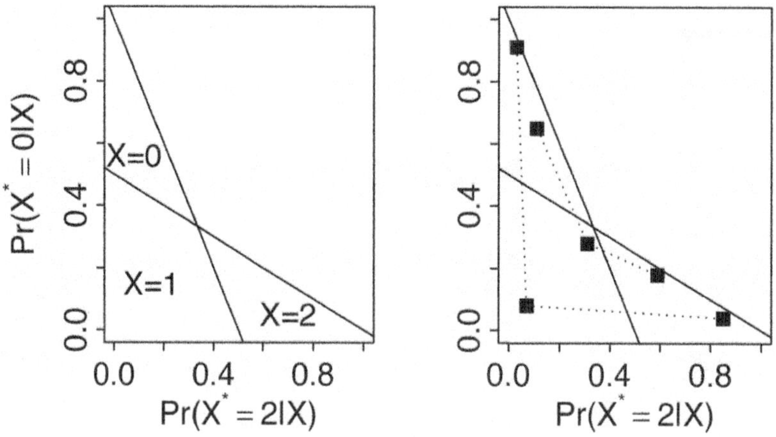


**FIGURE 4.2**
Visualization of misclassification parameters when $p = q = 3$. The left panel indicates the three disjoint regions to which $(\gamma_{i2}, \gamma_{i0})$ are restricted, for $i = 0, 1, 2$, presuming $\gamma$ is monotone. The right panel shows the two example matrices given in (4.3) and (4.4), with the former (involving very considerable misclassification) lying above the latter (involving much less misclassification).

Mimicking the previous section, we initially have a problem parameterized by $(\theta, \gamma)$. A simple prior specification is

$$\pi(\theta, \gamma) \quad \propto \quad I_P(\theta_{\cdot 0}) I_P(\theta_{\cdot 1}) I_M(\gamma), \tag{4.6}$$

where $P$ is the set of probability distributions on three elements, while $M$ is the set of monotone $3 \times 3$ classification matrices. Note that one can easily draw a Monte Carlo sample from this prior. (Particularly, for each row of $\gamma$ one can draw a Dirichlet$(1, 1, 1)$ realization, but reject this draw if it violates monotonicity.)

Next we can determine the limiting posterior distribution of $\gamma$ when the true parameter values are $(\theta^\dagger, \gamma^\dagger)$ (yielding $\phi^\dagger$ via (4.5)). This is simply the conditional prior distribution of $(\gamma \mid \phi = \phi^\dagger)$, having the form

$$\pi(\gamma \mid \phi) \quad \propto \quad \{h(\gamma)\}^{-2} I_M(\gamma) I_P\left(\left(\gamma^T\right)^{-1} \phi_{\cdot 0}\right) I_P\left(\left(\gamma^T\right)^{-1} \phi_{\cdot 1}\right). \tag{4.7}$$

We see immediately from this form that, as must be the case, a value of $\gamma$ is ruled out if it does not map the learned distribution of $(X^*|Y)$ back to a legitimate distribution for $(X|Y)$. The function $h()$ in (4.7), which arises from the Jacobian of the transformation, is determined to be

$$h(\gamma) \quad = \quad \gamma_{00}(\gamma_{11} - \gamma_{21}) + \gamma_{10}(\gamma_{21} - \gamma_{01}) + \gamma_{20}(\gamma_{01} - \gamma_{11}).$$

A convenient way to draw a Monte Carlo sample from the limiting posterior of $\gamma$ is via importance weighting of a sample drawn (using rejection sampling) from the uniform distribution over $M$.

In Figure 4.3 we display the true value $\gamma = \gamma^{\dagger}$, the prior mean of $\gamma$ and the limiting posterior mean of $\gamma$, for some example values of $(\theta^{\dagger}, \gamma^{\dagger})$. In particular, all four combinations arising from two settings for $\theta^{\dagger}$ and the two settings for $\gamma^{\dagger}$ in (4.3) and (4.4) are considered. Recalling the visualization of a classification matrix via two connected line segments, the figure indicates of the influence of the data on knowledge about the classification matrix, for given values of the underlying parameters. However, there is sufficient complexity that one cannot stare at the figure and draw a general conclusion about the learnability of the classification parameters. Thus we turn to an average-case analysis of the sort performed in the previous section.

The top row of Table 4.2 gives the average mean squared distance between the prior mean and true value of $\gamma$, and between the limiting posterior mean and the true value of $\gamma$. On the square-root scale, the latter is reduced by 20% compared to the former. For reference, the average mean squared distance between the prior and limiting posterior means is also reported.

Table 4.2 also gives results for a stronger prior specification. Whereas (4.6) restricts *rows* of the classification matrix to be unimodal with mode on the diagonal, we consider the stronger assertion that both rows and *columns* must have this property. Following the nomenclature of Ogburn and Vanderweele (2013), such classification matrices are referred to as *tapered.* Unsurprisingly, with sharper prior information, both $AMSE_{pri}$ and $AMSE_{lpst}$ are reduced. In fact, the relative improvement is similar to the monotone case, with a 20% reduction in RAMSE for the limiting posterior mean compared to the prior mean.

**TABLE 4.2**
Root-average-mean-squared error (RAMSE) when estimating $\gamma$ using (i), the prior mean, and (ii), the limiting posterior mean. The root-average-mean-squared distance (RAMSD) from the prior mean to the limiting posterior mean is also reported. Results are reported for the prior assertion that the classification is monotone, and for the prior assertion that the classification matrix is tapered. Entries are computed based on 100 Monte Carlo realizations from the prior distribution.

| | $RAMSE_{pri}$ | $RAMSE_{lpst}$ | $RAMSD$ |
|---|---|---|---|
| Monotone | 0.353 | 0.282 | 0.208 |
| Tapered | 0.326 | 0.248 | 0.196 |

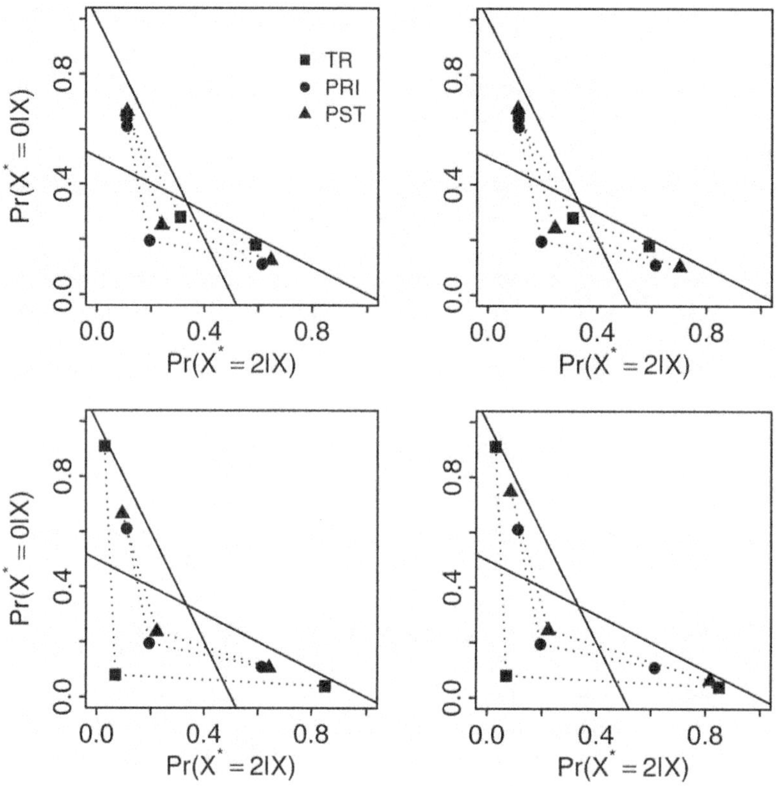


**FIGURE 4.3**
Visualization of learning about misclassification parameters when $p = q = 3$. Each panel depicts the true value of the misclassification parameters, the prior mean, and the limiting posterior mean. The true classification matrix $\gamma^{\dagger}$ is given by (4.3) in the top panels and (4.4) in the bottom panels. In the left panels, the underlying distribution of $X$ is given by $\theta^{\dagger}_{0\cdot} = (0.5, 0.3, 0.2)$ and $\theta^{\dagger}_{1\cdot} = (0.2, 0.3, 0.5)$. The right panels are based on $\theta^{\dagger}_{0\cdot} = (0.32, 0.33, 0.35)$ and $\theta^{\dagger}_{1\cdot} = (0.32, 0.11, 0.57)$.

## 4.4 The Case That $p = 2$ and $q = 3$

As a third and final situation we briefly consider the 'non-square' situation where $X$ is binary but $X^*$ is trinary. This could arise, for instance, in an epidemiological context involving a truly binary exposure status ascertained by a subject-area expert reviewing person-level documents (e.g., medical records, occupational history). The expert's classification scheme could result in a judgement that the individual is unlikely to be exposed

$(X^* = 0)$, possibly exposed $(X^* = 1)$, or likely exposed $(X^* = 2)$. Setting $\gamma_{ij} \doteq Pr(X^* = j|X = i)$ renders $\gamma$ as a $2 \times 3$ matrix with nonnegative entries and row sums equal to one.

As per Section 4.2, let $\theta$ parameterize $(X|Y)$ as $\theta_y \doteq Pr(X = 1|Y = y)$, for $y = 0, 1$. Consequently, presuming again that the misclassification is nondifferential, and taking $\phi_{ij} \doteq Pr(X^* = i|Y = j)$, we have $\phi_{\cdot j} = \gamma^T(1 - \theta_j, \theta_j)^T$, for $j = 0, 1$. The detailed mathematics of starting with a prior distribution on $(\theta, \gamma)$ and determining a posterior distribution, either for a finite sample or in the large-sample limit, is taken up in Wang, Shen and Gustafson (2012) and Gustafson (2015, Sec. 4.1). Here we simply wish to highlight a facet of this process, namely the form of the identification region for $\gamma$.

The notion of monotone misclassification from Section 4.4 can be imported to the present situation, by assuming the first row of $\gamma$ is non-increasing and the second row of $\gamma$ is non-decreasing. The consequent *a priori* restrictions to $(\gamma_{i2}, \gamma_{i0})$ for $i = 0, 1$ are visualized in the upper-left panel of Figure 4.4. The geometric narrative for determining the identification region is then illustrated in the upper-right figure panel, for given true values of the classification parameters ($\gamma^\dagger$, filled squares on the plot), and given true exposure prevalences ($\theta^\dagger$). The visualization proceeds by locating the points $(\phi^\dagger_{2j}, \phi^\dagger_{0j})$ for both $j = 0$ and $j = 1$ (open circles on the panel), and the line passing through these two points (dotted line). In the limit of observing infinite data we learn these values, and consequently learn that $(\gamma_{i2}, \gamma_{i0})$ must lie on this line, for both $i = 0$ and $i = 1$. Hence the intersection of this line with the prior region constitutes the identification region. Thus we learn that $(\gamma_{02}, \gamma_{00})$ lies on the thicker, solid line segment depicted in the northwest corner of the panel, and that $(\gamma_{12}, \gamma_{10})$ lies on the thicker, solid line segment depicted in the southeast corner of the panel.

The lower panels of Figure 4.4 again illustrate the identification region for $\gamma$, but for different underlying values of $(\theta^\dagger, \gamma^\dagger)$. Note particularly the variation in how much can be learned about $\gamma_{12} = Pr(X^* = 2|X = 2)$. In the upper-right case, data confirm that $\gamma_{12}$ is high, whereas in the lower-right case, the identification interval remains rather wide.

Generally, Figure 4.4 underscores a fundamental difference between this case and the 'square' classification cases of the previous sections. Now the identification region for the classification parameters is lower-dimensional than the *a priori* set of possible values. Explicitly, the prior support of $(\gamma_{i2}, \gamma_{i0})$ is a triangle in the unit square, whereas the limiting posterior support is a line segment. Thus there is a general sense of stronger learning about classification parameters in the present situation.

As a brief investigation of aggregate case performance, we consider how well the identification interval midpoint for $(\gamma_{12}, \gamma_{10})$ estimates the true value. The aggregation is taken with respect a uniform distribution over $(\theta, \gamma)$, bearing in mind that $\gamma$ is constrained to be monotone. Averaging over the appropriate region indicated in the top-left panel of Figure 4.4, $E\{(\gamma_{12}, \gamma_{10})\} = (11/18, 1/9)$. Using 250 Monte Carlo draws, we find the

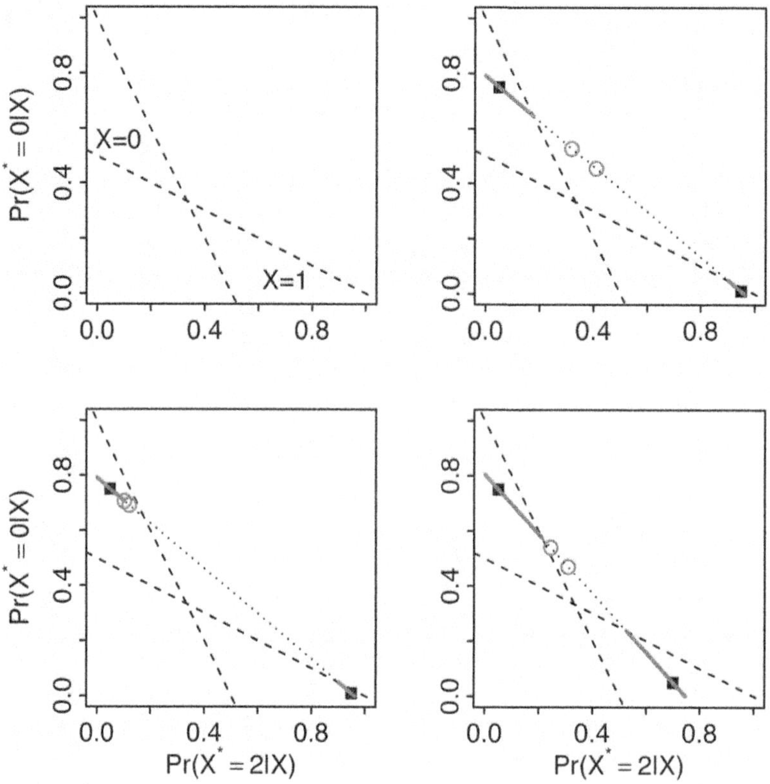


**FIGURE 4.4**
Visualization of learning about misclassification parameters when $p = 2$, $q = 3$. The top-left panel shows the prior regions for $(\gamma_{i2}, \gamma_{i0})$. In the other panels, the filled squares give the true values of these classification parameters, the open circles give the (learnable) values of $(\phi_{i2}, \phi_{i0})$, and the thicker, solid line segments give the identification regions for the classification parameters. The top-right panel is based on $(\gamma_{02}^{\dagger}, \gamma_{00}^{\dagger}) = (0.05, 0.75)$, $(\gamma_{12}^{\dagger}, \gamma_{10}^{\dagger}) = (0.95, 0.01)$, and $\theta^{\dagger} = (0.3, 0.4)$. The bottom-left panel modifies these initial settings with $\theta^{\dagger} = (0.06, 0.08)$. The bottom-right panel modifies the initial settings with $(\gamma_{12}^{\dagger}, \gamma_{10}^{\dagger}) = (0.7, 0.05)$.

root-mean-squared distance between this prior mean and the actual value of $(\gamma_{12}, \gamma_{10})$ to be $RAMSE_{pri} = 0.163$. Whereas, for the identification interval midpoint the root-mean-squared distance is reduced to $RAMSE_{mid} = 0.093$. This is indeed a much more substantial reduction than observed in the cases of square misclassification studied earlier.

## 4.5 Conclusion

As has been demonstrated in the literature, and as is reviewed later in this volume by Stamey and Seaman (2021), prior information about misclassification parameters can be incorporated into a Bayesian analysis. The posterior distribution arising from such an analysis integrates several levels of uncertainty, namely that $X$ is not observed, but also that $\gamma$ describing the relationship between $X$ and $X^*$ is not known exactly. And without validation data, we cannot expect to estimate $\gamma$ 'fully.' As stressed in this chapter, however, the opposite of 'fully' is not 'not at all.' There are no guarantees for a single dataset. However, in aggregate, meaning across different underlying values in the parameter space, we expect the posterior mean of $\gamma$ to be closer to the truth than the prior mean.

## References


Buonaccorsi, J. P. (2010). *Measurement Error: Models, Methods, and Applications.* Chapman and Hall, CRC Press.

Gustafson, P. (2004). *Measurement Error and Misclassification in Statistics and Epidemiology: Impact and Bayesian Adjustments.* Chapman & Hall, CRC Press.

Gustafson, P. (2006). Sample size implications when biases are modelled rather than ignored. *Journal of the Royal Statistical Society, Series A*, 169, 883-902.

Gustafson, P. (2014). Bayesian inference in partially identified models: Is the shape of the posterior distribution useful? *Electronic Journal of Statistics*, 8, 476-496.

Gustafson, P. (2015). *Bayesian inference for partially identified models: Exploring the limits of limited data.* Chapman and Hall, CRC Press.

Gustafson, P., Le, N. D. and Saskin, R. (2001). Case-control analysis with partial knowledge of exposure misclassification probabilities. *Biometrics*, 57, 598-609.

Ogburn, E. L. and Vanderweele, T. J. (2013). Bias attenuation results for nondifferentially mismeasured ordinal and coarsened confounders. *Biometrika*, 100(1), 241–248.

Sinha, S. (2021). Bayesian approaches for handling covariate measurement error. In G. Yi, A. Delaigle, and P. Gustafson (Eds.), *Handbook of Measurement Error Models.* Chapman and Hall, CRC Press, Chapter 24.

Stamey, J. and Seaman, J. (2021). Bayesian adjustment for misclassification. In G. Yi, A. Delaigle, and P. Gustafson (Eds.), *Handbook of Measurement Error Models.* Chapman and Hall, CRC Press, Chapter 23.

Wang, D., Shen, T., and Gustafson, P. (2012). Partial identification arising from nondifferential exposure misclassification: How informative are data on the unlikely, maybe, and likely exposed? *International Journal of Biostatistics*, 8, issue 1, article 31.

Yi, G. Y. (2017). *Statistical Analysis with Measurement Error or Misclassification.* Springer.

# 5

# *Using Instrumental Variables to Estimate Models with Mismeasured Regressors*

**Arthur Lewbel**

## CONTENTS



## 5.1 Introduction

This chapter discusses the use of intrumental variables (IV) methods for dealing with measurement errors in regression model covariates. In this context, an instrument is defined as an observed variable that correlates with the mismeasured variable, but does not correlate with the measurement error, and does not correlate with the model error. IV methods are used to deal with many sources of endogeneity (i.e., regressors that are correlated with model errors) in regression models, but this chapter will focus on their use with mismeasured regressors. IVs are used in many branches of statistics, but are particularly common in econometrics, where the information required for other methods of dealing with endogeneity is often unavailable. For example, in the case of mismeasured regressors, econometrics applications often lack information such as validation samples or knowledge of the error distribution.

DOI: 10.1201/9781315101279-5

There is some debate regarding the origins of IV methods. An early example of IV estimation was proposed by Sewall Wright (1925). Sewall's father, Philip Wright (1928) showed that Sewall's estimator could solve the problem of estimating the coefficient $b$ in a linear regression model $Y = a + bX^* + e$ where the observed $X^*$ and unobserved error $e$ are correlated (in his application of estimating the demand for pig iron, the correlation was due to simultaneity in the determination of $Y$ and $X^*$ rather than measurement error). More about the Wrights' work in this area can be found in Stock and Trebbi (2003), who also applied a stylometric analysis of their writing to verify that it was indeed Philip and not Sewall who composed this solution to this correlation problem.

Early analyses of regression coefficient estimation in the presence of measurement error are Adcock (1877, 1878) and Kummell (1879), who considered measurement errors in a Deming regression, as popularized in W. Edwards Deming (1943). This is a regression that minimizes the sum of squares of errors measured perpendicular to the fitted line. Gini (1921) gave an example of an estimator that deals with measurement errors in a standard linear regression, but early examples of what are essentially IV estimators are given by Frisch (1934), Koopmans (1937), and Durbin (1954).

## 5.2 The IV Idea

Consider estimation of the coefficient $b$ in the linear regression model

$$Y = a + Xb + U,$$

where $Y$ is an outcome variable, $a$ and $b$ are unknown constants, $X$ is a covariate of interest, and $U$ is a random mean zero error. Suppose we do not have a sample of observations of $Y$ and $X$, but our data does contain observations of $Y$ and $X^*$, where $X^* = X + V$. Here $X^*$ is a measure of $X$, where $X$ is the unobserved, correctly measured covariate of interest, and the random variable $V$ is measurement error in $X^*$. For now we maintain the classical measurement error and regression assumptions that $X$, $U$, and $V$ are mutually uncorrelated with each other.

Replacing $X$ with $X^* - V$ in the regression model gives $Y = a + X^*b + e$ where $e = U - Vb$. This linear regression of $Y$ on $X^*$ suffers from the endogeneity problem that $X^*$ and $e$ are correlated with each other, because both depend on $V$. In particular, $cov\left(X^*, e\right) = E\left[\left(X + V\right)\left(U - Vb\right)\right] = E\left(V^2\right)b$ which does not equal zero unless there is either no measurement error or the true coefficient $b$ is zero. If we had more information about the distribution of either $X$ or $V$, such as knowing the variance of either one (obtained perhaps from a validation sample), we could use that information along with the data on $Y$ and $X^*$ to recover a consistent estimate of $b$, based on suitably adjusting the ordinary least squares estimate of $b$.

To consistently estimate the coefficient $b$ without such distribution information regarding $X$ or $V$, assume that in addition to observations of $Y$ and $X^*$, we also observe a variable $Z$, which is the instrument. What makes $Z$ be an instrument is that it's assumed to be correlated with $X$ and uncorrelated with both $V$ and $U$. Just having observations of $Y$, $X^*$, and $Z$ does not provide enough information to recover observations of $X$, or to estimate the distribution of $X$, but it does enable estimation of $b$. In particular,

$$cov(Z,X^*) = cov(Z,X+V) = cov(Z,X) + cov(Z,V) = cov(Z,X)$$

and

$$cov(Z,Y) = cov(Z,Xb+U) = cov(Z,X)b + cov(Z,U) = cov(Z,X)b$$

so

$$\frac{cov(Z,Y)}{cov(Z,X^*)} = \frac{cov(Z,X)b}{cov(Z,X)} = b.$$

The key assumptions used for this derivation are the instrument properties $cov(Z,U) = 0$, $cov(Z,V) = 0$, and $cov(Z,X) \neq 0$. The associated IV estimator of $b$ just replaces these covariances with estimated covariances, so given $n$ observations $y_i, x_i, z_i$, the estimator is

$$\widehat{b} = \frac{\widehat{cov}(Z,Y)}{\widehat{cov}(Z,X^*)} = \frac{\sum_{i=1}^{n} z_i\,(y_i - \overline{y})}{\sum_{i=1}^{n} z_i\,(x_i - \overline{x})},$$

where $\overline{y}$ and $\overline{x}$ are the sample averages of $y$ and $x$. This $\widehat{b}$ will then be consistent as long as a law of large numbers can be applied. The constant $a$ can also be consistently estimated by $\widehat{a} = \overline{y} - \overline{x}\widehat{b}$.

Another way to think about the above construction is to write the model as $Y = a + X^*b + e$ where, as shown above, the unobserved error $e$ is given by $e = U - bV$. The assumption that $Z$ is uncorrelated with both the measurement error $V$ and the underlying model error $U$ means that $cov\,(e,Z) = 0$. Therefore,

$$cov(Z,Y) = cov(Z,X^*)b + cov(Z,e) = cov(Z,X^*)b,$$

and solving for $b$ gives $b = cov(Z,Y)/cov(Z,X^*)$ as before. The ordinary least squares estimator is just the special case of this IV estimator where $Z = X^*$, that is, when the regressor $X^*$ satisfies the conditions required to be an instrument.

This construction shows that the IV method does not just apply to models with measurement errors. Given any regression model $Y = a + bX^* + e$, all that is required for IV estimation is that we have $cov\,(Z,X^*) \neq 0$ and $cov\,(e,Z) = 0$. Measurement error in $X^*$ is just one situation where the endogeneity problem $cov\,(e,X^*) \neq 0$ arises, and therefore requires an alternative like IV estimation.

With any such endogeneity problem, we can say that a candidate instrument $Z$ is valid if $cov\,(e, Z) = 0$, and is useful if $cov\,(Z, X^*) \neq 0$. It is easy to find instruments that are merely valid (such as any $Z$'s drawn from a random number generator); the difficulty is finding useful instruments. An instrument $Z$ is defined to be weak if it's valid, but its correlation with $X^*$ is close to zero. Weak instruments will be discussed briefly in a later section. Generally, the stronger the instrument, meaning the higher is the correlation between the instument $Z$ and the true regressor $X$, the lower will be the variance of the IV estimated $\widehat{b}$.

Where do we find an instrument $Z$? It may be easiest to consider a specific example. Consider a model where $X$ is a person's true income, $X^*$ is his or her reported income, and $Y$ is how much the individual spends to buy food. One requirement of an instrument $Z$ is that it correlate with $X$. In this example, things we might observe that correlate with a person's income could be his or her wage rate, or wealth measures like indicators of whether the person owns a car or a house. A second requirement of $Z$ is that it not be correlated with the measurement error $V$. So in these examples, if income and wages or car and home ownership are all self reported by the individual being surveyed, we might be concerned that mismeasurement in both $X^*$ and $Z$ could be correlated, as with an individual who chooses to exaggerate both his or her income and his or her wealth. However, if, e.g., car or home ownership is observed by the surveyer, then that error in observation is unlikely to be correlated with a respondent's reporting error in income. As this example shows, it is permitted for both $X^*$ and $Z$ to be mismeasured, as long as the measurement errors in the two are not correlated. Finally, the third requirement is that $Z$ be uncorrelated with the model error $U$. So, e.g., if an individual's expenditures on food $Y$ correlate not only with his or her income but also with whether he or she owns a car (which could affect how often and where he or she shops), then car ownership would not be a valid instrument.

Another possible source of instruments is repeated measures. One measure of $X^*$ might serve as an instrument for another measure of $X^*$. In the above example, the same consumer might report his income both in a survey and on his tax form, yielding two potentially different measures of his income. Or the consumer might be asked his income in two different time periods. Even if his true income changes over time, one measure could still be a valid instrument for the other, since there is typically a high correlation between an individual's income in one time period and their income in the next. However, one concern with repeated measures is that, for one to be a valid instrument of the other, the errors in the two measures need to be uncorrelated. This condition might be violated if, e.g., the errors are due to making the same kind of reporting mistake in both periods, such as omitting some source of income in both, or purposely exaggerating one's income in both.

A convenient feature of IV estimation of the linear model is that instruments do not need to be continuously distributed. For example, an instrument

$Z$ can be both valid and useful even if $X^*$ is continuous and $Z$ is binary, as in the earlier example of car or home ownership instrumenting for income.

Suppose that we have more than one instument available, e.g., suppose both $Q$ and $R$ are valid instruments for $X^*$. Then letting $Z$ equal $Q$ or letting $Z$ equal $R$ gives two different possible estimators. Moreover, if we let $Z = c_0 + c_1Q + c_2R$ for any constants $c_0$, $c_1$, and $c_2$, then $Z$ will still generally be a valid instrument. What $Z$ (i.e., what values of $c_0$, $c_1$, and $c_2$) should we choose? The IV estimator is

$$\widehat{b} = \frac{\widehat{cov}(Z, a + Xb + U)}{\widehat{cov}(Z, X^*)} = \frac{\widehat{cov}(Z, a + (X^* - V)\,b + U)}{\widehat{cov}(Z, X^*)} = b + \frac{\widehat{cov}(Z, U - Vb)}{\widehat{cov}(Z, X^*)}.$$

This expression shows that, other things equal, the larger is the estimated covariance between $Z$ and $X^*$, the smaller is the error in the estimator $\widehat{b}$. This in turn suggests choosing the constants $c_0$, $c_1$, and $c_2$ to maximize $\widehat{cov}(Z, X^*)$. This in turn is equivalent to just linearly regressing $X^*$ on a constant, $Q$, and $R$ using ordinary least squares, and letting $Z$ be the fitted values from that regression. This estimator is called two stage least squares. Note that simply rescaling $Z$ to increase $\widehat{cov}(Z, X^*)$ is not helpful, because, e.g., doubling $Z$ would also double the unobserved sample covariance of $Z$ with $U - Vb$, leaving the estimation error $\widehat{b} - b$ unchanged.

## 5.3 Linear IV Models

The estimators of the previous section directly generalize to multiple regression with multiple mismeasured variables and multiple instruments. Consider the model $Y = X^*b + e$, where $Y$ is now an $n \times 1$ vector of observations of the dependent variable, $X^*$ is an $n \times k$ matrix of covariate observations (some or all of which may be mismeasured), $b$ is a $k \times 1$ vector of coefficients to be estimated, and $e$ is an $n \times 1$ vector of mean zero errors. Let $Z$ be an $n \times k$ matrix of instruments. Each column of $X^*$ and of $Z$ is a variable. Any variable that is not mismeasured can be an instrument for itself, that is, if a given column $j$ of $X^*$ is not mismeasured, then we can let column $j$ of $Z$ equal column $j$ of $X^*$. Note that the constant term, a vector of ones, would usually be included in both $X^*$ and $Z$.

The IV estimator of $b$ is then

$$\widehat{b} = (Z^T X^*)^{-1} Z^T Y.$$

Substituting in $X^*b + e$ for $Y$ shows immediately that the estimation error is $\widehat{b} - b = (Z^T X^*)^{-1} Z^T e$, so $\widehat{b}$ is consistent if $plim_{n\to\infty}\ (Z^T X^*)^{-1} Z^T e = 0$. Validity of the instrument matrix $Z$ is the assumption that $E(Z^T e) = 0$, and usefulness of $Z$ requires that $Z^T X^*$ be nonsingular. $\sqrt{n}-$ consistency and asymptotic normality of $\widehat{b}$ follows immediately as long as $plim_{n\to\infty}\, Z^T X^*/n$ is nonsingular and a central limit theorem can be applied to the average $Z^T e/n$. In particular, letting $\widehat{e} = Y - X^*\widehat{b}$, and assuming the elements of $e$ are IID (independently and identically distributed) then the limit distribution is

$$\sqrt{n}(\widehat{b} - b) \xrightarrow{d} N(0, \Psi);$$

$$\Psi = plim_{n\to\infty} \frac{\widehat{e}^T\widehat{e}}{n} \left(\frac{Z^T X^*}{n}\right)^{-1} \left(\frac{Z^T Z}{n}\right) \left(\frac{X^{*T} Z}{n}\right)^{-1}.$$

The IV estimator can alternatively be derived as a method of moments estimator. The moments we have are $E(Ze) = 0$. The method of moments replaces expectations with sample averages, giving

$$\frac{1}{n} Z(Y - X^*\widehat{b}) = 0,$$

which, when one solves for $\widehat{b}$, equals the IV estimator.

Suppose we have $L \geq k$ instruments. Let $Q$ be the $n \times L$ matrix of available instruments. Then the two stage least squares estimator is to first construct $Z$ by

$$Z = X^*(Q^T Q)^{-1} Q^T X^*,$$

and then let $\widehat{b} = (Z^T X^*)^{-1} Z^T Y$ as before. This construction of $Z$ is just the fitted values of a linear least squares regression of $X^*$ on $Q$.

In this model we have $L$ moments, given by $E(Qe) = 0$. When $L > k$, we have more moments than parameters, and so cannot directly apply the method of moments. However, we can instead apply Hansen's (1982) Generalized Method of Moments (GMM) estimator. That estimator takes the form

$$\widehat{b} = \arg\min \left[\frac{1}{n} Q^T \left(Y - X^*\widehat{b}\right)\right]^T \widehat{\Omega} \left[\frac{1}{n} Q^T \left(Y - X^*\widehat{b}\right)\right],$$

where $\widehat{\Omega}$ is an estimated $L \times L$ weight matrix that is chosen to minimize the asymptotic variance of $\widehat{b}$. When the errors $e$ (which are linear functions of both the model error and the measurement errors in $X^*$) are homoskedastic and uncorrelated across observations, the optimal GMM estimator is numerically identical to the two stage least squares estimator. More generally, GMM can be asymptotically more efficient than two stage least squares, though it may also perform worse in finite samples.

## 5.4 IV Estimators for Nonlinear Models with Measurement Error

Return to the case where $X$ is a scalar, but suppose now we have a quadratic model

$$Y = a + Xb + X^2c + U.$$

The goal now is to estimate the coefficients $a$, $b$, and $c$. We again observe scalars $Y$, $X^*$, and $Z$ where $X^* = X + V$, and $Z$ is an instrument. To deal with nonlinearity, we now strengthen the instrument validity and usefulness assumptions. Let $X = \gamma + Z\delta + W$ for some constants $\gamma$ and $\delta$ with $\delta \neq 0$, assume $U$, $V$ and $W$ have mean zero, and assume $U$, $V$, $W$, and $Z$ are mutually independent (these conditions are stronger than necessary but are convenient for illustrating the estimation method).

Let $S = \gamma + Z\delta$. Then

$$E(X^* \mid Z) = \gamma + Z\delta = S.$$

So we can linearly regress $X^*$ on a constant and on $Z$ using ordinary least squares, and the fitted value will be an estimate of $S$. Next, letting $\mu_j = E\left(W^j\right)$ where $j$ is a positive integer, observe that

$$\begin{aligned} E(Y \mid S) &= a + Sb + \left(S^2 + \mu_2\right)c \\ &= (a + \mu_2 c) + Sb + S^2 c. \end{aligned}$$

So if we linearly regress $Y$ on a constant, $S$, and $S^2$ using ordinary least squares, the coefficients will provide estimates of $(a + \mu_2 c)$, $b$, and $c$. This already gives us estimates of the desired coefficients $b$ and $c$. To obtain the remaining coefficient $a$, we have

$$X^*Y = Xa + X^2b + X^3c + UX + \left(a + Xb + X^2c + U\right)V$$

from which we can calulate

$$\begin{aligned} E(X^*Y \mid S) &= Sa + \left(S^2 + \mu_2\right)b + \left(S^3 + 3S\mu_2 + \mu_3\right)c \\ &= \zeta + S(a + 3\mu_2 c) + S^2 b + S^3 c; \end{aligned}$$

where $\zeta = \mu_2 b + \mu_3 c$. This shows that if we linearly regress $X^*Y$ on a constant, $S$, $S^2$, and $S^3$ using ordinary least squares, the coefficient of $S$ will provide an estimate of $a + 3\mu_2 c$, which along with the previous coefficient estimates allows us to recover an estimate of the remaining coefficient $a$. $\sqrt{n}-$ consistency and asymptotic normality of these estimators follows immediately from standard conditions that suffice for $\sqrt{n}-$ consistency of linear regression coefficients.

The above procedure of running repeated regressions is inefficient. To obtain more efficient estimates, we can recast the above equations as the following collection of unconditional moments

$$E\left[(X^* - \gamma - Z\delta)Z^j\right] = 0 \quad \text{for } j = 0, 1;$$

$$E\left[\left(Y-(a+\mu_2 c)-(\gamma+Z\delta)\,b-(\gamma+Z\delta)^2\,c\right)Z^j\right]=0 \text{ for } j=0,1,2;$$

$$E\left[\left(X^*Y-\zeta-(\gamma+Z\delta)\,(a+3\mu_2 c)-(\gamma+Z\delta)^2\,b-(\gamma+Z\delta)^3\,c\right)Z^j\right]=0$$
$$\text{for } j=0,1,2,3.$$

Under standard conditions we may then apply the GMM estimator to this set of nine moments to directly construct $\sqrt{n}-$ consistent, asymptotically normal estimates of the desired parameters $a$, $b$, and $c$, along with the additional parameters $\gamma$, $\delta$, $\mu_2$, and $\zeta$. The GMM estimator will also provide a consistent estimate of the asymptotic covariance matrix of these parameters.

In this quadratic regression case, the instrument $Z$ could not be binary, because we require $S$, $S^2$, and $S^3$ to not be perfectly correlated with each other. However, $Z$ and therefore $S$ could still be discretely distributed. We require $S$ and therefore $Z$ to take on at least four different values. Note that the above IV estimation method could be immediately extended to allow $Z$ to be a vector of instruments, by just letting $S=\gamma+Z^T\delta$ for a vector of coefficients $\delta$. So, e.g., if $Z$ was a two element vector where both elements were binary (such as the earlier example of an indicator of car ownership and an indicator of home ownership), then that would suffice to make $S$ four valued, as required.

This same IV methodology can be extended to identifying the coefficients of polynomials of any finite order. For details, see Hausman, Newey, Ichimura, and Powell (1991). This same idea can be further generalized to nonparametric estimation of regression functions as follows. Suppose we maintain the above uncorrelatedness assumptions about $X^*$, $U$, $V$, $W$, and $Z$, but now let $X=h(Z)+W$ and $Y=g(X)+U$ where $g$ and $h$ are unknown smooth functions. The goal is now estimation of the function $g$. Let $S=h(Z)$, which, given some regularity, can be consistently estimated by a nonparametric regression of $X^*$ on $Z$. Let $F(\cdot)$ be the distribution function of $W$. Then

$$E(Y\mid S)=\int g(S+w)\,dF(w);$$
$$E(X^*Y\mid Z)=\int (S+w)\,g(S+w)\,dF(w).$$

These are two integral equations in two unknown functions $g$ and $F$. Newey (2001) proposed using these equations to identify a parameterized $g$ function, Schennach (2007) and Zinde-Walsh (2014) provided conditions that suffice for nonparametric identification of $g$, and Schennach (2007) proposed a corresponding consistent estimator. Hu and Schennach (2008) further generalized this model by allowing for other forms of measurement error, for example, they allow $W$ to have median zero rather than mean zero. Lewbel and De Nadai (2016) extended this model to allow $X^*$ and $Y$ to both be mismeasured, with correlated measurement errors (as might result if, e.g., both are responses to questions in the same survey).

## 5.5 Additional Results and Issues

It was noted earlier that linear IV estimation allows the instrument $Z$ to be binary. There is a large literature devoted to the estimation of what is called a Local Average Treatment Effect (LATE), by applying the linear IV model when both $X^*$ and $Z$ are binary scalars. See Imbens and Angrist (1984). However, the properties that are required of an instrument $Z$ for LATE estimation are somewhat different from those needed for the estimators discussed in this chapter, and in particular do not apply when $X^*$ is mismeasured.

The estimators discussed here made the classical measurement error assumption that $X^* = X + U$ where the measurement error $U$ is uncorrelated with $X$. That assumption generally requires $X$ to be continuous (which is one reason why the assumptions for LATE do not apply to measurement error). Nevertheless, there do exist IV based estimators for regression models containing discrete mismeasured regressors. Examples include Mahajan (2006), Lewbel (2007), and Hu (2008).

Instruments $Z$ generally come from outside the model, as discussed earlier. However, there exist situations where instruments $Z$ can be constructed just from the observed variables $Y$ and $X^*$, if one is given some additional information regarding the structure of $Y$, $X^*$, and $X$. For example, return to the simple model where $Y$, $X^*$, and $X$ are scalars, $Y = a + bX + U$, $X^* = X + V$, and $U$, $V$, and $X$ are mutually independent. Suppose the measurement error $V$ is symmetrically distributed around zero and $X$ is asymmetrically distributed. Then $Z = [X^* - E(X^*)]^2$ is a valid and useful instrument, which can be estimated by replacing $E(X^*)$ with the sample average. See Lewbel (1997). Related results include Lewbel (2012), Erickson and Whited (2002), and Delaigle and Hall (2016).

A general problem that can arise in IV estimation is weak instruments, which occurs when the correlation of $X^*$ and $Z$ is close to zero. With weak instruments, in moderate sample sizes standard asymptotic theory provides poor approximations to finite sample distributions. For example, in the scalar case a weak instrument $Z$ causes both the numerator and denominator of $\widehat{b} = \widehat{cov}(Z, Y)/\widehat{cov}(Z, X^*)$ to be close to zero, making this estimated ratio very noisy. The corresponding elements in the asymptotic variance of $\widehat{b}$ will likewise be poorly estimated. To construct better asymptotic approximations in this case, assume that $X^* = \gamma_n Z + \varepsilon$ where $Z$ and $\varepsilon$ are uncorrelated, and $\gamma_n = \gamma n^{-1/2}$ for some constant $\gamma$. This drifting parameter model makes the covariance of $X^*$ and $Z$ shrink as the sample size $n$ grows, and so provides an asymptotic theory that embodies that idea that this covariance is relatively small, no matter how large the sample. See, e.g., Staiger and Stock (1997) and Andrews, Moreira and Stock (2006) on detecting weak instruments and on applying drifting parameter asymptotics to data with weak instruments.

## References

Adcock, R. J. (1877). Note on the method of least squares. *The Analyst (Annals of Mathematics)*, 4(6), 183-184.

Adcock, R. J. (1878). A problem in least squares. *The Analyst (Annals of Mathematics)*, 5(2), 53-54.

Andrews, D. W. K., Moreira, M. J., and Stock, J. H. (2006). Optimal two-sided invariant similar tests for instrumental variables regression. *Econometrica*, 74(3), 715-752.

Delaigle, A. and Hall, P. (2016). Methodology for non-parametric deconvolution when the error distribution is unknown. *Journal of the Royal Statistical Society series B*, 78, 231-252.

Deming, W. E. (1943), *Statistical Adjustment of Data.* Wiley, NY.

Durbin, J. (1954), Errors in variables. *Review of the International Statistical Institute*, 22(1), 23-32.

Erickson, T. and Whited, T. (2002), Two-step GMM estimation of the errors-in-variables model using high-order moments. *Econometric Theory*, 18(3), 776-799.

Frisch, R. (1934). *Statistical Confluence Analysis by Means of Complete Regression Systems.* Vol. 5, Universitetets Økonomiske Instituut.

Gini, C. (1921). Sull'interpoliazone di una retta quando i valori della variabile indipendente sono affetti da errori accidentali. *Metroeconomica*, 1, 63-82.

Hansen, L. P. (1982). Large sample properties of generalized method of moments estimators. *Econometrica*, 50(4), 1029-1054.

Hausman J., Newey, W., Ichimura, H., and Powell, J. (1991). Measurement errors in polynomial regression models. *Journal of Econometrics*, 50, 273-295.

Hu, Y. (2008). Identification and estimation of nonlinear models with misclassification error using instrumental variables: A general solution. *Journal of Econometrics*, 144, 27-61.

Hu, Y. and Schennach, S. M. (2008). Instrumental variable treatment of nonclassical measurement error models. *Econometrica*, 76, 195-216.

Imbens, G. W. and Angrist, J. D. (1994). Identification and estimation of local average treatment effects. *Econometrica*, 62, 467-475.

Koopmans, T. C. (1937). Linear regression analysis of economic time series. In DeErven F. Bohn (ed.), Haarlem, Netherlands.

Kummell, C. H. (1879). Reduction of observation equations which contain more than one observed quantity. *The Analyst (Annals of Mathematics)*, 6(4), 97-105.

Lewbel, A. (1997). Constructing instruments for regressions with measurement error when no additional data are available, with an application to patents and R&D. *Econometrica*, 65, 1201-1213.

Lewbel, A. (2007). Estimation of average treatment effects with misclassification. *Econometrica*, 75, 537-551.

Lewbel, A. (2012). Using heteroscedasticity to identify and estimate mismeasured and endogenous regressor models. *Journal of Business and Economic Statistics*, 30, 67-80.

Lewbel, A. and De Nadai, M. (2016). Nonparametric errors in variables models with measurement errors on both sides of the equation. *Journal of Econometrics*, 191(1), 19-32.

Mahajan, A. (2006). Identification and estimation of regression models with misclassification. *Econometrica*, 74(3), 631-665.

Newey (2001). Flexible simulated moment estimation of nonlinear errors-in-variables models. *Review of Economics and Statistics*, 83, 616-627.

Schennach, S. (2007). Instrumental variable estimation of nonlinear errors-in-variables models. *Econometrica*, 75, 201-239.

Staiger, D. O. and J. Stock, J. (1997). Instrumental variables regression with weak instruments. *Econometrica*, 65, 557-586.

Stock, J. H. and Trebbi, F. (2003). Retrospectives who invented instrumental variable regression? *Journal of Economic Perspectives*, 177-194.

Wright, P. G. (1915). Moore's economic cycles. *Quarterly Journal of Economics*, 29(4), 631-641.

Wright, P. G. (1928). *The Tariff on Animal and Vegetable Oils*. Macmillan, New York.

Wright, S. (1925). Corn and hog correlations. *U.S. Department of Agriculture Bulletin*, 1300, 1-60.

Zinde-Walsh, V. (2014). Measurement error and deconvolution in spaces of generalized functions. *Econometric Theory*, 30(6), 1207-1246.

# Part III

# General Methodology

# 6

# *Likelihood Methods with Measurement Error and Misclassification*

**Grace Y. Yi**

## CONTENTS



## 6.1 Introduction

The likelihood inference framework has been widely used to handle measurement error problems. Such a framework enjoys great generality and flexibility for handling various complex models. A variety of likelihood-based methods have been developed in the literature, and the discussion on this topic is available in research monographs including Chapter 8 of Carroll et al. (2006),

DOI: 10.1201/9781315101279-6

scattered sections of Fuller (1987), Buonaccorsi (2010), Yi (2017), and the references therein.

Suppose that $Y$ is the response variable and $\{X, Z\}$ are the associated covariates. The goal is to understand the relationship between $Y$ and $\{X, Z\}$ using the observed measurements of a sample. Let $h(y, x, z)$ denote the true probability density or mass function of $\{Y, X, Z\}$ which is unknown. In error-free settings we usually use the factorization

$$h(y, x, z) = h(y|x, z)h(x, z) \tag{6.1}$$

to guide us to introduce modeling strategies. Here $h(y|x, z)$ is the conditional probability density or mass function of $Y$ given $\{X, Z\}$ which is of primary interest, and $h(x, z)$ is the probability density or mass function of $X$ and $Z$. Often, we leave $h(x, z)$ unmodeled and focus on modeling $h(y|x, z)$, which can be done nonparametrically, semiparametrically, or parametrically. Such a procedure leads to the *conditional analysis* that has perhaps dominated the literature.

However, when the variables are involved with measurement error, such a conditional analysis may not be adequate to fully characterize stochastic changes in the associated variables. The inference framework has to be enlarged to facilitate the relevant information. In this chapter, we describe the likelihood inference strategy in general terms and outline some relevant issues, where the conditional distribution $h(y|x, z)$ is modeled parametrically with a class of models, indicated by $\{f(y|x, z; \beta) : \beta \in \Theta_\beta\}$. Here for $\beta \in \Theta_\beta$, $f(y|x, z; \beta)$ is a probability density or mass function, and $\Theta_\beta$ is the parameter space. With a reasonable model assumption, we hope that there is a parameter value, say $\beta_0 \in \Theta_\beta$, such that $f(y|x, z; \beta_0)$ recovers the true distribution $h(y|x, z)$.

Throughout the chapter, vectors are expressed as column vectors. Random variables or random vectors are represented in upper case letters and their realizations are denoted by the corresponding lower case letters. The symbol $h(\cdot)$ or $h(\cdot|\cdot)$ is reserved for the true (conditional) distribution for the random variables indicated by the corresponding arguments, and the notation $f(\cdot)$ or $f(\cdot|\cdot)$ is used to represent paremetric models for the associated true distribution $h(\cdot)$ or $h(\cdot|\cdot)$.

## 6.2 Measurement Error Mechanisms

Measurement error involved with present in any variables: it can be present in covariate variables alone, response variables alone, or both. Here we discuss general inference strategies which are differently formulated to reflect these features, following the lines of Yi (2017).

### 6.2.1 Measurement Error in Covariates

We first consider the case where some covariates are subject to measurement error. Suppose that $X$ is subject to mismeasurement and $Z$ is error-free. An additional variable, sometimes called a *surrogate*, $X^*$, comes along to represent the actual measurement of $X$ which may or may not differ from $X$. Unlike the error-free context which involves $h(y, x, z)$ alone, the joint probability density or mass function $h(y, x, z, x^*)$ for $\{Y, X, Z\}$ and $X^*$ serves as the basis for inferences in the context with measurement error in $X$. Because it is difficult to come up with a meaningful and transparent model to describe *simultaneous* stochastic changes in $\{Y, X, Z\}$ and $X^*$, we often factorize the joint distribution $h(y, x, z, x^*)$ into the product of a sequence of conditional distributions and a marginal distribution, each for a single type of variable.

A conventional scheme is to write

$$h(y, x, z, x^*) = h(y|x, z, x^*)h(x, z, x^*), \tag{6.2}$$

which treats the response variable $Y$ differently from the true covariates $\{X, Z\}$ and their observed versions $\{X^*, Z\}$. The factorization (6.2) allows us to employ various measurement error modeling strategies to describe $h(x, z, x^*)$, and hence conduct inferences by examining $h(y|x, z, x^*)$.

By comparing the conditional distribution $h(y|x, z, x^*)$ with the initially interesting conditional distribution $h(y|x, z)$, we introduce the following mechanisms that have been widely used in the literature of measurement error models. If

$$h(y|x, z, x^*) = h(y|x, z), \tag{6.3}$$

then we call it *nondifferential measurement error* (if $X$ is continuous), or *nondifferential misclassification* (if $X$ is discrete). Sometimes, the term "*non-differential (measurement) error mechanism*" is loosely used for both cases (Carroll et al., 2006). This mechanism says that $Y$ and $X^*$ are conditionally independent, given the true covariates $X$ and $Z$; the surrogate $X^*$ carries no information on inference about the response process, if the true covariates are being controlled. Assumption (6.3) is commonly adopted, explicitly or implicitly, for analysis of error-contaminated data, especially for those data arising from prospective observational studies.

In retrospective studies, such as case-control studies, the nondifferential error mechanism may be infeasible. If

$$h(y|x^*, x, z) \neq h(y|x, z), \tag{6.4}$$

then the corresponding mechanism is called the *differential measurement error mechanism* (if $X$ is continuous), or the *differential misclassification mechanism* (if $X$ is discrete). Occasionally, one may simply use *differential (measurement) error mechanism* to refer to both scenarios (Carroll et al., 2006).

In applications, rigourously verifying (6.3) is generally impossible because the associated distributions are unknown. Employing a measurement error mechanism, (6.3) or (6.4), is practically driven by the nature of data, the study background, the data collection process, and/or the domain knowledge. When parametric modeling is taken, these measurement error mechanisms are frequently phrased in terms of the associated models for the true distributions $h(y|x^*, x, z)$ and $h(y|x, z)$, such as

$$f(y|x, z, x^*) = f(y|x, z)$$

or

$$f(y|x, z, x^*) \neq f(y|x, z),$$

referring to nondifferential or differential error, where the parameters are suppressed in the notation.

### 6.2.2 Measurement Error in Response

Here we consider the case where only the response $Y$ is subject to mismeasurement and both covariates $X$ and $Z$ are error-free, and we let $Y^*$ denote the observed measurement, or a surrogate version, of $Y$.

To study the relationship between $Y$ and $\{X, Z\}$, we may start with the factorization of the joint distribution $h(y, y^*, x, z)$ of $\{Y, Y^*\}$ and $\{X, Z\}$,

$$h(y, y^*, x, z) = h(y^*, y|x, z)h(x, z),$$

which enables us to focus the discussion on the conditional distribution $h(y^*, y|x, z)$ and leave the distribution $h(x, z)$ of $\{X, Z\}$ unmodeled. Further factorizing $h(y^*, y|x, z)$ as

$$h(y^*, y|x, z) = h(y^*|y, x, z)h(y|x, z) \tag{6.5}$$

or

$$h(y^*, y|x, z) = h(y|y^*, x, z)h(y^*|x, z) \tag{6.6}$$

supplies us a separate way of modeling the response process and the mismeasurement process.

The factorization (6.5) shows that in the presence of response error alone, inference may be carried out by introducing an additional layer of modeling to reflect the conditional distribution $h(y^*|y, x, z)$ for $Y^*$ given $\{Y, X, Z\}$, in conjunction with using standard schemes to model the response process, featured by $h(y|x, z)$.

If

$$h(y^*|y, x, z) = h(y^*|x, z),$$

or equivalently,

$$h(y|y^*, x, z) = h(y|x, z), \tag{6.7}$$

we call this *nondifferential response measurement error*; and otherwise, *differential response measurement error*. When $Y$ is discrete, one may also refer to (6.7) as *nondifferential response misclassification*, otherwise *differential response misclassification* (Yi, 2017). This definition is analogous to the covariate measurement error mechanisms described in Section 6.2.1.

If response error is nondifferential, surrogate $Y^*$ and the true response $Y$ are conditionally independent, given covariates $\{X, Z\}$. In this instance, (6.5) and (6.6) are identical, showing that inference about $h(y|x, z)$ can be carried out using

$$h(y^*, y|x, z) = h(y|x, z)h(y^*|x, z),$$

where the mismeasurement process $h(y^*|x, z)$ can be characterized using the observed data on $Y^*$ and $\{X, Z\}$.

With differential response error, it is convenient to use (6.5) to conduct inference about $h(y|x, z)$, where modeling of $h(y^*|y, x, z)$ may be carried our using a regression model. An example is available in Chen et al. (2011) for binary variables $Y$ and $Y^*$.

Finally, we note that surrogate response variables may be defined distinctively for different contexts by different authors. For instance, in clinical settings without covariate measurement error, Prentice (1989) suggested a criterion for *outcome surrogacy* which requires that

$$h(y|y^*, x, z) = h(y|y^*).$$

This definition implies that the covariate effects of $\{X, Z\}$ on the outcome $Y$ would act solely through surrogate $Y^*$. If such a requirement is satisfied, then (6.6) yields

$$h(y^*, y|x, z) = h(y|y^*)h(y^*|x, z).$$

### 6.2.3 Measurement Error in Both Covariates and Response

When both the response and covariate variables are subject to measurement error, we let $Y^*$ denote the surrogate measurement of the response variable $Y$, let $X^*$ denote the surrogate measurement of the covariate vector $X$, and let $Z$ denote the vector of error-free covariates. We write the joint distribution of $Y, Y^*, X, X^*$ and $Z$ as

$$h(y, y^*, x, x^*, z) = h(y, y^*, x, x^*|z)h(z),$$

so that the conditional distribution $h(y, y^*, x, x^*|z)$ of $\{Y, Y^*, X, X^*\}$, given $Z$, is to be examined for inference about $h(y|x, z)$, with the marginal distribution $h(z)$ of $Z$ left unspecified.

Although there are multiple ways to examine $h(y, y^*, x, x^*|z)$, it is convenient to write $h(y, y^*, x, x^*|z)$ as

$$h(y, y^*, x, x^*|z) = h(y|y^*, x, x^*, z)h(y^*, x, x^*|z) \quad (6.8)$$

or

$$h(y, y^*, x, x^*|z) = h(y^*|y, x, x^*, z)h(y, x, x^*|z) \quad (6.9)$$

by viewing $Y$ and $Y^*$ differently based on varying conditioning variables.

These factorizations give us a basis to study the relationship between the true response $Y$ and true covariates $\{X, Z\}$. The choice of (6.8) or (6.9) is driven by the characteristics of measurement error. In the situation where

$$h(y|y^*, x, x^*, z) = h(y|x, z), \quad (6.10)$$

factorization (6.8) allows $h(y|x, z)$ to be spelled out explicitly, and we may perform inference about it by starting with usual modeling for error-free contexts. The only additional care is to be taken for $h(y^*, x, x^*|z)$ which is further factorized into conditional distributions pertinent to the response and covariate measurement error processes. Errors satisfying (6.10) are called *nondifferential errors-in-variables*, otherwise *differential errors-in-variables* (Yi, 2017, Ch.8).

On the other hand, factorization (6.9) allows us to examine $h(y, x, x^*|z)$ by invoking the strategies of handling covariate measurement error, similar to the way of studying (6.2) outlined in Section 6.2.1. In this instance, inference about $h(y|x, z)$ is conducted based on examining $h(y, x, x^*|z)$ which involves the covariate measurement error process only, coupled with $h(y^*|y, x, x^*, z)$ which facilitates the response measurement error process in terms of the true variables $\{Y, X, Z\}$ and the covariate surrogate $X^*$.

### 6.2.4 Discussion

The preceding discussion shows that in addition to modeling the relationship between $Y$ and $\{X, Z\}$ that is commonly conducted for error-free settings, analysis of error-contaminated data generally requires additional modeling of the measurement error process(es). In this section we describe different measurement error mechanisms which help us differentiate varying scenarios of measurement error, and ultimately guide us to call on different modeling schemes. The discussion here is directed to the contexts with measurement error alone. When other features, such as missing observations or censoring, are present in data, the current definition of measurement error mechanisms may become useless for simplifying modeling procedures. Sensible modifications are thereby needed. For settings with co-existing missing observations and covariate measurement error, new definitions of measurement error mechanisms were provided by Yi (2017, Ch.5). With error-prone censored data, modified measurement error mechanisms were discussed by Yi (2017, Ch.3).

Research on covariate measurement error has received extensive attention in the literature. In contrast, discussions on response measurement error have been relatively less though some methods were summarized in Fuller (1987), Carroll et al. (2006, Ch.15), Buonaccorsi (2010, Ch.10), and Yi (2017, Ch.6, Ch.8). Research on measurement error in both response and covariates, especially under the nonlinear model setup, remains fairly under-explored, while the work on this topic dated back to 1940 (e.g., Wald, 1940) or even earlier; some bibliographic note on this was given by Yi (2017, Sec.8.8).

In the following discussion, we confine our attention to the likelihood-based methods for handling measurement error in covariates only.

## 6.3 Induced Model and Bias Assessment

In this section we compare modeling for the conditional distribution of $Y$, given the observed covariates $\{X^*, Z\}$, to that for the conditional distribution of $Y$, given the true covariates $\{X, Z\}$. We consider the circumstance where only $X$ is subject to measurement error and the measurement error mechanism is nondifferential. In this instance, the conditional distribution of $Y$, given the observed covariates $\{X^*, Z\}$, can be modeled via

$$\begin{aligned} f(y|x^*, z; \theta) &= \int f(y, x|x^*, z; \theta)dx \\ &= \int f(y|x, z; \beta)f(x|x^*, z; \alpha)dx, \end{aligned} \tag{6.11}$$

where the integral is replaced by the summation over the sample space if $X$ is discrete; $f(y|x, z; \beta)$ and $f(x|x^*, z; \alpha)$, respectively, represent the models for the response and covariates process with distinct parameters $\beta$ and $\alpha$; and $\theta = (\beta^{\mathrm{T}}, \alpha^{\mathrm{T}})^{\mathrm{T}}$.

Model (6.11) is referred to as the *induced model* (e.g., Buonaccorsi, 2010, p.174; Yi, 2017, Sec. 2.5.1), which offers us the basis for conducting inferences in the presence of covariate measurement error. Implementations of this formulation are broadly available for a variety of settings (e.g., Zucker, 2005). We will elaborate on this strategy in Section 6.6. Here we use the following example to illustrate how the induced model may be connected with the original model for the conditional distribution of $Y$, given the true covariates $\{X, Z\}$.

**Example:** (Probit Regression)

Suppose that the response model is given by the probit regression model

$$P(Y = 1|X, Z) = \Phi(\beta_0 + \beta_x X + \beta_x Z), \tag{6.12}$$

where $Y$ is the binary response taking value 0 or 1, $X$ and $Z$ are scalar covariates, $\Phi(\cdot)$ is the cumulative distribution function for the standard normal distribution, and $\beta = (\beta_0, \beta_x, \beta_z)^{\mathrm{T}}$ is the vector of regression parameters.

Assume that the measurement error model is given by

$$X = \gamma_0 + \gamma_x X^* + \gamma_z Z + U \tag{6.13}$$

with the parameters $\gamma_0, \gamma_x$ and $\gamma_z$, where the error term $U$ follows a normal distribution with mean zero and variance $\sigma_U^2$.

Then by (6.11), the conditional model of $Y$ given the observed covariates $\{X^*, Z\}$ is given by

$$P(Y = 1|X^*, Z) = \Phi(\beta_0^* + \beta_x^* X^* + \beta_x^* Z),$$

where

$$\beta_0^* = \frac{\beta_0 + \beta_x \gamma_0}{\sqrt{1 + \beta_x^2 \sigma_U^2}}, \quad \beta_x^* = \frac{\beta_x \gamma_x}{\sqrt{1 + \beta_x^2 \sigma_U^2}}, \quad \text{and} \quad \beta_z^* = \frac{\beta_z + \beta_x \gamma_z}{\sqrt{1 + \beta_x^2 \sigma_U^2}}.$$

Relevant discussions can be found in Carroll et al. (1984) and Burr (1988).

This example shows that under the measurement error model (6.13), the induced model for the conditional distribution of $Y$, given the observed covariates $\{X^*, Z\}$, shares the same form as that of the conditional of $Y$, given the true covariates $\{X, Z\}$, which is given by the $\Phi(\cdot)$ function together with a linear function of the observed covariates $\{X^*, Z\}$ or the true covariates $\{X, Z\}$. The only differences lie in the coefficients of those linear functions.

On the other hand, the formulation (6.11) can also be used for bias analysis to characterize measurement error effects, especially for settings with regression models where modeling the mean structure of the response variable is of primary interest. The structure of the conditional mean of $Y$, given the observed covariates $\{X^*, Z\}$, may or may not share the same structure as that of the conditional mean of $Y$, given the true covariates $\{X, Z\}$. Indeed,

$$\begin{aligned}
E(Y|X^* = x^*, Z = z) &= \int y f(y|x^*, z) dy \\
&= \int y \left\{ \int f(y|x, z) f(x|x^*, z) dx \right\} dy \\
&= \int \left\{ \int y f(y|x, z) f(x|x^*, z) dy \right\} dx \\
&= \int \left\{ \int y f(y|x, z) dy \right\} f(x|x^*, z) dx \\
&= \int E(Y|x, z) f(x|x^*, z) dx \\
&= E\{E(Y|X, Z = z)|X^* = x^*, Z = z\}, \quad (6.14)
\end{aligned}$$

where the second identity is due to (6.11) and the third step comes from the exchangeability of the integrals. The dependence on the model parameters is suppressed in the notation for convenience.

Suppose that $X$ and $Z$ are $p_x \times 1$ and $p_z \times 1$ vectors of covariates, respectively. Assume that the measurement error model is given by a Berkson type regression model

$$X = \gamma_0 + \Gamma_x X^* + \Gamma_z Z + U, \qquad (6.15)$$

where the error term $U$ is independent of $\{Y, X^*, Z\}$ and has mean zero and covariance matrix $\Sigma_{\mathrm{U}}$, $\gamma_0$ is a $p_x \times 1$ vector, $\Gamma_x$ is a $p_x \times p_x$ matrix, and $\Gamma_z$ is a $p_x \times p_z$ matrix. Model (6.15) with $\gamma_0 = 0$, $\Gamma_x = I_{p_x \times p_x}$ and $\Gamma_z = 0$ is called a Berkson model (Berkson, 1950), where $I_{p_x \times p_x}$ stands for the $p_x \times p_x$ identify matrix, and 0 represents the real number zero, a zero vector, or a zero matrix whose meaning is given by the context.

To gain intuitive insights into the connection between the original model for $Y$, given $\{X, Z\}$, and the induced model for $Y$, given $\{X^*, Z\}$, we examine two regression models in the following examples.

**Example:** (Linear Regression)

Suppose that the response model is the linear regression model

$$Y = \beta_0 + \beta_x^{\mathrm{T}} X + \beta_x^{\mathrm{T}} Z + \epsilon, \tag{6.16}$$

where $\epsilon$ is independent of $\{X, Z\}$ as well as $X^*$ and $U$, and $\beta = (\beta_0, \beta_x^{\mathrm{T}}, \beta_z^{\mathrm{T}})^{\mathrm{T}}$ is the vector of regression parameters. Then (6.14) gives that

$$E(Y|X^*, Z) = \beta_0 + \beta_x^{\mathrm{T}} E(X|X^*, Z) + \beta_z^{\mathrm{T}} Z,$$

which equals, by (6.15),

$$E(Y|X^*, Z) = \beta_0^* + \beta_x^{*\mathrm{T}} X^* + \beta_z^{*\mathrm{T}} Z, \tag{6.17}$$

where

$$\beta_0^* = \beta_0 + \gamma_0^{\mathrm{T}} \beta_x, \ \beta_x^* = \Gamma_x^{\mathrm{T}} \beta_x, \text{ and } \beta_z = \Gamma_z^{\mathrm{T}} \beta_x + \beta_z.$$

This example shows that the mean structure of the induced model for $Y$, given the observed covariates $\{X^*, Z\}$, is identical to that of the original model of $Y$, given the true covariates $\{X, Z\}$, but their coefficients differ. Different to the previous example, the variance of the error term does not appear in the relations of those coefficients.

**Example:** (Linear Regression with Interaction and Quadratic Terms)

Suppose that the response model (6.16) is extended to including interaction and quadratic terms in error-prone covariates. For ease of exposition, we consider the case with $X = (X_1, X_2)^{\mathrm{T}}$ and no covariate $Z$ so the response model is given by

$$Y = \beta_0 + \beta_{x1} X_1 + \beta_{x2} X_2 + \beta_{x3} X_1^2 + \beta_{x4} X_2^2 + \beta_{x5} X_1 X_2 + \epsilon, \tag{6.18}$$

where $\epsilon$ is independent of $X$ as well as $X^*$ and $U$, and $\beta = (\beta_0, \beta_x^{\mathrm{T}})^{\mathrm{T}}$ is the vector of regression parameters with $\beta_x = (\beta_{x1}, \beta_{x2}, \beta_{x3}, \beta_{x4}, \beta_{x5})^{\mathrm{T}}$. Then (6.14) leads to

$$\begin{aligned} E(Y|X^*) \quad = \quad & \beta_0 + \beta_{x1} E(X_1|X^*) + \beta_{x2} E(X_2|X^*) + \beta_{x3} E(X_1^2|X^*) \\ & + \beta_{x4} E(X_2^2|X^*) + \beta_{x5} E(X_1 X_2|X^*). \end{aligned} \tag{6.19}$$

Now we closely examine (6.15) by using refined notation and dropping the term with $Z$. Write $\gamma_0 = (\gamma_{01}, \gamma_{02})^{\mathrm{T}}$, $\Gamma_x = \begin{pmatrix} \gamma_{x11} & \gamma_{x12} \\ \gamma_{x21} & \gamma_{x22} \end{pmatrix}$, and $\Sigma_{\mathrm{U}} = \begin{pmatrix} \sigma^2_{\mathrm{U}1} & \sigma_{\mathrm{U}12} \\ \sigma_{\mathrm{U}12} & \sigma^2_{\mathrm{U}2} \end{pmatrix}$. As a result, if writing $E(X_j|X^*) = \mu_j$ with $\mu_j = \gamma_{0j} + \gamma_{xj1}X_1^* + \gamma_{xj2}X_2^*$ for $j = 1, 2$, we have that

$$\begin{aligned} E(X_1X_2|X^*) &= \sigma_{\mathrm{U}12} + \mu_1\mu_2; \\ E(X_j^2|X^*) &= \sigma^2_{\mathrm{U}j} + \mu_j^2 \quad \text{for } j = 1, 2. \end{aligned} \tag{6.20}$$

Combining (6.19) and (6.20) gives that

$$\begin{aligned} E(Y|X^*) &= \beta_0^* + \beta_{x1}^*X_1^* + \beta_{x2}^*X_2^* \\ &\quad + \beta_{x3}^*X_1^{*2} + \beta_{x4}^*X_2^{*2} + \beta_{x5}^*X_1^*X_2^*, \end{aligned} \tag{6.21}$$

where

$$\begin{aligned} \beta_0^* &= \beta_0 + \beta_{x1}\gamma_{01} + \beta_{x2}\gamma_{02} + \beta_{x3}(\sigma^2_{\mathrm{U}1} + \gamma^2_{01}) + \beta_{x4}(\sigma^2_{\mathrm{U}2} + \gamma^2_{02}) \\ &\quad + \beta_{x5}(\sigma_{\mathrm{U}12} + \gamma_{01}\gamma_{02}); \\ \beta_{x1}^* &= \beta_{x1}\gamma_{x11} + \beta_{x2}\gamma_{x21} + 2\beta_{x3}\gamma_{01}\gamma_{x11} + 2\beta_{x4}\gamma_{02}\gamma_{x21} \\ &\quad + \beta_{x5}(\gamma_{x11}\gamma_{02} + \gamma_{x21}\gamma_{01}); \\ \beta_{x2}^* &= \beta_{x1}\gamma_{x12} + \beta_{x2}\gamma_{x22} + 2\beta_{x3}\gamma_{01}\gamma_{x12} + 2\beta_{x4}\gamma_{02}\gamma_{x22} \\ &\quad + \beta_{x5}(\gamma_{x12}\gamma_{02} + \gamma_{x22}\gamma_{01}); \\ \beta_{x3}^* &= \beta_{x3}\gamma^2_{x11} + \beta_{x4}\gamma^2_{x21} + \beta_{x5}\gamma_{x11}\gamma_{x21}; \\ \beta_{x4}^* &= \beta_{x3}\gamma^2_{x12} + \beta_{x4}\gamma^2_{x22} + \beta_{x5}\gamma_{x12}\gamma_{x22}; \\ \beta_{x5}^* &= 2\beta_{x3}\gamma_{x11}\gamma_{x12} + 2\beta_{x4}\gamma_{x21}\gamma_{x22} + \beta_{x5}(\gamma_{x11}\gamma_{x21} + \gamma_{x11}\gamma_{x22}). \end{aligned}$$

These expressions are available in Buonaccorsi (2010, Sec.6.7.2). The result (6.21) shows that even for a simple model, including interaction and quadratic terms of error-prone covariates can considerably complicate the expressions of the mean of the induced model, suggesting complex consequences of measurement error on changing the mean structure.

By the same principle, one may conduct bias analysis for other response models and measurement error models. For instance, Buonaccorsi (2010, Sec.6) summarized bias analysis for various models including the quadratic regression model, the log linear model, the logistic regression model, and the normal discriminant model. Discussions on other settings can be found in Wang (1998) and Carroll et al. (2006, Ch.4), among others.

Our illustrations here examine how measurement error in covariates may change the distribution form or the mean structure of the response model. When measurement error appears in response variables, or when measurement error is present in both response and covariate variables, one may follow the same principle to examine the measurement error effects on the change of the conditional distribution or the mean structure of $Y$, given the true covariates. Detailed discussions on this can be found in Neuhaus (1999), Neuhaus (2002), and Yi (2017, Ch.8), among others.

## 6.4 Functional and Structural Modeling Schemes

As discussed earlier, under the nondifferential measurement error mechanism, the factorization

$$h(y, x, x^*, z) = h(y|x, z)h(x, x^*, z)$$

offers us a convenient framework for conducting inferences about the distribution $h(y|x, z)$. It enables us to employ available modeling techniques developed for error-free settings to describe $h(y|x, z)$; the only extra work is to model the distribution $h(x, x^*, z)$ for the measurement error process. This additional modeling step distinguishes inferences with measurement error from usual inferences without measurement error.

To examine $h(x, x^*, z)$, one may factorize it as

$$h(x, x^*, z) = h(x^*|x, z)h(x, z) \tag{6.22}$$

or

$$h(x, x^*, z) = h(x|x^*, z)h(x^*, z) \tag{6.23}$$

to accommodate different modeling schemes for the measurement error process. Factorization (6.22) allows us to treat $\{X, Z\}$ as fixed and conduct inference by conditioning on $\{X, Z\}$, with the distribution $h(x, z)$ of $\{X, Z\}$ left unmodeled. This strategy is called the *functional method.* On the other hand, (6.23) emphasizes to view $X$ as a random variable whose conditional distribution $h(x|x^*, z)$, given $\{X^*, Z\}$, basically needs to be specified; this method is called the *structural modeling* scheme. When employing (6.22) or (6.23) in conjunction with parametric modeling, a tacit assumption is commonly made that parameters governing different models are *distinct.*

In contrast, under the differential error mechanism, the preceding factorizations do not necessarily offer us a quick way to simplify the problem. Gustafson (2004), Carroll et al. (2006), Buinaccorsi (2010), and Yi (2017) discussed strategies of handling differential measurement error for various settings. In the rest of this chapter we consider only the case with nondifferential measurement error.

While there are no definite rules on the choice of the functional or structural modeling strategy, opting for a particular modeling scheme may be driven by considerations related to the nature of the problem, the complexity of forming a valid inference procedure, and the intensity of computation; sometimes, this may be simply a matter of personal preference. Generally speaking, functional modeling is distribution-robust in the sense of no need for specifying the distribution of the true covarites, whereas structural modeling can be more efficient when there is good knowledge about the distribution of the true covariates. Structural modeling is typically required when inference is conducted within the Bayesian paradigm.

We note that in some measurement error problems, both functional and structural modeling schemes can be equally applicable. For example, Fuller (1987, Sec.1.2.3) compared these two strategies in terms of point estimation and variance estimation for the linear model parameters; the inference results and their interpretation are basically different.

With the structural modeling framework, the maximum likelihood method is often employed because of the straightforward formulation of the likelihood function. On the other hand, with the functional modeling framework, one may be tempted to apply the likelihood method by treating the $X$ variables as fixed parameters for all subjects in the sample. However, the resulting maximum likelihood estimators for the response model parameters cannot always be guaranteed to be consistent. Their consistency depends on the form of the response model (as well as the measurement error model), as illustrated in the following example, where the $Z$ covariate is not included for ease of exposition.

**Example:** Suppose that $\{(Y_i, X_i) : i = 1, \ldots, n\}$ is a random sample, where the $(Y_i, X_i)$ are independent and have same distribution as for $(Y, X)$ the measurement of the response variable $Y_i$ is precise, but the scalar covariate $X_i$ is error-corrupted. For $i = 1, \ldots, n$, let $X_i^*$ denote the surrogate measurement of $X_i$, and assume that

$$X_i^* = X_i + U_i,$$

where $U_i$ is independent of $\{Y_i, X_i\}$ and follows a normal distribution $N(0, \sigma_{\mathrm{U}}^2)$ with variance $\sigma_{\mathrm{U}}^2$. To highlight the idea, we assume that $\sigma_{\mathrm{U}}^2$ is known.

We now consider the functional modeling strategy for the following two response models, where we treat the true covariates $\{X_i : i = 1, \ldots, n\}$ as unknown model parameters in applying the likelihood method.

The first response model is given by

$$Y_i = \beta_0 + \beta_x X_i + \epsilon_i. \tag{6.24}$$

where $\epsilon_i$ is independent of $\{X_i, U_i\}$ and follows a normal distribution $N(0, \sigma^2)$ with variance $\sigma^2$.

Let $\theta = (\beta_0, \beta_x, \sigma^2)^{\mathrm{T}}$. Then the likelihood function for the model parameters $\theta$ and $(X_1, \ldots, X_n)^{\mathrm{T}}$ is

$$L(\theta, X_1, \ldots, X_n) = \prod_{i=1}^{n} (L_{\mathrm{Y}_i|\mathrm{X}_i} L_{\mathrm{X}_i}),$$

where

$$L_{\mathrm{Y}_i|\mathrm{X}_i} = \frac{1}{\sqrt{2\pi}\sigma} \exp\left\{-\frac{(Y_i - \beta_0 - \beta_x X_i)^2}{2\sigma^2}\right\}$$

and

$$L_{X_i} = \frac{1}{\sqrt{2\pi}\sigma_U} \exp\left\{-\frac{(X_i^* - X_i)^2}{2\sigma_U^2}\right\}.$$

Maximizing $L(\theta, X_1, \ldots, X_n)$ with respect to $\theta$ and $(X_1, \ldots, X_n)^T$ gives the estimators of $(\beta_0, \beta_x, \sigma^2, X_1, \ldots, X_n)^T$, given by

$$\widehat{\beta}_0 = \frac{1}{n}\sum_{i=1}^{n} Y_i - \frac{\widehat{\beta}_x}{n}\sum_{i=1}^{n} \widehat{X}_i, \quad \widehat{\beta}_x = \frac{\sum_{i=1}^{n} \widehat{X}_i(Y_i - \widehat{\beta}_0)}{\sum_{i=1}^{n} \widehat{X}_i^2},$$

$$\widehat{\sigma}^2 = \frac{1}{n}\sum_{i=1}^{n}(Y_i - \widehat{\beta}_0 - \widehat{\beta}_x\widehat{X}_i)^2, \quad \text{and} \quad \widehat{X}_i = \frac{\sigma_U^2\widehat{\beta}_x(Y_i - \widehat{\beta}_0) + \widehat{\sigma}^2 X_i^*}{\widehat{\beta}_x^2\sigma_U^2 + \widehat{\sigma}^2}.$$

Gleser (1981) showed that $\widehat{\beta}_0$ and $\widehat{\beta}_x$ are consistent estimators of $\beta_0$ and $\beta_x$, respectively.

However, if the response model (6.24) is replaced by a different model, say, the logistic regression model

$$\text{logit } P(Y_i = 1|X_i) = \beta_0 + \beta_x X_i \tag{6.25}$$

with the binary response $Y_i$ taking value 0 or 1, this likelihood method with $(X_1, \ldots, X_n)$ treated as parameters cannot ensure the resulting maximum likelihood estimators of $\beta_0$ and $\beta_x$ to be consistent anymore. In fact, Stefanski and Carroll (1987) showed that those estimators are inconsistent. The inconsistency of the maximum likelihood estimators of $\beta_0, \beta_x$ in this instance has the relevance to the diverging dimension of $(X_1, \ldots, X_n)^T$ as the sample size $n$ approaches infinity. This phenomenon was observed and discussed by Neyman and Scott (1948); a brief discussion on this can also be found in Yi (2017, pp.22-23).

## 6.5 Conditional Score Method

Section 6.4 demonstrates that under the functional modeling framework, although the likelihood method can be conceptually straightforward to implement by treating $\{X_1, \ldots, X_n\}$ as parameters together with the response model parameter $\beta$, this procedure does not ensure the consistency of the resulting estimator for $\beta$, except for some special response models such as linear regression. Furthermore, while it may be tempting to treat $(X_1, \ldots, X_n)^T$ as parameters in the same way as we regard the response model parameter $\beta$, it is useful to recognize their differences. The dimension of $(X_1, \ldots, X_n)^T$ goes to infinity when the sample size approaches infinity, whereas the dimension of $\beta$ is fixed regardless of the sample size. In the likelihood formulation, each component of $(X_1, \ldots, X_n)^T$ appears only once corresponding to a subject, i.e., it is subject-specific; on the contrary, each component of $\beta$ is shared by the likelihood contributions from all the subjects in the sample. Such a different nature is reflected by the notions of *structural* and *incidental* parameters (e.g., Neyman and Scott, 1948). The parameters *of interest*, $\beta$, are called *structural* parameters, and *nuisance* parameters $(X_1, \ldots, X_n)^{\mathrm{T}}$ are sometimes phrased as *incidental* parameters.

Despite such differences in $(X_1, \ldots, X_n)^{\mathrm{T}}$ and $\beta$, the likelihood method in Section 6.4 regards these two types of parameters equally when proceeding with estimation procedures, which is not ideal for us to put more emphasis on the parameters of interest than nuisance parameters. Motivated by these considerations, we take an alternative perspective to handle these parameters differently. We consider the *conditional score method* described by Stefanski and Carroll (1987). For ease of exposition, error-free covariates $Z$ are not included in the following discussion. The basic idea of this method is to start with the distribution of $Y$, given $X^*$, by taking $\beta$ as given and finding a complete sufficient statistic, say $\Delta(\beta)$, for $X$; then we use such a statistic to construct a conditional distribution of the response $Y$, given $\Delta(\beta)$ and the observed covariates, such that the distribution depends only on the observed data and $\beta$ but not on the unobserved $X$; and finally, we employ this conditional distribution to carry out inference about $\beta$.

To be specific, suppose that $X$ and $X^*$ are related via the classical additive measurement error model

$$X^* = X + U, \tag{6.26}$$

where the error term $U$ is independent of $\{Y, X\}$ and follows the normal distribution with mean zero and covariance matrix $\Sigma_{\mathrm{U}}$.

Suppose that given $X = x$, the response variable $Y$ has the probability density or mass function

$$f_{\mathrm{Y|X}}(y|x;\theta) = \exp\left\{\frac{y \times m(x;\beta) - b(m(x;\beta))}{a(\phi)} + c(y;\phi)\right\},$$

where $a(\cdot), b(\cdot)$ and $c(\cdot)$ are known functions, $m(x;\beta) = \beta_0 + \beta_x^{\mathrm{T}} x$ with $\beta = (\beta_0, \beta_x^{\mathrm{T}})^{\mathrm{T}}$, $\phi$ is the disperson parameter, and $\theta = (\beta^{\mathrm{T}}, \phi)^{\mathrm{T}}$.

Assume that $\Sigma_{\mathrm{U}}/a(\phi)$, denoted $\Sigma$, is known. Then the joint density of $Y$ and $X^*$, given $X$, is

$$f_{\mathrm{YX^*|X}}(y, x^*|x;\theta) = f_{\mathrm{Y|X}}(y|x;\theta) f_{\mathrm{X^*|X}}(x^*|x;\theta), \tag{6.27}$$

where

$$f_{\mathrm{X^*|X}}(x^*|x;\theta) = \frac{1}{\sqrt{(2\pi)^p|\Sigma_{\mathrm{U}}|}} \exp\left\{-\frac{1}{2}(x^* - x)^{\mathrm{T}}\Sigma_{\mathrm{U}}^{-1}(x^* - x)\right\}$$

is the probability density derived from the measurement error model (6.26).

Define

$$\Delta = X^* + Y\Sigma\beta_x.$$

If $X$ is regarded as a parameter with $\theta$ being given, then $\Delta$ is a sufficient statistic for $X$. That is, the conditional distribution of $Y$ given $\Delta$ depends only on $Y$, $X^*$ and $\theta$ but not on $X$. As a result, inference about $\beta$ can be carried out using this conditional distribution.

Specifically, let $f_{Y|\Delta}(y|\delta;\theta)$ denote the conditional distribution of $Y$ given $\Delta = \delta$, which is given by

$$f_{Y|\Delta}(y|\delta;\theta) = \exp\left[y\zeta - \frac{1}{2}y^2\beta_x^{\mathrm{T}}\Sigma\beta_x/a(\phi) + c(y;\phi) - \log d(\zeta,\beta_x,\phi)\right], \quad (6.28)$$

where $\delta = x^* + y\Sigma\beta_x$ is a realization of $\Delta$,

$$\zeta = (\beta_0 + \delta^{\mathrm{T}}\beta_x)/a(\phi),$$

and

$$d(\zeta,\beta_x,\phi) = \int \exp\left\{y\zeta - \frac{1}{2}y^2\beta_x^{\mathrm{T}}\Sigma\beta_x/a(\phi) + c(y;\phi)\right\} d\eta(y)$$

is the normalizing constant with respect to a $\sigma$-finite measure $\eta(\cdot)$. Thus, defining

$$\psi(y,x^*;\theta) = \left.\frac{\partial \log f_{Y|\Delta}(y|\delta;\theta)}{\partial\theta}\right|_{\delta=x^*+y\Sigma\beta_x},$$

we have that $\psi(y,x^*;\theta)$ is an unbiased estimating function of $\theta$. Then applying this function to the sample data, say $\{(y_i,x_i^*) : i = 1,\ldots,n\}$, and solving

$$\sum_{i=1}^{n}\psi(y_i,x_i^*;\theta) = 0$$

for $\theta$ yields a consistent estimator of $\theta$, provided regularity conditions hold.

Stefanski and Carroll (1987) discussed in detail the application of this method to generalized linear regression models. For example, with the logistic regression model

$$\text{logit } P(Y=1|X) = \beta_0 + \beta_x^{\mathrm{T}}X,$$

the conditional distribution of $Y$ given $\Delta = \delta$ is given by

$$P(Y=1|\Delta=\delta) = H\left\{\beta_0 + \left(\delta - \frac{1}{2}\Sigma\beta_x\right)^{\mathrm{T}}\beta_x\right\},$$

where $H(t) = 1/\{1+\exp(-t)\}$, and the resulting unbiased estimating function $\psi(y,x^*;\theta)$ is

$$\psi(y,x^*;\theta) = \left.\left\{y - H(\beta_0 + (\delta - \frac{1}{2}\Sigma\beta_x)^{\mathrm{T}}\beta_x)\right\}\begin{pmatrix}1\\ \delta - \Sigma\beta_x\end{pmatrix}\right|_{\delta=x^*+y\Sigma\beta_x}.$$

The implementation of the conditional score method is simple and does not require the specification of the distribution of the covariates $X$, thus it is robust in this sense. This method was developed by Stefanski and Carroll (1987) for the generalized linear model models where the response model is characterized by a distribution from the exponential family when measurement error is given by (6.26); an initiation of this scheme was available in Lindsay (1982). Extensions of this method are available for various settings (e.g., Carroll et al., 2006, Ch.7; Yi, 2017, Ch.2), including longitudinal error contaminated data (e.g., Pan et al. 2009), joint modeling of longitudinal and survival data with measurement error (e.g., Tsiatis and Davidian, 2001; Song et al., 2002), and case-control studies with error-contaminated data (e.g., McShane et al., 2001). In-depth discussions of the conditional score method can be found in Zucker (2021).

## 6.6 Observed Likelihood Method

As mentioned in Section 6.3, the *observed data likelihood*, also called the *induced likelihood*, may be used for inference about the model parameters associated with modeling the relationship between the response variable $Y$ and the true covariates $\{X, Z\}$. In this section we discuss this method and related issues.

Again, let $\{f(y|x, z; \beta) : \beta \in \Theta_\beta\}$ denote the parametric models for the conditional distribution of $Y$, given $\{X, Z\}$. Let $\{f(x^*, x|z; \alpha) : \alpha \in \Theta_\alpha\}$ represent the model for the measurement error process. Let $\theta = (\beta^{\mathrm{T}}, \alpha^{\mathrm{T}})^{\mathrm{T}}$ be the vector of model parameters, where $\beta$ is of interest, and $\alpha$ is the vector of nuisance parameters.

To perform likelihood estimation, we often start with constructing the conditional model for $\{Y, X^*\}$ given $Z$, given by

$$f(y, x^*|z; \theta) = \int f(y|x, z; \beta) f(x^*, x|z; \alpha) dx, \tag{6.29}$$

where the integral is replaced by the summation over the sample space if $X$ is discrete, and the nondifferential covariate measurement error mechanism is assumed.

### 6.6.1 Identifiability and Data Format

Suggested in Section 6.4, analysis of error-prone data often requires additional modeling of measurement error and/or the covariate processes, besides modeling the response process. This extra layer of modeling adds complications to inferential procedures. Parameter *identifiability* becomes a particular concern (e.g., Carroll et al., 2006, Sec. 8.1).

In contrast to the *model expansion* scheme discussed by Gustafson (2005), *model contraction* strategies are conventionally employed to handle nonidentifiability issues, where the prime goal is to reduce the parameter space. While imposing certain constraints on the associated parameters is frequently used to this end in error-free contexts (e.g., Carroll et al., 1997; Hung and Wang, 2013), in analyzing error-contaminated data it is common practice to call for additional data to help delineate the measurement error process.

Carroll et al. (2006, Ch.2), Buonaccorsi (2010, Ch.6) and Yi (2017, Ch.2) discussed several types of data sources used in analysis of error-contaminated data, including validation data, repeated measurements, and instrumental data. Depending on the measurement error mechanism, the requirement of additional data may be different. With nondifferential measurement error, it is possible to estimate parameter $\beta$ in the response model $f(y|x,z;\beta)$ even when the true covariates $X$ are not observable. This is, however, usually not true for differential error except for special cases, such as with linear models. In this case, a validation subsample which includes measurements of $X$ is often required. With the availability of repeated surrogate measurements, some specific forms, such as the classical additive measurement error model, are needed so that the parameters associated with the measurement error model can be consistently estimated from the replicates (Carroll et al., 2006). Broadly speaking, having a validation sample gives us the greatest flexibility in considering various kinds of measurement error models.

When nonidentifiability issues are present but we do not have additional data to facilitate estimation of parameters associated with the measurement error process, we may conduct *sensitivity analyses* to address measurement error effects. Typically, we take a number of candidate models for the measurement error process together with representative values specified for their parameters, and then apply a valid method which accommodates measurement error effects to perform inference about the response model parameters. It is then useful to assess how sensitive the results are to different specifications of measurement error models and to the degrees of measurement error or misclassification.

### 6.6.2 Likelihood Methods with Validation Data

To see how likelihood-based methods may be used to analyze error-contaminated data, here we consider the situation where a validation sample, either *internal* or *external*, is available together with the main study sample. In the main study/internal validation design (e.g., Spiegelman et al., 2001), available data include $\{(y_i, x_i^*, z_i) : i \in \mathcal{M}\}$ and $\{(y_i, x_i^*, x_i, z_i) : i \in \mathcal{V}\}$, where $\mathcal{M}$ and $\mathcal{V}$ contain $n$ and $m$ subjects, respectively; and $\mathcal{V}$ is a subset of $\mathcal{M}$.

On the contrary, in the main study/external validation design (e.g., Thurston et al., 2003), available data for the main study and the external study are, respectively, represented by $\{(y_i, x_i^*, z_i) : i \in \mathcal{M}\}$ and $\{(x_i^*, x_i, z_i) : i \in \mathcal{V}\}$, where $\mathcal{V}$ and $\mathcal{M}$ do not overlap, and there are no response measurements for the subjects in $\mathcal{V}$. With the main study/external validation design, it is often assumed that given $Z_i$, the conditional distribution of $\{X_i, X_i^*\}$ for $i \in \mathcal{V}$ is the same as that of $\{X_i, X_i^*\}$ for $i \in \mathcal{M}$; this assumption ensures that the information carried by the validation study $\mathcal{V}$ can be transported to the main study $\mathcal{M}$ when carrying out inferences. The feasibility of this assumption is justified by subject matter considerations. This assumption is typically reasonable for scenarios where both main and external validation studies are carried out for the same population.

Here we outline estimation procedures for the two designs. For ease of exposition, for subject $i$, let $L_{i\mathrm{M}}^*(\theta) = f(y_i, x_i^*|z_i;\theta)$, which is determined by applying (6.29) to subject $i$. Let $L_i(\beta) = f(y_i|x_i, z_i;\beta)$ and $L_{i\mathrm{V}}(\alpha) = f(x_i^*, x_i|z_i;\alpha)$ denote the conditional probability density or mass functions which model the conditional distribution of $Y_i$ given $\{X_i, Z_i\}$ and of $\{X_i^*, X_i\}$ given $Z_i$, respectively. Depending on how the measurement error process is modeled, $L_{i\mathrm{V}}(\alpha)$ can be equivalently expressed as $f(x_i^*|x_i, z_i;\alpha)f(x_i|z_i;\alpha)$ or $f(x_i|x_i^*, z_i;\alpha)f(x_i^*|z_i;\alpha)$, where associated modeling schemes are available in Carroll et al. (2006) and Yi (2017, Ch.2). Further, write $S_i(\beta) = \partial\{\log L_i(\beta)\}/\partial\beta$, $S_{i\mathrm{M}}^*(\theta) = \partial\{\log L_{i\mathrm{M}}^*(\theta)\}/\partial\theta$, and $S_{i\mathrm{V}}(\alpha) = \{\log L_{i\mathrm{V}}(\alpha)\}/\partial\alpha$.

The observed likelihood is formulated differently for subjects in the main study and the validation study, and the likelihood for the sample is also different for different study designs, as illustrated as follows (e.g., Yi et al., 2018).

With the main study/internal validation study design, the subjects in the main study contribute through the conditional distribution of $\{Y_i, X_i^*\}$ given $Z_i$ while the subjects in the validation study contribute through the conditional distribution of $\{Y_i, X_i, X_i^*\}$ given $Z_i$. Therefore, the observed likelihood contributed from the sample is given by

$$L_{\mathrm{INT}}(\theta) = \left\{\prod_{i\in\mathcal{M}\setminus\mathcal{V}} L_{i\mathrm{M}}^*(\theta)\right\} \times \left[\prod_{i\in\mathcal{V}}\{L_i(\beta)L_{i\mathrm{V}}(\alpha)\}\right].$$

Then maximizing $L_{\mathrm{INT}}(\theta)$ gives the maximum likelihood estimator of $\theta$, denoted $\widehat{\theta}_{\mathrm{INT}}$. Under regularity conditions and when the ratio $m/n$ approaches a positive constant, say $\rho$, as $n \to \infty$, $\widehat{\theta}_{\mathrm{INT}}$ is a consistent estimator of $\theta$, and $\sqrt{n}(\widehat{\theta}_{\mathrm{INT}} - \theta)$ has the asymptotic normal distribution with mean zero and covariance matrix $\Sigma_{\mathrm{INT}}$, given by

$$\Sigma_{\mathrm{INT}}^{-1} = (1-\rho)E\left(-\frac{\partial S_{i\mathrm{M}}^*(\theta)}{\partial\theta^{\mathrm{T}}}\right) + \rho\begin{pmatrix} E\left(-\frac{\partial S_i(\beta)}{\partial\beta^{\mathrm{T}}}\right) & 0 \\ 0 & E\left(-\frac{\partial S_{i\mathrm{V}}(\alpha)}{\partial\alpha^{\mathrm{T}}}\right)\end{pmatrix}.$$

On the contrary, under the main study/external validation study design, the likelihood function is given by

$$L_{\mathrm{EXT}}(\theta) = \left\{\prod_{i\in\mathcal{M}} L_{i\mathrm{M}}^*(\theta)\right\} \times \left\{\prod_{i\in\mathcal{V}} L_{i\mathrm{V}}(\alpha)\right\}.$$

Then maximizing $L_{\text{EXT}}(\theta)$ with respect to $\theta$ gives the maximum likelihood estimator of $\theta$, denoted $\widehat{\theta}_{\text{EXT}}$. Under regularity conditions and when the ratio $m/n$ approaches a positive constant, say $\rho$, as $n \to \infty$, $\widehat{\theta}_{\text{EXT}}$ is a consistent estimator of $\theta$, and $\sqrt{n}(\widehat{\theta}_{\text{EXT}} - \theta)$ has the asymptotic normal distribution with mean zero and covariance matrix $\Sigma_{\text{EXT}}$ given by $\Sigma_{\text{EXT}} = \frac{1}{1+\rho} A_{\text{EXT}}^{-1}$, where

$$A_{\text{EXT}} = \frac{1}{(1+\rho)} E\left(-\frac{\partial S_{i\text{M}}^*(\theta)}{\partial \theta^{\text{T}}}\right) + \frac{\rho}{1+\rho} \begin{pmatrix} 0 & 0 \\ 0 & E\left(-\frac{\partial S_{i\text{V}}(\alpha)}{\partial \alpha^{\text{T}}}\right) \end{pmatrix}.$$

### 6.6.3 Likelihood Method with Repeated Surrogate Measurements

In contrast to the availability of a validation sample considered in Section 6.6.2, we now consider the case where repeated surrogate measurements are available for avoiding potential nonidentifiability induced from the additional modeling of the measurement error process.

For subject $i$ with $i = 1, \ldots, n$, suppose that $Y_i$ is the response variable and $Z_i$ is the vector of error-free covariates, and that $X_i$ is the vector of error-prone covariates which are independently measured $m_i$ times with replicated surrogate measurements $X_{ij}^*$, where $j = 1, \ldots, m_i$. Assume the nondifferential measurement error mechanism

$$f(y_i|x_i, z_i, x_{i1}^*, \ldots, x_{im_i}^*) = f(y_i|x_i, z_i), \tag{6.30}$$

where the parameters are suppressed in the notation. Then the observed data likelihood can be written as

$$L_{\text{O}} = \prod_{i=1}^{n} \int f(y_i|x_i, z_i) f(x_{i1}^*, \ldots, x_{im_i}^*|x_i, z_i) f(x_i|z_i) dx_i, \tag{6.31}$$

where the dependence on the model parameters is suppressed in the notation, and the integral is replaced with the summation when $X_i$ is discrete.

When the three functions in the integrand of (6.31) are all normal density functions, it is straightforward to obtain the maximum likelihood estimator of the parameter $\beta$, illustrated by the following example discussed by Schafer and Purdy (1996, Sec.3).

**Example:** For $i = 1, \ldots, n$, suppose that

$$Y_i|(X_i, Z_i) \sim N(\beta_x^{\text{T}} X_i + \beta_z^{\text{T}} Z_i, \sigma^2)$$

and

$$X_i|Z_i \sim N(\Gamma Z_i, \Sigma_x),$$

where $\beta_x, \beta_z, \sigma^2$ are parameters, $\Gamma$ is a $p_x \times p_z$ matrix, and $\Sigma_x$ is a positive definite matrix. Assume (6.30) and suppose that the $X_{ij}^*$ are independent and that

$$X_{ij}^*|(X_i, Z_i) \sim N(X_i, \Sigma_{\mathrm{U}}) \quad \text{for } j = 1, \ldots, m_i,$$

where $\Sigma_{\mathrm{U}}$ is a positive definite matrix. Then the joint distribution of $Y_i$ and $\{X_{i1}^*, \ldots, X_{im_i}^*\}$, given $Z_i$, is a multivariate normal distribution with mean $\mu_i$ and covariance matrix $\Sigma_i^*$, where

$$\mu_i = \begin{pmatrix} \beta_z^{\mathrm{T}} Z_i + \beta_z^{\mathrm{T}} \Gamma Z_i \\ \Gamma Z_i \bigotimes 1_{m_i} \end{pmatrix},$$

$$\Sigma_i^* = \begin{pmatrix} \sigma^2 + \beta_x^{\mathrm{T}} \Sigma_x \beta_x & \beta_x^{\mathrm{T}} \Sigma_x \bigotimes 1_{m_i}^{\mathrm{T}} \\ \Sigma_x \beta_x \bigotimes 1_{m_i} & \Sigma_x \bigotimes 1_{m_i} 1_{m_i}^{\mathrm{T}} + \Sigma_{\mathrm{U}} \bigotimes I_{m_i \times m_i} \end{pmatrix},$$

$1_{m_i}$ is the $m_i \times 1$ unit vector, $I_{m_i \times m_i}$ is the $m_i \times m_i$ identity matrix, and $\bigotimes$ represents the Kronecker product. Consequently, the log likelihood function derived from (6.31) is

$$\log L_{\mathrm{O}} = \sum_{i=1}^{n} \left\{ -\frac{1}{2} \log |\Sigma_i^*| - \frac{1}{2} (V_i - \mu_i)^{\mathrm{T}} \Sigma_i^{*-1} (V_i - \mu_i) \right\}, \tag{6.32}$$

where $V_i = (Y_i, X_{i1}^{*\mathrm{T}}, \ldots, X_{im_i}^{*\mathrm{T}})^{\mathrm{T}}$. Estimation of the model parameters can then proceed with the maximization of (6.32).

Discussion on applying the likelihood method for settings with replicated surrogate measurements of $X_i$ can also be found in Buonaccorsi (2010, Sec.6.12.3).

## 6.7 Expectation-Maximization Algorithm

The observed likelihood (6.31), just like the conditional distribution (6.29) in Section 6.6.2, is the key for applying the likelihood method. In a special situation such as that all the associated distributions are normal, as aforementioned, or the case where the covariates $X$ are discrete (Carroll et al., 2006, Sec.8.3), calculation of (6.31) or (6.29) is straightforward; otherwise one needs to handle the associated integrals which can be difficult due to the lack of an analytical form. In this instance, one often invokes numerical techniques such as Gaussian quadrature rules, the Laplace approximation, or the Monte Carlo algorithm to approximate (6.31) or (6.29).

Alternatively, the problem can be handled using the *expectation-maximization* (EM) algorithm which, instead of integrating out the $X$ covariates from the integral (6.31) or (6.29), treats the $X$ covariates as "missing data" in the complete-data likelihood. The EM algorithm basically iterates between the expectation step (E-step) and the maximization step (M-step) until convergence of updated estimates of the parameters. For instance, in the case where replicates, $\{X_{i1}^*, \ldots, X_{m_i}^*\}$, of $X_i$ are available, the EM algorithm proceeds as follows. In the E-step of an iteration, say iteration $(t+1)$, we evaluate the conditional expectation of the logarithm of the complete-data likelihood (say, $L_C$), denoted $Q(\theta; \theta^{(t)}) = E(\log L_C | Y_i, X_{i1}^*, \ldots, X_{im_i}^*, Z_i; \theta^{(t)})$, where the conditional distribution of the unobserved variables, given the observed data, is evaluated at the parameter estimate $\theta^{(t)}$ at the previous iteration. In the M-step of this iteration, we maximize $Q(\theta; \theta^{(t)})$ with respect to $\theta$ and obtain a new update, $\theta^{(t+1)}$, of $\theta$. The E-step and M-step iterate until the convergence of $\theta^{(t+1)}$ for $t = 0, 1, \ldots$

To illustrate the usage of the EM algorithm, in the following example we describe the development of Schafer (1993) who considered the probit regression model with a scalar $X_i$.

**Example:** Suppose that the response variable $Y_i$ is binary which is defined to be 1 or 0 according to the sign of a latent variable $W_i$. Specifically, $Y_i = I(W_i > 0)$ and $W_i$ follows the distribution $N(\beta_x X_i + \beta_z^{\mathrm{T}} Z_i, 1)$, where $I(\cdot)$ is the indicator function, and $\beta_x$ and $\beta_z$ are parameters. Consequently, the response variable $Y_i$ and the covariates $\{X_i, Z_i\}$ can be expressed by the probit regression model

$$P(Y_i = 1 | X_i, Z_i) = \Phi(\beta_x X_i + \beta_z^{\mathrm{T}} Z_i).$$

Suppose that the conditional distribution of $X_i$, given $Z_i$, is $N(\alpha^{\mathrm{T}} Z_i, \sigma_x^2)$, and that the conditional distribution of $X_{ij}^*$, given $\{X_i, Z_i\}$, is $N(X_i, \sigma_{\mathrm{U}}^2)$ for $j = 1, \ldots, m_i$, where $\alpha, \sigma_x^2$ and $\sigma_{\mathrm{U}}^2$ are parameters.

To implement the EM algorithm, we first work out the complete-data likelihood

$$L_C = \prod_{i=1}^{n} f(w_i, y_i, x_i, x_{i1}^*, \ldots, x_{im_i}^* | z_i),$$

which can be written as $\prod_{i=1}^{n} f(y_i|w_i) f(w_i, x_{i1}^*, \ldots, x_{im_i}^* | x_i, z_i)$ by the definition of $Y_i$. Applying the given models to $L_C$ leads to the complete-data sufficient statistics, given by

$$S_{xw} = \sum_{i=1}^{n} X_i W_i, \; S_{zw} = \sum_{i=1}^{n} Z_i W_i, \; S_{zx} = \sum_{i=1}^{n} Z_i X_i,$$

$$S_{xx} = \sum_{i=1}^{n} X_i^2, \; S_{xx^*} = \sum_{i=1}^{n} \sum_{j=1}^{m_i} X_i X_{ij}^*, \; S_{x^*x^*} = \sum_{i=1}^{n} \sum_{j=1}^{m_i} X_{ij}^{*2},$$

$$\text{and } S_{xx}^* = \sum_{i=1}^{n} m_i X_i^2.$$

Then we implement the EM algorithm iteratively between the E-step and the M-step. Here, the "missing data" are $\{W_i, X_i\}$ and the observed data include $\{Y_i, X_i^*, Z_i\}$ with $X_i^* = (X_{i1}^*, \ldots, X_{im_i}^*)^{\mathrm{T}}$. The evaluation of the function $Q(\theta; \theta^{(t)}) = E(\log L_{\mathrm{C}} | Y_i, X_i^*, Z_i; \theta^{(t)})$ essentially involves calculations of the conditional expectation of the sufficient statistics, given the observed data $\{Y_i, X_i^*, Z_i\}$. Specifically, the expectation of the complete-data sufficient statistics is taken with respect to the joint distribution of the unobserved variables $\{W_i, X_i\}$, conditional on the observed data $\{Y_i, X_i^*, Z_i\}$, which may be handled using the double expectation property. For instance,

$$\begin{aligned} E(S_{xw}|\text{observed data}) &= \sum_{i=1}^{n} E(X_i W_i | Y_i, X_i^*, Z_i) \\ &= \sum_{i=1}^{n} E\{E(X_i | W_i, Y_i, X_i^*, Z_i) W_i | Y_i, X_i^*, Z_i\}. \end{aligned}$$

The inner conditional expectation $E(X_i|W_i, Y_i, X_i^*, Z_i)$ is free of $W_i$ and given by

$$\begin{aligned} E(X_i|W_i, Y_i, X_i^*, Z_i) &= E(X_i|Y_i, X_i^*, Z_i) \\ &= \alpha^{\mathrm{T}} Z_i + \frac{\sigma_x^2}{\sigma_{\mathrm{U}}^2(1 + \beta_x^2 \sigma_x^2) + m_i \sigma_x^2} \\ &\quad \times \left[ \beta_x \sigma_{\mathrm{U}}^2 \{w_i - (\beta_z + \beta_x \alpha)^{\mathrm{T}} Z_i\} + \sum_{j=1}^{m_i} (X_{ij}^* - \alpha^{\mathrm{T}} Z_i) \right]. \end{aligned}$$

The outer expectation is evaluated with respect to the conditional distribution of $W_i$ given $Y_i, Z_i$ and $X_i^*$, which is related to the truncated normal distribution with the mean and variance, given by

$$E(W_i|Y_i, Z_i, X_i^*) = \mu_i + v_i \phi(\omega_i) \left\{ \frac{Y_i}{\Phi(\omega_i)} - \frac{1 - Y_i}{\Phi(-\omega_i)} \right\}$$

and

$$\begin{aligned} \mathrm{var}(W_i|Y_i, Z_i, X_i^*) &= Y_i v_i^2 \left[ 1 - \frac{\omega_i \phi(\omega_i)}{\Phi(\omega_i)} - \left\{ \frac{\omega_i \phi(\omega_i)}{\Phi(\omega_i)} \right\}^2 \right] \\ &\quad + (1 - Y_i) v_i^2 \left[ 1 + \frac{\omega_i \phi(\omega_i)}{\Phi(-\omega_i)} - \left\{ \frac{\omega_i \phi(\omega_i)}{\Phi(-\omega_i)} \right\}^2 \right], \end{aligned}$$

respectively, where $\omega_i = \mu_i / v_i$, $\mu_i = (\beta_z + \beta_x \alpha)^{\mathrm{T}} Z_i + (\sigma_{\mathrm{U}}^2 + m_i \sigma_x^2)^{-1} \beta_x \sigma_x^2 \sum_{i=1}^{n} (X_{ij}^* - \alpha^T Z_i)$, $v_i^2 = 1 + \beta_x^2 \sigma_x^2 \sigma_{\mathrm{U}}^2 / (\sigma_{\mathrm{U}}^2 + m_i \sigma_x^2)$, and $\phi(\cdot)$ is the standard normal density function. More details can be found in Schafer (1993, Sec.3).

The implementation of the EM algorithm may not appear simpler than the observed likelihood method since it is still pertinent to both maximization and evaluation of integrals (involved in the E-step). However, this procedure differs from directly maximizing the observed data likelihood; we capitalize on the form of the complete-data likelihood which sometimes may be more convenient to handle than the observed data likelihood. General discussions on the EM algorithm can be found in McLachlan and Krishnan (1997) and the references therein.

## 6.8 Extensions and Discussion

Likelihood-based methods are conceptually simple and efficient in dealing with error-prone problems. In this chapter we discuss several strategies derived from the likelihood formulation to account for the measurement error effects. Those methods yield valid estimators in the sense that provided regularity conditions, they are consistent and possess asymptotic normal distributions, after a suitable transformation, usually by substracting the true parameter value from them and then being scaled by the square root of the sample size. The finite sample performance of those methods, however, can be quite different. For instance, Stefanski and Carroll (1996) compared estimates obtained from the conditional score approach and the maximum likelihood method for the logistic regression model. They found that the latter is more efficient when the measurement error is "large" or the logistic coefficient is "large". Considering settings with misclassified binary covariates, Yi et al. (2018) compared the relative performance of different methods under a unified framework.

We discuss the likelihood formulation for the cases with a validation subsample, regardless of being internal or external, as well as the case with repeated surrogate measurements (Buonaccorsi, 2010, Sec.6.12.3). When there is no information on a validation sample or replicates of surrogate measurements, the likelihood method is still a possible tool for inferences concerning data subject to measurement error. For instance, in the presence of instrumental variables, Fuller (1987, Sec.2.4) discussed the use of the likelihood method to perform estimation of the model parameters.

The main drawbacks of likelihood-based methods are related to the computational intensity and the sensitivity to model misspecification. When a direct likelihood approach is computationally intensive, one may use an approximate but simpler version to replace the likelihood function and proceed with the so-called *pseudo-likelihood* approach. For instance, Carroll et al. (1993) discussed a pseudo-likelihood method for handling case-control data where no $Z$ covariates are involved and error-prone $X$ is binary. The formulation (6.29) becomes

$$f(y, x^*; \theta) = \int f(y|x; \beta) f(x^*|x; \alpha) f(x) dx.$$

Rather than parametrically model the distribution of $X$ by giving a specific form for $f(x)$, Carroll et al. (1993) proposed to replace the marginal distribution of $X$ by its empirical estimate. The response model $f(y|x;\beta)$ was specified as a logistic model and $f(x^*|x;\alpha)$ was determined by a parametric model following the usual modeling schemes for measurement error models. Then the inference about the model parameters was carried out using the resulting pseudo-likelihood. The details can be found in Carroll et al. (1993) and (Yi 2017, Sec. 7.4).

To gain robustness of inference results, semiparametric methods or flexible parametric model forms are often employed. For example, Roeder et al. (1996) discussed a semiparametric approach to get around the difficulty of specifying the distribution of $X$, where a parametric model is used to characterize the measurement error process and a nonparametric mixture model is imposed to describe the marginal distribution of the true covariates $X$. In contrast, Pepe and Fleming (1991) described the measurement error process nonparametrically and used the empirical estimation of the likelihood to deal with the mismeasured covariate problem with validation data. When the likelihood formulation is deemed to be necessary but it is difficult to specify the distribution of $X$, nonparametric or semiparametric estimation is usually invoked to avoid specification of the distribution of $X$. Some details on this were outlined by Buonaccorsi (2010, Sec.10.2.3) who described the strategies concerning NPMLE, pseudo-nonparametric maximum likelihood estimation (NPMLE), and restricted NPMLE.

The discussion in this chapter focuses on the setting where measurement error occurs in covariates. When measurement error is involved with the response variable or is present in both response and covariate variables, one may adapt the preceding formulation and develop likelihood estimation procedures accordingly. This topic is touched on by Buonaccorsi (2010, Sec.6.12).

The likelihood-based methods in this chapter are directed to analyze data with a univariate response. The likelihood formulation can be applied to handle data with other features as well. For instance, when data possess multivariate outcomes such as arising from longitudinal studies or studies with clusters, modeling the response model as well as the measurement error and/or covariate processes is typically more complicated than the case with univeriate data. Generalized linear mixed models or nonlinear mixed effects models are usually used for such circumstances, and likelihood-based inferences can be carried out, where the observed likelihood needs to be modified to incorporate the random effects in the formulation. Discussions on this can be found in Carroll et al. (2006, Ch.11), Wu (2009, Ch.5), and the references therein.

When error-contaminated data contain incomplete observations, such as censored data that commonly arise in survival analysis or missing observations that are ubiquitous in many applications, the likelihood principle can be applied conveniently since it offers a viable tool to link multiple modeling processes each of which can reflect one feature of the data. Discussions on this are available in Carroll et al. (2006, Ch.14), Wu (2009, Ch.4, Ch.6), Yi (2017, Ch.3, Ch.5), and the references therein.

Finally, the discussion in this chapter merely focuses on the frequentist framework. Inference under the Bayesian paradigm has not been touched on here, but can be found in Gustafson (2004), Carroll et al. (2006, Ch.9), Sinha (2021), and Stamey and Seaman Jr. (2021).

## Acknowledgments

This reseach was supported by the Natural Sciences and Engineering Research Council of Canada (NSERC). Yi is Canada Research Chair in Data Science (Tier 1). Her research was undertaken, in part, thanks to funding from the Canada Research Chairs Program.

## Bibliography

Berkson, J. (1950). Are there two regressions? *Journal of the American Statistical Association*, 45, 164-180.

Buonaccorsi, J. P. (2010). *Measurement Error: Models, Methods, and Applications.* Chapman & Hall/CRC, Boca Baton, FL.

Burr., D. (1988). On errors-in-variables in binary regression-Berkson case. *Journal of the American Statistical Association*, 83, 739-743.

Carroll, R. J., Fan, Gijbels, J. I., and Wand, M. P. (1997). Generalized partially linear single-index models. *Journal of the American Statistical Association*, 92, 477-489.

Carroll, R. J., Gail, M. H., and Lubin, J. H. (1993). Case-control studies with errors in covariates. *Journal of the American Statistical Association*, 88, 185-199.

Carroll, R. J., Ruppert, D., Stefanski, L. A., and Crainiceanu, C. M. (2006). *Measurement Error in Nonlinear Models.* 2nd ed., Chapman & Hall/CRC.

Carroll, R. J., Spiegelman, C. H., Lan, K. K. G., Bailey, K. T., and Abbott, R. D. (1984). On errors-in-variables for binary regression models. *Biometrika*, 71, 19-25.

Chen, Z., Yi, G. Y., and Wu, C. (2011). Marginal methods for correlated binary data with misclassified responses. *Biometrika*, 98, 647-662.

Fuller, W. A. (1987). *Measurement Error Models.* Wiley, New York.

Gleser, L. J. (1981). Estimation in a multivariate 'errors in variables' regression model: Large sample results. *The Annals of Statistics*, 9, 24-44.

Gustafson, P. (2004). *Measurement Error and Misclassification in Statistics and Epidemiology.* Chapman & Hall/CRC, Boca Raton, Florida.

Gustafson, P. (2005). On model expansion, model contraction, identifiability and prior information two illustrative scenarios involving mismeasured variables. *Statistical Science*, 20, 111-140.

Hung, H. and Wang, C.-C. (2013). Matrix variate logistic regression model with application to eeg data. *Biostatistics*, 14, 189-202.

Lindsay, B. (1982). Conditional score functions: Some optimality results. *Biometrika*, 69, 503-512.

McLachlan, G. J. and Krishnan, T. (1997). *The EM Algorithm and Extensions.*

McShane, L. M., Midthune, D. N., Dorgan, J. F., Freedman, L. S., and Carroll, R. J. (2001). Covariate measurement error adjustment for matched case-control studies. *Biometrics*, 57, 62-73.

Neuhaus, J. M. (1999). Bias and efficiency loss due to misclassified responses in binary regression. *Biometrika*, 86, 843-855.

Neuhaus, J. M. (2002). Analysis of clustered and longitudinal binary data subject to response misclassification. *Biometrics*, 58, 675-683.

Neyman, J. and Scott, E. L. (1948). Consistent estimates based on partially consistent observations. *Econometrica*, 16, 1-32.

Pan, W., Zeng, D. and Lin, X. (2009). Estimation in semiparametric transition measurement error models for longitudinal data. *Biometrics*, 65, 728-736.

Pepe, M. S. and Fleming, T. R. (1991). A nonparametric method for dealing with mismeasured covariate data. *Journal of the American Statistical Association*, 86, 108-113.

Prentice, R. L. (1989). Surrogate endpoints in clinical trials: Definition and operational criteria. *Statistics in Medicine*, 8, 431-440.

Roeder, K., Carroll, R. J., and Lindsay, B. G. (1996). A semiparametric mixture approach to case-control studies with errors in covariables. *Journal of the American Statistical Association*, 91, 722-732.

Schafer, D. W. (1993). Likelihood analysis for probit regression with measurement errors. *Biometrika*, 80, 899-904.

Schafer, K. G. and Purdy, D. W. (1996). Likelihood analysis for errors-in-variables regression with replicate measurements. *Biometrika*, 83, 813-824.

Sinha, S. (2021). Bayesian approaches for handling covariate measurement error. In *Handbook of Measurement Error Models*, Yi, G. Y., Delaigle, A., and Gustafson, P. (Eds.), Chapman & Hall/CRC, Boca Raton, Florida, Chapter 24.

Song, X., Davidian, M., and Tsiatis, A. A. (2002). An estimator for the proportional hazards model with multiple longitudinal covariates measured with error. *Biostatistics*, 3, 511-528.

Spiegelman, D., Carroll, R. J., and Kipnis, V. (2001). Efficient regression calibration for logistic regression in main study/internal validation study designs. *Statistics in Medicine*, 29, 139-160.

Stamey, J. D. and W. Seaman Jr., J. W. (2021). Bayesian adjustment for misclassification. In *Handbook of Measurement Error Models*, Yi, G. Y., Delaigle, A., and Gustafson, P. (Eds.), Chapman & Hall/CRC, Boca Raton, Florida, Chapter 23.

Stefanski, L. A. and Carroll, R. J. (1987). Conditional scores and optimal scores for generalized linear measurement-error models. *Biometrika*, 74, 703-716.

Thurston, S. W., Spiegelman, D., and Ruppert, D. (2003). Equivalence of regression calibration methods in main study/external validation study designs. *Journal of Statistical Planning and Inference*, 113, 527-539.

Tsiatis, A. A. and Davidian, M. (2001). A semiparametric estimator for the proportional hazards model with longitudinal covariates measured with error. *Biometrika*, 88, 447-458.

Wald, A. (1940). The fitting of straight lines if both variables are subject to error. *The Annals of Mathematical Statistics*, 11, 284-300.

Wang, N., Lin, X., Gutierrez, R. G., and Carroll, R. J. (1998). Bias analysis and SIMEX approach in generalized linear mixed measurement error models. *Journal of the American Statistical Association*, 93, 249-261.

Wu, L. (2009). *Mixed Effects Models for Complex Data.* Chapman and Hall/CRC, Boca Raton, Florida.

Yi, G. Y. (2017). *Statistical Analysis with Measurement Error or Misclassification.* Springer Science+Business Media, LLC, New York.

Yi, G. Y., Yan, Y., Liao, X., and Spiegelman, D. (2018). Parametric regression analysis with covariate misclassification in main study/validation study designs. *The International Journal of Biostatistics*, 15, 1-24.

Zucker, D. M. (2005). A pseudo-partial likelihood method for semiparametric survival regression with covariate errors. *Journal of the American Statistical Association*, 100, 1264-1277.

Zucker, D. M. (2021). Conditional and corrected score methods. *In Handbook of Measurement Error Models*, Yi, G. Y., Delaigle, A., and Gustafson, P. (Eds.), Chapman & Hall/CRC, Boca Raton, Florida, Chapter 8.

# 7

# *Regression Calibration for Covariate Measurement Error*

**Pamela A. Shaw**

## CONTENTS



## 7.1 Introduction

Regression calibration is one of the first statistical methods introduced to address covariate measurement error. Despite its simplicity and approximate nature in non-linear models, regression calibration persists today as perhaps the single most popular method to address covariate measurement error in regression models. Its popularity stems not only from the simplicity and intuitiveness of this approach, but also because it has been observed to perform very well in many settings — often remaining competitive in terms of mean squared error with more complex, modern methods. In this chapter, we present the method of regression calibration. We begin with the mathematical justification of this method, which will also illustrate why this method is an exact fix in linear models and why this method so easily can be extended for non-linear problems, as an approximate fix to covariate measurement error. We illustrate the method with a few examples, which will highlight both its typical use and some of the challenges that can arise. We will discuss the performance of regression calibration in comparison to other methods. Finally, we will conclude the chapter with a few extensions to regression calibration,

DOI: 10.1201/9781315101279-7

which improve its performance in challenging settings, such as those with a high degree of non-linearity. We also discuss some applications of regression calibration to address error in the outcome.

## 7.2 The Regression Calibration Method

The ideal setting for regression calibration is the linear regression model, with normally distributed independent random error. When the outcome $Y$ and covariates $\{X, Z\}$ in the model are also normally distributed, one can derive the method as a simple application of the conditional mean of a multivariate normally distributed random variable. Normality will also allow for the choice of a moment-based or regression model based estimator. We will see in the sections that follow, that the method will perform well when on some scale approximate linearity holds and one can fit a regression model for the unobserved $X$ given an error prone version $X^*$ and other precisely observed covariates $Z$.

Formally, consider the outcome model

$$Y = \beta_0 + \beta_x^T X + \beta_z^T Z + \epsilon, \tag{7.1}$$

where $\{\beta_0, \beta_x, \beta_z\}$ are the unknown regression coefficients of interest and $\epsilon$ is random mean zero independent error term. Assume that instead of $X$, one observes the error prone version $X^*$ which is subject to linear measurement error. Thus, one has

$$X^* = \zeta_0 + \zeta_x^T X + \zeta_z^T Z + e, \tag{7.2}$$

where $\{\zeta_0, \zeta_x, \zeta_z\}$ are the error model parameters, $e$ is a Gaussian random variable with mean zero that is independent $\{Y, X, Z\}$. This is a common model assumed for measurement error seen in nutritional epidemiology (Prentice et al., 2002).

A common instrument in this setting, is the 24-hour recall, which through a subject interview or digital app, a study participant is asked about her diet in the last 24 hours. This type of self-report is subject to measurement error, as the diet is a complex exposure that varies from day-to-day and can be influenced by subject characteristics such as gender, age, or body mass index (BMI). Suppose for a given study, $X$ represents true energy intake, $Z = BMI - 30$ (BMI centered at 30 kg/m$^2$) and $X^* = -200 + 0.80X - 15Z + e$. The coefficient $\zeta_0$ represents location bias for someone with BMI=30, $\zeta_x$ represents scale bias, and $\zeta_z$ represents the change in location bias for every unit increase in BMI. In this case, a study participant with BMI=30 underestimates the amount of food she consumed by a fixed 200 calories in addition to underestimating the calories in her diet by 20%, and the fixed level of underreporting increases by an absolute 15 calories for every unit increase in BMI. Note in the special case that $\zeta_x = 1$ and $\zeta_z = 0$, one has the classical measurement error model $X^* = X + e$.

Even though it frequently makes sense to consider $X^*$ as the dependent variable and $X$ as the independent variable, due to mechanism driving the measurement error, mathematically it is more convenient for regression calibration to consider the model for $\mathrm{E}[X|X^*, Z]$. The linear relationship shown in equation (7.2) implies there exists a coefficient vector $\alpha = (\alpha_0, \alpha_x^T, \alpha_z^T)^T$ such that the following model also holds

$$X = \alpha_0 + \alpha_x^T X^* + \alpha_z^T Z + U, \tag{7.3}$$

where $U$ is an independent, mean zero error term. We will refer to this model for $\mathrm{E}[X|X^*, Z]$ as the calibration model. In the next section, we will discuss different settings for which the parameters are identifiable. Here, we present the principal motivation behind regression calibration method.

One first considers the regression of Y on the observed data $\{X^*, Z\}$, namely $\mathrm{E}[Y|X^*, Z]$, and then can apply the method of iterated expectation, together with the assumption of non-differential error, as follows

$$\begin{aligned} E[Y|X^*, Z] &= E[E[Y|X^*, Z, X]|X^*, Z] \\ &= E[E[Y|X, Z]|X^*, Z] \\ &= E[\beta_0 + \beta_x^T X + \beta_z^T Z|X^*, Z] \\ &= \beta_0 + \beta_x^T E[X|X^*, Z] + \beta_z^T Z. \end{aligned}$$

The last line justifies the regression calibration approach. The conditional expectation of $Y$ dependent on $\{X, Z\}$ is the same as its conditional expectation dependent on $\{\mathrm{E}[X|X^*, Z]$,Z$\}$. Thus, one simply needs to fit the linear model $Y$ that is a function of $\mathrm{E}[X|X^*, Z]$ and $Z$ and the parameter estimates will recover the same model coefficients as in the target outcome model (7.1). If the model for $\mathrm{E}[X|X^*, Z]$ is correct, so that as an estimator for $X$ has mean zero residual error that is independent of $\{X, Z\}$, then regression calibration will estimate the outcome model coefficient estimates consistently. In other words, $\hat{X} = \mathrm{E}[X|X^*, Z]$, as an estimate of $X$, has independent and non-differential, Berkson measurement error. The above derivation also highlights the importance of including all other covariates $Z$ from the outcome model in the calibration model, in order to recover the same model coefficients as in $\mathrm{E}[Y|X, Z]$, the original outcome model. This will be true even when the error in $X^*$ is classical measurement error. While this derivation assumed the model for $\mathrm{E}[Y|X, Z]$ is linear, regression calibration has been observed to perform well in other settings where linear a Taylor series argument can be used to justify a reasonable linear approximation (Carroll et al., 2006).

Regression calibration can be thought of as a 3-step method. First, one must fit a model $\mathrm{E}[X|X^*, Z]$. This model is then used to obtain predicted values for each individual, namely $\hat{X}$, and the outcome model is fit with covariates $\{\hat{X}, Z\}$. Finally the standard errors or confidence intervals for the model parameters in the outcome model must be obtained with a method that adjusts for uncertainty in both the calibration model and the outcome model. Variance estimation will be discussed in Section 7.4.

The regression calibration approach for the linear model was briefly discussed by Fuller (1987, pp. 261-262); however, the origin of the this method is often traced back to Prentice (1982) who introduced the approach an approximate method to address covariate measurement error in the Cox model for the rare event setting. Regression calibration has been thoroughly studied in the case of logistic regression (Rosner et al., 1989, 1990), failure time models (Prentice, 1982; Wang et al., 1997; Shaw and Prentice, 2012), generalized linear models (Armstrong, 1985), and more generally (Carroll and Stefanski, 1990). In several settings with non-linear outcome models, such as logistic or Cox regression, regression calibration has been observed to perform well for moderate levels $\beta_x$, rare events and moderate measurement error variance — all of which contribute to a more successful linear approximation. Regression calibration works less well in highly non-linear problems; Carroll et al. (2006), presented a good overview of methods that aim to improve the performance of regression calibration by addressing non-linearity. For the failure time outcome setting, Xie and Prentice (2001) proposed the extension *risk set regression* calibration, which refits the calibration equation within each riskset, and found this reduced bias for large hazard ratio parameters in the setting of classical measurement error. Shaw and Prentice (2012) further studied this method for a more general linear measurement error model.

## 7.3 Fitting the Calibration Model

Regression calibration can be applied whenever there is data to estimate the parameters in the regression model $\text{E}[X|X^*, Z]$. There are two basic settings for which this will be the case: on a subset of individuals, 1) the true $X$ will be simultaneously measured with $\{X^*, Z\}$ or 2) a second measure $X^{**}$ is obtained alongside $\{X^*, Z\}$ that contains only classical measurement error, i.e., $X^{**} = X + V$, where $V$ is independent of the random error term $U$ in equation (7.3), as well as {X, Z, Y}. The first case is often called a *validation subset* and the second case is often called a *calibration subset*. In the special case that $X^*$ has only classical measurement error, then replicates of $X^*$ on a subset will be sufficient. In this case, the calibration subset is often called the *replicate* or *reliability subset*.

On a validation subset, one observes $\{X, X^*, Z\}$ and thus can simply fit model (7.3) directly. With a calibration subset, one can obtain an estimate of the calibration model parameters by regressing $X^{**}$ on $\{X^*, Z\}$, since

$$E[X^{**}|X^*, Z] = E[X|X^*, Z] + E[V|X^*, Z] = E[X|X^*, Z]. \tag{7.4}$$

While convenient, the usual least-squares regression estimator for $\mathrm{E}[X^{**}|X^*, Z]$ using the calibration subset or $\mathrm{E}[X|X^*, Z]$ for the validation subset, may not be the most efficient estimator as it would only use the individuals on whom all variables in these regressions were observed. In the case where different individuals have differing amounts of information, an efficient estimator will take advantage of all measures available. A *best linear unbiased predictor* (BLUP) can be obtained by considering a method of moments estimator for the regression coefficients and replacing each moment with the estimator that uses all data available to estimate that moment. For example, Carroll et al. [2006], provided the BLUP for the case where $X^*$ has only classical measurement error and $k_i$ replicates are observed for individual $i = 1, \cdots, n$. In this case, one has

$$X^*_{ij} \;=\; X_i + V_{ij}, \text{ for } i = 1, \ldots n \text{ and } j = 1, \ldots, k_i,$$

and can estimate $E[X|X^*, Z]$ using the formula for the conditional mean of a multivariate normal distribution (best linear approximation), as follows:

$$\hat{X} = E[X|\bar{X}^*, Z] \approx \hat{\mu}_x + \begin{pmatrix}\hat{\Sigma}_{xx} & \hat{\Sigma}_{xz}\end{pmatrix} \begin{pmatrix}\hat{\Sigma}_{xx} + \hat{\Sigma}_{uu}/k & \hat{\Sigma}^t_{xz} \\ \hat{\Sigma}_{xz} & \hat{\Sigma}_{zz}\end{pmatrix}^{-1} \begin{pmatrix}\bar{X}^* - \hat{\mu}_{x^*} \\ Z - \hat{\mu}_z\end{pmatrix},$$

where $\hat{\mu}_z = \bar{Z}$ and $\hat{\Sigma}_{zz} = \widehat{\mathrm{var}}(Z)$ are the usual estimates; $\hat{\mu}_x = \hat{\mu}_{x^*} = \sum_{i=1}^n k_i \bar{X}^*_{i\cdot} / \sum_{i=1}^n k_i$, and

$$\begin{aligned}
\hat{\Sigma}_{uu} &= \frac{\sum_{i=1}^n \sum_{j=1}^n (X^*_{ij} - \bar{X}^*_{i\cdot})(X^*_{ij} - \bar{X}^*_{i\cdot})^t}{\sum_{i=1}^n (k_i - 1)}; \\
\hat{\Sigma}_{xz} &= \left\{ \sum_i k_i (\bar{X}^*_{i\cdot} - \hat{\mu}_{x^*})(Z_i - \hat{\mu}_z)^t \right\} / \nu; \\
\hat{\Sigma}_{xx} &= \left[ \left\{ \sum_{i=1}^n k_i (\bar{X}^*_{i\cdot} - \hat{\mu}_{x^*})(\bar{X}^*_{i\cdot} - \hat{\mu}_{x^*})^t \right\} - (n-1)\hat{\Sigma}_{uu} \right] / \nu,
\end{aligned}$$

with $\nu = \sum_{i=1}^n k_i - \sum_{i=1}^n k_i^2 / \sum_{i=1}^n k_i$.

Fitting the moments based on the available individuals assumes that membership into the validation/calibration and the total number of replicates available on an individual is randomly assigned. This relates to the issue of *transportability*, the assumption that the measurement error model (7.2) holds and the parameter values are the same in the subsample. Here, we must assume something stronger, that all moments must be consistently estimated on the subset. In an internal calibration subsample, this can be controlled by the sampling design, and if a design-based sample is taken the moments can be adjusted by inverse probability weighting. In an external calibration sample, this highlights why the measurement error correction itself is almost never transportable. For this to be the case, one would need not only the measurement error parameters, such as $\Sigma_{uu}$, to be the same across study populations; but also that the first and second moments of the covariates also to be the same.

## 7.4 Variance Estimation

The easiest and consequently the most common way to obtain confidence intervals or standard errors for parameter estimates following regression calibration, i.e., for a regression model with the true $X$ replaced with an estimate $\hat{X}$, is the bootstrap (Efron and Tibshirani, 1994). For each bootstrap sample of the data, one would refit the calibration model and then refit the outcome model with the new estimates of $E[X|X^*, Z]$. In many instances, the validation sample is fit on a subset of individuals on which extra data was collected to identify the parameters of the calibration model. In this instance, the bootstrap should be performed stratified on the validation/calibration subset indicator.

An alternative to the bootstrap is the sandwich estimator, which can be obtained using a stacked estimation approach (Stefanski and Boos, 2002). For this approach, one considers the estimating equation for each parameter in both the calibration and outcome models. These equations are solved for the associated parameters simultaneously and then the variance is obtained using the usual sandwich estimator. Carroll et al. (2006, Appendix B) described this approach in detail.

In many settings, the validation/calibration subset will be limited in size due to expense. Particularly for a binary or survival outcome, fitting the outcome model on the calibration subset may not be feasible. For the logistic settings where there is a sufficient sample to fit the target outcome model on the calibration subset, Spiegelman et al. (2001) provided an efficient estimator which uses an inverse-variance weighting of the two estimates: one from the calibration subset and one from the main cohort. Generalized raking is another robust approach that can be used in combination with regression calibration to efficiently combine information from the calibration and main study measurements when outcomes are available on the calibration sample (Lumley et al., 2011).

## 7.5 Example

Regression calibration is a popular approach in nutritional epidemiology. One recent review found this method was used by nearly all articles surveyed [Shaw et al., 2018] The typical setting is a prospective cohort study in which diet is assessed at baseline using a self-reported instrument, such as the food frequency questionnaire (FFQ) or 24-hour dietary recall. The cohort is followed up longitudinally for an outcome of interest, such as time to a cancer diagnosis. For some nutrients, there are biomarkers that capture intake with only classical measurement error. Examples of these biomarkers, known as recovery biomarkers, include doubly-labeled water for total energy (Schoeller, 1988) and urinary nitrogen for protein (Bingham and Cummings, 1985). The Women's Health Initiative is one such cohort in which the main instrument for diet was the food frequency questionnaire, and these biomarkers, were measured in a subset of individuals. Prentice et al. (2009) report on the hazard ratio associated with increased intake energy, protein and percent energy for protein associated for several cancer outcomes. The calibration model was fit by regressing the biomarker value on the self-report and other characteristics on the calibration subset (Neuhouser et al., 2008). Standard errors for the outcome model following regression calibration were obtained using the bootstrap. These authors compared the naive approach, one that ignores the measurement error in the FFQ assessment, with those using regression calibration. In all cases the calibrated coefficients were notably further away from the null; however, the uncertainty in the parameter estimates was dramatically increased.

This example highlights a few of the challenges of implementing regression calibration. The first is the confidence intervals are noticeably wider than those from the naive regression. This additional uncertainty is a true reflection of the loss of information from using the observed $X^*$ in place of $X$, due to the measurement error. Lagakos (1988) showed that the asymptotic relative efficiency compared to the model without error in many settings is inversely proportional to $\rho^2$, where $\rho = \text{cor}(X^*, X)$. Thus, if $N$ was the sample size needed to achieve a certain power for a test of the null hypothesis for the coefficient of a precisely observed $X$, then $N/\rho^2$ is the necessary sample size for a similar regression on $X^*$. A second practical challenge, noted by Prentice et al. (2009) is that BMI was both a potential confounder and potential mediator along the causal pathway between excess energy intake and increased cancer risk; BMI was also an important predictor in the measurement error model. From Section 7.2, it was shown that BMI should be included in the calibration and outcome model. If BMI mediates the association between energy and cancer risk, then including BMI in the outcome model could remove or substantially weaken this association. Prentice et al. (2009) presented results with and without BMI in the outcome model and results varied substantially. Huang and Prentice (2011) further discussed potential ways to address this issue.

## 7.6 Conclusion

Regression calibration is a flexible method to address covariate measurement error that has been applied in many regression model settings. While this method is generally only an approximate solution for nonlinear regression models, its performance has compared favorably to other methods — particularly in settings where approximate linearity holds (Han et al., 2019) and where calibration subsets are small (Shepherel et al., 2012). Messer and Natarajan (2008) also found regression calibration performed in comparison to a likelihood approach and multiple imputation well when sample sizes were small and the measurement error was not too large. Freedman et al. (2008) found that in settings where outcome information is also available on the calibration subset, the efficient version of regression calibration (Spiegelman et al., 2001) was seen to be competitive or outperform multiple imputation and moment reconstruction for binary outcomes. Limited work has applied regression calibration to other settings with outcome measurement error in linear (Shaw et al., 2018) or failure time outcomes (Oh et al., 2018). Though efforts are needed to understand the level of bias when regression calibration is applied in the non-linear setting; given its simplicity, regression calibration is a good first approach and may be a practical solution in settings where more complex measurement error adjustments are not feasible.

## Bibliography

Armstrong, B. (1985). Measurement error in the generalised linear model. *Communications in Statistics-Simulation and Computation*, 14(3), 529-544.

Bingham, S. A. and Cummings, J. H. (1985). Urine nitrogen as an independent validatory measure of dietary intake: a study of nitrogen balance in individuals consuming their normal diet. *The American Journal of Clinical Nutrition*, 42(6), 1276-1289.

Carroll, R. J., Ruppert, D., Stefanski, L. A. and Crainiceanu, C. M. (2006). *Measurement Error in Nonlinear Models: A Modern Perspective.* CRC Press.

Carroll, R. J. and Stefanski, L. A. (1990). Approximate quasi-likelihood estimation in models with surrogate predictors. *Journal of the American Statistical Association*, 85(411), 652-663.

Efron, B. and Tibshirani, R. J. (1994). *An Introduction to the Bootstrap.* CRC Press.

Freedman, L. S., Midthune, D., Carroll, R. J., and Kipnis, V. (2008). A comparison of regression calibration, moment reconstruction and imputation for adjusting for covariate measurement error in regression. *Statistics in medicine*, 27(25), 5195-5216.

Fuller, W. A. (1987). *Measurement Error Models.* John Wiley & Sons.

Han, K., Shaw, P. A., and Lumley, T. (2019). Combining multiple imputation with raking of weights in the setting of nearly-true models. *arXiv preprint arXiv:1910.01162*.

Lagakos, S. (1988). Effects of mismodelling and mismeasuring explanatory variables on tests of their association with a response variable. *Statistics in Medicine*, 7(1-2), 257-274.

Lumley, T., Shaw, P., and Dai, J. (2011). Connections between survey calibration estimators and semiparametric models for incomplete data. *International Statistical Review*, 79(2), 200-220.

Messer, K. and Natarajan, L. (2008). Maximum likelihood, multiple imputation and regression calibration for measurement error adjustment. *Statistics in Medicine*, 27(30), 6332-6350.

Neuhouser, M. L., Tinker, L., Shaw, P. A., Schoeller, D., Bingham, S. A., Van Horn, L., Beresford, S. A. A., Caan, B., Thompson, C., Satterfield, S., Kuller, L., Heiss, G., Smit, E., Sarto, G., Ockene, J., Stefanick, M. L., Assaf, A., Runswick, S., and Prentice, R. L. (2008). Use of recovery biomarkers to calibrate nutrient consumption self-reports in the Women's Health Initiative. *American Journal of Epidemiology*, 167(10), 1247-1259.

Oh, E. J., Shepherd, B. E., Lumley, T., and Shaw, P. A. (2018). Considerations for analysis of time-to-event outcomes measured with error: Bias and correction with SIMEX. *Statistics in Medicine*, 37(8), 1276-89.

Prentice, R. L. (1982). Covariate measurement errors and parameter estimation in a failure time regression model. *Biometrika*, 69, 331-342.

Prentice, R. L. and Huang, Y. (2011). Measurement error modeling and nutritional epidemiology association analyses. *Canadian Journal of Statistics*, 39(3), 498-509.

Prentice, R. L., Shaw, P. A., Bingham, S. A., Beresford, S. A., Caan, B., Neuhouser, M. L., Patterson, R. E., Stefanick, M. L., Satterfield, S., Thomson, C. A., et al. (2009). Biomarker-calibrated energy and protein consumption and increased cancer risk among postmenopausal women. *American Journal of Epidemiology*, 169(8), 977-989.

Prentice, R. L., Sugar, E., Wang, C., Neuhouser, M., and Patterson, R. (2002). Research strategies and the use of nutrient biomarkers in studies of diet and chronic disease. *Public Health Nutrition*, 5(6A), 977-984.

Rosner, B., Spiegelman, D., and Willett, W. (1990). Correction of logistic regression relative risk estimates and confidence intervals for measurement error: the case of multiple covariates measured with error. *American Journal of Epidemiology*, 132(4), 734-745.

Rosner, B., Willett, W., and Spiegelman, D., (1989). Correction of logistic regression relative risk estimates and confidence intervals for systematic within-person measurement error. *Statistics in Medicine*, 8(9), 1051-1069.

Schoeller, D. A. (1988). Measurement of energy expenditure in free-living humans by using doubly labeled water. *Journal of Nutrition*, 118, 1278-1289.

Shaw, P., He, J. and Shepherd, B. (2018). Regression calibration to correct correlated errors in outcome and exposure. *arXiv preprint arXiv:1811.10147.*

Shaw, P. A. and Prentice, R. L. (2012). Hazard ratio estimation for biomarker-calibrated dietary exposures. *Biometrics*, 68(2), 397-407.

Shepherd, B. E., Shaw, P. A., and Dodd, L. E. (2012). Using audit information to adjust parameter estimates for data errors in clinical trials. *Clinical Trials*, 9(6), 721-729.

Spiegelman, D., Carroll, R. J., and Kipnis, V. (2001). Efficient regression calibration for logistic regression in main study/internal validation study designs with an imperfect reference instrument. *Statistics in Medicine*, 20(1), 139-160.

Stefanski, L. A. and Boos, D. D. (2002). The calculus of M-estimation. *The American Statistician*, 56(1), 29-38.

Wang, C., Hsu, L., Feng, Z., and Prentice, R. L. (1997). Regression calibration in failure time regression. *Biometrics*, 131-145.

Xie, S. X., Wang, C. Y., and Prentice, R. L. (2001). A risk set calibration method for failure time regression by using a covariate reliability sample. *Journal of the Royal Statistical Society, Series B*, 63(4), 855-870.

# 8

## Conditional and Corrected Score Methods

**David M. Zucker**

## CONTENTS



## 8.1 Introduction

This chapter presents measurement error correction approaches based on modifications to the likelihood score function. The methods presented include the conditional score approach and the corrected score approach. Both approaches are functional modeling approaches.

We begin by reviewing the concept of the likelihood score function. At this stage, we work in the context of a generalized linear model (GLM). The theory of GLM's is presented in McCullagh and Nelder (1989), where proofs of basic facts about GLM's may be found. Suppose we have observations on $n$ independent individuals, with the data on individual $i$ consisting of a response variable $Y_i$ and a $p$-vector of covariates $W_i$ (where, in models with an intercept term, $W_i$ includes an element that is equal to 1 for every $i$). We assume that the conditional probability mass or density function of $Y_i$ given $W_i$ takes the form

$$f_{Y_i|W_i}(y|w) = \exp\{\phi^{-1}[y\gamma(\beta^T w) - b(\gamma(\beta^T w))] + c(y, \phi)\} \tag{8.1}$$

DOI: 10.1201/9781315101279-8

where $\gamma, b$, and $c$ are known functions, $\beta$ is a vector of regression coefficients that we wish to estimate, and $\phi$ is a parameter that may be known or unknown.

Under the model (8.1), we have $E[Y_i|W_i = w] = b'(\gamma(\beta^T w))$ and $\text{Var}(Y|X_i = w) = \phi b''(\gamma(\beta^T w))$. Letting $q$ denote the inverse function of $b'$, the function $g(\mu) = \gamma^{-1}(q(\mu))$, which describes the relationship between $E[Y_i|W_i = w]$ and the linear predictor $\beta^T x$ and $E[Y_i|W_i = w]$, is called the *link function*. The *canonical link* is obtained when $\gamma$ is the identity function.

Some key special cases are listed below:

- *Classical Linear Regression*: $\gamma(\eta) = \eta, b(\xi) = \xi^2/2, q(\mu) = \mu$, $c(y, \phi) = -y^2/(2\phi) - \log(2\pi\phi)/2, E[Y_i|W_i = w] = \beta^T w, \text{Var}(Y|W_i = w) = \phi$;

- *Classical Nonlinear Regression*: $\gamma(\eta) = \psi(\eta), b(\xi) = \xi^2/2, q(\mu) = \mu, a(\phi) = \phi, c(y, \phi) = -y^2/(2\phi) - \log(2\pi\phi)/2, E[Y_i|W_i = w] = \psi(\beta^T w), \text{Var}(Y|W_i = w) = \phi$;

- *Poisson Regression With Log Link*: $\gamma(\eta) = \eta, b(\xi) = e^{\xi}, q(\mu) = \log\mu, a(\phi) = \phi, \phi \equiv 1, c(y, \phi) = \log y!, E[Y_i|W_i = w] = e^{\beta^T w}, \text{Var}(Y|W_i = w) = e^{\beta^T w}$;

- *Logistic Regression*: $\gamma(\eta) = \eta, b(\xi) = \log(1 + e^{\xi}), q(\mu) = \log(\mu/(1 - \mu)), a(\phi) = \phi, \phi \equiv 1, c(y, \phi) = 0, E[Y_i|W_i = w] = e^{\beta^T w}/(1 + e^{\beta^T w}), \text{Var}(Y|W_i = w) = e^{\beta^T w}/(1 + e^{\beta^T w})^2$;

- *Probit Regression*: $\gamma(\eta) = \log(\Phi(\eta)/(1 - \Phi(\eta)), b(\xi) = \log(1 + e^{\xi}), q(\mu) = \log(\mu/(1 - \mu)), a(\phi) = \phi, \phi \equiv 1, c(y, \phi) = 0, E[Y_i|W_i = w] = \Phi(\beta^T w), \text{Var}(Y|W_i = w) = \Phi(\beta^T w)(1 - \Phi(\beta^T w))$.

Writing $\theta = (\beta, \phi)$, the log-likelihood of the data is

$$\mathcal{L}(\theta) = \sum_{i=1}^{n} \ell(Y_i, W_i; \theta), \tag{8.2}$$

where

$$\begin{aligned}\ell(Y_i, W_i; \theta) &\equiv \log f_{Y_i|W_i}(Y_i|W_i; \theta)\\ &= \phi^{-1} \sum_{i=1}^{n} [Y_i \gamma(\beta^T W_i) - b(\gamma(\beta^T W_i)) + c(Y_i, \phi)].\end{aligned}$$

The *score function* is defined as $U(\theta) = \nabla_\theta \mathcal{L}(\theta)$, where $\nabla$ denotes the gradient (vector of first derivatives). We can write

$$U(\theta) = \sum_{i=1}^{n} u_i(W_i; \theta), \tag{8.3}$$

where $u_i(w; \theta) = u(Y_i, W_i; \theta)$ with $u(y, w; \theta) = \nabla_\theta \log f(y|w; \theta)$. The maximum likelihood estimate of $\theta$ is obtained by solving the equation $U(\theta) = 0$.

Letting $\theta^\circ$ denote the true value of $\theta$, we have $E[U(\theta^\circ)] = 0$. The portion of the score function corresponding to the derivatives with respect to the components of $\beta$ is given by

$$U^{(\beta)}(\theta) = \sum_{i=1}^{n} u^{(\beta)}(Y_i, W_i; \theta)$$

with

$$u^{(\beta)}(y, w; \theta) = \phi^{-1}\gamma'(\beta^T w)w[y - b'(\gamma(\beta^T w))]. \tag{8.4}$$

As an alternative to maximum likelihood, $\theta$ can be estimated using a maximum quasi-likelihood approach, based on solving the equations $U^{(\beta)}(\theta) = 0$ and $H(\theta) = \sum_{i=1}^{n} h(Y_i, W_i; \theta) = 0$ with

$$h(y, w; \theta) = \left(\frac{n-p}{n}\right)\phi - \frac{(y - b'(\beta^T w))^2}{b''(\beta^T w)}. \tag{8.5}$$

Note that $E[H(\theta^\circ)] = 0$. In some cases, the maximum quasi-likelihood estimate coincides with the maximum likelihood estimate.

In the measurement error setting, the covariate vector $W_i$ consists of two parts, an error-prone part $X_i$ and an error-free part $Z_i$ (where, for models with an intercept term, the vector $Z_i$ contains an element which is equal to 1 for all $i$). Thus, the linear predictor $\beta^T w$ takes the form $\beta_x^T x + \beta_z^T z$. Instead of observing $X$, we observe a surrogate version $X^*$. Unless mentioned otherwise, we impose throughout the surrogacy assumption that $Y$ and $X^*$ are conditionally independent given $X$ and $Z$, i.e., that if we know $X$ and $Z$, then the value of $X^*$ provides no additional information about $Y$.

## 8.2 Conditional Score Approach

The conditional score approach was introduced by Stefanski and Carroll (1987). In this approach, the true covariate vector $X_i$ is regarded as a vector of unknown nuisance parameters. We construct the joint likelihood $L(\theta, X_1, \ldots, X_n)$, we find a sufficient statistic for the $X_i$'s, and we then eliminate $X_i$'s from the problem by conditioning on the sufficient statistic. Conditioning is a well-known method of eliminating nuisance parameters. One example is conditional logistic regression, where conditioning is used to eliminate intercept parameters. The application of conditioning here, however, is non-standard in that the sufficient statistic for $(X_1, \ldots, X_n)$ is derived assuming temporarily that $\theta$ and the measurement error model parameters are known.

The conditional score approach was developed for the case where the link function in the GLM is the canonical link ($\gamma$ is the identity function) and the measurement error model is the classical additive error model $X^* = X + \epsilon$, with $\epsilon \sim N(0, \Sigma_\epsilon)$ independent of $X$. In this case, the joint likelihood $L(\theta, X_1, \ldots, X_n)$ can be written as $L(\theta, X_1, \ldots, X_n) = \exp(\mathcal{A} + \mathcal{B})$, where

$$\mathcal{A} = \phi^{-1} \sum_{i=1}^{n} [Y_i(\beta_0 + \beta_x^T X_i + \beta_z^T Z_i) - b(\beta_0 + \beta_x^T X_i + \beta_z^T Z_i) + c(Y_i, \phi)];$$

$$\mathcal{B} = -(np/2)\log(2\pi) - \frac{n}{2}\log\det(\Sigma_\epsilon) - \frac{1}{2}\sum_{i=1}^{n}(X_i^* - X_i)^T \Sigma_\epsilon^{-1}(X_i^* - X_i).$$

Suppose temporarily that $\theta$ and $\Sigma_\epsilon$ are known. With some algebraic manipulation, we find that $L(\theta; X_1, \ldots, X_n) = L_1 L_2 L_3$, where

$$L_1(\theta; X_1, \ldots, X_n) = \exp\left(\sum_{i=1}^{n} X_i^T \Sigma_\epsilon^{-1}[X_i^* + \phi^{-1} Y_i \Sigma_\epsilon \beta_x]\right);$$

$$L_2(\theta; X_1, \ldots, X_n) = \exp\left(\phi^{-1}\sum_{i=1}^{n}[Y_i(\beta_0 + \beta_z^T Z_i) + c(Y_i, \phi)]\right) \times \exp\left(-\frac{1}{2}\sum_{i=1}^{n} X_i^{*T}\Sigma_\epsilon^{-1} X_i^*\right);$$

$$L_3(\theta; X_1, \ldots, X_n) = \exp\left(-\phi^{-1}\sum_{i=1}^{n} b(\beta_0 + \beta_x^T X_i + \beta_z^T Z_i)\right) \times \exp\left(-(np/2)\log(2\pi) - \frac{n}{2}\log\det(\Sigma_\epsilon) - \frac{1}{2}X_i^T \Sigma_\epsilon^{-1} X_i\right).$$

Note that $L_2$ depends only on the $Y_i$'s, the $X_i^*$'s, and known quantities, while $L_3$ depends only on the $X_i$'s and known quantities. Thus, defining $\Delta(x^*, y; \theta) = x^* + \phi^{-1} y \Sigma_\epsilon \beta_x$, the quantity $\Delta(X_i^*, Y_i; \theta)$ is sufficient for $X_i$.

It can be shown that the conditional distribution of $Y_i$ given $(Z_i, \Delta_i) = (z, \delta)$ takes the GLM form

$$f_{Y_i|Z_i,\Delta_i}(y|z,\delta) = \exp\{\phi^{-1}[(y\eta_* - b_*(\eta_*, \beta_x^T \Sigma_\epsilon \beta_x))]/\phi + c_*(y, \phi, \beta_x^T \Sigma_\epsilon \beta_x)\}),$$

where

$$\eta_* = \eta_*(\delta, z) = \beta_x^T \delta + \beta_z^T z,$$
$$c_*(y, \phi, \beta_x^T \Sigma_\epsilon \beta_x) = c(y, \phi) - (1/2)(y/\phi)^2 \beta_x^T \Sigma_\epsilon \beta_x,$$
$$b_*(\eta_*, \beta_x^T \Sigma_\epsilon \beta_x) = \phi \log \int \exp(y\eta_*/\phi + c_*(y, \phi, \beta_x^T \Sigma_\epsilon \beta_x))dy,$$

and the integral in the definition of $b_*$ is interpreted as an integral if $Y$ is continuous and as a sum if $Y$ is discrete.

The estimator is then obtained by solving estimation equations that are defined by analogy to the estimating equations described previously for GLM models. That is, we solve the equations

$$U_*^{(\beta)}(\theta) = \sum_{i=1}^{n} u_*^{(\beta)}(Y_i, X_i^*, Z_i; \theta) = 0;$$

$$H_*(\theta) = \sum_{i=1}^{n} h_*(Y_i, , X_i^*, Z_i; \theta) = 0,$$

where $u_*^{(\beta)}(y, x, z; \theta)$ and $h_*(y, x^*, z; \theta)$ are modified versions of the quantities $u^{(\beta)}(y, x, z; \theta)$ and $h(y, w; \theta)$ defined in (8.4) and (8.5). The derivatives $b'$ and $b''$ in (8.4) and (8.5) are replaced by $b'_* = \partial b_* / \partial \eta_*$ and $b''_* = \partial^2 b_* / \partial \eta_*^2$. The definition in (8.4) changes to

$$u_*^{(\beta)}(y, x_*, z; \theta) = \phi^{-1} \begin{pmatrix} \Delta(x_*, y; \theta) \\ z \end{pmatrix} \left[ y - b'_*(\beta_x^T \Delta(x^*, y; \theta) + \beta_z^T z) \right]$$

with $\gamma$ no longer appearing because we are now working with the canonical link, with $\gamma$ being the identity function. Similarly, we have

$$h(y, x^*, z; \theta) = \left( \frac{n - p}{n} \right) \phi - \frac{\left( y - b'_* \left( \beta_x^T \Delta(x^*, y; \theta) + \beta_z^T z \right) \right)^2}{b''_* \left( \beta_x^T \Delta(x^*, y; \theta) + \beta_z^T z \right)}.$$

It can be shown, under suitable regularity conditions, that the estimating equations defined in this manner yield consistent estimators.

For more information about the conditional score approach, the reader is referred to Carroll et al. (2006, Ch. 7). It appears that there has not been much development of the conditional score approach subsequent to the publication of Carroll et al. (2006).

## 8.3 Corrected Score Approach

### 8.3.1 Introduction

The corrected score approach was introduced by Stefanski (1989) and Nakamura (1990). The idea of the approach is to find a function $\bar{u}(y, x^*, z; \theta)$ such that

$$E[\bar{u}(Y_i, X_i^*, Z_i; \theta) | X_i, Z_i, Y_i] = u(Y_i, X_i, Z_i; \theta). \tag{8.6}$$

We define $\bar{u}_i(x^*; \theta) = \bar{u}(Y_i, x^*, Z_i; \theta)$, and then use the modified likelihood score function

$$\bar{U}(\theta) = n^{-1} \sum_{i=1}^{n} \bar{u}_i(X_i^*; \theta) \tag{8.7}$$

in place of $U(\theta)$ as the basis for estimation. The estimation equation thus becomes $\bar{U}(\theta) = 0$. The relation (8.6) implies that

$$E[\bar{U}(\theta)|\{X_i, Z_i, Y_i\}_{i=1}^n] = U(\theta), \tag{8.8}$$

which in turn implies that $E[\bar{U}(\theta^\circ)] = E[U(\theta^\circ)] = 0$, where, as before $\theta^\circ$ denotes the true value of $\theta$.

The corrected score approach can also be defined in terms of the concept of corrected likelihood, as as described in Nakamura (1990). We seek a function $\bar{\ell}(y, x^*, z; \theta)$ such that

$$E[\bar{\ell}(Y_i, X_i^*, Z_i; \theta)|X_i, Z_i, Y_i] = \ell(Y_i, X_i, Z_i; \theta), \tag{8.9}$$

and work with

$$\bar{\mathcal{L}}(\theta) = \sum_{i=1}^n \bar{\ell}(Y_i, W_i; \theta).$$

Under typical regularity conditions, if $\bar{\ell}(y, x^*, z; \theta)$ satisfies (8.9) then its gradient with respect to $\theta$ will satisfy (8.6).

Stefanski (1989) studied the case where $X_i^* = X_i + \epsilon_i$ with $\epsilon_i \sim N(0, \sigma_\epsilon^2)$. For this case, he showed that a necessary condition for the existence of an exact corrected score is that the function $u(y, x, z; \theta)$, as a function of $x$ is an entire function in the complex plane, i.e., admits an infinite power series representation at all points of the complex plane.

Nakamura (1990) presented general theory for the corrected score function approach. In particular, he showed, under certain conditions, that the estimator $\hat{\theta}$ based on the corrected score is consistent and the $\sqrt{n}(\hat{\theta} - \theta^\circ)$ is asymptotically mean-zero normal, with covariance matrix that can be estimated using the sandwich type-estimator

$$D(\hat{\theta})^{-1} \left( n^{-1} \sum_i \bar{u}_i(X_i^*, \hat{\theta}) \bar{u}_i(X_i^*; \theta)^T \right) (D(\hat{\theta})^{-1})^T,$$

where

$$D(\theta) = \frac{1}{n} \sum_{i=1}^n \nabla_\theta \bar{u}_i(X_i^*; \theta).$$

### 8.3.2 Corrected Score for General Linear Models

Nakamura (1990) derived corrected score functions for several generalized linear model settings. One setting he considered is linear regression with classical additive error. Here, $Y_i = \beta_0 + \beta_X^T X_i + \beta_Z^T Z_i + \eta_i$ with $\eta_i \sim N(0, \sigma^2)$ and $X_i^* = X_i + \epsilon_i$, with $\epsilon_i$ having mean 0 and covariance matrix $\Sigma_\epsilon$, and with $\epsilon_i$ uncorrelated with $X_i$ and $Z_i$. In this case,

$$u^{(\beta_x)}(y, x, z; \theta) = \sigma^{-2}[xy - x(\beta_0 + x^T \beta_x + x^T \beta_z)],$$
$$u^{(\beta_z)}(y, x, z; \theta)(\theta) = \sigma^{-2}[zy - z(\beta_0 + x^T \beta_x + z^T \beta_z)],$$

and a $\bar{u}$ satisfying (8.6) is given by

$$\bar{u}^{(\beta_x)}(y, x^*, z; \theta) = \sigma^{-2}[x^* y - x^*(\beta_0 + (x^*)^T \beta_x + z^T \beta_z)], +n\sigma^{-2}\Sigma_\epsilon \beta_x;$$
$$\bar{u}^{(\beta_z)}(y, x^*, z; \theta) = \sigma^{-2}[zy - z(\beta_0 + (x^*)^T \beta_x + z^T \beta_z)].$$

The fact that the above $\bar{u}$ satisfies (8.6) is easily seen using the relations $E[X_i\epsilon_i] = 0$, $E[Z_i\epsilon_i] = 0$, and $E[\epsilon_i\epsilon_i^T] = \Sigma_\epsilon$. The above $\bar{u}$ leads to the estimator

$$\begin{pmatrix} \hat{\beta}_x \\ \hat{\beta}_z \end{pmatrix} = \begin{pmatrix} \sum_{i=1}^n X_i^*(X_i^*)^T - n\Sigma_\epsilon & \sum_{i=1}^n X_i^* Z_i^T \\ \sum_{i=1}^n Z_i (X_i^*)^T & \sum_{i=1}^n Z_i Z_i^T \end{pmatrix}^{-1} \begin{pmatrix} \sum_{i=1}^n Y_i X_i^* \\ \sum_{i=1}^n Y_i Z_i \end{pmatrix}.$$

which coincides with the traditional error-corrected estimator for this setting.

Another setting Nakamura (1990) considered is Poisson regression with normally distributed classical additive error, which was also studied by Stefanski (1989). Here, $Y_i \sim \text{Poi}(\lambda_i)$ with $\lambda_i = \exp(\beta_0 + \beta_X^T X_i + \beta_Z^T Z_i)$, and $X_i^* = X_i + \epsilon_i$, with $\epsilon_i \sim N(0, \Sigma_\epsilon)$, independent of $X_i$ and $Z_i$. We have

$$u^{(\beta_x)}(y, x, z; \theta) = xy - x\exp(\beta_0 + x^T \beta_x + z^T \beta_z);$$
$$u^{(\beta_z)}(y, x, z; \theta) = zy - z\exp(\beta_0 + x^T \beta_x + z^T \beta_z).$$

It follows from the assumptions on $\epsilon_i$ and known properties of the normal distribution that the following relations hold:

$$E[\exp(\beta_x^T X_i^*)|X_i, Z_i] = \exp(\beta_x^T X_i + \beta_x^T \Sigma_\epsilon \beta/2);$$
$$E[X_i^* \exp(\beta_x^T X_i^*)|X_i, Z_i] = (X_i + \Sigma_\epsilon \beta_x)\exp(\beta_x^T X_i + \beta_x^T \Sigma_\epsilon \beta/2);$$
$$E[X_i^*(X_i^*)^T \exp(\beta_x^T X_i^*)|X_i, Z_i] = [\Sigma_\epsilon + (X_i + \Sigma_\epsilon \beta_x)(X_i + \Sigma_\epsilon \beta_x)^T] \times \exp(\beta_x^T X_i + \beta_x^T \Sigma_\epsilon \beta/2).$$

Using these relations, it can be seen that a $\bar{u}$ satisfying (8.6) is given by

$$\bar{u}^{(\beta_x)}(y, x^*, z; \theta) = x^* y - (x^* - \Sigma_\epsilon \beta_x)\exp(\beta_0 + (x^*)^T \beta_x + z^T \beta_z - \beta_x^T \Sigma_\epsilon \beta_x/2);$$
$$\bar{u}^{(\beta_z)}(y, x^*, z; \theta) = zy - z\exp(\beta_0 + (x^*)^T \beta_x + z^T \beta_z - \beta_x^T \Sigma_\epsilon \beta/2).$$

### 8.3.3 Corrected Score for the Cox Regression Model

Nakamura (1992) studied application of the corrected score approach to the Cox (1972) regression model for right-censored time to event data, where the hazard function is modeled as $\lambda(t|x, z) = \lambda_0(t)\exp(\beta_x^T x + \beta_z^T z)$, with the form of $\lambda_0(t)$ left unspecified. Cox proposed a method for estimating the regression parameters in this model based on the concept of partial likelihood. The partial likelihood score function in the Cox model is given by

$$U^{(\beta_x)}(\beta_x, \beta_z) = \sum_{i=1}^n \delta_i \left[ X_i - \frac{\sum_{j=1}^n Y_j(T_i) X_j \exp(\beta_x^T X_j + \beta_z^T Z_j)}{\sum_{j=1}^n Y_j(T_i)\exp(\beta_x^T X_j + \beta_z^T Z_j)} \right];$$
$$U^{(\beta_z)}(\beta_x, \beta_z) = \sum_{i=1}^n \delta_i \left[ Z_i - \frac{\sum_{j=1}^n Y_j(T_i) X_j \exp(\beta_x^T X_j + \beta_z^T Z_j)}{\sum_{j=1}^n Y_j(T_i)\exp(\beta_x^T X_j + \beta_z^T Z_j)} \right];$$

where $T_i$ denotes the follow-up time on individual $i$, $\delta_i$ is a 0–1 variable indicating whether the time to event for individual $i$ was observed ($\delta_i = 1$) or censored ($\delta_i = 0$), and $Y_i(t) = I(T_i \geq t)$. It is known that, under standard conditions, $E[U^{(\beta_x)}(\beta_x^\circ, \beta_z^\circ)] = 0$ and $E[U^{(\beta_z)}(\beta_x^\circ, \beta_z^\circ)] = 0$ and that the estimator based on setting $U^{(\beta_x)}(\beta_x, \beta_z) = 0$ and $U^{(\beta_z)}(\beta_x, \beta_z) = 0$ yields a consistent asymptotically normal estimator (Tsiatis, 1981; Andersen and Gill, 1982).

Throughout this subsection, we will assume that survival time and the censoring time are conditionally independent given $X$ and $Z$. In addition, we will assume that the measurement error is conditionally independent of the survival and censoring times given $X$ and $Z$. We will also subsume $Z$ within $X$, with the block of $\Sigma_\epsilon$ corresponding to $\text{Cov}(Z)$ taken to be zero.

Nakamura (1992) worked under the classical error model $X_i^* = X_i + \epsilon_i$ with $\epsilon_i \sim N(0, \Sigma_\epsilon)$, independent of $X_i$. We can write the Cox partial likelihood score as

$$U(\beta) = \sum_{i=1}^{n} \delta_i \left[ X_i - \frac{S_1(\beta)}{S_0(\beta)} \right]$$

with

$$S_0(\beta) = \frac{1}{n} \sum_{j=1}^{n} Y_j(T_i) \exp(\beta^T X_j);$$

$$S_1(\beta) = \frac{1}{n} \sum_{j=1}^{n} Y_j(T_i) X_j \exp(\beta^T X_j).$$

The theory in Stefanski (1989) implies that an exact corrected score for the Cox partial likelihood score does not exist. Nakamura therefore developed an approximate corrected score based on Taylor expansion. Note that, using the normality assumption on $\epsilon$, we have

$$E[e^{\beta^T \epsilon}] = \exp(\beta^T \Sigma_\epsilon \beta / 2); \tag{8.10}$$

$$E[\epsilon e^{\beta^T \epsilon}] = \exp(\beta^T \Sigma_\epsilon \beta / 2) \Sigma_\epsilon \beta. \tag{8.11}$$

Write

$$E(X, \beta, t) = \frac{\sum_{j=1}^{n} Y_j(t) X_j \exp(\beta^T X_j)}{\sum_{j=1}^{n} Y_j(t) \exp(\beta^T X_j)};$$

$$\bar{E}(X^*, \beta, t) = \frac{\sum_{j=1}^{n} Y_j(t) X_j^* \exp(\beta^T X_j^*)}{\sum_{j=1}^{n} Y_j(t) \exp(\beta^T X_j^*)}.$$

First-order Taylor expansion shows that

$$\bar{E}(X^*, \beta, t) \approx E(X, \beta, t) + \Sigma_\epsilon \beta.$$

This leads to the corrected score

$$\bar{U}(\beta) = \sum_{i=1}^{n} \delta_i [X_i^* - \bar{E}(X^*, \beta, T_i) + \Sigma_\epsilon \beta].$$

In simulation studies, Nakamura (1992) found that the resulting estimator had reduced bias relative to the naive estimate ignoring the measurement error, but the bias was still appreciable. He therefore proposed a refined method based on second-order Taylor expansion. Denoting

$$S(X^*, \beta, t) = \sum_{j=1}^{n} Y_j(t) \exp(\beta^T X_j^*),$$

the corrected score is given by

$$\bar{U}'(\beta) = \sum_{i=1}^{n} \delta_i \left[ [X_i^* - \bar{E}(X^*, \beta, T_i) + \left(1 - \frac{S(X^*, 2\beta, T_i)}{S(X^*, \beta, T_i)^2}\right) \Sigma_\epsilon \beta \right].$$

Nakamura (1992) found that this corrected score led to better simulation results. Later, Kong and Gu (1999) proved that the estimator based on the first-order approximate corrected score is consistent and asymptotically normal.

Huang and Wang (2000b) developed a corrected score method for the Cox regression model with replicate measurement data. The method is nonparametric in the sense that it does not assume a specific distribution (e.g., normal) for the measurement error. It is, however, assumed that the measurement error is additive and independent of $X$. For simplicity, we will describe the method for the case where each individual has exactly two replicates. Thus, we have measurements $X_{ij}^* = X_i + \epsilon_{ij}$, $j = 1, 2$, where the $\epsilon_{ij}$'s are identically distributed with zero expectation, are independent of $X_i$ and of each other, and are also independent of the survival time and the censoring. The proposed corrected score is given by

$$\bar{U}(\beta) = \sum_{i=1}^{n} \delta_i \left[ \frac{X_{i1}^* + X_{i2}^*}{2} - \frac{S_1^*(\beta)}{S_0^*(\beta)} \right],$$

with

$$S_0^*(\beta) = \frac{1}{n} \sum_{j=1}^{n} Y_j(T_i)[\exp(\beta^T X_{j1}^*) + \exp(\beta^T X_{j2}^*)]/2;$$

$$S_1^*(\beta) = \frac{1}{n} \sum_{j=1}^{n} Y_j(T_i)[X_{j1}^* \exp(\beta^T X_{j2}^*) + X_{j2}^* \exp(\beta^T X_{j1}^*)]/2.$$

We can write

$$\bar{U}(\beta) = \sum_{i=1}^{n} \delta_i \left[ X_i - \frac{S_1^*(\beta)}{S_0^*(\beta)} \right] + \sum_{i=1}^{n} \delta_i (\epsilon_{i1} + \epsilon_{i2})$$

with the second sum having expectation zero. Further, using the independence assumptions and the fact that the $\epsilon_{ij}'s$ have expectation zero, we have

$$
\begin{aligned}
&E[Y_j(T_i)X_{j1}^* \exp(\beta^T X_{j2}^*)] \\
&\quad = E[Y_j(T_i)(X_j + \epsilon_{j1}) \exp(\beta^T (X_j + \epsilon_{j2}))] \\
&\quad = E[\exp(\beta^T \epsilon_{j2})] \left(E[Y_j(T_i)X_j \exp(\beta^T X_j)] + E[Y_j(T_i)\epsilon_{j1} \exp(\beta^T X_j)]\right) \\
&\quad = M(\beta) \left(E[Y_j(T_i)X_j \exp(\beta^T X_j)] + E[Y_j(T_i) \exp(\beta^T X_j)]E[\epsilon_{j1}]\right) \\
&\quad = M(\beta)E[Y_j(T_i)X_j \exp(\beta^T X_j)],
\end{aligned}
$$

where $M(\beta) = E[\exp(\beta^T \epsilon_{j1})]$. Similarly,

$$E[Y_j(T_i) \exp(\beta^T X_{j1}^*)] = M(\beta)E[Y_j(T_i) \exp(\beta^T X_j)].$$

We thus have

$$\frac{E[S_1^*(\beta)]}{E[S_0^*(\beta)]} = \frac{M(\beta)E[S_1(\beta)]}{M(\beta)E[S_0(\beta)]} = \frac{E[S_1(\beta)]}{E[S_0(\beta)]}. \tag{8.12}$$

It follows that the asymptotic limit of $n^{-1}\bar{U}(\beta)$ is the same as that of $n^{-1}U(\beta)$, and, in particular, the asymptotic limit of $n^{-1}\bar{U}(\beta^\circ)$ is zero. Given this result, Huang and Wang show, under regularity conditions, that the estimator based on $n^{-1}\bar{U}(\beta)$ is consistent and asymptotically mean zero normal. They provide a sandwich-type estimate for the asymptotic covariance matrix. The argument leading to (8.12) argument depends crucially on the assumed structure of the measurement error.

For the case where the number of replicates differs across individuals (but with at least two replicates for each individual), the corrected score function is defined by averaging over all possible pairs of replicates.

Song and Huang (2005) discuss a related estimator, including a refinement that improves finite-sample performance.

Yi and Lawless (2007) proposed an alternative corrected score method for the Cox model. Their approach differs from the above-described approaches in their handling of the baseline hazard $\lambda_0(t)$. Instead of leaving $\lambda_0(t)$ completely unspecified, they work with a piecewise exponential model, which serves as a flexible parametric model. Augustin (2004) presented a similar method. Thus, we have

$$\lambda_0(t) = \sum_{k=1}^{K} I(t \in [\tau_{k-1}, \tau_k))\lambda_{0k},$$

where $\tau_1, \ldots, \tau_{K-1}$ are pre-specified cutpoints, $\tau_0 = 0, \tau_K = \infty$, and $\lambda_{01}, \ldots, \lambda_{0K}$ The corresponding cumulative baseline hazard hazard is

$$\Lambda_0(t) = \sum_{k=1}^{K} \lambda_{0k}(\min(t, t_k) - t_{k-1})_+,$$

where $u_+ = \max(u, 0)$. The measurement error takes the form $X^* = X + \epsilon$, where $\epsilon$ is a mean-zero random variable which is independent of $X$ and of the survival and censoring times. The distribution of $\epsilon$ is assumed known; it is straightforward to extend to the case where the distribution of $\epsilon$ follows a known parametric model and estimates of the parameters are available.

When $X$ is observed, the likelihood score $U(\theta)$ is of the form (8.3) with

$$u(t, \delta, x; \theta) = \delta \log \lambda_0(t) + \delta\beta^T x - \Lambda_0(t)e^{\beta^T x}.$$

A corrected score $\bar{U}(\theta)$ is given by (8.7)

$$\bar{u}(t, \delta, x^*; \theta) = \delta \log \lambda_0(t) + \delta x^* - \Lambda_0(t)e^{\beta^T x - \Omega(\beta)},$$

where $\Omega(b) = \log E[e^{b^T \epsilon}]$ is the cumulant generating function of $\epsilon$.

Yi and Lawless (2012) extend this method to recurrent events data.

### 8.3.4 Misclassification

Akazawa, Kinukawa and Nakamura (1998) discussed corrected score estimation for discrete covariates subject to misclassification. Thus, $X$ is discrete, while $Z$ may include any combination of discrete and continuous variables. Denote the possible values of $X$ by $x_1, \ldots, x_K$, assume that $X^*$ has the same range of possible values, and define $A_{kl} = \Pr(X^* = x_l | X = x_k)$. Denote $B = A^{-1}$, so that $AB = I$, where $I$ is the identity matrix. For simplicity, we assume that the conditional distribution of $X^*$ given $X$ does not depend on $Z_i$, although this assumption can be relaxed. We define

$$\bar{u}(y, x_k, z; \theta) = \sum_{l=1}^{K} B_{kl} u(y, x_l, z; \theta). \tag{8.13}$$

Let $k(i)$ denote the value of $k$ such that $X_i = x_k$. We then have

$$\begin{aligned}
E[\bar{u}(Y_i, X_i^*, Z_i; \theta) | Y_i, X_i, Z_i] &= \sum_{m=1}^{K} Pr(X^* = x_m | X_i) \sum_{l=1}^{K} B_{ml} u(Y_i, x_l, Z_i; \theta) \\
&= \sum_{m=1}^{K} A_{k(i)m} \sum_{l=1}^{K} B_{ml} u(Y_i, x_l, Z_i; \theta) \\
&= \sum_{l=1}^{K} \left( \sum_{m=1}^{K} A_{k(i)m} B_{ml} \right) u(Y_i, x_l, Z_i; \theta) \\
&= \sum_{l=1}^{K} (AB)_{k(i)l} u(Y_i, x_l, Z_i; \theta) \\
&= u(Y_i, x_{k(i)}, Z_i; \theta) \\
&= u(Y_i, X_i, Z_i; \theta),
\end{aligned}$$

so that $\tilde{u}$ satisfies (8.6). Akazawa, Kinukawa and Nakamura (1998) introduced this device for the case of logistic regression with covariate misclassification. Zucker and Spiegelman (2008) applied this approach for the case of Cox survival regression with covariate misclassification. Akazawa, Kinukawa and Nakamura (1998) assumed the classification probabilities to be known, whereas Zucker and Spiegelman (2008) allowed them to be estimated, and derived corrections to the estimated covariance matrix of the parameter estimates that reflect the error in estimating the classification probabilities.

### 8.3.5 Huang and Wang Modified Corrected Score

Huang and Wang (2000b) provide a modified corrected score estimator for logistic regression. They work in the setting where $X_i^* = X_i + \epsilon_i$ with $\epsilon_i$ independent of $X_i$ and $Y_i$. They do not assume any specific distribution for $\epsilon_i$, and they do not assume that $E[\epsilon_i] = 0$. Arbitrary dependence is allowed among the components of $\epsilon_i$ for a given $i$. We again subsume $Z$ within $X$. We will also write the intercept term explicitly, with the model represented as $\Pr(Y = 1|X = x) = \exp(\alpha + \beta^T x)/(1 + \exp(\alpha + \beta^T x))$.

Recall that in the case with $X$ known, the likelihood score function is given by

$$U(\alpha, \beta) = \sum_{i=1}^{n} u(Y_i, X_i, \alpha, \beta)$$

with

$$u(y, x, \alpha, \beta) = \left[\begin{array}{c} 1 \\ x \end{array}\right] \left( y_i - \frac{e^{\alpha+\beta^T x}}{1 + e^{\alpha+\beta^T x}} \right).$$

As mentioned previously, this score function is not an entire function in the complex plane, and therefore a corresponding exact corrected score function does not exist. The idea behind the proposed method is to introduce weights into the score function to obtain a modified score function for which a corresponding corrected score exists. Thus, instead of working with $U(\beta)$, we work with

$$\tilde{U}(\alpha, \beta) = \sum_{i=1}^{n} w(\alpha + \beta^T X_i) u(Y_i, X_i, \alpha, \beta)$$

for some weight function $w$. Clearly we have $\tilde{U}(\alpha^\circ, \beta^\circ) = 0$.

Huang and Wang (2001) focus on two possible choices of the weight function $w$: $w_1(u) = 1 + e^u$ and $w_2(u) = 1 + e^{-u}$. Let us consider first $w_1(u) = (1 + e^u)$. We then get

$$\tilde{U}^{(1)}(\alpha, \beta) = \sum_{i=1}^{n} \tilde{u}^{(1)}(Y_i, X_i, \alpha, \beta)$$

with

$$\tilde{u}^{(1)}(y, x, \alpha, \beta) = \left[\begin{array}{c} 1 \\ x \end{array}\right] (y + (y-1)e^{\alpha+\beta^T x}).$$

The score function $\tilde{U}^{(2)}(\alpha, \beta)$ corresponding to $w_2(u)$ can be defined in a similar way.

Huang and Wang (2001) begin with the case where the distribution of $\epsilon_i$ is known. The corrected score $\bar{U}^{(1)}(\alpha, \beta)$ corresponding to $\tilde{U}^{(1)}(\alpha, \beta)$ is

$$\bar{U}^{(1)}(\alpha, \beta) = \sum_{i=1}^{n} \bar{u}^{(1)}(Y_i, X_i^*, \alpha, \beta)$$

with

$$\bar{u}^{(1)}(y, x^*, \alpha, \beta) = y \begin{bmatrix} 1 \\ x^* - E[\epsilon_i] \end{bmatrix} + \frac{(y-1)e^{\alpha+\beta x^*}}{E[e^{\beta^T \epsilon_i}]} \begin{bmatrix} 1 \\ x^* - E[\epsilon_i e^{\beta^T \epsilon_i}]/E[e^{\beta^T \epsilon_i}] \end{bmatrix}.$$

Using the independence between $\epsilon_i$ and $(X_i, Y_i)$, it is easily verified that $E[\bar{u}^{(1)}(Y_i, X_i^*, \alpha, \beta)|Y_i, X_i] = \tilde{u}^{(1)}(Y_i, X_i, \alpha, \beta)$. The corrected score $\bar{U}^{(2)}(\alpha, \beta)$ corresponding to $\tilde{U}^{(2)}(\alpha, \beta)$ is constructed similarly.

Huang and Wang's (2001) final estimator is constructed as follows. Define

$$\bar{U}(\alpha, \beta) = \begin{bmatrix} \bar{U}^{(1)}(\alpha, \beta) \\ \bar{U}^{(2)}(\alpha, \beta) \end{bmatrix}.$$

Let $\hat{M}(\alpha, \beta)$ be an empirical estimate of the covariance matrix of $\bar{U}(\alpha, \beta)$. The proposed estimator is then the minimizer of $\bar{U}(\alpha, \beta)^T \hat{M}(\hat{\alpha}_{ini}, \hat{\beta}_{ini})\bar{U}(\alpha, \beta)$, where $(\hat{\alpha}_{ini}, \hat{\beta}_{ini})$ is a preliminary consistent estimate of $(\alpha, \beta)$, such as the solution to $\bar{U}^{(1)}(\alpha, \beta) = 0$ or the solution to $\bar{U}^{(2)}(\alpha, \beta) = 0$.

If $\epsilon$ is mean-zero normal, the expressions case be simplified using (8.10) and (8.11).

The procedure generalizes immediately to the case where the distribution of $\epsilon_i$ is known up to a set of parameters for which estimates are available. In this case, the estimated covariance matrix has to be adjusted to account for the error in estimating these parameters.

Huang and Wang (2001) then discuss the case where the distribution of the measurement error is unknown, but there are replicate measurements $X_{ij}^* = X_i + \epsilon_{ij}$, $j = 1, \ldots, J_i$, where the $\epsilon_{ij}$'s are identically distributed, are independent of $X_i$ and of each other, and are also independent of $Y_i$. They deal with this case using the same approach that they used in their nonparametric corrected score method for the Cox survival model. Assume for simplicity that $J_i = 2$ for all $i$. We then define

$$\begin{aligned} \bar{u}^{(1)}(y, x_1^*, x_2^*, \alpha, \beta) &= \frac{1}{2} \begin{bmatrix} 1 \\ x_1^* \end{bmatrix} (y + (y-1)e^{\alpha+\beta^T x_2^*}) \\ &+ \frac{1}{2} \begin{bmatrix} 1 \\ x_2^* \end{bmatrix} (y + (y-1)e^{\alpha+\beta^T x_1^*}). \end{aligned}$$

Using the arguments that Huang and Wang (2000) used for the Cox model, it can be shown that $E[\bar{u}^{(1)}(Y_i, X_i^*, \alpha, \beta)|Y_i, X_i] = \tilde{u}^{(1)}(Y_i, X_i, \alpha_+, \beta)$, where

$\alpha_+ = \alpha - \log E[e^{\beta\epsilon_{ij}}]$. Similarly, with $\bar{u}^{(2)}(y, x_1^*, x_2^*, \alpha, \beta)$ defined in a parallel manner, we get $E[\bar{u}^{(2)}(Y_i, X_i^*, \alpha, \beta)|Y_i, X_i] = \tilde{u}^{(2)}(Y_i, X_i, \alpha_-, \beta)$, where $\alpha_- = \alpha + \log E[e^{-\beta\epsilon_{ij}}]$. It follows that an estimator based on $\bar{U}^{(1)}(\alpha, \beta)$ and $\bar{U}^{(2)}(\alpha, \beta)$, along the lines described above, will yield an consistent and asymptotically normal estimator of $(\alpha_+, \alpha_-, \beta)$. In general, $\alpha$ is not identifiable, but if $\epsilon_{ij}$ is assumed to be symmetric around 0 then $\alpha$ is identifiable and can be estimated by $\hat{\alpha} = (\hat{\alpha}_- + \hat{\alpha}_+)/2$. Again, the arguments supporting the asymptotic theory depend crucially on the assumed structure of the measurement error.

For the case where the distribution of the measurement error is known, Chen, Hanfelt and Huang (2015) presented a similar estimator based on the single modified score function

$$\tilde{U}(\alpha, \beta) = \sum_{i=1}^{n} w(\alpha + \beta^T X_i) u(Y_i, X_i, \alpha, \beta)$$

with $w(u) = \cosh u$. A corresponding corrected score is defined, and shown to lead to a consistent and asymptotically normal estimator of $\alpha$ and $\beta$.

### 8.3.6 Complex Variable Simulation Extrapolation

Novick and Stefanski (2002) presented a corrected score method based on complex variable simulation extrapolation. This method was developed for the classical error model $X_i^* = X_i + \epsilon_i$ with $\epsilon_i \sim N(0, \Sigma_\epsilon)$, independent of $X_i$. The theoretical development involves complex variable theory and assumes that the function $u(y, x, z; \theta)$, as a function of $x$, is an entire function in the complex plane. Suppose $\zeta_i, i = 1, \ldots, n$ are i.i.d. $N(0, \Sigma_\epsilon)$ random vectors independent of all other random variables in the model. Define $\tilde{X}_i^* = X_i^* + \iota\zeta_i$, where $\iota = \sqrt{-1}$. Stefanski and Cook (1995) show that for any entire function $g$ we have $E[\text{Re}(g(\tilde{X}_i^*))|X_i] = g(X_i)$, where $\text{Re}(\alpha)$ denotes the real part of the complex number $\alpha$. Thus, the function $\bar{u}(y, x, z; \theta) = E[\text{Re}(u(y, \tilde{X}_i^*, z; \theta))|X_i = x]$ satisfies (8.6). In simple situations, the expectation $E[\text{Re}(u(y, \tilde{X}_i^*, z; \theta))|X_i = x]$ can be evaluated analytically. This is the case for linear regression and Poisson regression, for which evaluation of the expectation leads to the corrected score functions presented by Nakamura (1990) and described in Section 8.3.2. For situations where the expectation cannot be evaluated analytically, Novick and Stefanski proposed evaluating it by simulation. Let $J$ be a user-specified large integer, and let $\zeta_{ij}, i = 1, \ldots, n, j = 1, \ldots, J$ be i.i.d. $N(0, \Sigma_\epsilon)$ random vectors independent of all other random variables in the model. The $\zeta_{ij}$ can be generated using standard algorithms for generating multivariate normal random vectors. Define $\tilde{X}_{ij}^* = X_i^* + \iota\zeta_{ij}$. With these definitions, Novick and Stefanski (2002) proposed using the corrected score function

$$\bar{u}(Y_i, X_i^*, Z_i; \theta, J) = \frac{1}{J} \sum_{j=1}^{J} \text{Re}(\bar{u}(Y_i, \tilde{X}_{ij}^*, Z_i; \theta)),$$

which satisfies (8.6). The real part $\text{Re}(\bar{u}(Y_i, \tilde{X}^*_{ij}, Z_i; \theta))$ can be evaluated either analytically or by using complex arithmetic, which is available in many programming languages, including R.

In the case of logistic regression, the score function $u(y, x, z; \theta)$ is not entire in $x$ because it has singularities in the complex plane. Thus, in this case, the theory underlying Novick and Stefanski's method does not apply. However, Novick and Stefanski presented simulation results showing that their method nonetheless performs well in this case.

### 8.3.7 Regularization Extrapolation Corrected Score

Zucker et al. (2013) proposed an approximate corrected score method, which they called the regularization extrapolation corrected score (RECS) method, based on the Tikhonov regularization for integral equations (Delves and Mohamed, 1985, Section 12.3; Kress, 1989, Ch. 16). This method is designed for continuous error-prone covariates. We present here a sketch of the method and refer the reader to Zucker et al. (2013) for implementation details.

Suppose for simplicity that there is a single error-prone covariate. Let $a_i(x, x^*)$ denote the conditional density of $X_i^*$ given $X_i = x$, with the subscript $i$ indicating possible dependence on $Z_i$ and $Y_i$. The condition (8.6) can then be written in integral equation form as

$$\int a_i(x, x^*)\bar{u}_{ij}(y, x^*, Z_i)dx^* = u_{ij}(y, x, Z_i),$$

where we suppress the argument $\theta$. The idea of the RECS method is to forego trying to find an exact solution to the above integral equation (which may not exist, as in the case of logistic regression), and instead seek an approximate solution via Tikhonov regularization.

Define the integral operator $A_i g(x) = \int a_i(x, w)g(w)dw$. Write $\Delta_{ij}(x) = u_{ij}(x) - A_i u_{ij}(x)$ and $\bar{\Delta}_{ij}(x) = \bar{u}_{ij}(x) - u_{ij}(x)$. We can then write the above integral equation as $A_i\bar{\Delta}_{ij} = \Delta_{ij}$. We seek the $\bar{\Delta}_{ij}(\cdot; \theta, \alpha)$ that minimizes the penalized loss function

$$\mathcal{L}_{ij}(\bar{\Delta}_{ij}) = \|A_i\bar{\Delta}_{ij} - \Delta_{ij}\|_2^2 + \alpha\|_2\bar{\Delta}_{ij}\|_2^2, \tag{8.14}$$

where $\|g\|_2^2$ denotes the weighted squared $L_2$ norm $\|g\|_2^2 = \int c(v)g(v)^2dv$ (for a specified weight function $c(v)$) and $\alpha > 0$ is a penalty factor. The penalty is introduced in order to avoid ill-conditioning and ensure existence of a solution. After obtaining $\bar{\Delta}_{ij}(\cdot; \theta, \alpha)$, we use $\bar{u}_{ij}(x; \theta, \alpha) = u_{ij}(x) + \bar{\Delta}_{ij}(x; \theta, \alpha)$ as a corrected score term.

For numerical implementation, Zucker et al. (2013) proposed representing the solution $\bar{\Delta}_{ij}(\cdot; \theta, \alpha)$ in a basis expansion

$$\bar{\Delta}_{ij}(x; \theta, \alpha) = \sum_{m=1}^{M} d_{ijm}(\alpha)\psi_m(x), \tag{8.15}$$

where the $\psi_m$ are specified basis functions, chosen to be which are orthonormal with respect to the weight function $c$. Denote $\phi_{im}(x) = A_i\psi_m(x)$ and $d_{ij} = [d_{ij1} \ldots d_{ijM}]^T$ (suppressing the argument $\alpha$ in $d_{ijm}$ for the time being). We then can express the objective function $\mathcal{L}_{ij}(\bar{\Delta}_{ij})$ as

$$\mathcal{L}_{ij}(\bar{\Delta}_{ij}) = \| \sum_{m=1}^{M} d_{ijm}\phi_{im} - \Delta_{ij}\|_2^2 + \alpha\, d_{ij}^T d_{ij},$$

where $\|\bar{\Delta}_{ij}\|_2^2 = d_{ij}^T d_{ij}$ because of the orthonormality of the $\psi_m$ functions. We now approximate the $L^2$ norm in the first term on the right side via the quadrature approximation

$$\int \varphi(v)g(v)dv \doteq \sum_{k=1}^{K} q_k g(x_k), \tag{8.16}$$

where for specified quadrature points and weights $x_k$ and $q_k$. Given the approximation (8.16), we can express the objective function as

$$\begin{aligned}\mathcal{L}_{ij}(\bar{\Delta}_{ij}) &= \sum_{k=1}^{K} q_k \left[\sum_{m=1}^{M} d_{ijm}\phi_{im}(x_k) - \Delta_{ij}(x_k)\right]^2 + \alpha\, d_{ij}^T d_{ij} \\ &= \sum_{k=1}^{K} \left[\sum_{m=1}^{M} d_{ijm}\tilde{\phi}_{imk} - \tilde{\Delta}_{ijk}\right]^2 + \alpha\, d_{ij}^T d_{ij},\end{aligned}$$

where $\tilde{\phi}_{imk} = \sqrt{q_k}\phi_m(x_k)$ and $\tilde{\Delta}_{ijk} = \sqrt{q_k}\Delta_{ij}(x_k)$. Next, define the matrix $\tilde{\Phi}_i$ by $\tilde{\Phi}_{ikm} = \tilde{\phi}_{imk}$ and the vector $\tilde{\Delta}_{ij} = [\tilde{\Delta}_{ij1} \ldots \tilde{\Delta}_{ijK}]$. We obtain $\mathcal{L}_{ij}(\bar{\Delta}_{ij}) = (\tilde{\Phi}_i d_{ij} - \tilde{\Delta}_{ij})^T\ (\tilde{\Phi}_i d_{ij} - \tilde{\Delta}_{ij}) + \alpha\, d_{ij}^T d_{ij}$. We then find, by standard least squares theory, that the vector $d_{ij}(\alpha)$ that minimizes the above quantity is given by $d_{ij}(\alpha) = C(\alpha)\tilde{\Delta}_{ij}$, where $C(\alpha) = (\tilde{\Phi}^T\tilde{\Phi} + \alpha I)^{-1}$, which does not depend on $\theta$. Finally, we define $\bar{u}_{ij}(w;\theta,\alpha) = u_{ij}(w;\theta) + \bar{\Delta}_{ij}(w;\theta,\alpha)$, where $\bar{\Delta}_{ij}(w;\theta,\alpha)$ is given by (8.15) with $d_{ijm}(\alpha)$ as just described. Then, as indicated in the preceding section, we put $\bar{U}(\theta,\alpha) = n^{-1}\sum_i \bar{u}_i(W_i;\theta,\alpha)$ and define the estimator $\hat{\theta}^{(\alpha)}$ to be the solution to $\bar{U}(\theta,\alpha) = 0$.

Zucker et al. (2013) showed that, for fixed $\alpha$, the resulting estimator of $\theta$ converges almost surely to a limit $\tilde{\theta}^{(\alpha)}$ and is asymptotically normal. They gave an expression for the asymptotic covariance matrix. They showed further that as $\alpha$ decreases to 0, $\tilde{\theta}^{(\alpha)}$ converges to $\theta^{\circ}$. They discussed selection of $\alpha$ based on the generalized cross validation (GCV) criterion (Hansen, 1994, 2007), and they presented simulation results under the logistic regression model.

The main advantage of the RECS approach is its great flexibility. The method can handle both internal and external validation designs. It can handle the replicate measures design as well, with the overall surrogate measurement defined as the sample mean (or other summary measure) of the available measurements on the individual. Moreover, the method can handle arbitrary measurement error structures, in contrast with other methods which require independent additive error, often with an additional assumption of normality. Differential measurement error, where the measurement error depends on the response and possibly also background covariates, is also covered. Thus, the surrogacy assumption required for most other methods can be dropped. The main disadvantage is that it can be hard to implement when there are more than two error-prone covariates. There is no limitation, however, on the number of error-free covariates.

### 8.3.8 Trend Constrained Corrected Score Method

Huang (2014) proposed a variation on the corrected score method, called the trend constrained corrected score method. This method is aimed at addressing problems that arise with the corrected score method under a high degree of measurement error.

Huang presents his method in the context of count data with a log-linear model for the expected count. That is, subsuming $Z$ within $Z$, the model specifies that

$$E[Y|X] = \exp(\alpha + \beta^T X). \tag{8.17}$$

If in addition $Y$ has a Poisson distribution, then the log-likeihood is given by (8.2) with

$$\ell(y, x; \theta) = y(\alpha + \beta^T x) - \exp(\alpha + \beta^T x).$$

Without the Poisson assumption, maximizing $\ell(\theta)$ defined in this way still yields a consistent estimator of $\theta$. We will proceed without the Poisson assumption.

Suppose now that we measure $X^* = X + \epsilon$, where $\epsilon$ is independent of $(X, Y)$. We assume that the distribution of $\epsilon$ is known; it is straightforward to extend to the case where the distribution of $\epsilon$ has a known parametric form and estimates of the parameters are available. A corrected likelihood can then be constructed taking

$$\bar{\ell}(y, x^*; \theta) = y(\alpha + \beta^T(x^* - \Omega'(0))) - \exp(\alpha + \beta^T x^* - \Omega(\beta)),$$

where $\Omega(b) = \log E[e^{b^T \epsilon}]$ is the cumulant generating function of $\epsilon$ and $\Omega'(b)$ is its gradient. The corresponding corrected score is based on

$$\bar{u}(y, x*; \theta) = y \begin{bmatrix} 1 \\ x^* - \Omega'(0) \end{bmatrix} - \exp(\alpha + \beta^T x - \Omega(\beta)) \begin{bmatrix} 1 \\ x^* - \Omega'(\beta) \end{bmatrix}.$$

The log-likelihood $\ell(\theta)$ with observed $X$ has a unique maximum and correspondingly the likelihood score function $U(\theta)$ has a unique root at which the Jacobian of $U$ (which is the Hessian of $\mathcal{L}$) is negative definite. By contrast, the corrected score $\bar{U}(\theta)$ can sometimes have a single root which is not a local maximum of $\bar{\ell}$ or multiple roots. Such behavior often occurs when the measurement error variance is large.

Huang's proposed solution for dealing with problem is to introduce an additional estimating equation and use an empirical likelihood approach. It is easy to see that under (8.17) and the structure of the measurement error we have that for $r, s = 1, \ldots p$

$$E\left[Y\left\{\frac{\partial^2}{\partial\beta_r\partial\beta_s}\exp(\beta^T X^* - \Omega(\beta))\right\}\bigg|_{\beta=0} - \left\{\frac{\partial^2}{\partial\beta_r\partial\beta_s}\exp(\alpha + \beta^T X^* - \Omega(\beta))\right\}\bigg|_{\beta=\beta^\circ}\right] = 0.$$

This motivates empirical likelihood estimation of the joint distribution function $F(x, y; \theta)$ of $(Y_i, X_i^*)$ subject to the constraints

$$E_F[\bar{u}(Y, X^*; \theta) = 0$$
$$E_F\left[Y\left\{\frac{\partial^2}{\partial\beta_r\partial\beta_s}\exp(\beta^T X^* - \Omega(\beta))\right\}\bigg|_{\beta=0} - \left\{\frac{\partial^2}{\partial\beta_r\partial\beta_s}\exp(\alpha + \beta^T X^* - \Omega(\beta))\right\}\bigg|_{\beta=\beta^\circ}\right] = 0 \quad \text{for all } r, s.$$

The empirical likelihood $\mathcal{L}_{emp}(\theta)$ at a given $\theta$ is given by the global maximum over $w_1, \ldots, w_n$ of

$$\prod_{i=1}^n nw_i,$$

subject to the constraints

$$\sum_{i=1}^n w_i = 1, \quad w_i \geq 0 \text{ for all } i; \tag{8.18}$$

$$\sum_{i=1}^n w_i \bar{u}(Y_i, X_i^*; \theta) = 0; \tag{8.19}$$

$$\sum_{i=1}^n w_i\left[Y_i\left\{\frac{\partial^2}{\partial\beta_r\partial\beta_s}\exp(\beta^T X_i^* - \Omega(\beta))\right\}\bigg|_{\beta=0} - \left\{\frac{\partial^2}{\partial\beta_r\partial\beta_s}\exp(\alpha + \beta^T X_i^* - \Omega(\beta))\right\}\bigg|_{\beta=\beta}\right] = 0 \quad \text{for all } r, s. \tag{8.20}$$

Huang shows that the constraints (8.20) force the estimated expected Jacobian of $\bar{u}(Y_i, X_i^*; \theta)$ to be negative definite. The estimator of $\theta$ is then the global maximizer of $\mathcal{L}_{emp}(\theta)$. Owen (2001) presents computational algorithms. According to established empirical likelihood theory (Qin and Lawless, 1994), this estimator is consistent and asymptotically normal with asymptotic covariance that can be estimated by a sandwich estimator. Huang presents simulation results in the Poisson regression setting showing that the proposed method performs substantially better than the ordinary corrected score estimator. Extension of the method to other models such as logistic regression and Cox regression remains an open problem.

## Bibliography


Akazawa, K., Kinukawa, N., and Nakamura, T. (1998). A note on the corrected score function corrected for misclassification. *Journal of the Japan Statistical Society*, 28, 115-123.

Andersen, P. K. and Gill, R. D. (1982). Cox's regression model for counting processes: a large sample study. *Annals of Statistics*, 10, 1100-1120.

Augustin, T. (2004). An exact corrected log-likelihood function for Cox's proportional hazards model under measurement error and some extensions. *Scandinavian Journal of Statistics*, 31, 43-50.

Carroll, R. J., Ruppert, D., Stefanski, L. A. and Crainiceanu, C. M. (2006). *Measurement Error in Nonlinear Models: A Modern Perspective*, 2nd ed. Chapman and Hall/CRC, Boca Raton.

Chen, J., Hanefelt, J. J., and Huang, Y. (2015). A simple corrected score for logistic regression with errors-in-covariates. *Communications in Statistics - Theory and Methods*, 44, 2024-2036.

Cox, D. R. (1972). Regression models and life tables (with discussion). *Journal of the Royal Statistical Society, Series B*, 34, 187-200.

Huang, Y. (2014). Corrected score with sizable covariate measurement error: pathology and remedy. *Statistica Sinica*, 24, 357-374.

Huang, Y. and Wang, C. Y. (2000a). Consistent functional methods for logistic regression with errors in covariates. *Journal of the American Statistical Association*, 96, 1469-1482.

Huang, Y. and Wang, C. Y. (2000b). Cox regression with accurate covariates unascertainable: a nonparametric-correction approach. *Journal of the American Statistical Association*, 95, 1209-1219.

Kong, F. H. and Gu, M. (1999). Consistent estimation in Cox proportional hazards model with covariate measurement errors. *Statistica Sinica*, 9, 953-969.

McCullagh, P. and Nelder, J. A. (1989). *Generalized Linear Models*, 2nd ed. Chapman and Hall/CRC, Boca Raton.

Nakamura, T. (1990). Corrected score function of errors-in-variables models: methodology and application to generalized linear models. *Biometrika*, 77, 127-137.

Nakamura, T. (1992). Proportional hazards model with covariates subject to measurement error. *Biometrics*, 48, 829-838.

Novick, S. J. and Stefanski, L. A. (2002). Corrected score estimation via complex variable simulation extrapolation. *Journal of the American Statistical Association*, 97, 472-481.

Owen, A. B. (2001). *Empirical Likelihood.* Chapman and Hall/CRC, Boca Raton.

Qin, J. and Lawless, J. (1994). Empirical likelihood and general estimating equations. *Annals of Statistics*, 22, 300-325.

Song, X. and Huang, X. (2005). On corrected score approach for proportional hazards model with covariate measurement error. *Biometrics*, 61, 702-714.

Stefanski, L. (1989). Unbiased estimation of a nonlinear function of a normal mean with application to measurement-error models. *Communications in Statistics, Theory and Methods*, 18, 4335-4358.

Stefanski, L. A. and Carroll, R. J. (1987). Conditional scores and optimal scores for generalized linear measurement-error models. *Biometrika*, 74, 703-716.

Stefanski, L. A. and Cook, J. R. (1995). Simulation-extrapolation: the measurement error jackknife. *Journal of the American Statistical Association*, 90, 1247-1256.

Tsiatis, A. A. (1981). A large sample study of Cox's regression model. *Annals of Statistics*, 9, 93-108.

Yi, G. Y. and Lawless, J. F. (2007). A corrected likelihood method for the proportional hazards model with covariates subject to measurement error. *Journal of Statistical Planning and Inference*, 137, 1816-1828.

Yi, G. Y. and Lawless, J. F. (2012). Likelihoodbased and marginal inference methods for recurrent event data with covariate measurement error. *Canadian Journal of Statistics*, 40, 530-549.

Zucker, D. M. and Spiegelman, D. (2008). Corrected score estimation in the proportional hazards model with misclassified discrete covariates. *Statistics in Medicine*, 27, 1911-1933.

Zucker, D. M., Gorfine, M., Li, Y., Tadesse, M., and Spiegelman, D. (2013). A regularization corrected score method for nonlinear regression models with covariate error. *Biometrics*, 69, 80-90.

# 9

# *Semiparametric Methods for Measurement Error and Misclassification*

**Yanyuan Ma**

## CONTENTS



## 9.1 Introduction

A measurement error model typically contains two components, the regression component and the error component. The simplest regression component is probably the linear model, where the response ($Y$) and the covariate ($X$) are linked via the simple linear regression $Y = \beta_c + X\beta_1 + \epsilon$, and the regression error $\epsilon$ has a normal distribution with mean zero and variance $\sigma^2$. For simplicity, let us even assume $\sigma^2$ is known and only $\beta \equiv (\beta_c, \beta_1)^{\mathrm{T}}$ is the unknown parameter to be estimated. The simplest error component is probably the additive normal model, where $X^* = X + U$, and $U$ has a normal distribution with mean zero variance $\sigma_U^2$. For simplicity, we also assume $\sigma_U^2$ is known. Of course, being a measurement error model, $X$ is not observed, and what is observable is $(X_i^*, Y_i), i = 1, \ldots, n$, which are independent and identically distributed (iid) for a sample of the size $n$. The goal is to use the observations and the model assumption to estimate $\beta$ and make inference.

DOI: 10.1201/9781315101279-9

Even though we started with a completely parametric model to describe the relation of $Y$ and $X$, and also a completely known model to link $X^*$ and $X$, we in fact are handling a semiparametric model as we now explain. We first write down the joint probability density function (pdf) of the $i$th observation $(X_i^*, Y_i)$ as

$$f_{X^*,Y}(x_i^*, y_i, \beta, \eta) = \int \frac{1}{\sigma}\phi\left(\frac{y_i - \beta_c - x\beta_1}{\sigma}\right)\frac{1}{\sigma_U}\phi\left(\frac{x_i^* - x}{\sigma_U}\right)\eta(x)dx. \quad (9.1)$$

Here, $\phi(t) = (2\pi)^{-1/2}\exp(-t^2/2)$ is the standard normal pdf, and we use $\eta(\cdot)$ to denote the pdf of the unobservable covariate $X$. In the functional measurement error model context, we do not make any specific parametric assumption on the distribution of the unobservable covariate $X$. The only thing we know about $\eta$ is that it is a valid pdf. Thus, (9.1) is in fact a semiparametric model, in the sense that the model contains two types of parameters, $\beta$ and $\eta$. The parameter of interest is $\beta$, which is of finite dimension (dimension 2 in our example), while the nuisance parameter is $\eta$, which is a function itself and is thus an infinite dimensional parameter.

Of course, there is nothing special about the simple linear regression model and the normal additive error model considered above. Generally speaking, if we are considering a parametric regression model that links the response $Y$ to the covariates $X$, we can always write the model into the form $f_{Y|X}(Y, X, \beta)$, where $\beta$ contains all the unknown parameters involved in the regression. Likewise, we can consider a general error model of the form $f_{X^*|X}(x^*, x)$. Then the joint pdf of $(X_i^*, Y_i)$ is

$$f_{X^*,Y}(x_i^*, y_i, \beta, \eta) = \int f_{Y|X}(y_i, x, \beta) f_{X^*|X}(x_i^*, x)\eta(x)dx, \quad (9.2)$$

which is still a semiparametric model with parameter of interest $\beta$ and nuisance parameter $\eta$.

To make the model in (9.2) more general, we now consider adding a vector of categorical covariates $Z$, which is subject to misclassification. For example, when $Z$ contains only one binary variable, we can think of $Z$ to have values 0 or 1. Instead of observing $Z$, we only observe $T$, which is also a binary variable and is linked to $Z$ via $\text{pr}(T = 1 \mid Z = 1) = p_1$ and $\text{pr}(T = 0 \mid Z = 0) = p_0$. In general, we can think of a known relation between $T$ and $Z$ described through $f_{T|Z}(\mathbf{t}, z)$. Now let the regression be $f_{Y|X,Z}(y, x, z, \beta)$, and the observations be $(X_i^*, T_i, Y_i), i = 1, \ldots, n$. Then the joint pdf of $(X_i^*, T_i, Y_i)$ is

$$\begin{aligned} & f_{X^*,T,Y}(x_i^*, \mathbf{t}_i, y_i, \beta, \boldsymbol{\alpha}, \eta) \\ = & \sum_z \int f_{Y|X,Z}(y_i, x, z, \beta) f_{X^*|X}(x_i^*, x) f_{T|Z}(\mathbf{t}_i, z)\eta(x, z) f_Z(z, \boldsymbol{\alpha})dx, \end{aligned}$$

where $\eta(x, z)$ represents the pdf of $X$ conditional on $Z$, $f_Z(z, \boldsymbol{\alpha})$ is the probability mass function (pmf) of $Z$. Note that we made the surragacy assumption here, i.e. we have assumed $X^*$ is independent of $Y, Z, T$ given $X$, $T$ is independent of $Y, X, X^*$ given $Z$, and $Y$ is independent of $T, X^*$ given $X, Z$. Because $Z$ is categorical, hence its pmf, although completely unknown, depends only on finitely many parameters which we capture with $\boldsymbol{\alpha}$. The summation $\sum_z$ is across all possible supporting values of the random vector $Z$.

Our final generalization is to further allow a covariate vector $S$ in the regression model that is precisely observed. This leads us to the model

$$\begin{aligned} & f_{X^*,T,Y|S}(x_i^*, \mathbf{t}_i, s_i, y_i, \beta, \boldsymbol{\alpha}, \eta) \qquad (9.3) \\ = & \sum_z \int f_{Y|X,Z,S}(y_i, x, z, s_i, \beta) f_{X^*|X}(x_i^*, x) f_{T|Z}(\mathbf{t}_i, z) \eta(x, z) f_Z(z, \boldsymbol{\alpha}) dx. \end{aligned}$$

We point out that for simplification, we have assumed $X^*$ to be independent of $S$ given $X$, and $T$ to be independent of $Z$ given $S$, and $(X^{\mathrm{T}}, Z^{\mathrm{T}})^{\mathrm{T}}$ to be independent of $S$. Allowing dependence on $S$ of these quantities will not cause conceptual difficulties, but will increase notational complexity. Similarly, relaxing the surrogacy assumption also does not cause fundamental difference, as long as one can still ensure the identifiability of the problem. In the following, we mainly focus on analyzing the models in (9.2) and (9.3).

## 9.2 Semiparametrics

Our approach to analyzing (9.2) and (9.3) is through a geometric treatment in semiparametrics. This approach was first proposed in Bickel et al. (1993), and was then popularized by Tsiatis (2006). The general idea is to take advantage of the relation between an estimator and its influence function, and to find estimators through finding influence functions. Because parametric models are familiar to most people, we frequently refer to parametric models to illustrate the corresponding concept in semiparametric models in our subsequent explanation.

In a parametric model, the maximum likelihood estimator (MLE) or a method of moment estimator (MME) can be written as the solution of an estimating equation $\sum_{i=1}^n g(O_i, \beta) = 0$. Here $\beta \in \mathcal{R}^p$ is the parameter to be estimated, we use $O_i$ to denote the $i$th observation, and we call $g(\cdot) \in \mathcal{R}^p$ the estimating function. Clearly, at the true parameter value $\beta_0$, $E\{g(O_i, \beta_0)\} = 0$, while at the estimated parameter value $\widehat{\beta}$, $n^{-1}\sum_{i=1}^n g(O_i, \widehat{\beta}) = 0$. Standard

Taylor expansion of the estimating equation around $\beta_0$ then leads to

$$\begin{aligned} 0 &= n^{-1}\sum_{i=1}^{n} g(O_i, \widehat{\beta}) \\ &= n^{-1}\sum_{i=1}^{n} g(O_i, \beta_0) + \left\{ n^{-1}\sum_{i=1}^{n} \frac{\partial g(O_i, \beta_0)}{\partial \beta^{\mathrm{T}}} + o_p(1) \right\} (\widehat{\beta} - \beta_0) \\ &= n^{-1}\sum_{i=1}^{n} g(O_i, \beta_0) + \left[ E\left\{ \frac{\partial g(O_i, \beta_0)}{\partial \beta^{\mathrm{T}}} \right\} + o_p(1) \right] (\widehat{\beta} - \beta_0), \end{aligned}$$

where $\partial g(O_i, \beta_0)/\partial \beta^{\mathrm{T}}$ represents $\partial g(O_i, \beta)/\partial \beta^{\mathrm{T}}$ evaluated at $\beta = \beta_0$. Hence, noting that $n^{-1}\sum_{i=1}^{n} \phi(O_i, \beta_0) = O_p(n^{-1/2})$, we get

$$\widehat{\beta} - \beta_0 = n^{-1}\sum_{i=1}^{n} \phi(O_i, \beta_0) + o_p(n^{-1/2}), \tag{9.4}$$

where $\phi(O_i, \beta) = -[E\{\partial g(O_i, \beta)/\partial \beta^{\mathrm{T}}\}]^{-1} g(O_i, \beta)$ is named the influence function of the corresponding MLE or MME. In fact, many other estimators also have the type of expression described in (9.4) and we name such estimator regular asymptotically linear (RAL) estimator.

The same analysis applies to semiparametric models as well. For a semiparametric model with parameter of interest $\beta$ and nuisance parameter $\eta$, any RAL estimator $\widehat{\beta}$ can be expressed as

$$\widehat{\beta} - \beta_0 = n^{-1}\sum_{i=1}^{n} \phi(O_i, \beta_0, \eta_0) + o_p(n^{-1/2}), \tag{9.5}$$

where $\phi(O_i, \beta_0, \eta_0)$ is an influence function. Here, $\eta_0$ represents the true parameter value of $\eta$. One way to use the influence function $\phi$ is to construct estimators. Indeed, given an influence function $\phi$, we can form an estimating equation $\sum_{i=1}^{n} \phi(O_i, \beta, \eta_0) = 0$ and solve it to obtain $\widehat{\beta}$. The properties of influence function will ensure the resulting estimator $\widehat{\beta}$ to be a RAL estimator that satisfies (9.5). Based on such intrinsic relation of RAL estimators and influence functions, it is natural to look for estimators through finding influence functions.

To characterize the influence functions associated with a semiparametric model, say $f(O, \beta, \eta)$, we now return to the geometric description by Bickel et al. (1993). Consider the Hilbert space $\mathcal{H}$ formed by all the mean zero, finite variance, $p$ component functions of $O$, where the mean and variance are evaluated with respect to $f(O, \beta_0, \eta_0)$, and $p$ is the dimension of $\beta$. The inner product of the Hilbert space $\mathcal{H}$ is defined as the covariance of two functions, i.e. $\langle g_1, g_2 \rangle = E(g_1^{\mathrm{T}} g_2)$.

Now consider a subspace of $\mathcal{H}$ named the nuisance tangent space, denoted $\Lambda$. The elements of $\Lambda$ have the form $\mathbf{A}\partial \log f(O, \beta_0, \gamma_0)/\partial \gamma_0$, where $\gamma_0 \in$

$\mathcal{R}^q$, where $q$ is a positive integer, and $\mathbf{A}$ can be any $p \times q$ matrix. Here, $f(O, \beta_0, \gamma_0)$ is what is termed a parametric submodel, implying two properties. First, $f(O, \beta, \gamma)$ is a smaller model contained in the original semiparametric model $f(O, \beta, \eta)$. In other words, a special choice of $\eta$ would yield the model that contains parameter $\gamma$. For example, in (9.1), replacing the unspecified pdf $\eta(X)$ with a special parametric model $(1 - \gamma)\eta_0(x) + \gamma\phi(x)$ would generate a submodel index by parameter $\gamma$. Here, $\eta_0(x)$ is the true pdf of $X$. Note that the parametric form $(1-\gamma)\eta_0(x)+\gamma\phi(x)$ is a valid pdf, which is all that $\eta(\cdot)$ has to satisfy, hence it is indeed a submodel. Second, $f(O, \beta, \gamma)$ must contain the true model. In other words, there is $\gamma_0$, so that $f(O, \beta_0, \gamma_0)$ is indeed the true pdf of the data generation process. This seemingly innocent requirement is in fact a very stringent one. Imagine that if one can indeed identify a parametric submodel that contains the true data generation pdf, then there is in fact no need to work with the semiparametric model. One should simply work with the more specific, more structured and more informative parametric model $f(O, \beta, \gamma)$, instead of the vague and harder to deal with semiparametric model $f(O, \beta, \eta)$. Indeed, the parametric submodel example $(1 - \gamma)\eta_0(x) + \gamma\phi(x)$ we provided is unrealistic, because it requires the knowledge of the true pdf $\eta_0(x)$. Regardless whether a submodel is practically obtainable or not, conceptually it can be formulated, and this formulation leads to the nuisance tangent space described above. Strictly speaking, the nuisance tangent space $\Lambda$ is defined as the subspace of $\mathcal{H}$ that is formed by all the functions of the form

$$\mathbf{A}\{\partial \log f(O, \beta_0, \gamma_0)/\partial\gamma_0\},$$

and their linear combinations as well as the mean squared closure, where $\mathbf{A} \in \mathcal{R}^{p\times q}$. Note that $q \equiv \dim(\gamma)$ and can change when we consider $\gamma$ of different length. The definition of $\Lambda$ is key. With $\Lambda$ well defined, we can subsequently define $\Lambda^\perp$, which, as its notation suggests, is the orthogonal complement of $\Lambda$ in $\mathcal{H}$.

Having properly defined $\Lambda^\perp$, we are now ready to characterize the influence functions. For a function $\phi(\cdot)$ to be a valid influence function, it simply needs to satisfy two requirements, namely $\phi(\cdot) \in \Lambda^\perp$ and $E(\phi S_\beta^{\mathrm{T}}) = \mathbf{I}_p$, where $S_\beta = \partial \log f(O, \beta, \eta)/\partial\beta$ evaluated at $\beta = \beta_0$ and $\eta = \eta_0$. We now elaborate on these two requirements. The first requirement indicates that an influence function must belong to the nuisance tangent space orthogonal complement. This is a quite fundamental requirement that erases the possible effect of the nuisance parameter estimation on the parameter of interest. If given an arbitrary mean zero function $\mathbf{h}$, we can project it onto the nuisance tangent space and retain the orthogonal residual to obtain a function that belongs to $\Lambda^\perp$. The second requirement is in fact only a normalization requirement and is less crucial. Given any function $\mathbf{h}$ in $\Lambda^\perp$, we can easily normalize it to obtain $\{E(\mathbf{h}S_\beta^{\mathrm{T}})\}^{-1}\mathbf{h}$ which satisfies the second requirement.

Such characterization of the influence function provides a route to identify influence functions, hence identify RAL estimators. Note that for the purpose of constructing estimating equations, the second normalization requirement of the influence functions is not essential or even necessary. Using the unnormalized "influence functions", we can construct the estimating equations that generate the same RAL estimators as using the properly normalized influence functions.

Among all the influence functions, the one with the smallest variance will lead to the most efficient RAL estimator. This is obvious from the expression in (9.5), which indicates that to the leading order, the variance of an RAL estimator is the same as the variance of its corresponding influence function, i.e. $\text{var}(\widehat{\beta}) = \text{var}\{\phi(O_i, \beta_0, \eta_0)\}/n + o(n^{-1})$. The influence function with the smallest variance is termed the efficient influence function, and we now describe it in detail. The efficient influence function can be viewed as the orthogonal projection of the score function $S_\beta$ onto the nuisance tangent space orthogonal complement $\Lambda^\perp$, i.e. $S_{\text{eff}} = \Pi(S_\beta \mid \Lambda^\perp)$, where $\Pi(S_\beta \mid \Lambda^\perp)$ represents the orthogonal projection of $S_\beta$ onto the space $\Lambda^\perp$. This leads to the efficient influence function $\phi_{\text{eff}} = \{E(S_{\text{eff}} S_\beta^{\text{T}})\}^{-1} S_{\text{eff}} = \{E(S_{\text{eff}} S_{\text{eff}}^{\text{T}})\}^{-1} S_{\text{eff}}$. To see that the efficient influence function $\phi_{\text{eff}}$ is indeed efficient, we can verify that

$$
\begin{aligned}
\text{var}(\phi) - \text{var}(\phi_{\text{eff}}) &= E\{(\phi + \phi_{\text{eff}})(\phi - \phi_{\text{eff}})^{\text{T}}\} \\
&= E\{(\phi - \phi_{\text{eff}})(\phi - \phi_{\text{eff}})^{\text{T}}\} + 2E\{\phi_{\text{eff}}(\phi - \phi_{\text{eff}})^{\text{T}}\} \\
&= \text{var}(\phi - \phi_{\text{eff}}) + 2\{E(S_{\text{eff}} S_\beta^{\text{T}})\}^{-1} E\{S_{\text{eff}}(\phi - \phi_{\text{eff}})^{\text{T}}\} \\
&= \text{var}(\phi - \phi_{\text{eff}}) + 2\{E(S_{\text{eff}} S_\beta^{\text{T}})\}^{-1} E\{S_\beta(\phi - \phi_{\text{eff}})^{\text{T}}\} \\
&= \text{var}(\phi - \phi_{\text{eff}}) + 2\{E(S_{\text{eff}} S_\beta^{\text{T}})\}^{-1} (\mathbf{I}_p - \mathbf{I}_p) \\
&= \text{var}(\phi - \phi_{\text{eff}}),
\end{aligned}
$$

hence it is positive. In the above, the fourth equality is because the difference between $S_{\text{eff}}$ and $S_\beta$ is an element in $\Lambda$, which is orthogonal to any influence function, and the fifth equality is because $E(S_\beta \phi^{\text{T}}) = \mathbf{I}_p$ for any influence function.

The above derivation implies that not only we can find all the RAL estimators through identifying all the influence functions, we can also identify the most efficient RAL estimator through constructing the efficient influence function or the efficient score function.

## 9.3 Semiparametrics in Measurement Error Model

### 9.3.1 Basic Semiparametric Derivations

We now analyze (9.2) using the semiparametrics tools discussed in Section 9.2. Consider the parametric submodel $(1-\gamma)\eta_0(x) + \gamma f_X(x)$, where $f_X(x)$ is a valid yet arbitrary pdf of $X$. This leads to

$$
f_{X^*,Y}(x^*, y, \beta, \gamma) = \int f_{Y|X}(y, x, \beta) f_{X^*|X}(x^*, x)\{(1-\gamma)\eta_0(x) + \gamma f_X(x)\} dx,
$$

hence we get

$$\begin{aligned}
&\frac{\partial \log f_{X^*,Y}(x^*, y, \beta, \gamma)}{\partial \gamma} \\
&= \frac{\int f_{Y|X}(y, x, \beta) f_{X^*|X}(x^*, x)\{f_X(x) - \eta_0(x)\}dx}{f_{X^*,Y}(x^*, y, \beta, \gamma)} \\
&= \int \frac{f_{Y|X}(y, x, \beta) f_{X^*|X}(x^*, x)\{(1-\gamma)\eta_0(x) + \gamma f_X(x)\}}{f_{X^*,Y}(x^*, y, \beta, \gamma)} \\
&\quad \frac{f_X(x) - \eta_0(x)}{(1-\gamma)\eta_0(x) + \gamma f_X(x)} dx \\
&= E\left\{ \frac{f_X(X) - \eta_0(X)}{(1-\gamma)\eta_0(X) + \gamma f_X(X)} \middle| x^*, y \right\}.
\end{aligned}$$

At $\beta = \beta_0, \boldsymbol{\gamma} = \gamma_0 = 0$, we further get

$$\left.\frac{\partial \log f_{X^*,Y}(x^*, y, \beta, \gamma)}{\partial \gamma}\right|_{\beta=\beta_0, \boldsymbol{\gamma}=0} = E\left\{ \frac{f_X(X) - \eta_0(X)}{\eta_0(X)} \middle| x^*, y \right\}.$$

Note that because $f_X(x)$ can be any pdf, the only property about $\{f_X(x) - \eta_0(x)\}/\eta_0(x)$ appears to be that $E[\{f_X(X) - \eta_0(X)\}/\eta_0(X)] = \int\{f_X(x) - \eta_0(x)\}dx = 0$. Treating $\{f_X(x) - \eta_0(x)\}/\eta_0(x)$ as a single function, say $a(x)$, considering that there are many different choices of $f_X(x)$, each corresponding to a different $a(x)$, we conjecture that the nuisance tangent space of the model (9.2) is

$$[E\{\mathbf{a}(X) \mid x^*, y\} : E\{\mathbf{a}(X)\} = 0, \mathbf{a}(x) \in \mathcal{R}^p]. \tag{9.6}$$

We now formally show that the space described in (9.6) is indeed the nuisance tangent space of the model in (9.2). For notational convenience, we denote the space defined in (9.6) $\Gamma$, and aim at showing that $\Gamma = \Lambda$. We first show that $\Gamma \subset \Lambda$. To this end, for any arbitrary element in $\Gamma$ with the corresponding $\mathbf{a}(x)$, consider the parametric submodel $\eta_0(x) + \boldsymbol{\gamma}^{\mathrm{T}}\mathbf{a}(x)\eta_0(x)$, which satisfies $\int\{\eta_0(x) + \boldsymbol{\gamma}^{\mathrm{T}}\mathbf{a}(x)\eta_0(x)\}dx = 1$ by the property of $\mathbf{a}(x)$ required by $\Gamma$. Here $\boldsymbol{\gamma}$ is a vector of the same length as $\mathbf{a}(x)$. The nuisance score function of this parametric submodel is

$$\begin{aligned}
&\frac{\partial \log f_{X^*,Y}(x^*, y, \beta, \boldsymbol{\gamma})}{\partial \gamma} \\
&= \frac{\int f_{Y|X}(y, x, \beta) f_{X^*|X}(x^*, x)\mathbf{a}(x)\eta_0(x)dx}{\int f_{Y|X}(y, x, \beta) f_{X^*|X}(x^*, x)\{\eta_0(x) + \boldsymbol{\gamma}^{\mathrm{T}}\mathbf{a}(x)\eta_0(x)\}dx} \\
&= \int \frac{f_{Y|X}(y, x, \beta) f_{X^*|X}(x^*, x)\{\eta_0(x) + \boldsymbol{\gamma}^{\mathrm{T}}\mathbf{a}(x)\eta_0(x)\}}{f_{X^*,Y}(x^*, y, \beta, \boldsymbol{\gamma})} \\
&\quad \frac{\mathbf{a}(x)\eta_0(x)}{\eta_0(x) + \boldsymbol{\gamma}^{\mathrm{T}}\mathbf{a}(x)\eta_0(x)} dx \\
&= E\left\{ \frac{\mathbf{a}(X)\eta_0(X)}{\eta_0(X) + \boldsymbol{\gamma}^{\mathrm{T}}\mathbf{a}(X)\eta_0(X)} \middle| x^*, y \right\}.
\end{aligned}$$

At $\gamma = \gamma_0 = 0$, this leads to $\partial \log f_{X^*,Y}(x^*, y, \beta, \gamma)/\partial\gamma = E\{\mathbf{a}(X) \mid x^*, y\}$. Thus $E\{\mathbf{a}(X) \mid x^*, y\} \in \Lambda$. Thus, we have shown that $\Gamma \subset \Lambda$.

Now, to show $\Lambda \subset \Gamma$, consider an arbitrary element of $\Lambda$, which by definition of $\Lambda$, can be expressed as $\sum_{k=1}^{K} \mathbf{A}_k \partial \log f_{X^*,Y}(x^*, y, \beta, \gamma_k)/\partial\gamma_k$, where the $k$th submodel of $\eta(x)$ can be generally written as $\eta_k(x, \gamma_k)$. Using the form of $f_{X^*,Y}(x^*, y, \beta, \gamma_k)$, we obtain

$$
\begin{aligned}
& \sum_{k=1}^{K} \mathbf{A}_k \frac{\partial \log f_{X^*,Y}(x^*, y, \beta, \gamma_k)}{\partial \gamma_k} \bigg|_{\gamma_k=\gamma_{k0}} \\
= & \sum_{k=1}^{K} \mathbf{A}_k \frac{\int f_{Y|X}(y, x, \beta) f_{X^*|X}(x^*, x) \partial \eta_k(x, \gamma_k)/\partial \gamma_k dx}{\int f_{Y|X}(y, x, \beta) f_{X^*|X}(x^*, x) \eta_k(x, \gamma_k) dx} \bigg|_{\gamma_k=\gamma_{k0}} \\
= & \sum_{k=1}^{K} \mathbf{A}_k \int \frac{f_{Y|X}(y, x, \beta) f_{X^*|X}(x^*, x) \eta_k(x, \gamma_k)}{f_{X^*,Y}(x^*, y, \beta, \gamma_k)} \frac{\partial \eta_k(x, \gamma_k)/\gamma_k}{\eta_k(x, \gamma_k)} dx \bigg|_{\gamma_k=\gamma_{k0}} \\
= & E\left\{ \sum_{k=1}^{K} \mathbf{A}_k \frac{\partial \eta_k(X, \gamma_k)/\partial \gamma_k}{\eta_k(X, \gamma_k)} \mid x^*, y \right\} \bigg|_{\gamma_k=\gamma_{k0}} .
\end{aligned}
$$

Now we can verify that

$$
\begin{aligned}
E\left\{ \sum_{k=1}^{K} \mathbf{A}_k \frac{\partial \eta_k(X, \gamma_k)/\partial \gamma_k}{\eta_0(X)} \bigg|_{\gamma_k=\gamma_{k0}} \right\} &= \sum_{k=1}^{K} \mathbf{A}_k \int \frac{\partial \eta_k(x, \gamma_k)}{\partial \gamma_k} \bigg|_{\gamma_k=\gamma_{k0}} dx \\
&= \sum_{k=1}^{K} \mathbf{A}_k \frac{\partial \int \eta_k(x, \gamma_k) dx}{\partial \gamma_k} \bigg|_{\gamma_k=\gamma_{k0}} \\
&= 0.
\end{aligned}
$$

Thus,

$$
\sum_{k=1}^{K} \mathbf{A}_k \frac{\partial \eta_k(x, \gamma_k)/\partial \gamma_k}{\eta_0(x)} \bigg|_{\gamma_k=\gamma_{k0}}
$$

is a qualified $\mathbf{a}(x)$ described in $\Gamma$, hence $\Lambda \subset \Gamma$. Thus, we indeed verified $\Lambda = \Gamma$.

We now continue to characterize the nuisance tangent space $\Lambda^{\perp}$. The form of the elements of $\Lambda$ in (9.6) directly leads to the fact that for any element $\underline{(}x^*, y) \in \mathcal{H}$, $\underline{(}x^*, y) \in \Lambda$ is equivalent to

$$
\begin{aligned}
0 &= E[\underline{(}X^*, Y)^{\mathrm{T}} E\{\mathbf{a}(X) \mid X^*, Y\}] \\
&= E[E\{\underline{(}X^*, Y) \mid X\}^{\mathrm{T}} \mathbf{a}(X)]
\end{aligned}
$$

for all mean zero $\mathbf{a}(x)$, which is further equivalent to $E\{\underline{(}X^*, Y) \mid X\} = 0$. This is because we can simply set $\mathbf{a}(x) = E\{\underline{(}X^*, Y) \mid x\}$, which has mean zero because $(x^*, y) \in \mathcal{H}$, and it will lead to non-zero of $E[E\{(X^*, Y) \mid X\}^{\mathrm{T}}\mathbf{a}(X)]$. Thus, the nuisance tangent space is

$$\Lambda^{\perp} = [(x^*, y) \in \mathcal{R}^p : E\{(X^*, Y) \mid X\} = 0]. \tag{9.7}$$

Note that the requirement $E\{(X^*, Y) \mid X\} = 0$ automatically ensures $E\{(X^*, Y)\} = 0$, which guarantees that $(x^*, y) \in \mathcal{H}$.

We now proceed to construct the efficient score function and subsequently the efficient influence function. We first calculate the score function $S_\beta$. Simple calculation leads to

$$\begin{aligned}
& S_\beta(x^*, y, \beta, \eta) \\
= \; & \frac{\log f_{X^*,Y}(x^*, y, \beta, \eta)}{\partial \beta} \\
= \; & \frac{\int \{\partial f_{Y|X}(y, x, \beta)/\partial \beta\} f_{X^*|X}(x^*, x)\eta(x)dx}{f_{X^*,Y}(x^*, y, \beta, \eta)} \\
= \; & \frac{1}{f_{X^*,Y}(x^*, y, \beta, \eta)} \int \frac{\partial f_{Y|X}(y, x, \beta)/\partial \beta}{f_{Y|X}(y, x, \beta)} f_{Y|X}(y, x, \beta) f_{X^*|X}(x^*, x)\eta(x)dx \\
= \; & E\{\partial \log f_{Y|X}(y, X, \beta)/\partial \beta \mid x^*, y\}.
\end{aligned}$$

We now project the score function $S_\beta$ onto $\Lambda^{\perp}$ to calculate $S_{\text{eff}}$. To do this, based on the description of $\Lambda$ and $\Lambda^{\perp}$, we write the orthogonal projection of $S_\beta$ to $\Lambda$ as $E\{\mathbf{a}(X) \mid x^*, y\}$ for some $\mathbf{a}(x)$, and the difference $S_\beta - E\{\mathbf{a}(X) \mid x^*, y\}$ must be in $\Lambda^{\perp}$, hence it has to satisfy $E[S_\beta - E\{\mathbf{a}(X) \mid X^*, Y\} \mid x] = 0$. Unfortunately, we are unable to obtain a more explicit description of the efficient score $S_{\text{eff}}$ due to our inability to solve for an explicit form of $\mathbf{a}(x)$. In other words, the only description we can prescribe for $S_{\text{eff}}$ is that

$$S_{\text{eff}}(x^*, y, \beta_0, \eta_0) = S_\beta(x^*, y, \beta_0, \eta_0) - E\{\mathbf{a}(X) \mid x^*, y\}, \tag{9.8}$$

where $\mathbf{a}(x)$ is a function that satisfies

$$E\{S_\beta(X^*, Y, \beta_0, \eta_0) \mid x\} = E[E\{\mathbf{a}(X) \mid X^*, Y\} \mid x]. \tag{9.9}$$

It is worth pointing out that as long as our problem is identifiable in the sense that there exists at least one RAL estimator, then there must exists an efficient RAL estimator, hence there must exists the efficient score. Thus, as part of the description of the efficient score function, (9.9) must have a solution $\mathbf{a}(x)$. However, in general, there is no guarantee of uniqueness. Thus, there could be several $\mathbf{a}(x)$ that solve the equation (9.9). This however does not pose a problem for our purpose since $\mathbf{a}(x)$ is not our final quantity of interest. We only use $\mathbf{a}(x)$ to construct the efficient score in (9.8), which will lead to unique efficient score. Having characterized the efficient score function $S_{\text{eff}}$, we then normalized it to obtain the efficient influence function if desired.

### 9.3.2 Feasibility and Alteration

Recall that our original purpose is to identify influence functions and the efficient influence function so that we can construct RAL estimators and the efficient RAL estimator. Since we have identified the efficient score function (the unnormalized efficient influence function), our intention is to utilize the result to form the efficient estimating equation. However, when we get to this step, we face a great hurdle. The description of the efficient score $S_{\text{eff}}$ contains the true form of the nuisance parameter $\eta$, which prevents us from performing any calculation in practice. In fact, looking at the description of $S_{\text{eff}}$ in (9.8) and (9.9), $\eta_0$ appears in the description of the score function $S_\beta$ as well as the conditional expectation calculation $E(\cdot \mid x^*, y)$. Without the availability of $\eta_0$, we are unable to calculate either of these two, hence the efficient score calculation is not feasible.

A natural way to get around this issue is to estimate the nuisance parameter $\eta$, and then carry out the efficient score calculation under the estimated version of $\eta$, say $\widehat{\eta}$, instead of the truth $\eta_0$. This may work, even though it is not necessarily easy to estimate $\eta$. Note that $\eta$ is the pdf of an unobservable covariate $X$, and its estimation is typically through deconvolution and is known to have very slow rate (Carroll and Hall, 1988). When the estimation of $\eta$ is tangled together with the unknown $\beta$ of the model, the estimation procedure may further involve iteration or profiling steps and the resulting convergence property may be harder to analyze. This will further affect the convergence property of the estimation of the parameter of interest $\beta$. It is the potential complexity of both the implementation and the theoretical analysis that triggered us to find an alternative approach while bypassing the estimation of $\eta$.

It is beneficial to stress that if we have a nondegenerate $p$-component consistent estimating function $g(x^*, y, \beta)$ which satisfies $E\{g(X_i^*, Y_i, \beta_0)\} = 0$, then we can construct consistent estimating equations $\sum_{i=1}^n g(X_i^*, Y_i, \beta) = 0$ and solve it to obtain a consistent estimator for $\beta$, even if $g$ is not an influence function or not even in the nuisance tangent space orthogonal complement $\Lambda^\perp$. In other words, our analysis of semiparametrics earlier provides a way to construct consistent estimating function, but it is not necessarily the only way. We thus inspect the results provided in (9.8) and (9.9) and see how to take advantage of them to construct an unbiased estimating function that is not necessarily in $\Lambda^\perp$.

Because the difficulty in utilizing (9.8) to form estimating function lies in the unavailability of $\eta_0$ and in the complexity of estimating $\eta$, the only option left is to adopt a working model of $\eta$ that may not be correct. To reflect the difference between a parameter $\eta$ and a working model of it, we denote the working model $\eta^*$. Note that a working model is a fully specified model and it does not contain any unknown component. If we are bold enough to construct the "efficient score" under the working model, what we obtain will be

$$S_{\text{eff}}^*(x^*, y, \beta) = S_\beta^*(x^*, y, \beta) - E^*\{\mathbf{a}(X) \mid x^*, y\}, \tag{9.10}$$

where $\mathbf{a}(x)$ is a function that satisfies

$$E\{S_\beta^*(X^*, Y, \beta) \mid x\} = E[E^*\{\mathbf{a}(X) \mid X^*, Y\} \mid x]. \tag{9.11}$$

Here, all the functions and operations that are affected by the replace of $\eta$ with $\eta^*$ has been notified with an extra $^*$. For example, the pdf of the observation is

$$f_{X^*,Y}^*(x^*, y, \beta) = \int f_{Y|X}(y, x, \beta) f_{X^*|X}(x^*, x)\eta^*(x)dx,$$

and the score function is

$$\begin{aligned} & S_\beta^*(x^*, y, \beta) \\ = & \frac{\int \partial f_{Y|X}(y, x, \beta)/\partial\beta f_{X^*|X}(x^*, x)\eta^*(x)dx}{\int f_{Y|X}(y, x, \beta) f_{X^*|X}(x^*, x)\eta^*(x)dx} \\ = & \frac{1}{f_{X^*,Y}^*(x^*, y, \beta)} \int \frac{\partial f_{Y|X}(y, x, \beta)/\partial\beta}{f_{Y|X}(y, x, \beta)} f_{Y|X}(y, x, \beta) f_{X^*|X}(x^*, x)\eta^*(x)dx \\ = & E^*\{\partial \log f_{Y|X}(y, X, \beta)/\partial\beta \mid x^*, y\}. \end{aligned}$$

Similarly, $E^*(\mathbf{a}(X) \mid x^*, y\}$ is calculated as

$$E^*\{\mathbf{a}(X) \mid x^*, y\} = \frac{\int \mathbf{a}(x) f_{Y|X}(y, x, \beta) f_{X^*|X}(x^*, x)\eta^*(x)dx}{f_{X^*,Y}^*(x^*, y, \beta)}.$$

A closer inspection of (9.11) reveals a key observation: the unbiasedness of (9.10) is guaranteed by (9.11) alone, regardless of whether $\eta^*$ is the true $\eta_0$ or not. This is clear since the expectation of $S_{\text{eff}}^*$ is directly written as the expectation of the conditional expectation of $S_{\text{eff}}^*$ given $X$, which is guaranteed to vanish because of the requirement (9.11), i.e.,

$$\begin{aligned} E\{S_{\text{eff}}^*(X_i^*, Y_i, \beta_0)\} &= E[E\{S_{\text{eff}}^*(X_i^*, Y_i, \beta_0) \mid X\}] \\ &= E(E\{S_\beta^*(X^*, Y, \beta_0) \mid x\} - E[E^*\{\mathbf{a}(X) \mid X^*, Y\} \mid x]) \\ &= 0. \end{aligned}$$

In fact, the requirement (9.11) directly ensures that $S_{\text{eff}}^*(x^*, y, \beta_0)$ is an element in $\Lambda^\perp$ even though we did not insist this property in our relaxation.

We therefore can devise a practically feasible estimator that is consistent based on the above observation. The procedure is the following.

**Algorithm for measurement error model**

1. Select a working model $\eta^*(x)$ to describe the distribution of $X$. Treat the working model $\eta^*(x)$ as if it were the true pdf of $X$, denote all the quantities or operations affected by the replacement of $\eta_0$ by $\eta^*$.

2. Construct the working score function $S^*_\beta(x^*, y, \beta)$ from $S^*_\beta(x^*, y, \beta) = \partial \log \int f_{Y|X}(y, x, \beta) f_{X^*|X}(x^*, x)\eta^*(x)dx/\partial\beta$.
3. Construct the working efficient score function $S^*_{\text{eff}}$ by forming $S^*_{\text{eff}}(x^*, y, \beta) = S^*_\beta(x^*, y, \beta) - E^*\{\mathbf{a}(X) \mid x^*, y\}$, where $\mathbf{a}(x)$ is a function that satisfies (9.11).
4. Form the estimating equation $\sum_{i=1}^n S^*_{\text{eff}}(x_i^*, y_i, \beta) = 0$ and solve it to obtain the root $\widehat{\beta}$.

### 9.3.3 Implementation

While the algorithm in Section 9.3.2 is clear conceptually, its implementation is not straightforward. The nontrivial component is in extracting the working efficient score function, which does not have an explicit form. In fact, its calculation involves obtaining $\mathbf{a}(x)$ first from solving (9.11), which is a so called Fredholm integral equation of the first type Kress (1999), and is known to be an ill posed problem. Note that solving for $\mathbf{a}(x)$ from (9.11) is a pure numerical analysis problem and it does not involve data.

Our approach to solving (9.11) is through discretization. To this end, we pretend that $\mathbf{a}(x)$ is only supported on a finite set of grid points $x_1, \ldots, x_m$, with weights $\mathbf{a}_1, \ldots, \mathbf{a}_m$ to be determined. We also approximate any integration $\int f(x)\eta^*(x)dx$ using a finite sum $\sum_{j=1}^m f(x_j)\eta^*(x_j)$. Under this approximation, (9.11) is equivalently written as

$$
\begin{aligned}
& E\{S^*_\beta(X^*, Y, \beta) \mid x\} \\
= \quad & E\left\{ \left. \frac{\int \mathbf{a}(x)\eta^*(x) f_{Y|X}(Y, x, \beta) f_{X^*|X}(X^*, x)dx}{\int \eta^*(x) f_{Y|X}(Y, x, \beta) f_{X^*|X}(X^*, x)dx} \right| x \right\} \\
\approx \quad & E\left\{ \left. \frac{\sum_{j=1}^m \mathbf{a}_j \eta^*(x_j) f_{Y|X}(Y, x_j, \beta) f_{X^*|X}(X^*, x_j)}{\sum_{j=1}^m \eta^*(x_j) f_{Y|X}(Y, x_j, \beta) f_{X^*|X}(X^*, x_j)} \right| x \right\} \\
\approx \quad & \sum_{j=1}^m \mathbf{a}_j E\left\{ \left. \frac{\eta^*(x_j) f_{Y|X}(Y, x_j, \beta) f_{X^*|X}(X^*, x_j)}{\sum_{j=1}^m \eta^*(x_j) f_{Y|X}(Y, x_j, \beta) f_{X^*|X}(X^*, x_j)} \right| x \right\}.
\end{aligned}
$$

The above equality holds at all $x$, and thus holds certainly at $x = x_1, \ldots, x_m$. Letting $x = x_1, \ldots, x_m$, we obtain

$$
\begin{aligned}
& \sum_{j=1}^m \mathbf{a}_j E\left\{ \left. \frac{\eta^*(x_j) f_{Y|X}(Y, x_j, \beta) f_{X^*|X}(X^*, x_j)}{\sum_{j=1}^m \eta^*(x_j) f_{Y|X}(Y, x_j, \beta) f_{X^*|X}(X^*, x_j)} \right| x_k \right\} \\
\approx \quad & E\{S^*_\beta(X^*, Y, \beta) \mid x_k\}.
\end{aligned}
$$

This is in fact a linear system of the typical form $\mathbf{aA} = \mathbf{b}$, where $\mathbf{A}$ is an $m \times m$ matrix with its $(j,k)$ entry

$$\mathbf{A}(j,k) = E\left\{ \frac{\eta^*(x_j) f_{Y|X}(Y, x_j, \beta) f_{X^*|X}(X^*, x_j)}{\sum_{j=1}^m \eta^*(x_j) f_{Y|X}(Y, x_j, \beta) f_{X^*|X}(X^*, x_j)} \bigg| x_k \right\},$$

$\mathbf{a} \equiv (\mathbf{a}_1, \ldots, \mathbf{a}_m)$ is an unknown $p \times m$ matrix, and $\mathbf{b} \equiv (\mathbf{b}_1, \ldots, \mathbf{b}_m)$ is a known $p \times m$ matrix with its $k$th column $\mathbf{b}_k = E\{S_\beta^*(X^*, Y, \beta) \mid x_k\}$. We can then easily construct $\mathbf{A}$ and $\mathbf{b}$ and obtain $\mathbf{a} = \mathbf{A}^{-1}\mathbf{b}$. We then insert $\mathbf{a}$ into the working efficient score function to form

$$\begin{aligned} S_{\text{eff}}^*(x_i^*, y_i, \beta) &= S_\beta^*(x_i^*, y_i, \beta) - E^*\{\mathbf{a}(X) \mid x_i^*, y_i\} \\ &= S_\beta^*(x_i^*, y_i, \beta) - \frac{\sum_{j=1}^m \mathbf{a}_j \eta^*(x_j) f_{Y|X}(y_i, x_j, \beta) f_{X^*|X}(x_i^*, x_j)}{\sum_{j=1}^m \eta^*(x_j) f_{Y|X}(y_i, x_j, \beta) f_{X^*|X}(x_i^*, x_j)}, \end{aligned}$$

and subsequently to form and solve the resulting estimating equations. We point out here that the paremeter $\beta$ not only appears in $S_\beta^*$, but also affects the construction of $\mathbf{A}$, $\mathbf{b}$ and subsequently $\mathbf{a}$ and the calculation of $E^*\{\mathbf{a}(X) \mid x^*, y\}$. Thus, in solving the estimating equation via, say Newton Raphson procedure, when evaluating the estimating equation at a candidate $\beta^{(t)}$ value, we have to resolve the linear system and recalculate all these quantities at the current $\beta^{(t)}$ in each iteration.

We have mentioned the ill posedness of the type I Fredholm integral equation. The consequence of the ill poseness is that although more supporting points $m$ indicates a closer approximation to the true function $\mathbf{a}(x)$, we do not necessarily want to use a very large value of $m$. This is because a very large value of $m$ will lead to a linear system that is closer to singularity, a direct consequence of the ill posed problems, which will require further numerical treatment such as penalization, etc. that we will not discuss here. On the other hand, a very small value of $m$ will lead to crude approximation and affect the integrity to the original integral equation. Deciding a suitable $m$ is a difficult problem and is highly problem-dependent. In the limited examples we have handled, $m$ between 10 and 30 usually leads to good results.

### 9.3.4 Theoretical Consequence of the Working Model

The fact that even though we constructed the working efficient score function under a likely misspecified working model $\eta^*$, the resulting estimating function still belongs to the authentic nuisance tangent space orthogonal complement $\Lambda^\perp$ proves to be very useful. It directly results in a simple asymptotic analysis of the estimator devised in Section 9.3.3. Specifically, a direct Taylor expansion leads to

$$\begin{aligned}
0 &= n^{-1/2}\sum_{i=1}^{n} S_{\text{eff}}^{*}(x_i^*, y_i, \widehat{\beta}) \\
&= \frac{1}{\sqrt{n}}\sum_{i=1}^{n} S_{\text{eff}}^{*}(x_i^*, y_i, \beta_0) + \left\{\frac{1}{n}\sum_{i=1}^{n}\frac{\partial S_{\text{eff}}^{*}(x_i^*, y_i, \beta_0)}{\partial \beta^{\text{T}}} + o_p(1)\right\}\sqrt{n}(\widehat{\beta}-\beta_0) \\
&= \frac{1}{\sqrt{n}}\sum_{i=1}^{n} S_{\text{eff}}^{*}(x_i^*, y_i, \beta_0) + \left[E\left\{\frac{\partial S_{\text{eff}}^{*}(X_i^*, Y_i, \beta_0)}{\partial \beta^{\text{T}}}\right\} + o_p(1)\right]\sqrt{n}(\widehat{\beta}-\beta_0) \\
&= \frac{1}{\sqrt{n}}\sum_{i=1}^{n} S_{\text{eff}}^{*}(x_i^*, y_i, \beta_0) - \{E(S_{\text{eff}}^{*}S_{\beta}^{\text{T}}) + o_p(1)\}\sqrt{n}(\widehat{\beta}-\beta_0),
\end{aligned}$$

where the last equality is because $\int S_{\text{eff}}^{*}(x^*, y, \beta)f(x^*, y, \beta)dx^*dy = 0$ for all $\beta$, hence

$$\begin{aligned}
0 &= \frac{\partial}{\partial \beta^{\text{T}}}\int S_{\text{eff}}^{*}(x^*, y, \beta)f(x^*, y, \beta)dx^*dy \\
&= \int \frac{\partial S_{\text{eff}}^{*}(x^*, y, \beta)}{\partial \beta^{\text{T}}}f(x^*, y, \beta)dx^*dy + \int S_{\text{eff}}^{*}(x^*, y, \beta)\frac{\partial f(x^*, y, \beta)}{\partial \beta^{\text{T}}}dx^*dy \\
&= E\left\{\frac{\partial S_{\text{eff}}^{*}(x^*, y, \beta)}{\partial \beta^{\text{T}}}\right\} + E\{S_{\text{eff}}^{*}(x^*, y, \beta)S_{\beta}^{\text{T}}(X^*, Y, \beta)\}.
\end{aligned}$$

We thus have

$$\sqrt{n}(\widehat{\beta}-\beta_0) = n^{-1/2}\sum_{i=1}^{n}\{E(S_{\text{eff}}^{*}S_{\beta}^{\text{T}})\}^{-1} S_{\text{eff}}^{*}(x_i^*, y_i, \beta_0) + o_p(1). \tag{9.12}$$

Because $S_{\text{eff}}^{*}(x_i^*, y_i, \beta_0) \in \Lambda^{\perp}$, $\{E(S_{\text{eff}}^{*}S_{\beta}^{\text{T}})\}^{-1}S_{\text{eff}}^{*}(x_i^*, y_i, \beta_0)$ is indeed an influence function, although it may not be the efficient influence function. The expansion in (9.12) immediately leads to the asymptotic properties of $\widehat{\beta}$ in Theorem 1 below.

**Theorem 1** *When $n \to \infty$, the estimator $\widehat{\beta}$ constructed in Section 9.3.2 satisfies $\sqrt{n}(\widehat{\beta}-\beta_0) \to \text{Normal}(0, V)$ in distribution, where $\mathbf{V} = \{E(S_{\text{eff}}^{*}S_{\beta}^{\text{T}})\}^{-1}var\{S_{\text{eff}}^{*}(X_i^*, Y_i, \beta_0)\}\{E(S_{\beta}S_{\text{eff}}^{*\,\text{T}})\}^{-1}$. When the working model $\eta^* = \eta_0$, $\mathbf{V} = [var\{S_{\text{eff}}(X_i^*, Y_i, \beta_0)\}]^{-1}$ and the estimator is efficient.*

The result of Theorem 1 is more or less self evident hence we skip a formal proof. The efficient result in Theorem 1 makes use of the fact that $E(S_{\text{eff}}^{*}S_{\beta}^{\text{T}}) = E(S_{\text{eff}}^{*}S_{\text{eff}}^{\text{T}})$ since $S_{\text{eff}}^{*} \in \Lambda^{\perp}$. In practice, to perform inference, such as construct confidence intervals and perform hypothesis testing, we need to assess the asymptotic variance $\mathbf{V}$. This can be easily done via

$$\widehat{\mathbf{V}} = \{\widehat{E}(S_{\text{eff}}^{*}S_{\beta}^{\text{T}})\}^{-1}\widehat{\text{var}}\{S_{\text{eff}}^{*}(X_i^*, Y_i, \beta_0)\}\{\widehat{E}(S_{\beta}S_{\text{eff}}^{*\,\text{T}})\}^{-1},$$

where

$$\widehat{E}(S^*_{\text{eff}} S^{\text{T}}_\beta) = n^{-1} \sum_{i=1}^{n} S^*_{\text{eff}}(x^*_i, y_i, \widehat{\beta}) S^{\text{T}}_\beta(x^*_i, y_i, \widehat{\beta});$$

$$\widehat{\text{var}}\{S^*_{\text{eff}}(X^*_i, Y_i, \beta_0)\} = n^{-1} \sum_{i=1}^{n} S^*_{\text{eff}}(x^*_i, y_i, \widehat{\beta}) S^*_{\text{eff}}(x^*_i, y_i, \widehat{\beta})^{\text{T}}.$$

Theorem1 clearly states that regardlessof whether the working model $\eta^*$ equals $\eta_0$ or not, the resulting estimator is always root-$n$ consistent. In addition, it has the added property that if $\eta^* = \eta_0$, the estimator will be efficient. We name such an estimator a locally efficient estimator. In other words, a locally efficient estimator is simply a consistent estimator that has the potential of being efficient.

### 9.3.5 An Example

We now illustrate the performance of the semiparametric approach to measurement error models through a concrete example extracted from Tsiatis and Ma (2004).

Considering a simple regression model, where the binary response $Y$ depends on a single covariate $X$ through a quadratic logistic regression model

$$\text{pr}(Y = 1 \mid X) = \frac{\exp(\beta_c + \beta_1 X + \beta_2 X^2)}{1 + \exp(\beta_c + \beta_1 X + \beta_2 X^2)}.$$

Being a measurement error model, $X$ is not observable, and we observe $X^* = X + U$, where $U$ is independent of $Y$ and $X$ and has a normal distribution with mean zero and variance $\sigma^2_U = 0.4^2$. The parameter of interest is $\beta = (\beta_c, \beta_1, \beta_2)^{\text{T}}$. In generating the data $(x^*_i, y_i)$, we first generate $x_i$ from a normal distribution with mean and variance both 1, and then generate $y_i$ and $x^*_i$ according to the models described above. Note that with $X$ distributed as $N(1, 1)$, $U$ represents a substantial amount of measurement errors. We generated 500 observations to form each data set and repeated the study 1000 times.

To show the performance of the semiparametric estimation procedures in comparison with other approaches, we implemented several estimators. First, we implemented the naive estimator, where we simply ignored the issue of measurement error and treated $x^*_i$ as $x_i$ and performed a straightforward MLE to fit the quadratic logistic model. We then also implemented the regression calibration estimation procedures. A regression calibration requires to replace $x_i, x_i^2$ with $E(X_i \mid x^*_i)$, $E(X^2_i \mid x^*_i)$ and then treat $E(X_i \mid x^*_i)$, $E(X^2_i \mid x^*_i)$ as the covariate and its square and perform a quadratic logistic regression based on $\{E(X_i \mid x^*_i), E(X^2_i \mid x^*_i), y_i\}, i = 1, \ldots, n$. It is easy to see that to calculate $E(X_i \mid x^*_i)$ and $E(X^2_i \mid x^*_i)$, one needs a model for $\eta(x)$ since $E(X_i \mid x^*_i) = \int x\eta(x) f_{X^*|X}(x^*_i, x)dx / \int \eta(x) f_{X^*|X}(x^*_i, x)dx$ and

$E(X_i^2 \mid x_i^*) = \int x^2\eta(x)f_{X^*|X}(x_i^*, x)dx / \int \eta(x)f_{X^*|X}(x_i^*, x)dx$. We thus experimented with two working models of $\eta$. In the first case, we set the working model to be identical to the truth, i.e. $\eta^* = \eta_0$, which is the normal distribution with mean and variance both 1, while in the second case, we set the working model to be a uniform distribution supported on $[-2, 4]$. Finally, we also implemented the semiparametric methods. Recall that the semiparametric methods also require a working model $\eta^*$, and we experimented exactly the same two working models as in the regression calibration estimators. In the implementation of the semiparametric methods, we used $m = 15$ discretization points evenly distributed on Carroll and Hall (1988) and Tsiatis (2006), which is 3 times standard deviations from the center. In fact, we found the results to be insensitive to the number of discretization points $m$ as long as $m$ is between 7 and 20. In order to construct $\mathbf{A}$ and $\mathbf{b}$ in Section 9.3.3, we also have to evaluate the integrals with respect to $w$, which we calculated via Hermite quadrature methods. The final results of the $\beta$ estimation are presented in the left half of Table 9.1, where the values in the parentheses are the true parameter values.

We further extended the simulation by considering an exponential measurement $U$ with mean $\mu_U = 0.4$. This allows investigation of the consequences of an asymmetric measurement error, which is also a substantial amount given that $X \sim N(1, 1)$. All other aspects of the data generation are identical to the normal measurement error case. In performing the estimation, we still used $m = 15$ discretization points, while we used Laguerre quadrature to evaluate the integrals in order to adapt to the exponential measurement error. The results of the simulation are given in the right half of Table 9.1.

In Table 9.1, the covariance matrix of the semiparametric estimator was estimated using the results presented in Theorem 1, and the 95% confidence intervals were constructed using the estimate $\pm$ 1.96 estimated standard error. Similar approaches were used to calculate the estimated variances and 95% confidence interval coverage rates for the naive and both regression calibration estimators.

The results of the simulations summarized in Table 9.1 are encouraging and unsurprising. The naive estimators for $\beta$ are severely biased whereas the semiparametric estimators all provide good results. These estimators exhibit little bias, the average of the estimated variances closely approximates the Monte-Carlo variance, and the percentage of times that the estimated 95% confidence interval covers the true value is close to the nominal level. Of particular interest is that the results appear insensitive to misspecification of $\eta(x)$. The efficiency when using the misspecified uniform distribution is virtually identical to that when using the correct normal distribution for the normal measurement error example, and there is only a slight loss of efficiency for the exponential error example. We found this to be the case in all of the many simulations we conducted. When we used the correct distribution for $X$, the regression calibration estimators showed a slight bias. However, use of the same misspecification for the distribution of $X$ as that for the

**TABLE 9.1**
Bias, variance and coverage probabilities of the naive, regression calibration and locally efficient semiparametric estimators for the quadratic logistic regression model with normal and exponential measurement error

| | $\beta_0$(-1) | $\beta_1$(0.7) | $\beta_2$(0.7) | $\beta_0$(-1) true | $\beta_1$(0.7) | $\beta_2$(0.7) |
|---|---|---|---|---|---|---|
| true | -1 | 0.7 | 0.7 | -1 | 0.7 | 0.7 |
| | naive estimator | | | | | |
| | normal errors | | | exponential errors | | |
| mean | -0.970 | 0.400 | 0.480 | -0.990 | 0.370 | 0.480 |
| var | 0.021 | 0.028 | 0.007 | 0.022 | 0.033 | 0.008 |
| $\widehat{\text{var}}$ | 0.020 | 0.027 | 0.007 | 0.020 | 0.022 | 0.006 |
| 95%CI | 94.0% | 53.0% | 24.0% | 93.0% | 40.0% | 25.0% |
| | regression calibration (true) | | | | | |
| | normal errors | | | exponential errors | | |
| mean | -0.970 | 0.630 | 0.640 | -0.990 | 0.640 | 0.660 |
| var | 0.023 | 0.046 | 0.012 | 0.022 | 0.048 | 0.013 |
| $\widehat{\text{var}}$ | 0.022 | 0.046 | 0.012 | 0.022 | 0.045 | 0.012 |
| 95%CI | 94.0% | 94.0% | 89.0% | 95.0% | 93.0% | 90.0% |
| | regression calibration (mis) | | | | | |
| | normal errors | | | exponential errors | | |
| mean | -1.030 | 0.440 | 0.490 | -1.070 | 0.370 | 0.480 |
| var | 0.021 | 0.027 | 0.007 | 0.022 | 0.031 | 0.008 |
| $\widehat{\text{var}}$ | 0.020 | 0.029 | 0.007 | 0.021 | 0.022 | 0.006 |
| 95%CI | 94.0% | 64.0% | 31.0% | 92.0% | 40.0% | 24.0% |
| | semiparametric estimator (true) | | | | | |
| | normal errors | | | exponential errors | | |
| mean | -1.000 | 0.720 | 0.720 | -1.010 | 0.690 | 0.700 |
| var | .026 | 0.068 | 0.022 | 0.024 | 0.064 | 0.017 |
| $\widehat{\text{var}}$ | 0.026 | 0.070 | 0.022 | 0.026 | 0.070 | 0.018 |
| 95%CI | 95.0% | 96.0% | 95.0% | 95.0% | 94.0% | 94.0% |
| | semiparametric estimator (mis) | | | | | |
| | normal errors | | | exponential errors | | |
| mean | -1.000 | 0.720 | 0.720 | -1.000 | 0.680 | 0.690 |
| var | 0.027 | 0.068 | 0.022 | 0.023 | 0.073 | 0.020 |
| $\widehat{\text{var}}$ | 0.026 | 0.070 | 0.022 | 0.024 | 0.077 | 0.021 |
| 95%CI | 94.0% | 96.0% | 95.0% | 95.0% | 94.0% | 93.0% |

rc (true) and rc (mis) denote the regression calibration estimators derived under the true distribution and misspecified distribution of $X$, respectively; semi (true) and semi(mis) denote the locally efficient semiparametric estimators derived under the true distribution and misspecified distribution of $X$, respectively; var is the empirical Monte-Carlo variance of the estimators; $\widehat{\text{var}}$ is the average of the estimated variances; CI is the proportion of the simulations whose estimated 95% confidence intervals cover the true value of the parameters.

semiparametric estimators resulted in regression calibration estimators that were severely biased.

Finally, we point out that we used a quadratic logistic model to illustrate the usefulness of the semiparametric method, because in this case, prior to the semiparametric estimation, there is no consistent estimator in the literature as far as we are aware. This reflects the utility and promise of the semiparametric approach to measurement error models.

## 9.4 Measurement Error and Misclassification

Having understood the semiparametric treatment to the measurement error model in (9.2), it is then straightforward to adapt the similar semiparametric ideas to handle the additional misclassification issue in (9.3). To this end, let $\boldsymbol{\theta} = (\beta^{\mathrm{T}}, \boldsymbol{\alpha}^{\mathrm{T}})^{\mathrm{T}}$ and treat $\boldsymbol{\theta}$ in (9.3) as the parameter of interest, with its role similar to that of $\beta$ in (9.2). We then proceed with the similar type of analysis as in Section 9.3.

More specifically, taking a parametric submodel of $\eta(x,z)$, say $(1-\gamma)\eta_0(x,z)+\gamma f_{X|Z}(x,z)$, where $f_{X|Z}(x,z)$ is an arbitrary valid pdf of $X$ conditional on $Z$, leads to a nuisance score function of the form

$$\frac{\partial \log f_{X^*,T,Y|S}(x^*,\mathbf{t},s,y,\boldsymbol{\theta},\gamma)}{\partial\gamma} = \frac{\begin{array}{l}\sum_z \int f_{Y|X,Z,S}(y,x,z,s,\beta) f_{X^*|X}(x^*,x) f_{T|Z}(\mathbf{t},z)\{f_{X|Z}(x,z) \\ \quad -\eta_0(x,z)\} f_Z(z,\boldsymbol{\alpha})dx\end{array}}{f_{X^*,T,Y|S}(x^*,\mathbf{t},s,y,\boldsymbol{\theta},\gamma)}.$$

At $\gamma=\gamma_0=0$, this leads to $\partial \log f_{X^*,T,Y|S}(x^*,\mathbf{t},s,y,\boldsymbol{\theta},\gamma)/\partial\gamma = E[\{f_{X|Z}(X,Z)/\eta_0(X,Z)-1\} \mid x^*,\mathbf{t},s,y]$. Given that $f_{X|Z}(x,z)$ can be any conditional pdf, the general form of the nuisance tangent space is then conjectured to be

$$\Gamma \equiv [E\{\mathbf{a}(X,Z)\mid x^*,\mathbf{t},s,y\} : E\{\mathbf{a}(X,Z)\} = E\{\mathbf{a}(X,Z)\mid S\} = 0].$$

Through adopting a specific parametric submodel $\eta_0(x,z)\{1+\gamma^{\mathrm{T}}\mathbf{a}(x,z)\}$, we can then show that $\Gamma \subset \Lambda$ in a similar way as in Section 9.3.1. On the other hand, for any element $\sum_{k=1}^K \mathbf{A}_k \partial \log f_{X^*,T,Y|S}(x^*,\mathbf{t},s,y,\beta,\gamma_k)/\partial\gamma_k$ in $\Lambda$, we can also show that the element is a valid member of $\Gamma$ hence show $\Lambda \subset \Gamma$. We thus can establish $\Lambda = \Gamma$. It is also not difficult to verify that the nuisance tangent space orthogonal complement in this case is

$$\Lambda^{\perp} = [\underline{(X^*,T,S,Y)} : E\{\underline{(X^*,T,S,Y)} \mid X,Z,S\} = 0].$$

We subsequently calculate the score function and the efficient score function to be

$$S_{\boldsymbol{\theta}}(x^*, \mathbf{t}, s, y, \boldsymbol{\theta}, \eta) = E\{\partial \log\{f_{Y|X,Z,S}(y, X, Z, s, \beta) f_Z(Z, \boldsymbol{\alpha})\}/\partial\boldsymbol{\theta} \mid x^*, \mathbf{t}, s, y\}$$
$$S_{\text{eff}}(x^*, \mathbf{t}, s, y, \boldsymbol{\theta}, \eta) = S_{\boldsymbol{\theta}}(x^*, \mathbf{t}, s, y, \boldsymbol{\theta}, \eta) - E\{\mathbf{a}(X, Z) \mid x^*, \mathbf{t}, s, y\},$$

where $\mathbf{a}(X, Z)$ satisfies

$$E\{S_{\boldsymbol{\theta}}(X^*, T, S, Y, \boldsymbol{\theta}, \eta) \mid x, z, s\} = E[E\{\mathbf{a}(X, Z) \mid X^*, T, S, Y\} \mid x, z, s]. \quad (9.13)$$

We skip the details of these calculations as they are very similar to those in Section 9.3.1.

Also as in Section 9.3.1, we carry out all the calculation above under a working model $\eta^*(x, z)$ in order to facilitate the implementation. We can show that this results in a locally efficient semiparametric estimator. This estimator will remain consistent regardless of the working model, and will be efficient if the working model is identical to the true $\eta_0(x, z)$. The implementation procedure is however somewhat different from the one described in Section 9.3.3 due to the presence of $T$ and $S$ as we now describe.

**Algorithm for measurement error model with misclassification**

1. Select a working model $\eta^*(x, z)$ to describe the distribution of $X$ given $z$. Because $z$ is categorical, this in fact implies select $q$ working models, each corresponding to the different vector value that $Z$ can be. Here $q$ is the total number of different vector values $Z$ can be.

   Treat the working model $\eta^*(x, z)$ as if it were the true pdf of $X$ conditional on $Z$, denote all the quantities or operations affected by the replacement of $\eta_0$ by $\eta^*$.

2. Construct the "score function" $S^*_{\boldsymbol{\theta}}(x^*, \mathbf{t}, s, y, \boldsymbol{\theta})$ from $S^*_{\boldsymbol{\theta}}(x^*, \mathbf{t}, s, y, \boldsymbol{\theta}) = \partial \log \sum_z \int f_{Y|X,Z,S}(y, x, z, s, \beta) f_{X^*|X}(x^*, x) \eta^*(x, z) f_Z(z, \boldsymbol{\alpha}) dx / \partial\boldsymbol{\theta}$.

3. Construct the "efficient score function" $S^*_{\text{eff}}$ by forming $S^*_{\text{eff}}(x^*, \mathbf{t}, s, y, \boldsymbol{\theta}) = S^*_{\boldsymbol{\theta}}(x^*, \mathbf{t}, s, y, \boldsymbol{\theta}) - E^*\{\mathbf{a}(X, Z) \mid x^*, \mathbf{t}, s, y\}$, where $\mathbf{a}(x, z)$ is a function that satisfies (9.13).

   The integral equation described in (9.13) needs to be solved separately at each observed $s_i$ value at each iteration of $\boldsymbol{\theta}$.

4. Form the estimating equation $\sum_{i=1}^n S^*_{\text{eff}}(x_i^*, \mathbf{t}_i, s_i, y_i, \boldsymbol{\theta}) = 0$ and solve it to obtain the root $\widehat{\boldsymbol{\theta}}$.

The computation cost of the procedure is relatively high, mostly because we have to solve $n$ integral equations corresponding to the $n$ different $s_i$ values in each Newton-Raphson iteration when solving for $\boldsymbol{\theta}$, where $n$ is the sample size. Note that at each fixed $s$ value, we solve the integral equation (9.13) separately while such equations at other $s$ values, hence a better notation of $\mathbf{a}(X, Z)$ is $\mathbf{a}(X, Z, s)$. When $S$ is categorical, some simplification may be possible by considering the different vector values that $S$ can be and compare it with the sample size $n$ and opt for the smaller one.

We now highlight an example given originally in Yi et al. (2015) to demonstrate the performance of the semiparametric estimators. For comparison, we included two pseudo-MLE and also include two approximate methods, augmented regression calibration and augmented SIMEX. The pseudo MLE, the augmented regression calibration as well as the semiparametric estimators all need a working model for $\eta(X, Z)$. We set these working models to be both correct and misspecified models $\eta^*(x, z)$ that are identical in all these constructions for fair comparison. The sample size is taken as $n = 1000$. One thousand simulations are run for each parameter configuration.

The true covariates $X_i$ were independently generated from the uniform distribution on $[-3.0, 4.0]$, and the discrete variables $Z_i$ and $S_i$ were independently simulated from a Bernoulli distribution with success probability 0.5. We generated $X_i^*$ from the model $X_i^* = X_i + U_i$, where $X_i^*$ is a centered normal random error with standard deviation half of that of $X_i$, and we generated $T_i$ from the Bernoulli distribution with the probability of misclassification 0.2 under both $Z_i = 0$ and $Z_i = 1$. We generated the response $Y_i$ from the logistic regression model

$$\text{logit}\{\text{pr}(Y_i = 1 \mid X_i, Z_i, S_i)\} = \beta_0 + \beta_z Z_i + \beta_x X_i + \beta_s S_i, \tag{9.14}$$

with the true parameter values set as $\beta = (\beta_0, \beta_z, \beta_x, \beta_s)^{\text{T}} = (0.1, -1.0, 0.7, 0.5)^{\text{T}}$, $i = 1, \cdots, n$. We then discarded $(X_i, Z_i), i = 1, \ldots, n$. Thus, the simulated data included data $\{(Y_i, X_i^*, T_i, S_i) : i = 1, \cdots, n\}$. Because $Z_i$ is binary, the parameter $\alpha$ is simply the probability of $Z_i = 1$. For simplicity, we set $\alpha = 0.5$ to be known.

The results of the above mentioned seven different methods are reported in Figure 9.1 and Table 9.2, where the estimated standard errors ($\widehat{\text{sd}}$) were calculated using asymptotic results similar to those given in Theorem 1, with all the associated quantities evaluated at the estimated parameter values. From these results, we can see that when the latent variable distribution model $\eta(x, z)$ is correctly specified, the pseudo-likelihood method has the best performance in terms of both estimation bias and variability. However, as soon as this model was misspecified, for example, here we misspecified the uniform distribution as normal, the pseudo-likelihood method showed severe bias. In contrast, the semiparametric method retained a small bias regardless of the correctness of the model specification, and the inference results were also quite precise judging from the close match between the sample and estimated standard deviations and the 95% confidence interval coverage rate and its nominal value. The two approximate methods, augmented regression calibration and augmented SIMEX, both reduced the estimation bias somewhat, but did not fully produce a consistent estimator, judging from the nontrivial sample biases.

The second half of the example is similar to the first half, except that we now generate the latent variable from a normal distribution, and we increased

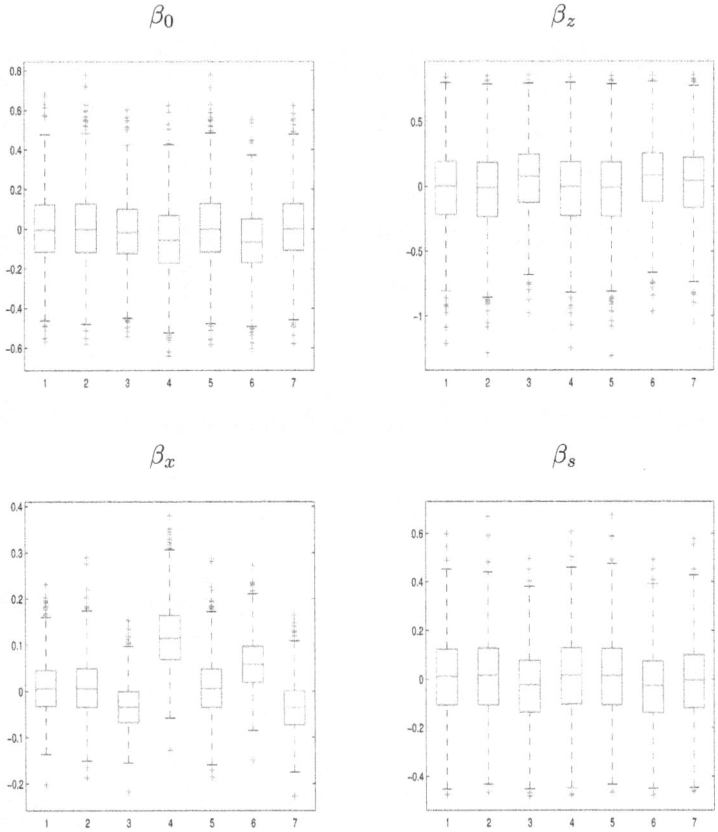


**FIGURE 9.1**
Boxplots of the biases of the seven estimators for $\beta_0$, $\beta_z$, $\beta_x$ and $\beta_s$ in first half simulation of Section 9.4. The seven estimators are respectively pseudo-likelihood (1) , estimating function (2) and regression calibration (3) estimators under uniform distribution model for $X$, pseudo-likelihood (4), estimating function (5) and regression calibration (6) estimators under normal distribution model for $X$, and SIMEX estimator (7).

**TABLE 9.2**

Results in first half simulation of Section 9.4 based on 1,000 data sets, $m = 500, n = 1000$ and $X$ is normal. Mean (est), standard deviation (sd), the average of the estimated standard deviation ($\widehat{\text{sd}}$) and 95% confidence interval coverage are reported for likelihood methods, estimating function methods, regression calibration methods, all based on both uniform and normal latent variable distribution models. SIMEX estimation results are reported in the left last block. The true latent variable distribution is uniform.

| | $\beta_0$ | $\beta_z$ | $\beta_x$ | $\beta_s$ | $\beta_0$ | $\beta_z$ | $\beta_x$ | $\beta_s$ |
|---|---|---|---|---|---|---|---|---|
| true | 0.1 | -1.0 | 0.7 | 0.5 | 0.1 | -1.0 | 0.7 | 0.5 |
| | maximum likelihood | | | | | | | |
| | uniform | | | | normal | | | |
| est | 0.101 | -1.012 | 0.707 | 0.511 | 0.049 | -1.019 | 0.818 | 0.516 |
| sd | 0.184 | 0.303 | 0.060 | 0.170 | 0.184 | 0.305 | 0.073 | 0.172 |
| $\widehat{\text{sd}}$ | 0.183 | 0.299 | 0.060 | 0.166 | 0.184 | 0.300 | 0.073 | 0.168 |
| 95%CI | 95.2% | 94.8% | 95.7% | 95.4% | 94.1% | 94.9% | 67.3% | 95.4% |
| | estimating function | | | | | | | |
| | uniform | | | | normal | | | |
| est | 0.107 | -1.027 | 0.709 | 0.511 | 0.107 | -1.027 | 0.709 | 0.511 |
| sd | 0.194 | 0.313 | 0.064 | 0.176 | 0.194 | 0.314 | 0.066 | 0.176 |
| $\widehat{\text{sd}}$ | 0.185 | 0.300 | 0.063 | 0.174 | 0.185 | 0.300 | 0.063 | 0.174 |
| 95%CI | 93.8% | 94.5% | 95.6% | 95.8% | 93.8% | 94.4% | 95.2% | 95.9% |
| | regression calibration | | | | | | | |
| | uniform | | | | normal | | | |
| est | 0.088 | -0.936 | 0.666 | 0.472 | 0.039 | -0.930 | 0.759 | 0.472 |
| sd | 0.170 | 0.277 | 0.050 | 0.157 | 0.168 | 0.274 | 0.058 | 0.157 |
| $\widehat{\text{sd}}$ | 0.169 | 0.273 | 0.050 | 0.153 | 0.167 | 0.270 | 0.057 | 0.153 |
| 95%CI | 95.2% | 93.4% | 88.3% | 94.9% | 93.2% | 93.3% | 84.4% | 94.8% |
| | simulation extrapolation | | | | | | | |
| est | 0.103 | -0.970 | 0.665 | 0.495 | 0.103 | -0.970 | 0.665 | 0.495 |
| sd | 0.178 | 0.287 | 0.055 | 0.165 | 0.178 | 0.287 | 0.055 | 0.165 |

the measurement error in $X_i$ so that the standard deviation of $U$ is about 90% of that of $X_i$. All other aspects of the data generation procedure remain unchanged. The corresponding results are given in Figure 9.2 and Table 9.3. As it can be clearly seen, similar conclusions can be drawn as in the first half.

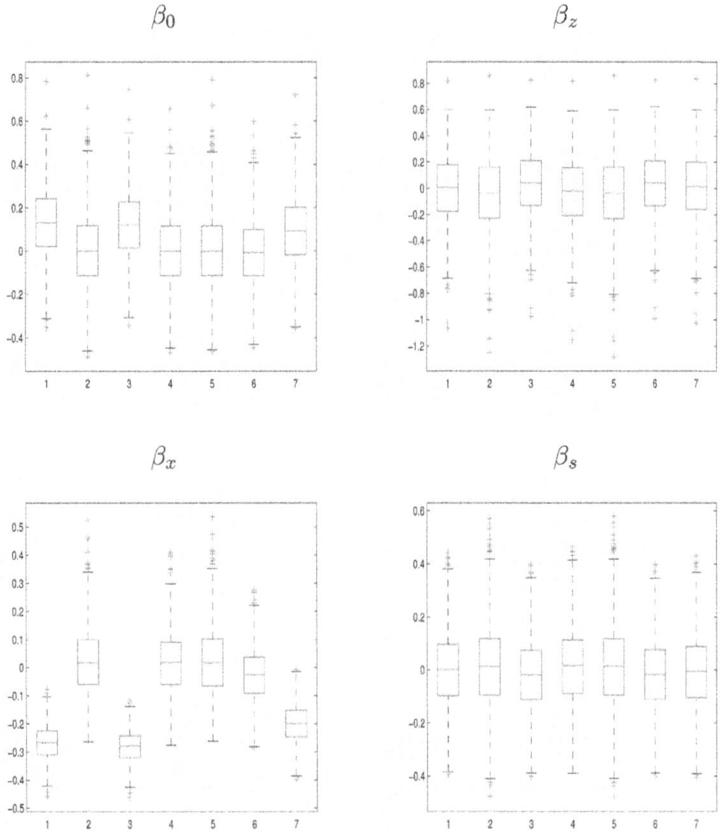


**FIGURE 9.2**

Boxplots of the biases of the seven estimators for $\beta_0$, $\beta_z$, $\beta_x$ and $\beta_s$ in second half simulation of Section 9.4. The seven estimators are respectively pseudo-likelihood (1) , estimating function (2) and regression calibration (3) estimators under uniform distribution model for $X$, pseudo-likelihood (4), estimating function (5) and regression calibration (6) estimators under normal distribution model for $X$, and SIMEX estimator (7).

**TABLE 9.3**
Results in second half simulation of Section 9.4 based on 1,000 data sets, $m = 500, n = 1000$ and $X$ is uniform. Mean (est), standard deviation (sd), the average of the estimated standard deviation ($\widehat{\text{sd}}$) and 95% confidence interval coverage are reported for likelihood methods, estimating function methods, regression calibration methods, all based on both uniform and normal latent variable distribution models. SIMEX estimation results are reported in the left last block. The true latent variable distribution is normal.

| | $\beta_0$ | $\beta_z$ | $\beta_x$ | $\beta_s$ | $\beta_0$ | $\beta_z$ | $\beta_x$ | $\beta_s$ |
|---|---|---|---|---|---|---|---|---|
| true | 0.1 | -1.0 | 0.7 | 0.5 | 0.1 | -1.0 | 0.7 | 0.5 |
| | maximum likelihood | | | | | | | |
| | uniform | | | | normal | | | |
| est | 0.231 | -1.008 | 0.433 | 0.500 | 0.100 | -1.034 | 0.721 | 0.514 |
| sd | 0.158 | 0.256 | 0.061 | 0.146 | 0.166 | 0.265 | 0.113 | 0.151 |
| $\widehat{\text{sd}}$ | 0.161 | 0.257 | 0.060 | 0.146 | 0.167 | 0.266 | 0.109 | 0.150 |
| 95%CI | 89.6% | 96.0% | 1.8% | 94.7% | 95.8% | 96.1% | 95.3% | 94.5% |
| | estimating function | | | | | | | |
| | uniform | | | | normal | | | |
| est | 0.104 | -1.049 | 0.723 | 0.513 | 0.104 | -1.049 | 0.724 | 0.514 |
| sd | 0.177 | 0.284 | 0.122 | 0.166 | 0.178 | 0.284 | 0.129 | 0.167 |
| $\widehat{\text{sd}}$ | 0.170 | 0.271 | 0.118 | 0.161 | 0.170 | 0.272 | 0.118 | 0.161 |
| 95%CI | 94.5% | 95.9% | 95.7% | 94.8% | 94.1% | 95.7% | 93.9% | 94.6% |
| | regression calibration | | | | | | | |
| | uniform | | | | normal | | | |
| est | 0.221 | -0.968 | 0.419 | 0.480 | 0.093 | -0.967 | 0.675 | 0.481 |
| sd | 0.152 | 0.244 | 0.055 | 0.140 | 0.156 | 0.244 | 0.094 | 0.140 |
| $\widehat{\text{sd}}$ | 0.155 | 0.245 | 0.054 | 0.140 | 0.156 | 0.245 | 0.088 | 0.140 |
| 95%CI | 90.2% | 95.5% | 0% | 94.1% | 95.9% | 95.5% | 91.6% | 94.2% |
| | simulation extrapolation | | | | | | | |
| est | 0.191 | -0.992 | 0.500 | 0.492 | 0.191 | -0.992 | 0.500 | 0.492 |
| sd | 0.157 | 0.252 | 0.068 | 0.145 | 0.157 | 0.252 | 0.068 | 0.145 |

## 9.5 Conclusion

A geometric approach to the semiparametric model analysis is a rather universal and powerful tool. Our illustration has shown its usefulness in handling measurement error models with or without misclassifications. Here we point out that measurement error models can be viewed as a special case of the latent variable models, hence it is not surprising that the method may also work in more general latent variable models. Nonetheless, general as the approach might be, its development in a specific problem often involves mathematical treatment which can sometimes be quite technical. The success of the approach often requires nontrivial analytic tools and problem-specific insight. Such a process can be challenging and rewarding simultaneously, and is something that makes research entertaining and exciting.

## Bibliography

Bickel, P. J., Klaassen, C. A., Ritov, Y. and Wellner, J. A. (1993). *Efficient and Adaptive Estimation for Semiparametric Models.* Johns Hopkins University Press, Baltimore, MD.

Carroll, R. J. and Hall, P. (1988). Optimal rates of convergence for deconvolving a density. *Journal of American Statistical Association*, 83, 1184-1186.

Kress, R. (1999). *Linear Integral Equation.* Springer, New York.

Tsiatis, A. A. (2006). *Semiparametric Theory and Missing Data.* Springer, New York, NY.

Tsiatis, A. A. and Ma, Y. (2004). Locally efficient semiparametric estimators for functional measurement error models. *Biometrika*, 91, 835-848.

Yi, G. Y., Ma, Y., Spiegelman, D. and Carroll, R. J. (2015). Functional and structural methods with mixed measurement error and misclassification in covariates. *Journal of the American Statistical Association*, 110, 681-696.

# Part IV

# Nonparametric Inference

# 10

# *Deconvolution Kernel Density Estimation*

**Aurore Delaigle**

## CONTENTS



DOI: 10.1201/9781315101279-10

## 10.1 Introduction

In this chapter, we consider nonparametric estimation of the density $f_X$ of a variable $X$ which is observed with an independent additive noise $U$ of known distribution. This problem has received a lot of attention in the literature, and the most popular estimator is the deconvolution kernel density estimator. In this chapter, we introduce this estimator and study some of its theoretical and practical properties. We also discuss some extensions and related problems. Alternative nonparametric procedures of density deconvolution are discussed in Chapter 11 (Kang and Qiu, 2021) and the case where the error distribution is unknown is studied in Chapter 12 (Delaigle and Van Keilegom, 2021). The regression case is discussed in Chapter 14 (Apanasovich and Liang, 2021).

This chapter is organised as follows. We introduce the classical measurement error model in Section 10.2 and the deconvolution kernel density estimator in Section 10.3. In Section 10.4 we discuss some of its $L_2$ theoretical properties. These depend heavily on the smoothness of the error distribution, and we introduce two types of errors usually considered in the literature: ordinary smooth and supersmooth errors. We compute the mean integrated squared error of the estimator for the two types of errors and study its rates of convergence for various levels of smoothness of the density $f_X$. Computing the deconvolution kernel density estimator in practice requires to choose a kernel function and a smoothing parameter called bandwidth. We discuss the impact of those choices in Section 10.5, where we also present some of the numerical issues that can be encountered when computing the deconvolution kernel density estimator. The choice of the bandwidth is particularly important: in order for the estimator to work well, the bandwidth must be selected in a carefully designed data-driven way. We dedicate Section 10.6 to several data-driven procedures of bandwidth selection. Finally, we discuss generalisations of the classical problem in Section 10.7 to the cases where the data are dependent or multivariate, where the measurement errors are not identically distributed and the characteristic function of the errors vanishes at some isolated points. We also show that in some cases, it is possible to compute the estimator using a simple analytic formula.

## 10.2 Model and Data

In the classical measurement error problem, we are interested in a variable $X$ but can only observe independent and identically distribution (i.i.d.) data $X_1^*, \ldots, X_n^*$ from a noisy version $X^*$ of $X$. The variable $X^*$ comes from the classical measurement error model

$$X^* = X + U\,, \tag{10.1}$$

where $U$ represents a measurement error independent of $X$, and which has density $f_U$. There are many applications where it is reasonable to assume that the noisy data come from (10.1), but often the model holds after transformation. For example, (10.1) is often employed for measured food consumption in nutrition studies. In those studies, food intake is often obtained from 24 hour recalls, where individuals report their food intake of the last 24 hours. It is common to assume that the model at (10.1) holds for $X^* = \log(\text{reported intake from 24 hour recalls})$. There, $X$ is the logarithm of the usual intake, which can be roughly described as the average intake of an individual over a long period of time. In this chapter, we follow the literature on nonparametric deconvolution and ignore such transformations; that is, we assume that the data come directly from (10.1). For comprehensive reviews of the measurement error problem and techniques in the parametric context, see Carroll et al. (2006) and Buonaccorsi (2010).

Throughout this chapter we assume that the error density $f_U$ is known and is an even function. It is possible to deal with the case where $f_U$ is unknown, as long as it can be estimated nonparametrically, either from a sample from $f_U$ (Diggle and Hall, 1993; Neumann, 1997), from replicated noisy measurements of all or some of the individuals (Delaigle et al., 2008), or even without additional data but under some conditions that permit its identifiability (Delaigle and Hall, 2016); it will be the topic of Chapter 12 (Delaigle and Van Keilegom, 2021), where we will also discuss parametric and semiparametric procedures for estimating $f_U$.

## 10.3 Deconvolution Kernel Density Estimator

In measurement error problems, it is often of interest to estimate the density $f_X$ of $X$ from data $X_1^*, \ldots, X_n^*$ coming from (10.1). For example, if $X$ represents the usual intake of a nutrient, knowing its density can help understand the food consumption of individuals in a population. The most popular nonparametric estimator of $f_X$ in this context is the deconvolution kernel density estimator of Stefanski and Carroll (1990) and Carroll and Hall (1988). It is constructed by noting that under (10.1), we have

$$\varphi_{X^*} = \varphi_X\, \varphi_U\,,$$

where throughout this chapter we use $\varphi_T(t) = E(e^{iTt})$ to denote the characteristic function of a variable $T$ or the Fourier transform $\int e^{itx} T(x)\, dx$ of an absolutely integrable function $T$, and $i$ denotes the complex number such that

$i^2 = -1$. Therefore, if $\varphi_U(t) \neq 0$ for all $t \in \mathbb{R}$, then $\varphi_X = \varphi_X^*/\varphi_U$, and by the Fourier inversion theorem, we deduce that

$$f_X(x) = \frac{1}{2\pi}\int e^{-itx}\varphi_X(t)\,dt = \frac{1}{2\pi}\int e^{-itx}\frac{\varphi_X^*(t)}{\varphi_U(t)}\,dt\,. \tag{10.2}$$

Since $f_U$ is known, then $\varphi_U$ is known and the only unknown in the second integral at (10.2) is $\varphi_X^*(t)$, which can be easily estimated by the empirical characteristic function $\hat{\varphi}_{X^*}(t) = n^{-1}\sum_{j=1}^n e^{itX_j^*}$. It is tempting to construct an estimator of $f_X(x)$ by plugging $\hat{\varphi}_{X^*}$ into that integral. However, $\hat{\varphi}_{X^*}(t)$ is very unreliable in the tails, i.e., for large $|t|$, whereas $\varphi_U(t) \to 0$ as $|t| \to \infty$; as a result, $\hat{\varphi}_X^*(t)/\varphi_U(t)$ is not integrable. To overcome these unreliable tail fluctuations, Stefanski and Carroll (1990) and Carroll and Hall (1988) introduced a weight function $w(t)$, which is such that $w(t)$ is close to one when $\hat{\varphi}_X^*(t)$ is reliable, and close to zero elsewhere. Specifically, they took

$$\hat{f}_X(x) = \frac{1}{2\pi}\int e^{-itx}\frac{\hat{\varphi}_X^*(t)w(t)}{\varphi_U(t)}\,dt\,,$$

where $w(t) = \varphi_K(ht)$, with a smoothing parameter $h > 0$, called bandwidth, and a univariate smooth function $K$ that integrates to 1, called kernel.

Thus, the deconvolution kernel density estimator of Stefanski and Carroll (1990) and Carroll and Hall (1988) is defined by

$$\hat{f}_X(x;h) = \frac{1}{2\pi}\int e^{-itx}\hat{\varphi}_X^*(t)\frac{\varphi_K(ht)}{\varphi_U(t)}\,dt \tag{10.3}$$

$$= \frac{1}{nh}\sum_{j=1}^n K_U\Big(\frac{x - X_j^*}{h}\Big)\,, \tag{10.4}$$

where the deconvolution kernel $K_U$ is defined by

$$K_U(x) = \frac{1}{2\pi}\int e^{-itx}\frac{\varphi_K(t)}{\varphi_U(t/h)}\,dt\,. \tag{10.5}$$

The following conditions guarantee that this estimator is well defined:

$$\varphi_U(t) \neq 0 \text{ for all } t\,; \tag{10.6}$$

$$\int |\varphi_X(t)|\,dt < \infty; \tag{10.7}$$

$$\sup_{t\in\mathbb{R}} |\varphi_K(t)/\varphi_U(t/h)| < \infty \quad \text{and} \quad \int |\varphi_K(t)/\varphi_U(t/h)|\,dt < \infty\,. \tag{10.8}$$

Liu and Taylor (1989) discussed a variant of this estimator where they truncated the domain of the integral at (10.5) to an interval $[-M_n, M_n]$, where $M_n \to \infty$ as $n \to \infty$. However, such truncation is not needed when $\varphi_K$ is compactly supported (something very common in the deconvolution problem, see Section 10.5.2), in which case their estimator reduces to the deconvolution kernel density estimator. Even when $\varphi_K$ is not compactly supported, the advantage of using two parameters ($h$ and $M_n$) is unclear, as reflected by the numerical results in Liu and Taylor (1990), who found that better results were often obtained by taking $h = 0$ when $M_n$ was positive. Another variant of the deconvolution kernel estimator that is consistent under the $L_1$ norm was introduced by Devroye (1989), and Zhang (1990) studied a closely related problem of estimation of mixing densities.

Although in principle the weight function $w(t)$ above could take various forms, taking $w(t) = \varphi_K(ht)$ has several useful interpretations. First, when $U \equiv 0$, that is when there are no errors and $\varphi_U(t) = 1$ for all $t$, this estimator reduces to the standard kernel density estimator; indeed, in that case (10.3) reduces to $\hat{f}_X(x;h) = \hat{f}_X^*(x;h)$, where

$$\hat{f}_X^*(x;h) = \frac{1}{2\pi}\int e^{-itx}\hat{\varphi}_X^*(t)\varphi_K(ht)\,dt = \frac{1}{nh}\sum_{j=1}^{n} K\Big(\frac{x - X_j^*}{h}\Big) \tag{10.9}$$

is the standard kernel density estimator of $f_X^*(x)$. Second, by Fourier inversion of (10.9), we have $\varphi_{\hat{f}_X^*(\cdot;h)}(t) = \hat{\varphi}_X^*(t)\varphi_K(ht)$. Comparing with (10.3), we see that the deconvolution kernel estimator at (10.3) is nothing but the estimator of $f_X(x)$ obtained by replacing $\varphi_{X^*}$ in the second integral at (10.2) by the Fourier transform of the kernel density estimator of $f_{X^*}$. See also Delaigle (2014) for a discussion of main principles of deconvolution, including a description of the general unbiased score technique for deconvolution that also leads to the estimator at (10.4).

## 10.4 Overview of Some Theoretical Properties

In this section we review some of the most important theoretical properties of the deconvolution kernel density estimator. As we shall see, they depend heavily on the smoothness of the error distribution. In Section 10.4.1 we introduce two types of error distributions (ordinary smooth and supersmooth) typically encountered in the deconvolution literature. We describe the mean integrated squared error (MISE) of the estimator in Section 10.4.2 and its asymptotic expression in Section 10.4.3. As we shall see, standard convergence based on the this asymptotic expression is often slow. However, such rates are developed under the assumption that $f_X$ only has a finite number of derivatives. In Section 10.4.4 we will see that by studying the MISE of the estimator in the Fourier domain, it is possible to show that if $f_X$ is infinitely differentiable then the convergence rates are considerably faster. Finally, in Section 10.4.5 we mention some other useful theoretical properties that have been established in the literature.

While we will mention some of the important conditions, in this section, to keep the text readable, we will not list all the technical conditions required to write the results we present. We refer to the original papers and to Meister (2009a) for a deep and rigourous account of theoretical properties.

### 10.4.1 Error Type

The rate of convergence of $\hat{f}_X$ to $f_X$ depends on the smoothness of the error distribution, which is characterised by the rate of decay of its characteristic function in the tails. Following the terminology in Fan (1991a, 1991b, 1991c), one typically distinguishes between two classes of errors called supersmooth and ordinary smooth. An error $U$ is supersmooth of order $\beta$ if, for some constants $\beta_0 \leq \beta_1$, $0 < d_0 \leq d_1$, $\beta > 0$ and $\gamma > 0$,

$$d_0|t|^{\beta_0} \exp(-|t|^{\beta}/\gamma) \leq |\varphi_U(t)| \leq d_1|t|^{\beta_1} \exp(-|t|^{\beta}/\gamma) \quad \text{for large } |t|\,; \quad (10.10)$$

for example, normal and Cauchy distributions are supersmooth. As noted by Butucea and Tsybakov (2008a, 2008b), most densities in this class that are well known and can be expressed in a closed form are such that $\beta \leq 2$.

An error $U$ is ordinary smooth of order $\beta$ if, for some constants $0 < d_0 \leq d_1$ and $\beta > 0$,

$$d_0|t|^{-\beta} \leq |\varphi_U(t)| \leq d_1|t|^{-\beta} \quad \text{for large } |t|\,; \quad (10.11)$$

for example, a Laplace distribution is ordinary smooth.

We will see that supersmooth errors make the deconvolution problem much more difficult than ordinary smooth errors.

### 10.4.2 Mean Integrated Squared Error

Theoretical properties of $\hat{f}_X$ are usually assessed via the mean integrated square error defined by

$$\text{MISE}(h) = \int \text{Bias}^2\{\hat{f}_X(x;h)\}\,dx + \int \text{var}\{\hat{f}_X(x;h)\}\,dx\,,$$

where we follow the usual approach in the literature and omit the dependence on the kernel $K$ in the notation.

It follows from the conditional unbiased score property

$$E\{K_U(x - X_j^*)|X_j\} = E\{K(x - X_j)\},$$

which is at the heart of the deconvolution kernel technique (Delaigle, 2014; Stefanski and Carroll, 1990) that the bias of the deconvolution kernel density estimator is the same as that of the error-free kernel density estimator:

$$\text{Bias}\{\hat{f}_X(x;h)\} = E\{\hat{f}_X(x;h)\} - f_X(x) = K_h * f_X(x) - f_X(x)\,,$$

where $K_h(x) = K(x/h)/h$ and $f * g(x) = \int f(x-u)g(u)\,du$ denotes the convolution product of two functions $f$ and $g$. In particular, the MISE of the deconvolution kernel estimator computed from the contaminated $X_j^*$'s differs from that of the standard kernel density estimator computed from the error-free $X_j$'s only through its variance.

The integrated variance of the deconvolution kernel density estimator is equal to (Stefanski and Carroll, 1990; Stefanski, 1990)

$$\int \text{var}\{\hat{f}_X(x;h)\}\,dx = \frac{1}{2\pi nh}\int \frac{|\varphi_K(t)|^2}{|\varphi_U(t/h)|^2}\,dt - n^{-1}\int (K_h * f_X)^2(x)\,dx\,.$$

More formally, Stefanski and Carroll (1990) showed that under Conditions (10.6) to (10.8) and if $K$ is integrable, we have

$$\begin{aligned}\text{MISE}(h) =& \frac{1}{2\pi nh}\int \frac{|\varphi_K(t)|^2}{|\varphi_U(t/h)|^2}\,dt + (1-n^{-1})\int (K_h * f_X)^2(x)\,dx \\ &+ \int f_X^2(x)\,dx - 2\int K_h * f_X(x) f_X(x)\,dx\,.\end{aligned}$$

### 10.4.3 Asymptotic Mean Integrated Squared Error

As in the error-free case, the MISE is difficult to interpret, and it is standard to analyse instead its asymptotically dominating part. For this, it is useful to recall that a $k$th order kernel $K$ is a kernel whose moments satisfy

$$\mu_{K,j} = \int x^j K(x)\,dx = \begin{cases} 1 & \text{for } j = 0 \\ 0 & \text{for } j = 1,\ldots,k-1 \\ c & \text{for } j = k\,, \end{cases}$$

where $c \neq 0$ is a finite constant. As usual with kernel density estimation, $K$ is almost always chosen to be symmetric around zero, so that $k$ is even (indeed, for $k$ odd we could not have $\mu_{K,k} = c \neq 0$). Using a Taylor expansion, Stefanski and Carroll (1990) showed that under (10.6) to (10.8), if $K$ is a $k$th order kernel such that $\int |x^{k+1}K(x)|\,dx < \infty$, $f_X$ has $k+1$ continuous and bounded derivatives, $f_X^{(k)}$ is square integrable and $h \to 0$ and $nh \to \infty$ as $n \to \infty$, then $\text{MISE}(h) = \text{AMISE}(h) + O(n^{-1}) + o(h^{2k})$, where

$$\text{AMISE}(h) = \frac{h^{2k}}{(k!)^2}\mu_{K,k}^2 \int \{f_X^{(k)}(x)\}^2\,dx + \frac{1}{2\pi nh}\int \frac{|\varphi_K(t)|^2}{|\varphi_U(t/h)|^2}\,dt\,. \quad (10.12)$$

We learn from this expression that the rate of convergence of $\hat{f}_X$ to $f_X$ depends on the smoothness of $f_X$ and the smoothness of the error distribution; see Carroll and Hall (1988), Stefanski and Carroll (1990), and Fan (1991b, 1991c) for detailed calculations and asymptotic results. In particular, those authors have shown that, under sufficient conditions, in the ordinary smooth error case at (10.11), $\int |\varphi_K(t)|^2|\varphi_U(t/h)|^{-2}\,dt \sim h^{-2\beta}$, so that AMISE$(h) \sim c_1h^{2k}+c_2/(nh^{2\beta+1})$, where $c_1$ and $c_2$ are positive constants. Thus, in the ordinary smooth error case, if we use a $k$th order kernel and $f_X$ is smooth enough, the estimator $\hat{f}_X$ converges the fastest by taking $h \sim n^{-1/(2\beta+2k+1)}$, which results in MISE$(h) \sim$ AMISE$(h) \sim n^{-2k/(2\beta+2k+1)}$. Fan (1991c) showed that, under sufficient smoothness conditions, these rates are optimal. Fan (1991a) also established asymptotic normality of the estimator.

Things are more involved in the supersmooth error case at (10.10), where the fast decay of $\varphi_U$ in its tails makes it difficult to find kernels for which the integral $\int |\varphi_K(t)|^2|\varphi_U(t/h)|^{-2}\,dt$ exists, except if we take kernels for which $\varphi_K$ is compactly supported; the choice of the kernel will be discussed in Section 10.5.2. Furthermore, it is difficult to obtain an explicit expression for the integrated variance term, for which we typically only have upper bounds. Despite these complications, following Fan (1991a, 1991b, 1991c), it is possible to find bandwidths for which the rate of the AMISE$(h)$ is the smallest possible. Specifically, if we choose $K$ such that $\varphi_K$ is supported on $[-B, B]$ for some $0 < B < \infty$, then we have $\int |\varphi_K(t)|^2|\varphi_U(t/h)|^{-2}\,dt = O\{h^{2\beta_0}\exp(2|B/h|^{\beta}/\gamma)\}$, which is of order $O\{n^{d^{-\beta}-1}(\log n)^{(-2\beta_0+1)/\beta}\}$, if we take $h = dB(2/\gamma)^{1/\beta}(\log n)^{-1/\beta}$, with $d > 1$. With the same choice of $h$, the integrated squared bias term is of exact order $(\log n)^{-2k/\beta}$, so that MISE$(h) \sim$ AMISE$(h) \sim (\log n)^{-2k/\beta}$, since the integrated variance term is negligible compared to the integrated bias term.

Despite the pessimistic very slow convergence rates in the supersmooth case, deconvolution in practice works reasonably well even if the error is supersmooth. This has partly to do with the fact that these traditional asymptotic results do not take the variance of the errors into account, whereas these play an important role in the success of a deconvolution procedure. To take the magnitude of the error variance into account, several authors have developed a double asymptotic procedure where the error variance is assumed to tend to zero as $n \to \infty$. See for example Fan (1992), Carroll and Hall (2004), Delaigle (2008), Van Es and Gugushvili (2010), and Delaigle and Van Keilegom (2021). Fan (1991c) showed that if $f_X$ has a finite number of continuous derivatives, these rates are optimal. However, if $f_X$ is very smooth, then using a finite order kernel can give rise to considerably suboptimal results, as we show in Section 10.4.4.

### 10.4.4 Fourier Domain and Supersmooth Distributions of $X$

The asymptotic analysis in Section 10.4.3 and the rates of convergence discussed there only exploit the fact that $f_X$ has a finite number, $k$, of derivatives. However, many densities have an infinite number of derivatives; for those, the convergence rate of the estimator, and that of alternative estimators (Pensky et al., 1999) is considerably faster if we use a so-called infinite order kernel. Specifically, convergence rates can be much faster if, as in Butucea (2004b) and Butucea and Tsybakov (2008a, 2008b), $f_X$ is such that

$$(2\pi)^{-1}\int|\varphi_X(t)|^2\exp(2\alpha|t|^{\beta_X})\,dt\le L\,, \tag{10.13}$$

with $L>0$, $\alpha>0$ and where $\beta_X>0$ are finite constants.

To understand why, using Parseval's identity, we express the MISE in the Fourier domain as (Stefanski, 1990)

$$\begin{aligned}\text{MISE}(h)=&\frac{1}{2\pi nh}\int\frac{|\varphi_K(t)|^2}{|\varphi_U(t/h)|^2}\,dt+\frac{(1-n^{-1})}{2\pi}\int|\varphi_X(t)|^2|\varphi_K(ht)|^2\,dt\\&+\frac{1}{2\pi}\int|\varphi_X(t)|^2\,dt-\frac{1}{\pi}\int|\varphi_X(t)|^2\varphi_K(ht)\,dt\,.\end{aligned} \tag{10.14}$$

In the particular case of the sinc kernel $K$ defined by $\varphi_K(t)=I\{|t|\le1\}$, where $I\{\cdot\}$ is the indicator function (see Section 10.5.2 for a detailed discussion of kernels), this reduces to

$$\text{MISE}(h)=\frac{1}{2\pi nh}\int_{-1}^{1}\frac{1}{|\varphi_U(t/h)|^2}\,dt+\frac{1}{2\pi}\int_{|t|>1/h}|\varphi_X(t)|^2\,dt+O(n^{-1})\,.$$

Now, using (10.13), we have

$$\begin{aligned}\frac{1}{2\pi}\int_{|t|>1/h}|\varphi_X(t)|^2\,dt=&\frac{1}{2\pi}\int_{|t|>1/h}|\varphi_X(t)|^2\exp(2\alpha|t|^{\beta_X})\exp(-2\alpha|t|^{\beta_X})\,dt\\\le&\frac{e^{-2\alpha h^{-\beta_X}}}{2\pi}\int_{|t|>1/h}|\varphi_X(t)|^2\exp(2\alpha|t|^{\beta_X})\,dt\\\le&L\exp(-2\alpha h^{-\beta_X})\,.\end{aligned}$$

On the other hand, we know from Section 10.4.3 that $\int|\varphi_U(t/h)|^{-2}\,dt=O\{h^{2\beta_0}\exp(2h^{-\beta}/\gamma)\}$ if $U$ is supersmooth of order $\beta$, and $\int|\varphi_U(t/h)|^{-2}\,dt\sim h^{-2\beta}$ if $U$ is ordinary smooth of order $\beta$. Thus, if $U$ is ordinary smooth of order $\beta$ then

$$\text{MISE}(h)\le L\exp(-2\alpha h^{-\beta_X})+c_1h^{-2\beta-1}n^{-1}+O(n^{-1})\,,$$

with $c_1>0$ a constant; taking $h=\{\log n/(2\alpha)\}^{-1/\beta_X}$ as in Butucea (2004b), we deduce that $\text{MISE}(h)=O(n^{-1})+O\{n^{-1}(\log n)^{(2\beta+1)/\beta_X}\}=O\{n^{-1}(\log n)^{(2\beta+1)/\beta_X}\}$, which is only slightly slower than the parametric $n^{-1}$ rate, and faster than the rate $n^{-2k/(2\beta+2k+1)}$ obtained when assuming only that $f_X$ has $k$ smooth derivatives.

If $U$ is supersmooth of order $\beta$, then we have

$$\text{MISE}(h)\le L\exp(-2\alpha h^{-\beta_X})+c_1n^{-1}h^{2\beta_0-1}\exp(2h^{-\beta}/\gamma)+O(n^{-1})\,. \tag{10.15}$$

In that case too, Butucea and Tsybakov (2008a, 2008b) showed that it is possible to choose a more precise bandwidth than the one suggested in Section 10.4.3, such that the rates are faster than the slow logarithmic rates obtained when assuming only that $f_X$ has $k$ smooth derivatives. Indeed, if we take $h \leq d(\log n)^{-1/\beta_X}$ for some constant $d > 0$, then the first term of (10.15) is of order $n^{-a}$ for some $a > 0$, and if we take $h = d(2/\gamma)^{1/\beta}(\log n)^{-1/\beta}$ with $d > 1$, then we have seen in the previous section that the second term of (10.15) is of order $O\{n^{d^{-\beta}-1}(\log n)^{(-2\beta_0+1)/\beta}\}$. Thus, if $\beta \leq \beta_X$, then by taking $h = d(2/\gamma)^{1/\beta}(\log n)^{-1/\beta}$ with $d > 1$, the estimator converges at polynomial rates. The case where $\beta_X < \beta$ was studied by Butucea and Tsybakov (2008a, 2008b), who proposed a more precise choice of $h$. They showed that, using that bandwidth, the bias contribution dominates the variance contribution, and that again the rate is faster than the one obtained when assuming that $f_X$ has only a finite number $k$ of derivatives.

### 10.4.5 Further Reading

Stefanski (1990) established strong uniform consistency of the estimator, and Liu and Taylor (1989) established strong uniform consistency for their truncated estimator. Devroye (1989) established $L_1$ consistency of his modified kernel estimator and Song (2010) studied moderate deviations in the ordinary smooth error case. Asymptotic normality for supersmooth errors of order $\beta$ was studied by Van Es and Uh (2004, 2005), who noted that, when considering pointwise properties of the estimator, the case where $\beta < 1$ behaves differently from that where $\beta > 1$; see also Butucea and Tsybakov (2008a) for a similar remark and Holzmann and Boysen (2006) for the asymptotic distribution of the integrated squared error of the estimator in the supersmooth error case, which corrects a result from Butucea (2004a). Finally, Zu (2015) established asymptotic normality with a logarithmic chi-square error.

## 10.5 Computing the Estimator in Practice

In practice, some care needs to be taken when computing the deconvolution kernel density estimator. First, computing the estimator requires the choice of a bandwidth and a kernel. We discuss these issues in Sections 10.5.1 and 10.5.2. Second, often the estimator has no analytic expression and needs to be computed numerically; we discuss issues related to this in Section 10.5.3.

### 10.5.1 Importance of the Bandwidth

As in the error-free case, the choice of the bandwidth $h$ is crucial for the empirical success of $\hat{f}_X$: a too small $h$ will result in a too variable, wiggly, estimator, and a too large $h$ will result in a biased, oversmoothed, estimator. In theory, the best choice of $h$ is the one that minimises the distance between $f_X$ and $\hat{f}_X$. There are many ways to choose such a distance. For example, a distance can be global (distance between the whole curves $f_X$ and $\hat{f}_X$), or local (distance between $f_X(x)$ and $\hat{f}_X(x)$ at each $x$ of interest). The two most popular global distances are the MISE or its asymptotic approximation AMISE, and the most popular local distance is the mean squared error

$$\text{MSE}(x; h) = E\big[\{\hat{f}_X(x; h) - f_X(x)\}^2\big] = \text{Bias}^2\{\hat{f}_X(x; h)\} + \text{var}\{\hat{f}_X(x; h)\}$$

or its asymptotic version $\text{AMSE}(x; h)$.

We choose $h$ by minimising a global distance when we intend to use the same bandwidth $h$ at each $x$ where we compute the estimator $\hat{f}_X$; such a bandwidth is called a global bandwidth. For example, the MISE and the AMISE bandwidths are defined by, respectively,

$$h_{\text{MISE}} = \text{argmin}_h \text{MISE}(h) \text{ and } h_{\text{AMISE}} = \text{argmin}_h \text{AMISE}(h)\,.$$

We choose $h$ by minimising a local distance if we wish to use a different bandwidth $h(x)$ at each $x$; such a bandwidth is called a local bandwidth. For example, the MSE and the AMSE bandwidths are defined by, respectively,

$$h_{\text{MSE}}(x) = \text{argmin}_h \text{MSE}(x; h) \text{ and } h_{\text{AMISE}}(x) = \text{argmin}_h \text{AMSE}(x; h)\,.$$

A local bandwidth is preferable when $f_X$ has sharp features (e.g., is very wiggly) in some parts of its domain and is very smooth (e.g., non wiggly) elsewhere. There, ideally $h$ should be smaller in wiggly areas and larger elsewhere.

In practice, we cannot compute any of those theoretically optimal bandwidths since they all depend on the unknown $f_X$ that we are trying to estimate. In Section 10.6 we will discuss various methods that have been developed in the literature for approximating them in practice.

### 10.5.2 Importance of the Kernel

As in standard kernel density estimation problems without measurement errors, the choice of the kernel function $K$ is less important than the choice of the bandwidth $h$. However, in order for the estimator at (10.3) to work well in practice, the kernel $K$ needs to be a smooth and unimodal function that integrates to 1 (so that $\hat{f}_X$ integrates to 1 too). Moreover, in order for the estimator at (10.3) to be well defined, the integral at (10.5) needs to exist. Therefore, $K$ has to be such that $\varphi_K(t)$ tends to zero faster than $\varphi_U(t/h)$ as $|t| \to \infty$, which often makes it impossible to use kernels that are frequently used in the error-free case such as the Epanechnikov kernel, defined by $K(x) = 3/4\,(1 - x^2) \cdot I\{|x| \leq 1\}$, or the standard normal kernel, defined by $K = \phi$, the standard normal density.

To understand why standard kernels such as the Epanechnikov kernel can often not be used in the error case, note that the Fourier transform of the Epanechnikov kernel is given by $\varphi_K(t) = 3(\sin t - t\cos t)/t^3$, which, for large $|t|$, behaves like $|t|^{-2}$. Thus, for ordinary smooth errors satisfying (10.11), we can only guarantee that the integral at (10.5) exists if $\beta \leq 1$, which is not even satisfied by Laplace errors, for which $\beta$ in (10.11) is equal to 2. It is easy to see that this integral cannot exist in the supersmooth error case.

On the other hand, the standard normal kernel can be used with ordinary smooths at (10.11). Indeed, in this case we have $\varphi_K(t) = \exp(-t^2/2)$, which tends to zero much faster than $|t|^{-\beta}$, so that the integral at (10.5) exists. An advantage of this kernel in this case is that its associated $K_U$ has an explicit (analytic) formula, and so do various quantities required to compute a data-driven bandwidth. For supersmooth errors at (10.10) however, with this kernel, the integral at (10.5) exists only if $\beta < 2$, or if $\beta = 2$ and $h > \gamma^{-1/2}$. This is only possible for $n$ small, since the estimator at (10.3) is only consistent if $h \to 0$ as $n \to \infty$. Therefore, this kernel is not used for supersmooth errors.

To guarantee that the integral at (10.5) exists for both supersmooth and ordinary smooth errors, it is common to use kernels whose Fourier transform is compactly supported. Two kernels are commonly employed: the sinc kernel $K_1(x) = \sin(x)/(\pi x)$, whose Fourier transform is equal to $\varphi_K(t) = I\{|t| \leq 1\}$ and the kernel $K_2$, defined through its characteristic function by $\varphi_{K_2}(t) = (1-t^2)^3 I\{|t| \leq 1\}$. A drawback of these kernels is that often they do not produce an analytic formula for $K_U$, which has to be computed by numerical integration; see Section 10.5.3.

While the sinc kernel $K_1$ is not absolutely integrable, it has the advantage that it is an infinite order kernel: it automatically adapts to the smoothness of $f_X$, which, in simple terms, is the number of smooth and bounded derivatives that $f_X$ has. As in the error-free case, this means that, with this kernel, the deconvolution kernel density estimator of $f_X$ tends to have a smaller bias and is able to better capture sharp features of $f_X$, sometimes much better than finite order kernels; see Section 10.4.4. However, this typically comes at the cost of pronounced unattractive negative wiggles in the tail of the estimator.

Lütkenöner (2015) proposed a family of kernels whose Fourier transform is of the form

$$\varphi_K(t) = \{\cos(\pi t/2)\}^{\kappa} I\{|t| \leq 1\},$$

where $\kappa \geq 0$. For example, when $\kappa = 0$, $\varphi_K(t) = I\{|t| \leq 1\}$ corresponds to the sinc kernel, which does not have a single finite moment. When $\kappa \geq 2$ (resp., $\kappa \geq 4$), the corresponding kernels have at least 2 (resp., at least 4) finite moments. Lütkenöner (2015) showed that the advantage of using these kernels is that in the normal error case where $U \sim N(0, \sigma^2)$, for $\kappa > 0$, we can write $K_U$ explicitly as

$$K_U(x) = \frac{1}{2^k} \sum_{k=0}^{\kappa} \binom{\kappa}{k} K_0\{x - (\kappa/2 - k)\pi\},$$

where $K_0$ corresponds to $K_U$ for the sinc kernel:

$$K_0(x) = \frac{-\lambda}{\sqrt{2\pi}} e^{1/(2\lambda^2)} \mathbb{I}\big[\exp(-i|x|) w\{(i\lambda|x| - 1/\lambda)/\sqrt{2}\}\big],$$

with $\mathbb{I}$ denoting the imaginary part, $i^2 = -1$, $\lambda = h/\sigma$, and $w(z) = e^{-z^2}\text{erfc}(-iz)$, with erfc the complementary error function. As pointed by Lütkenöner (2015), $w$ is known as the Faddeeva function and there exist efficient algorithms to evaluate it numerically.

In the case without measurement errors, an optimal kernel of order $k$ is sometimes defined to be a kernel of order $k$ that minimises the MISE of the standard kernel estimator. Since that problem is degenerate (it does not have a unique solution), Granovsky et al. (1995) and Granovsky and Müller (1989, 1991) proposed to choose the $k$th order kernel that minimises the MISE and satisfies a number of additional side constraints, such as having $k - 2$ sign changes. Delaigle and Hall (2006) argued that these side constraints are not appropriate in the case with measurement errors, where kernels chosen in that way result in much poorer practical performance, compared to the kernels discussed above. They also showed that the choice of the kernel is much more important in the error case than in the error-free case, in that it influences much more the value of the MISE and the practical performance of the estimator.

### 10.5.3 Computing the Estimator in Practice

In general, computing the deconvolution kernel density estimator is not straightforward as it requires computing an inverse Fourier transform through $K_U$, which often does not have an analytic formula.

In some cases, it is possible to express the deconvolution kernel density estimator analytically without going through the Fourier domain. For example, in the case where $U$ is a Laplace($\sigma$) random variable, we have $\varphi_U(t) = 1/(1 + \sigma^2 t^2)$, so that

$$K_U(x) = \frac{1}{2\pi}\int e^{-itx}\varphi_K(t)\,dt + \frac{\sigma^2}{h^2}\cdot\frac{1}{2\pi}\int e^{-itx}t^2\varphi_K(t)\,dt = K(x) - \frac{\sigma^2}{h^2}K''(x).$$

Thus, the deconvolution kernel density estimator can be expressed as

$$\hat{f}_X(x;h) = \hat{f}_{X^*}(x;h) - \sigma^2 \hat{f}''_{X^*}(x;h), \tag{10.16}$$

where $\hat{f}_{X^*}(x;h)$ is the standard kernel density estimator at (10.9) and $\hat{f}''_{X^*}(x;h)$ is its second derivative with respect to $x$; see Section 10.7.1 for other examples.

In those simple cases, we can use a standard kernel of the same type as those used in the error-free case, for example the standard normal kernel, and the deconvolution kernel density estimator can be computed using this simple analytic formula. It is important to note that if we choose kernels with a compactly supported Fourier transform equal to a polynomial on its domain (e.g., $K_1$ or $K_2$ introduced in Section 10.5.2), then even if $K_U$ has an analytic expression such as the one derived above, that expression often cannot be used directly as it can cause dramatic cancellation. For a detailed discussion of this issue, see Delaigle and Gijbels (2007), who also proposed a solution to this problem. However, if we bypass completely the computation of $K_U$ and compute $\hat{f}_X$ directly, then we can avoid such problems; for example in the Laplace case we can avoid this problem if we compute $\hat{f}_{X^*}(x;h)$ and $\hat{f}''_{X^*}(x;h)$, and then take $\hat{f}_X(x;h) = \hat{f}_{X^*}(x;h) - \sigma^2 \hat{f}''_{X^*}(x;h)$.

More generally, and especially in the supersmooth error case, there is often no analytic formula for $K_U$ and $\hat{f}_X$ has to be computed numerically. If we use (10.4) to compute $\hat{f}_X$, at each $x$ we need to evaluate $n$ integrals (one for each version of $K_U$ in (10.4)). Delaigle and Gijbels (2007) have shown that computing $K_U$ numerically is also quite difficult. Indeed, the periodic oscillations inside the integral at (10.5) can cause the integral to be poorly approximated if standard fast iterative integration algorithms are employed, such as the Romberg method. While a more accurate approximation can be obtained by the fast Fourier transform or the trapezoidal rule on a fine grid, the calculation of $K_U$ can be bypassed entirely if we compute $\hat{f}_X$ numerically through the formula at (10.3). The latter only requires to evaluate one integral numerically for each $x$ at which we compute $\hat{f}_X$.

As noted in Section 10.5.2 for the sinc kernel, the deconvolution kernel density estimator typically has some negative wiggles in the tail, although these vanish as $n \to \infty$ (recall that the estimator is consistent). More generally, even if we use a kernel $K$ that is a density, the deconvolution kernel $K_U$ is typically not a density (it integrates to 1 but has negative wiggles, whose magnitude increases to as $h$ decreases and/or $\sigma^2$ increases). In the error-free case, it is sometimes advocated that a density estimator $\hat{f}$ that takes negative values should be truncated to zero and rescaled to integrate to 1 (Hall and Murison, 1993), that is, take

$$\tilde{f}(x) = \max\{\hat{f}(x), 0\} \Big/ \int \max\{\hat{f}(y), 0\}\, dy\,.$$

However, since $K_U$ often has big negative wiggles, the negative wiggles in the tails of $\hat{f}_X$ in the error case can be much larger than those in the error-free case. Therefore, rescaling the estimator as above is not necessarily a good idea: as $\hat{f}_X$ (with its negative wiggles) integrates to 1, rescaled its truncated version will often introduce a large bias. Instead, in the error case, it is often more appropriate to take

$$\tilde{f}_X(x;h) = \max\{\hat{f}_X(x;h), 0\}\,,$$

without rescaling, even though this often implies that $\tilde{f}_X$ is not a density since it does not integrate exactly to 1.

## 10.6 Bandwidth Selection in Practice

In Section 10.5.1 we highlighted the importance of the choice of $h$ for the empirical success of the estimator $\hat{f}_X$. There we defined some theoretical bandwidths that result in good practical performance, but none of them can be computed in practice since they all depend on the unknown $f_X$. In this section, we discuss several strategies for approximating those bandwidths from the data. As we shall see, some (e.g., cross-validation, bootstrap, and SIMEX) are based on the MISE, and others (e.g., plug-in) are based on asymptotic expressions such as the AMISE at (10.12).

It is important to note that the AMISE at (10.12) relies on the kernel to have a finite number $k$ of moments, and $f_X$ to be at least $k$ times differentiable. Therefore, techniques based on the AMISE cannot be employed for the sinc kernel. We will see that the cross-validation, the bootstrap and the SIMEX bandwidths can all be used with the sinc kernel. Most of the techniques discussed in this section are available in the R package `deconvolve` (Delaigle et al., 2020), while Matlab codes are available on Delaigle's webpage.

### 10.6.1 Cross-Validation Bandwidth

The first data-driven procedure for selecting $h$ in practice was proposed by Stefanski and Carroll (1990). It was originally developed for normal errors but it can be applied more generally (Hesse, 1999). As in the standard error-free case, it is designed to provide an estimator of the bandwidth that minimises the integrated squared error $\text{ISE}(h) = \int \{\hat{f}_X(x) - f_X(x)\}^2\, dx$, or equivalently, which minimises

$$\text{ISE}(h) - \int \{f_X(x)\}^2\, dx = \int \{\hat{f}_X(x)\}^2\, dx - 2\int \hat{f}_X(x) f_X(x)\, dx\,. \quad (10.17)$$

In the Fourier domain, the first term on the right hand side of (10.17) can be expressed as $(2\pi)^{-1}\int |\varphi_K(ht)|^2|\hat{\varphi}_{X^*}(t)|^2|\varphi_U(t)|^{-2}\, dt$. Stefanski and Carroll (1990) showed that the second term has the same expectation as a cross-validation quantity that can be rewritten as $\{\pi(n-1)\}^{-1}\int \varphi_K(-ht)\{n|\hat{\varphi}_{X^*}(t)|^2 - 1\}|\varphi_U(t)|^{-2}\, dt$. Motivated by this, they defined the cross-validation bandwidth by

$$\hat{h}_{\text{CV}} = \text{argmin}_h \text{CV}(h)\,, \quad (10.18)$$

where $\text{CV}(h)$ is the cross-validation criterion defined by

$$\text{CV}(h) = \frac{1}{2\pi}\int \frac{|\varphi_K(ht)|^2|\hat{\varphi}_{X^*}(t)|^2 - 2(n-1)^{-1}\varphi_K(-ht)\{n|\hat{\varphi}_{X^*}(t)|^2 - 1\}}{|\varphi_U(t)|^2}\, dt\,.$$

Theoretical properties of this bandwidth were studied by Hesse (1999) and Youndjé and Wells (2002) in the ordinary smooth error case; the authors showed that an advantage of the cross-validation bandwidth is that it relies on very few smoothness assumptions, unlike the plug-in technique introduced in the next section. However, in practice the CV bandwidth has a tendency to select too small bandwidths, which is useful for capturing sharp features such as sharp peaks, but it often comes at the price of an estimator that is too variable. Moreover, as in the error-free case, the cross-validation bandwidth is not always uniquely defined, and in that case it is not clear which local solution of (10.18) should be chosen; Delaigle and Gijbels (2004b) recommended to choose among them the smallest bandwidth for which the estimator appears visually smooth enough, or if this is not possible, to choose the largest solution.

In the particular case of the sinc kernel, CV simplifies into

$$\mathrm{CV}(h) = \frac{1}{2\pi(n-1)} \int_{-1/h}^{1/h} \frac{2-(n+1)|\hat{\varphi}_{X^*}(t)|^2}{|\varphi_U(t)|^2}\, dt \tag{10.19}$$

so that

$$\mathrm{CV}'(h) = \frac{1}{\pi(n-1)h^2} \frac{(n+1)|\hat{\varphi}_{X^*}(1/h)|^2 - 2}{|\varphi_U(1/h)|^2}.$$

Since $\hat{h}_{\mathrm{CV}}$ is a solution of $\mathrm{CV}'(h) = 0$, in this case it can be found by solving $|\hat{\varphi}_{X^*}(1/h)|^2 = 2/(n+1)$. Interestingly, as pointed by Stefanski and Carroll (1990), since the bandwidth chosen by cross-validation does not depend on the error distribution, we see that in this case, it is the same for estimating $f_X$ and for estimating $f_{X^*}$. As we will see later, this is generally not true for the approaches based on a finite order kernel.

As shown by Stefanski and Carroll (1990) the CV bandwidth can be viewed as an estimator of the bandwidth $h_{\mathrm{MISE}}$ that minimises the MISE. For example, in the case of the sinc kernel, using (10.14) and recalling that $\varphi_X = \varphi_{X^*}/\varphi_U$, we have

$$\mathrm{MISE}(h) = \frac{1}{2\pi n} \int_{-1/h}^{1/h} \frac{1-(n+1)|\varphi_{X^*}(t)|^2}{|\varphi_U(t)|^2}\, dt + \frac{1}{2\pi}\int |\varphi_X(t)|^2\, dt. \tag{10.20}$$

(Note that the last term does not depend on $h$). Therefore,

$$\mathrm{MISE}'(h) = \frac{1}{\pi n h^2} \frac{(n+1)|\varphi_{X^*}(1/h)|^2 - 1}{|\varphi_U(1/h)|^2}.$$

Since $h_{\mathrm{MISE}}$ satisfies $\mathrm{MISE}'(h) = 0$, in the particular case of the sinc kernel, $h_{\mathrm{MISE}}$ is a solution of $|\varphi_{X^*}(1/h)|^2 = 1/(n+1)$. This equation uniquely identifies $h$ under some conditions (Stefanski and Carroll, 1990) and is the same as the equation for finding the CV bandwidth given above, except that the unknown $\varphi_{X^*}$ is replaced by its estimator $\hat{\varphi}_{X^*}$, and $-2$ is replaced here by $-1$ (this is to remove some of the bias of the estimator $|\hat{\varphi}_{X^*}|^2$ of $|\varphi_{X^*}|^2$).

### 10.6.2 Plug-in and Normal Reference Bandwidths

When we can reasonably assume that the density $f_X$ has at least $k$ smooth derivatives, and we use a $k$th order kernel, with $k$ even, instead of using the cross-validation bandwidth we can use instead the plug-in (PI) bandwidth (Delaigle and Gijbels, 2004b). As in the error-free case, this bandwidth is quite popular because it often works well in practice and is much faster to compute than the cross-validation bandwidth. We also discuss another bandwidth called the normal reference bandwidth, which is even simpler to compute but usually gives rather poor practical performance.

The plug-in bandwidth is obtained by plugging, in the AMISE expression, a kernel estimator of the unknown quantity, and then minimise the resulting estimator of the AMISE with respect to $h$. Specifically, recalling the AMISE expression from (10.12), the only unknown is $\theta_k \equiv \int \{f_X^{(k)}(x)\}^2\,dx$, which is estimated by $\hat{\theta}_k \equiv \int \{\hat{f}_X^{(k)}(x;h_k)\}^2\,dx$, where

$$\hat{f}_X^{(k)}(x;h_k) = \frac{1}{nh_k^{k+1}}\sum_{j=1}^{n} K_U^{(k)}\Big(\frac{x-X_j^*}{h_k}\Big) = \frac{1}{2\pi}\int (-it)^k e^{-itx}\frac{\hat{\varphi}_X^*(t)\varphi_K(h_k t)}{\varphi_U(t)}\,dt$$

is the $k$th derivative of $\hat{f}_X(x;h_k)$ at (10.4) computed with a bandwidth $h_k$ (Delaigle and Gijbels, 2002) and $K_U^{(k)}(x) = (2\pi)^{-1}\int(-it)^k e^{-itx}\varphi_K(t)/\varphi_U(t/h)\,dt$ is the $k$th derivative of $K_U$. As mentioned earlier, the kernel $K$ is almost always taken to be symmetric so that its order $k$ is even; in that case, $(-i)^k = (-1)^{k/2}$.

Using Parseval's identity, $\hat{\theta}_k$ can be expressed as

$$\hat{\theta}_k = (2\pi)^{-1}\int t^{2k}|\hat{\varphi}_X^*(t)|^2|\varphi_K(h_k t)|^2|\varphi_U(t)|^{-2}\,dt\,,$$

which leads to the following estimator $\widehat{\text{AMISE}}(h)$ of AMISE$(h)$:

$$\frac{\mu_{K,k}^2}{(k!)^2}\frac{h^{2k}}{2\pi h_k^{2k+1}}\int t^{2k}\frac{|\hat{\varphi}_X^*(t/h_k)|^2|\varphi_K(t)|^2}{|\varphi_U(t/h_k)|^2}\,dt + \frac{1}{2\pi nh}\int\frac{|\varphi_K(t)|^2}{|\varphi_U(t/h)|^2}\,dt\,.$$

Then, the bandwidth is chosen by minimising $\widehat{\text{AMISE}}(h)$ with respect to $h$. If the error density is unknown and estimated from data as in Delaigle and Van Keilegom (2021), what often works well in practice is to replace $\varphi_U$ in this expression by its estimator $\hat{\varphi}_U$.

To compute $\widehat{\text{AMISE}}(h)$, we need to choose the bandwidth $h_k$ used to compute $\hat{\theta}_k$. Here, $h_k$ should be chosen to estimate $\theta_k$ the best way possible. Delaigle and Gijbels (2002, 2004b) suggest choosing $h_k$ to minimise (an estimator of) the mean squared error (MSE) of $\hat{\theta}_k$, and doing this typically results in $h_k$ different from $h$. For example, it leads to $h_k \sim n^{-1/(2\beta+3k+1)}$ if $U$ is ordinary smooth of order $\beta$, whereas we saw in Section 10.4.3 that the bandwidth $h$ that minimises the MISE of $\hat{f}_X$ is of order $h \sim n^{-1/(2\beta+2k+1)}$. Thus, in this case case, $h_k$ is an order of magnitude larger than $h$.

If the error is supersmooth of order $\beta$, Delaigle and Gijbels (2002) showed that if $\varphi_K$ is supported on $[-B, B]$, the optimal convergence rate for estimating $\theta_k$ is obtained by taking $h = dB(2/\gamma)^{1/\beta}(\log n)^{-1/\beta}$ with $d > 1$. This is also the bandwidth found in Section 10.4.3 for computing $f_X$ at the best possible rate. Thus in theory, in the supermsooth error case we could take $h_k = h = dB(2/\gamma)^{1/\beta}(\log n)^{-1/\beta}$ with $d > 1$. However, the value of $d$ influences the practical success of the estimator and it is not clear how to choose $d$. Instead, as in the ordinary smooth error case, taking $h$ and $h_k$ to minimise an estimator of the AMISE of $\hat{f}_X$ and of the MSE of $\hat{\theta}_k$, respectively, often gives good results; see Delaigle and Gijbels (2004b).

The MSE of $\hat{\theta}_k$, used to choose $h_k$, also contains some unknowns that need to be estimated from the data. This is done via an iterative process; see Delaigle and Gijbels (2002, 2004b). The plug-in bandwidth often performs significantly better than the CV bandwidth, which tends to be too small. An exception to this is when the $f_X$ has very sharp features, in which case its deconvolution kernel density estimator with the PI bandwidth tends to oversmooth those features, whereas the estimator computed with the CV bandwidth is often able to capture them better.

As in the error-free case, we can also compute a quick and dirty bandwidth called the normal reference bandwidth (Delaigle and Gijbels, 2004b). It consists in estimating $\theta_k$ by pretending that $f_X$ is a normal density, that is, in estimating $\theta_k$ by $\hat{\theta}_k = (2k)!/\{(2\hat{\sigma}_X)^{2k+1}k!\sqrt{\pi}\}$, where $\hat{\sigma}_X^2 = \max\{1/n, \hat{\sigma}_{X^*}^2 - \text{var}(U)\}$ is an estimator of the variance of $X$, with $\hat{\sigma}_{X^*}^2$ the empirical variance of the $X_i^*$'s. The normal reference bandwidth is obtained by minimising the resulting estimator of AMISE$(h)$. Since it is obtained under the assumption that $f_X$ is normal, it is often too large and makes the estimator of $f_X$ oversmoothed. Delaigle and Gijbels (2004b) also developed an alternative plug-in bandwidth called the solve-the-equation bandwidth but found it had little practical advantage compared to their main plug-in bandwidth introduced above.

In practice, since we usually do not know how smooth $f_X$ is, it is common to take $k = 2$ and use a second order kernel. As in the error-free case, even if we had the information that $f_X$ had more than 2 derivatives using a kernel of order $k > 2$ would produce more wiggly estimators, although it would capture sharp features better (taking $k$ larger means taking $h$ smaller and thus having a smaller bias but a larger variance). See also our discussion about the sinc kernel in Section 10.6.1. Note that the sinc kernel does not have a finite number $k$ of moments and cannot be used with the plug-in or the normal reference bandwidths.

### 10.6.3 Bootstrap Bandwidth

Delaigle and Gijbels (2004a) proposed a bootstrap bandwidth that directly attempts to minimise an estimator of the MISE. Recalling the expression at

(10.14), and noting that $\int |\varphi_X(t)|^2\,dt$ does not depend on $h$, they propose to choose $h$ by minimising

$$\begin{aligned}\mathrm{MISE}_2^*(h) =& \frac{1}{2\pi nh}\int \frac{|\varphi_K(t)|^2}{|\varphi_U(t/h)|^2}\,dt + \frac{(1-n^{-1})}{2\pi}\int |\hat{\varphi}_{X,\tilde{h}}(t)|^2|\varphi_K(ht)|^2\,dt \\ &- \frac{1}{\pi}\int |\hat{\varphi}_{X,\tilde{h}}(t)|^2\varphi_K(ht)\,dt\,,\end{aligned}$$

where $\hat{\varphi}_{X,\tilde{h}}(t) = \hat{\varphi}_{X^*}(t)\varphi_K(\tilde{h}t)/\varphi_U(t)$ is the Fourier transform of the deconvolution kernel density estimator at (10.3), computed with a bandwidth $\tilde{h}$. Although Delaigle and Gijbels (2004a) originally motivated this approach by bootstrap ideas, it does not require to generate any bootstrap sample. The bandwidth $\tilde{h}$ is generally not taken to be equal to $h$, and in the case of a kernel of a finite order $k$, Delaigle and Gijbels (2004a) suggested choosing $\tilde{h}$ equal to the bandwidth $h_k$ used to compute the plug-in bandwidth introduced in Section 10.6.2. In their numerical investigation, Delaigle and Gijbels (2004b) found that the bootstrap bandwidth was often outperformed by the plug-in bandwidth.

In the particular case of the sinc kernel, if we take $\tilde{h} \geq h$, we have

$$\mathrm{MISE}_2^*(h) = \frac{1}{2\pi n}\int_{-1/h}^{1/h} \frac{1-(n+1)|\hat{\varphi}_{X^*}(t)|^2}{|\varphi_U(t)|^2}\,dt\,,$$

which is an estimator of the first term of (10.20) (recall that the second term of (10.20) does not depend on $h$), where $|\varphi_{X^*}(t)|^2$ is estimated by $|\hat{\varphi}_{X^*}(t)|^2$. This is almost identical to the cross-validation criterion at (10.19), with 2 there replaced by 1 here; see our discussion about this in the last paragraph of Section 10.6.1.

### 10.6.4 SIMEX Bandwidth

The procedures introduced above are all targeted at the estimation of the density $f_X$. Delaigle and Hall (2008) introduced a more general SIMEX (simulation extrapolation) procedure that can be applied in a wide class of deconvolution problems. Their procedure applies to the bandwidth selection context, the SIMEX procedure developed by Cook and Stefanski (1994) and Stefanski and Cook (1995). A preliminary version of the SIMEX bandwidth, that used only one level of simulated data, was proposed by Delaigle and Meister (2007) in a heteroscedastic errors-in-variables regression context. The two-level SIMEX described here was proposed by Delaigle and Hall (2008). In this section we assume that the error density $f_U$ is known; see Delaigle and Hall (2008) for a variant of the SIMEX bandwidth in the case where $f_U$ is unknown but replicated data are available.

The main idea of SIMEX is as follows: suppose we want to estimate a curve, $g$ say, that depends on a variable $X$ that we cannot observe directly.

For example, in the density estimation problem, $g = f_X$ and in the regression estimation problem, $g(x) = E(Y|X = x)$, where $Y$ is a dependent variable. Instead of observing a sample $X_1, \ldots, X_n \sim f_X$, we observe $X_1^*, \ldots, X_n^*$ coming from the classical measurement error model at (10.1). Let $\hat{g}$ denote a nonparametric estimator of $g$ based on the contaminated $X_i^*$, which requires the choice of one or several smoothing parameters, and let $\hat{g}_{EF}$ denote the a nonparametric estimator of $g$ that we would use if we could observe the $X_i$'s (here EF stands for error-free). For example, in the density estimation case, $\hat{g}$ could be the deconvolution kernel density estimator $\hat{f}_X$ introduced earlier, which requires the choice of a bandwidth $h$, and $\hat{g}_{EF}$ could be the standard error-free kernel density estimator computed from the $X_i$'s. In the errors-in-variables regression case, $\hat{g}$ could be the local constant errors-in-variables estimator of Fan and Truong (1993) computed from a sample of $(X_i^*, Y_i)$'s distributed as $(X^*, Y)$, or the more general local polynomial errors-in-variables estimator of Delaigle et al. (2009), both of which require the choice of a bandwidth $h$ and, optionally, of a ridge parameter $\rho$; $\hat{g}_{EF}$ could be the standard error-free local polynomial estimator of $g$ computed from a sample of $(X_i, Y_i)$'s distributed as $(X, Y)$.

Let $H$ denote the smoothing parameters required to compute $\hat{g} \equiv \hat{g}(\cdot; H)$. For example, in the density estimation problem, $H = h$, the bandwidth. In the regression estimation problem, $H = (h, \rho)$. If we were able to compute $\hat{g}$ and $\hat{g}_{EF}$, an approach we could take to choose $H$ would be to choose

$$\hat{H} = \text{argmin}_H D\{\hat{g}(\cdot;, H), \hat{g}_{EF}\}, \tag{10.21}$$

where $D$ denotes a distance, for example, a weighted integrated squared error

$$D(\hat{g}, \hat{g}_{EF}) = \int \{\hat{g}(x; H) - \hat{g}_{EF}(x)\}^2 w(x),$$

with $w$ a weight function of our choice. In general, such a procedure is justified because the convergence rate of $\hat{g}_{EF}$ to $g$ is faster than that of $\hat{g}$ to $g$, so that choosing $H$ that minimises the distance above is asymptotically equivalent to choosing $H$ that minimises $D\{\hat{g}(\cdot;, H), g\}$. In the density case, we can take $w(x) = 1$; in the regression case, since nonparametric regression estimators are not able to estimate a regression curve well at the tails of the distribution of the explanatory variable, we can take $w(x) = 1_{[a,b]}(x)$ with $a$ and $b$ some finite values, for example, a lower and an upper quantile of $X$.

Of course, we cannot compute (10.21) in practice since we do not observe the $X_i$'s and so we cannot compute $\hat{g}_{EF}$. The idea of SIMEX is to simulate artificial data which mimic the data we cannot observe, and use them to approximate the bandwidth $\hat{H}$ at (10.21). To do this, first we simulate data $X_1^{**}, \ldots, X_n^{**}$ and $X_1^{***}, \ldots, X_n^{***}$ from the following two error models:

$$X_i^{**} = X_i^* + U_i^*\ ,\ X_i^{***} = X_i^{**} + U_i^{**}\,, \tag{10.22}$$

where $U_i^* \sim f_U$ and $U_i^{**} \sim f_U$ are independent. Let $g^*$ and $g^{**}$ denote the versions of $g$ with $X$ replaced by $X^*$ and $X_i^{**}$, respectively. For example, in the density case, $g^* = f_{X^*}$ and $g^{**} = f_{X^{**}}$ and in the regression case, $g^*(x) = E(Y|X^* = x)$ and $g^{**}(x) = E(Y|X^{**} = x)$. Since we observe the $X_i^*$'s and we generate the $U_i^*$'s and the $U_i^{**}$'s, then in the two error models at (10.22), we observe the contaminated variables $X_i^{**}$ and $X_i^{***}$, as well as their non contaminated version $X_i^*$ and $X_i^{**}$, respectively. Therefore, we can compute the deconvolution estimators $\hat{g}^*$ and $\hat{g}^{**}$ of $g^*$ and $g^{**}$, based on the $X_i^{**}$'s and the $X_i^{***}$'s, respectively, but we can also compute the standard estimators $\hat{g}_{EF}^*$ and $\hat{g}_{EF}^{**}$ of $g^*$ and $g^{**}$, based on the $X_i^*$'s and $X_i^{**}$'s, respectively. Therefore, we are able to compute the versions of (10.21) that correspond to those more contaminated data. That is, we can compute

$$\hat{H}^* = \text{argmin}_H D\{\hat{g}^*(\cdot;, H), \hat{g}_{EF}^*\}\ ,\ \hat{H}^{**} = \text{argmin}_H D\{\hat{g}^{**}(\cdot;, H), \hat{g}_{EF}^{**}\}\,.$$

Of course, such $\hat{H}^*$ and $\hat{H}^{**}$ depend heavily on the particular $X_i^{**}$'s and $X_i^{***}$'s generated at (10.22). To reduce this dependence, we simulate repeated, say $B$, samples $X_{b,1}^{**}, \ldots, X_{b,n}^{**}$ and $X_{b,1}^{***}, \ldots, X_{b,n}^{***}$ in the same way as at (10.22), for $b = 1, \ldots, B$, and take

$$\hat{H}^* = \text{argmin}_H B^{-1} \sum_{b=1}^{B} D\{\hat{g}_b^*(\cdot;, H), \hat{g}_{EF}^*\}\,,$$
$$\hat{H}^{**} = \text{argmin}_H B^{-1} \sum_{b=1}^{B} D\{\hat{g}_b^{**}(\cdot;, H), \hat{g}_{b,EF}^{**}\}\,,$$

where we used the index $b$ to indicate that an estimator was computed from the $b$th sample; $\hat{g}_{EF}^*$ does not have an index $b$ since only one sample from $X^*$ is available.

Next, since $X^{***}$ (resp., $X^{**}$) measures $X^{**}$ (resp., $X^*$) in the same way as $X^*$ measures $X$, it is reasonable to think that when $H$ is a single parameter (typically a bandwidth), the relationship between $\hat{H}^{**}$ and $\hat{H}^*$ approximates reasonably well the relationship between $\hat{H}^*$ and $\hat{H}$. This suggests that $\hat{H}/\hat{H}^* \approx \hat{H}^*/\hat{H}^{**}$, which suggests approximating $\hat{H}$ by

$$\hat{H} \approx (\hat{H}^*)^2/\hat{H}^{**}\,.$$

In the case where $H$ is multivariate, the approximation needs to be done with more thought as the relationship between the various components of $H$ may be important. For example, in the regression case where $H = (h, \rho)$, the values of $h$ and $\rho$ influence each other; see Delaigle and Hall (2008).

In general, since the errors used in the models at (10.22) have the same distribution as the $U_i$'s, then when $H = h$ is a bandwidth, the SIMEX bandwidth $\hat{h}$ converges to zero at the same speed as the optimal bandwidth corresponding to the distance used at (10.21). For example, for the deconvolution kernel density estimator, in the ordinary smooth error case, if $h_{\text{MISE}} \sim c_1 n^{-1/(2\beta+2k+1)}$, then $\hat{h} \sim c_2 n^{-1/(2\beta+2k+1)}$, but in general $c_2 \neq c_1$. That is, the SIMEX bandwidth is not a consistent estimator of the optimal bandwidth. However, in general too, $c_2$ is good approximation of $c_1$. This is contrast with the bandwidths introduced in the previous sections, which were consistent estimators of an optimal bandwidth. In cases where it is possible to compute a consistent estimator of the optimal bandwidth, it is often preferable to use such a consistent estimator, and dedicate SIMEX to more complex problems where such a bandwidth cannot be computed easily enough.

### 10.6.5 Further Reading

In the case where the error density $f_U$ is unknown and estimated from direct data generated from $f_U$, and $K$ is the sinc kernel, Diggle and Hall (1993) and Barry and Diggle (1995) proposed regression-based practical bandwidths.

Achilleos and Delaigle (2012) developed a local Empirical Bias Bandwidth Selector (EBBS) and a local integrated plug-in approach, both based on estimating the asymptotically dominating part of the MSE of $\hat{f}_X$ (the AMSE). They also proposed a local SIMEX approach based on the MSE. They showed that their plug-in and EBBS methods give good practical results and perform considerably better than global bandwidths in cases where $f_X$ has sharp features, without degrading much the quality of estimators (compared to using a global bandwidth) when $f_X$ is very smooth. R codes for those bandwidths are available on Delaigle's webpage.

## 10.7 Generalisations

Over the last three decades, a lot of effort has been dedicated to various problems related to nonparametric kernel density deconvolution, so much that it is not possible to present them all here, and we discuss only a few extensions. In Section 10.7.1, we show that in some cases, it is possible to perform the deconvolution explicitly without having to go through the Fourier domain. In Section 10.7.2, we discuss the case where the characteristic function of the errors vanishes and in Section 12.2.3 we discuss that where the errors are not identically distributed. In Section 10.7.4 we discuss multivariate extensions. We conclude with Section 10.7.5, where we briefly summarise some other related work developed in the literature.

### 10.7.1 Settings with Analytic Inversion Formulae

One of the difficulties of estimating a density from data measured with classical errors is that it involves a complex inversion process. Often, this deconvolution process can only be written analytically in the Fourier domain, as reflected by the Fourier approach taken by the deconvolution kernel density estimator. However, in some cases, it is possible to express $f_X$ analytically in terms of $f_{X^*}$ and thus to deconvolve without going through Fourier transforms.

Van Es and Kok (1998) considered two such particular cases. The first is when $U = \lambda_1 E_1 + \ldots + \lambda_m E_m$, where the $E_j$'s are independent standard exponential random variables, $m$ is a known positive integer and the $\lambda_j$'s are known constants; the second is when $U = \lambda_1 L_1 + \ldots + \lambda_m L_m$, where the $L_j$'s are independent standard Laplace random variables and the $\lambda_j$'s are known constants. They showed that in the exponential case we can write $F_X(x) = F_{X^*}(x) + \sum_{j=1}^m e_j f_{X^*}^{(j-1)}(x)$ and $f_X(x) = f_{X^*}(x) + \sum_{j=1}^m e_j f_{X^*}^{(j)}(x)$, where $e_j = \sum_{1\le i_1<\cdots<i_j\le m} \lambda_{i_1}\cdots\lambda_{i_j}$; in the Laplace case we have $F_X(x) = F_{X^*}(x)+\sum_{j=1}^m(-1)^j\ell_j f_{X^*}^{(2j-1)}(x)$ and $f_X(x) = f_{X^*}(x)+\sum_{j=1}^m(-1)^j\ell_j f_{X^*}^{(2j)}(x)$, where $\ell_j = \sum_{1\le i_1<\cdots<i_j\le m} \lambda_{i_1}^2\cdots\lambda_{i_j}^2$. Therefore, in the exponential we can estimate $F_X(x)$ and $f_X(x)$ by

$$\hat{F}_X(x) = \hat{F}_{X^*}(x) + \sum_{j=1}^m e_j \hat{f}_{X^*}^{(j-1)}(x)\,, \quad \hat{f}_X(x) = \hat{f}_{X^*}(x) + \sum_{j=1}^m e_j \hat{f}_{X^*}^{(j)}(x)\,,$$

and in the Laplace case we can take

$$\hat{F}_X(x) = \hat{F}_{X^*}(x)+\sum_{j=1}^m(-1)^j\ell_j \hat{f}_{X^*}^{(2j-1)}(x), \hat{f}_X(x) = \hat{f}_{X^*}(x)+\sum_{j=1}^m(-1)^j\ell_j \hat{f}_{X^*}^{(2j)}(x),$$

where $\hat{F}_{X^*}$ is a standard error-free kernel estimator of $F_{X^*}$ and $\hat{f}_{X^*}^{(j)}$ is the $j$th derivative of the standard kernel density estimator of $f_{X^*}$, all constructed from the $X_i^*$'s. In the Laplace case, the estimator is identical to the deconvolution kernel density estimator (see our example at (10.16) in Section 10.5.3). However, in the exponential case, the deconvolution kernel density estimator does not exist because $\varphi_U$ has some zeros; see Section 10.7.2.

Another particular case was considered by Groeneboom and Jongbloed (2003), who studied the case where $U$ follows a uniform distribution on $[0,1]$ and $f_X$ is supported on $[0,\infty)$ (the extension to a uniform $[0,b]$ error distribution is straightforward and obtained by simple rescaling). In that case,

$$f_{X^*}(x) = F_X(x) - F_X(x-1)\,, \tag{10.23}$$

a relationship that can be exploited to construct a nonparametric maximum likelihood estimator (NPMLE) $\hat{F}_X$ of $F_X$. This estimator is uniquely defined; it can only assign masses to points in the set $\{X_i^*, \ldots, X_n^*\}$. From there, a continuous estimator of $f_X(x)$ can be obtained by taking $\hat{f}_X(x) = \int K_h(x-y)\,d\hat{F}_X(y)\,dy$. As usual with kernel estimators, if $f_X$ is not continuous at 0, then $\hat{f}_X$ suffers from boundary problems which can be corrected by standard boundary correction techniques.

These authors discussed an alternative kernel smoothing approach for estimating $f_X$. Its construction is based on a recursive application of the relationship $F_X(x) = F_X(x-1) + f_{X^*}(x)$, which follows from (10.23). Together with the fact that for all $x \in \mathbb{R}$, $F_X(x-j) = 0$ when $j > x$, it leads to

$$F_X(x) = \sum_{j=0}^{\infty} f_{X^*}(x-j) \text{ and } f_X(x) = \sum_{j=0}^{\infty} f'_{X^*}(x-j), \tag{10.24}$$

where the second equality is obtained by differentiation of the first. This suggests estimating $f_X(x)$ by $\hat{f}_X(x) = \sum_{j=0}^{\infty} \hat{f}'_{X^*}(x-j)$, where $\hat{f}'_{X^*}$ denotes the first derivative of the standard kernel density estimator of $f_{X^*}$ (or a boundary corrected version if $f_X$ is not continuous as 0). Here too we cannot apply the deconvolution kernel density estimator since we have $\varphi_U(t) = (e^{it}-1)/(it)$, and thus $\varphi_U(t) = 0$ for $t = 2k\pi$, for all $k \in \mathbb{Z}_0$; see Section 10.7.2.

Delaigle and Meister (2011) considered a more general setting than the uniform case. Assuming that the distribution of $X$ has a finite left endpoint $a$, they considered error distributions whose characteristic function $\varphi_U$ has periodic isolated zeros, namely, where zeros of $\varphi_U$ can only be of the form $t = k\lambda$ for a fixed $\lambda$, where $k \in \mathbb{Z}_0$. For example, the ordinary smooth error case can be generalised by allowing $\varphi_U$ to satisfy

$$|\varphi_U(t)| \geq d_0 |\sin(t\pi/\lambda)|^{\nu} |t|^{-\beta} \quad \text{for large } |t| \tag{10.25}$$

and the supersmooth error case can be generalised by allowing $\varphi_U$ to satisfy

$$|\varphi_U(t)| \geq d_0 |\sin(t\pi/\lambda)|^{\nu} |t|^{\beta_0} \exp(-|t|^{\beta}/\gamma) \quad \text{for large } |t|. \tag{10.26}$$

This includes symmetric uniform distributions, their self convolutions, and their convolution with ordinary smooth or supersmooth distributions.

For such error distributions, we cannot estimate $\varphi_X(t)$ by $\hat{\varphi}_{X^*}(t)/\varphi_U(t)$ for all $t$ since $\varphi_U$ has zeros. To overcome this difficulty, instead of directly estimating $\varphi_X(t)$, Delaigle and Meister (2011) considered estimating first

$$\varphi_p(t) \equiv \big\{\exp(2it\pi/\lambda) - 1\big\}^{\nu} \varphi_X(t).$$

The term $\{\exp(2it\pi/\lambda) - 1\}^{\nu}$ is introduced to compensate for the term $|\sin(t\pi/\lambda)|^{\nu}$ term at (10.25) and (10.26). It is such that $\lim_{t\to k\lambda} |\exp(2it\pi/\lambda) - 1|^{\nu} |\sin(t\pi/\lambda)|^{-\nu}$ is finite, so that dividing by $\varphi_U$ no longer causes difficulties. In particular we can estimate $\varphi_p(t)$ by

$$\hat{\varphi}_p(t) = \begin{cases} \big\{\exp(2it\pi/\lambda) - 1\big\}^{\nu} \hat{\varphi}_{X^*}(t)/\varphi_U(t) & \text{if } t \neq k\lambda, k \in \mathbb{Z}_0 \\ c_k & \text{if } t = k\lambda, k \in \mathbb{Z}_0, \end{cases}$$

where $c_k = \lim_{t\to k\lambda} \hat{\varphi}_p(t)$ if it exists and 0 otherwise.

To deduce an estimator of $f_X$, let $p(x) = (2\pi)^{-1} \int e^{itx} \varphi_p(t)\, dt$. If $f_X$ is supported on $[a, \infty)$ with $a$ finite, then for all $J \geq \lambda(x-a)/(2\pi)$ we can write

$f_X(x) = \sum_{k=0}^{J} \eta_k \, p(x - 2k\pi/\lambda)$, where $(\eta_0, \ldots, \eta_J) = (1, 0, \ldots, 0)\mathbf{\Gamma}^{-1}$ and $\mathbf{\Gamma}$ is an upper triangular matrix whose component $(j, k)$, above the diagonal, is equal to $\binom{\nu}{k-j}(-1)^{\nu-k+j}$. Letting $\hat{p}(x) = (2\pi)^{-1} \int e^{itx} \varphi_K(ht)\hat{\varphi}_p(t)\, dt$ with $K$ a kernel and $h$ a bandwidth, and taking $J = J(x) = \lceil \lambda(x-a)/(2\pi) \rceil$, or taking $J = \lceil \lambda(b-a)/(2\pi) \rceil$ if $f_X$ is supported on $[a, b]$ with $b$ finite, we can estimate $f_X(x)$ by

$$\hat{f}_X(x) = \sum_{k=0}^{J} \eta_k \, \hat{p}(x - 2k\pi/\lambda) \cdot I\{a \leq x < \infty\}.$$

Delaigle and Meister (2011) showed that this estimator can be expressed in a form very similar to the deconvolution kernel density estimator.

### 10.7.2 When the Fourier Transform Vanishes

As we discussed in Section 10.7.1, since it involves dividing by $\varphi_U(t)$, the deconvolution kernel density estimator cannot be used when $\varphi_U(t)$ vanishes at some $t$. Since compactly supported distributions have a characteristic function that vanishes at some points, there are many important cases where this estimator cannot be used. In Section 10.7.1 we discussed simple alternative procedures that can be used in particular cases where $f_X$ can be expressed analytically in terms of $f_{X^*}$ without the need to work in the Fourier domain. In this section we discuss other procedures that can be used even when no such analytic expressions are available.

Devroye (1989) was one of the first to consider this problem. He showed that if $\varphi_U$ vanishes on a set of measure zero, we can still construct a consistent estimator of $f_X$. He proposed to modify the deconvolution kernel density estimator by replacing $\varphi_U^{-1}(t)$ at (10.3) by $\varphi_U^{-1}(t) \cdot I\{|\varphi_U(t)| \leq \rho\}$, for some small parameter $\rho > 0$. In other words, he proposed to remove, from the integration domain, the regions where $|\varphi_U|$ is too small. Instead of removing these regions from the integration domain, Meister (2007) proposed to replace $\hat{\varphi}_{X^*}(t)/\varphi_U(t)$ in those regions by using a polynomial approximation obtained from nearby points.

In the same context where $\varphi_U$ has isolated zeros, Hall and Meister (2007) proposed to use a ridge procedure, where they replace $\varphi_U$ by a ridge function when $|\varphi_U|$ gets too small. Using the fact that $\varphi_{X*}(t) = \varphi_X(t)\varphi_U(t)$ can be expressed as $\varphi_{X*}(t)\varphi_U(-t) = \varphi_X(t)|\varphi_U(t)|^2$, we could estimate $\varphi_X(t)$ by

$$\hat{\varphi}_X(t) = \frac{\hat{\varphi}_{X*}(t)\varphi_U(-t)}{\max\{|\varphi_U(t)|, \rho(t)\}^2},$$

where $\rho(t) > 0$ is a ridge function that prevents the denominator from getting too close to zero. The advantage of multiplying the numerator and the denominator by $\varphi_U(-t)$ before ridging is that unlike $\varphi_U(t)$, $|\varphi_U(t)|$ is guaranteed to be nonnegative, so that $\rho(t)$ can be restricted to be positive.

More generally, they write $\varphi_{X*}(t)\varphi_U(-t)|\varphi_U(t)|^r = \varphi_X(t)|\varphi_U(t)|^{r+2}$ for some $r \geq 0$ and propose to estimate $\varphi_X(t)$ by

$$\hat{\varphi}_X(t) = \frac{\hat{\varphi}_{X*}(t)\varphi_U(-t)|\varphi_U(t)|^r}{\max\{|\varphi_U(t)|, \rho(t)\}^{r+2}}.$$

Then assuming that $|\varphi_U(t)|^{r+1}$ is integrable, they estimate $f_X(x)$ by

$$\hat{f}_X(x) = \frac{1}{2\pi}\int e^{-itx}\frac{\hat{\varphi}_{X*}(t)\varphi_U(-t)|\varphi_U(t)|^r}{\max\{|\varphi_U(t)|, \rho(t)\}^{r+2}}\,dt.$$

Since the integral exists for all $x$, this approach does not require a kernel function, although Hall and Meister (2007) showed that the estimator can actually be expressed in a kernel form. See Hall and Meister (2007) for how to choose the ridge function $\rho(t)$ in practice using cross-validation. They studied the convergence rates of this estimator under various settings and showed that in some cases, those rates are the same as when $\varphi_U$ does not vanish anywhere (i.e., the same as those from Section 10.4). However, for errors as at (10.25), those rates are slower whereas the method proposed by Delaigle and Meister (2011) (see Section 10.7.1) has the same rates as when $\varphi_U$ does not vanish anywhere.

Meister and Neumann (2010) considered the case where $\varphi_U$ has some zeros and some replicated contaminated measurements are observed. Exploiting the replicates, they were able to propose yet another procedure.

### 10.7.3 Heteroscedatic Errors

Delaigle and Meister (2008) considered the density estimation problem in cases where the errors are not identically distributed. There, the observations $X_1^*, \ldots, X_n^*$ are independent and for $i = 1, \ldots, n$, $X_i^* = X_i + U_i$ where $X_i$ and $U_i$ are independent, $X_i \sim f_X$ for all $i$, but $U_i \sim f_{U_i}$, where the $f_{U_i}$'s are not necessarily identical. In that case, for $j = 1, \ldots, n$ we have $\varphi_{X_j^*}(t) = \varphi_X(t)\varphi_{U_j}(t)$ so that $\sum_{j=1}^n \varphi_{X_j^*}(t) = \varphi_X(t)\sum_{j=1}^n \varphi_{U_j}(t)$. Using Fourier inversion, if $\sum_{j=1}^n \varphi_{U_j}$ never vanishes we have

$$f_X(x) = \frac{1}{2\pi}\int e^{-itx}\frac{\sum_{j=1}^n \varphi_{X_j^*}(t)}{\sum_{j=1}^n \varphi_{U_j}(t)}\,dt.$$

Mimicking the deconvolution kernel estimation procedure at (10.3), this suggests that we could estimate $f_X(x)$ by

$$\hat{f}_X(x) = \frac{1}{2\pi}\int e^{-itx}\frac{\hat{\varphi}_{X^*}(t)\varphi_K(ht)}{n^{-1}\sum_{j=1}^n \varphi_{U_j}(t)}\,dt,$$

where $\hat{\varphi}_{X^*}(t) = n^{-1}\sum_{j=1}^n e^{itX_j^*}$ and with $K$ and $h$ as in Section 10.3.

While this approach is simple, Delaigle and Meister (2008) showed that faster convergence rates can be obtained by exploiting the relationship $\varphi_{X_j^*}(t)\varphi_{U_j}(-t) = \varphi_X(t)|\varphi_{U_j}(t)|^2$. Then if $\sum_{j=1}^n |\varphi_{U_j}(t)|^2 \neq 0$ for all $t \in \mathbb{R}$,

$$f_X(x) = \frac{1}{2\pi}\int e^{-itx}\frac{\sum_{j=1}^n \varphi_{X_j^*}(t)\varphi_{U_j}(-t)}{\sum_{j=1}^n |\varphi_{U_j}(t)|^2}\,dt\,,$$

which suggests estimating $f_X(x)$ by

$$\hat{f}_X(x) = \frac{1}{2\pi}\int e^{-itx}\frac{\sum_{j=1}^n e^{itX_j^*}\varphi_{U_j}(-t)}{\sum_{j=1}^n |\varphi_{U_j}(t)|^2}\varphi_K(ht)\,dt\,.$$

They generalised their procedure to the case where the error densities are unknown but the noisy observations are replicated; see Section 12.2 in Delaigle and Van Keilegom (2021). McIntyre and Stefanski (2011) also considered this problem in the case where the $U_{ij}$'s are normally distributed. Hesse (1995, 1996) considered a related setting where only a fraction of the observations are contaminated by errors and the others are observed without noise.

### 10.7.4 Multivariate and Dependent Cases

In Masry (1991), the observations are a univariate sample $X_1^*, \ldots, X_n^*$ from the classical error model at (10.1), but the $X_i$'s and the $U_i$'s are allowed the have a dependence structure, whereas the $X_i$'s remain independent of the $U_i$'s. For $\mathbf{T} = \mathbf{X}$ and $T_j = X_j$, $\mathbf{T} = \mathbf{X}^*$ and $T_j = X_j^*$, and $\mathbf{T} = \mathbf{U}$ and $T_j = U_j$, with $j = 1, \ldots, p$, let $f_{\mathbf{T}}$ and $\varphi_{\mathbf{T}}$ denote, respectively, the density and the characteristic function of $\mathbf{T} = (T_1, \ldots, T_p)$, where $p < n$. For simplicity we omit the explicit dependence on $p$ and all vectors in this section are assumed to be of size $p$. Assuming that the process $\{X_i\}_{i=-\infty}^{\infty}$ is stationary, the goal in Masry (1991) is to estimate $f_{\mathbf{X}}$ from the univariate data $X_1^*, \ldots, X_n^*$.

Masry (1991) generalised the deconvolution kernel estimator to this $p$-variate case, as follows. Since $\varphi_{\mathbf{X}^*}(\mathbf{t}) = \varphi_{\mathbf{X}}(\mathbf{t})\varphi_{\mathbf{U}}(\mathbf{t})$, if $\varphi_{\mathbf{U}}(\mathbf{t}) \neq 0$ for all $\mathbf{t}$ and all integrals below are well defined, by Fourier inversion we have

$$f_{\mathbf{X}}(\mathbf{x}) = \frac{1}{(2\pi)^p}\int e^{-i\mathbf{t}\cdot\mathbf{x}}\varphi_{\mathbf{X}^*}(\mathbf{t})/\varphi_{\mathbf{U}}(\mathbf{t})\,d\mathbf{t}\,,$$

where $\mathbf{t}\cdot\mathbf{x} = \sum_{j=1}^p t_j x_j$. This suggests extending the deconvolution kernel density estimator to the $p$-variate case by taking

$$\hat{f}_{\mathbf{X}}(\mathbf{x}) = \frac{1}{(2\pi)^p}\int e^{-i\mathbf{t}\cdot\mathbf{x}}\varphi_{\mathbf{K}}(\mathbf{t}h)\frac{\hat{\varphi}_{\mathbf{X}^*}(\mathbf{t})}{\varphi_{\mathbf{U}}(\mathbf{t})}\,d\mathbf{t}\,,$$

where $\mathbf{K}$ is a $p$-variate kernel function, $h > 0$ is a bandwidth, and $\hat{\varphi}_{\mathbf{X}^*}(\mathbf{t}) = (n-p+1)^{-1}\sum_{j=1}^{n-p+1} e^{i\mathbf{t}\mathbf{X}_j^*}$, with $\mathbf{X}_j^* = (X_j^*, \ldots, X_{j+p-1}^*)$. Letting $\mathbf{K}_{\mathbf{U}}(\mathbf{x}) =$

$(2\pi)^{-p}\int e^{-i\mathbf{t}\cdot\mathbf{x}}\varphi_{\mathbf{K}}(\mathbf{t})/\varphi_{\mathbf{U}}(\mathbf{t}/h)\,d\mathbf{t}$, we can express this estimator as

$$\hat{f}_{\mathbf{X}}(\mathbf{x}) = \frac{1}{(n-p+1)h^p}\sum_{j=1}^{n-p+1}\mathbf{K}_{\mathbf{U}}\Big(\frac{\mathbf{x}-\mathbf{X}_j^*}{h}\Big).$$

This definition uses a single bandwidth $h$, but as in the error-free case, we could also define a more general version with a $p$-variate bandwidth matrix.

Masry (1991) studied $L_2$ properties of this estimator and derived a number of technical results that are useful for more general deconvolution problems. Asymptotic normality, strong consistency and further properties were derived in Masry (1993a, 1993b, 2003) in the particular case where the $U_k$'s are i.i.d. In that case, if $\varphi_U$ denotes the common characteristic function of the $U_k$'s, and we take $\varphi_{\mathbf{K}}(\mathbf{t}) = \prod_{k=1}^p \varphi_K(t_k)$ where $K$ is a univariate kernel, we can write

$$\hat{f}_{\mathbf{X}}(\mathbf{x}) = \frac{1}{(n-p+1)h^p}\sum_{j=1}^{n-p+1}\prod_{k=0}^{p-1}K_U\Big(\frac{x_j - X_{j+k}^*}{h}\Big),$$

with $K_U$ at (10.5). In a related work where $p = 1$, Kulik (2008) studied properties of the deconvolution kernel density and distribution estimators in the case where the $X_i$'s are dependent and the errors are ordinary smooth, and showed that the order of the bandwidth and central limit theorems can be influenced by the strength of the dependence.

Youndjé and Wells (2008) considered a related multivariate density estimation problem. There, the observations are i.i.d. $p$-vectors $\mathbf{X}_1^*,\ldots,\mathbf{X}_n^*$, where for $i = 1,\ldots,n$, $\mathbf{X}_i^* = \mathbf{X}_i + \mathbf{U}_i$ and the $p$-variate $\mathbf{X}_i$'s are independent of the $p$-variate $\mathbf{U}_i$'s. This setting is different from the one above since here, for $\mathbf{T}_i = \mathbf{X}_i$ and $T_{ij} = X_{ij}$, $\mathbf{T}_i = \mathbf{X}_i^*$ and $T_{ij} = X_{ij}^*$, and $\mathbf{T}_i = \mathbf{U}_i$ and $T_{ij} = U_{ij}$, with $j = 1,\ldots,p$, the $\mathbf{T}_i$'s are defined by $\mathbf{T}_i = (T_{i1},\ldots,T_{ip})$, so that the $\mathbf{T}_i$'s are independent; for $i = 1,\ldots,n$ and $\mathbf{T} = \mathbf{X}$, $\mathbf{X}^*$ and $\mathbf{U}$, we use $f_{\mathbf{T}}$ and $\varphi_{\mathbf{T}}$ to denote, respectively, the density and the characteristic function of $\mathbf{T}_i$. An estimator of $f_{\mathbf{X}}$ can essentially be constructed as above but with a different estimator of $\varphi_{\mathbf{X}^*}$. Specifically, we take $\hat{\varphi}_{\mathbf{X}^*}(\mathbf{t}) = n^{-1}\sum_{j=1}^n e^{i\mathbf{t}\mathbf{X}_j^*}$ and estimate $f_{\mathbf{X}}(\mathbf{x})$ by

$$\hat{f}_{\mathbf{X}}(\mathbf{x}) = \frac{1}{(2\pi)^p}\int e^{-i\mathbf{t}\cdot\mathbf{x}}\varphi_{\mathbf{K}}(\mathbf{t}h)\hat{\varphi}_{\mathbf{X}^*}(\mathbf{t})/\varphi_{\mathbf{U}}(\mathbf{t})\,d\mathbf{t} = \frac{1}{nh^p}\sum_{j=1}^n \mathbf{K}_{\mathbf{U}}\Big(\frac{\mathbf{x}-\mathbf{X}_j^*}{h}\Big),$$

with $\mathbf{K}_{\mathbf{U}}$ as above. In the particular case where the $U_{ij}$'s are i.i.d. and we take $\varphi_{\mathbf{K}}(\mathbf{t}) = \prod_{j=1}^p \varphi_K(t_j)$, this estimator simplifies into

$$\hat{f}_{\mathbf{X}}(\mathbf{x}) = \frac{1}{nh^p}\sum_{j=1}^n\prod_{k=1}^p K_U\Big(\frac{x_k - X_{jk}^*}{h}\Big),$$

with $K_U$ at (10.5).

### 10.7.5 Further Reading

Hall and Lahiri (2008) considered the estimation of a cumulative distribution function, its moments and its quantiles, when the contaminated data come from the classical error model. Minimax properties of the distribution estimation problem were studied by Dattner et al. (2011) in the ordinary smooth error case; the quantile estimation problem was also considered by Dattner et al. (2016).

Rachdi and Sabre (2000) considered the problem of mode estimation of a density in the nonparametric deconvolution problem. Zhang and Karunamuni (2000) and Zhang and Karunamuni (2009) considered deconvolution kernel density estimation in the case where $f_X$ has a compact support, and Hall and Simar (2002), Goldenshluger and Tsybakov (2004), Delaigle and Gijbels (2006a, 2006b), Meister (2006), Aarts et al. (2007), and Kneip et al. (2015) proposed ways to estimate the boundary of this support.

Holzmann et al. (2007) and Butucea et al. (2009) considered general tests of hypothesis on the density $f_X$; Meister (2009b) considered tests of local monotonicity and Carroll et al. (2011) considered estimating and testing shape-constrained nonparametric density and regression with measurement errors. Their tilting technique consists in assigning weights $p_i$ to each $X_i^*$, such that $p_i \geq 0$ and $\sum_{i=1}^n p_i = 1$ (whereas the standard deconvolution kernel estimator assigns the same weight $1/n$ to each observation), where the $p_i$'s are chosen so that the density estimator satisfies the desired shape constraint. In a related work, Hazelton and Turlach (2009) proposed a weighted kernel density estimator $\hat{f}_X$ which assigns positive weights $p_i$ to each observation, but uses a standard kernel $K$ instead of the deconvolution kernel $K_U$. To choose the weights, they proposed to minimise the $L_2$ distance between the standard kernel density estimator of $f_{X^*}$ computed from the $X_i^*$'s and $\hat{f}_{X^*} = \hat{f}_X * f_U$. They also proposed a multivariate version of their procedure.

Hazelton and Turlach (2010) considered a semiparametric kernel estimator that avoids the use of a deconvolution technique by incorporating some parametric information in the construction; they extended their technique to the multivariate case. Delaigle and Hall (2014) considered a parametrically assisted version of the deconvolution kernel density estimator, where some a priori parametric information is included in the estimation technique. Potgieter (2020) considered a related deconvolution problem in the case where we can reasonably assume that $X$ has a generalised skew-symmetric distribution.

Some related work was also developed for other variants of the classical measurement error model. This includes Delaigle (2007), who considered kernel density estimation of a density contaminated by classical and Berkson errors, and Camirand Lemyre et al. (2021), who considered the kernel deconvolution problem with excess zeros. There, the interest is in a continuous random variable, typically representing the long term intake $X$ of a nutrient, and the measured variables are either equal to a contaminated version $X^*$ of $X$, if the measurement was taken on a consumption day, or to zero if the observed individual did not eat the nutrient on the day where the measurement was taken.

## Acknowledgment

Delaigle acknowledges support from the Australian Research Council (DP170102434).

## Bibliography

Aarts, L., Groeneboom, P., and Jongbloed, G. (2007). Estimating the upper support point in deconvolution. *Scandinavian Journal of Statistics*, 34(3), 552-568.

Achilleos, A. and Delaigle, A. (2012). Local bandwidth selectors for deconvolution kernel density estimation. *Statistics and Computing*, 22(2), 563-577.

Apanasovich, T. and Liang, H. (2021). Nonparametric measurement errors models for regression. In *Handbook of Measurement Error Models*, G. Y. Yi, A., Delaigle, and P. Gustafson (Eds.), CRC, Chapter 14.

Barry, J. and Diggle, P. (1995). Choosing the smoothing parameter in a Fourier approach to nonparametric deconvolution of a density estimate. *Journal of Nonparametric Statistics*, 4(3), 223-232.

Buonaccorsi, J. P. (2010). *Measurement Error: Models, Methods, and Applications.* CRC Press.

Butucea, C. (2004a). Asymptotic normality of the integrated square error of a density estimator in the convolution model. *SORT: Statistics and Operations Research Transactions*, 28(1), 9-26.

Butucea, C. (2004b). Deconvolution of supersmooth densities with smooth noise. *Canadian Journal of Statistics*, 32(2), 181-192.

Butucea, C., Matias, C., and Pouet, C. (2009). Adaptive goodness-of-fit testing from indirect observations. In *Annales de l'ihp probabilités et statistiques* Volume 45, pp. 352-372.

Butucea, C. and Tsybakov, A. B. (2008a). Sharp optimality in density deconvolution with dominating bias. *Theory of Probability & Its Applications*, 52(1), 24-39.

Butucea, C. and Tsybakov, A. B. (2008b). Sharp optimality in density deconvolution with dominating bias. *Theory of Probability & Its Applications*, 52(1), 237-249.

Camirand Lemyre, F., Carroll, R. J., and Delaigle, A. (2021). Semiparametric estimation of the distribution of episodically consumed foods measured with error. *Journal of the American Statistical Association.* doi: 10.1080/01621459.2020.1787840.

Carroll, R. J., Delaigle, A., and Hall, P. (2011). Testing and estimating shape-constrained nonparametric density and regression in the presence of measurement error. *Journal of the American Statistical Association*, 106(493), 191-202.

Carroll, R. J. and Hall, P. (1988). Optimal rates of convergence for deconvolving a density. *Journal of the American Statistical Association*, 83(404), 1184-1186.

Carroll, R. J. and Hall, P. (2004). Low order approximations in deconvolution and regression with errors in variables. *Journal of the Royal Statistical Society: Series B*, 66(1), 31-46.

Carroll, R. J., Ruppert, D., Stefanski, L. and Crainiceanu, C. (2006). *Measurement Error in Nonlinear Models: A Modern Perspective.* CRC Press.

Cook, J. R. and Stefanski, L. A. (1994). Simulation-extrapolation estimation in parametric measurement error models. *Journal of the American Statistical association*, 89(428), 1314-1328.

Dattner, I., Goldenshluger, A., and Juditsky, A. (2011). On deconvolution of distribution functions. *The Annals of Statistics*, 39:2477-2501.

Dattner, I., Reiß, M., and Trabs, M. (2016). Adaptive quantile estimation in deconvolution with unknown error distribution. *Bernoulli*, 22(1), 143-192.

Delaigle, A. (2007). Nonparametric density estimation from data with a mixture of Berkson and classical errors. *Canadian Journal of Statistics*, 35(1), 89-104.

Delaigle, A. (2008). An alternative view of the deconvolution problem. *Statistica Sinica*, 18, 1025-1045.

Delaigle, A. (2014). Nonparametric kernel methods with errors-in-variables: constructing estimators, computing them, and avoiding common mistakes. *Australian & New Zealand Journal of Statistics*, 56(2), 105-124.

Delaigle, A., Fan, J., and Carroll, R. J. (2009). A design-adaptive local polynomial estimator for the errors-in-variables problem. *Journal of the American Statistical Association*, 104(485), 348-359.

Delaigle, A. and Gijbels, I. (2002). Estimation of integrated squared density derivatives from a contaminated sample. *Journal of the Royal Statistical Society: Series B*, 64(4), 869-886.

Delaigle, A. and Gijbels, I. (2004a). Bootstrap bandwidth selection in kernel density estimation from a contaminated sample. *Annals of the Institute of Statistical Mathematics*, 56(1), 19-47.

Delaigle, A. and Gijbels, I. (2004b). Practical bandwidth selection in deconvolution kernel density estimation. *Computational statistics & data analysis*, 45(2), 249-267.

Delaigle, A. and Gijbels, I. (2006a). Data-driven boundary estimation in deconvolution problems. *Computational Statistics & Data Analysis*, 50(8), 1965-1994.

Delaigle, A. and Gijbels, I. (2006b). Estimation of boundary and discontinuity points in deconvolution problems. *Statistica Sinica*, 16, 773-788.

Delaigle, A. and Gijbels, I. (2007). Frequent problems in calculating integrals and optimizing objective functions: a case study in density deconvolution. *Statistics and Computing*, 17(4), 349-355.

Delaigle, A. and Hall, P. (2006). On optimal kernel choice for deconvolution. *Statistics & Probability Letters*, 76(15), 1594-1602.

Delaigle, A. and Hall, P. (2008). Using SIMEX for smoothing-parameter choice in errors-in-variables problems. *Journal of the American Statistical Association*, 103(481), 280-287.

Delaigle, A. and Hall, P. (2014). Parametrically assisted nonparametric estimation of a density in the deconvolution problem. *Journal of the American Statistical Association*, 109(506), 717-729.

Delaigle, A. and Hall, P. (2016). Methodology for non-parametric deconvolution when the error distribution is unknown. *Journal of the Royal Statistical Society: Series B*, 78, 231-252.

Delaigle, A., Hall, P. and Meister, A. (2008). On deconvolution with repeated measurements. *The Annals of Statistics*, 36(2), 665-685.

Delaigle, A., Hyndman, T., and Wang, T. (2020). Deconvolve: Deconvolution tools for measurement error problems. R package version 0.1.0.

Delaigle, A. and Meister, A. (2007). Nonparametric regression estimation in the heteroscedastic errors-in-variables problem. *Journal of the American Statistical Association*, 102, 1416-1426.

Delaigle, A. and Meister, A. (2008). Density estimation with heteroscedastic error. *Bernoulli*, 14, 562-579.

Delaigle, A. and Meister, A. (2011). Nonparametric function estimation under Fourier-oscillating noise. *Statistica Sinica*, 21, 1065-1092.

Delaigle, A. and Van Keilegom, I. (2021). Deconvolution with unknown error distribution. In *Handbook of Measurement Error Models*, G. Y. Yi, A. Delaigle, and P. Gustafson (Eds.), CRC, Chapter 12.

Devroye, L. (1989). Consistent deconvolution in density estimation. *The Canadian Journal of Statistics*, 17, 235-239.

Diggle, P. and Hall, P. (1993). A Fourier approach to nonparametric deconvolution of a density estimate. *Journal of the Royal Statistical Society: Series B*, 55(2), 523-531.

Fan, J. (1991a). Asymptotic normality for deconvolution kernel density estimators. *Sankhyā: The Indian Journal of Statistics, Series A*, 53, 97-110.

Fan, J. (1991b). Global behavior of deconvolution kernel estimates. *Statistica Sinica*, 1, 541-551.

Fan, J. (1991c). On the optimal rates of convergence for nonparametric deconvolution problems. *The Annals of Statistics*, 19, 1257-1272.

Fan, J. (1992). Deconvolution with supersmooth distributions. *Canadian Journal of Statistics*, 20(2), 155-169.

Fan, J. and Truong, Y. K. (1993). Nonparametric regression with errors in variables. *The Annals of Statistics*, 21, 1900-1925.

Goldenshluger, A. and Tsybakov, A. (2004). Estimating the endpoint of a distribution in the presence of additive observation errors. *Statistics & Probability Letters*, 68(1), 39-49.

Granovsky, B. L. and Müller, H.-G. (1989). On the optimality of a class of polynomial kernel functions. *Statistics & Risk Modeling*, 7(4), 301-312.

Granovsky, B. L. and Müller, H.-G. (1991). Optimizing kernel methods: a unifying variational principle. *International Statistical Review/Revue Internationale de Statistique*, 59, 373-388.

Granovsky, B. L., Müller, H.-G., and Pfeifer, C. (1995). Some remarks on optimal kernel functions. *Statistics & Risk Modeling*, 13(2), 101-116.

Groeneboom, P. and Jongbloed, G. (2003). Density estimation in the uniform deconvolution model. *Statistica Neerlandica*, 57(1), 136-157.

Hall, P. and Lahiri, S. N. (2008). Estimation of distributions, moments and quantiles in deconvolution problems. *The Annals of Statistics*, 36(5), 2110-2134.

Hall, P. and Meister, A. (2007). A ridge-parameter approach to deconvolution. *The Annals of Statistics*, 35(4), 1535-1558.

Hall, P. and Murison, R. D. (1993). Correcting the negativity of high-order kernel density estimators. *Journal of Multivariate Analysis*, 47(1), 103-122.

Hall, P. and Simar, L. (2002). Estimating a changepoint, boundary, or frontier in the presence of observation error. *Journal of the American statistical Association*, 97(458), 523-534.

Hazelton, M. L. and Turlach, B. A. (2009). Nonparametric density deconvolution by weighted kernel estimators. *Statistics and Computing*, 19(3), 217-228.

Hazelton, M. L. and Turlach, B. A. (2010). Semiparametric density deconvolution. *Scandinavian Journal of Statistics*, 37(1), 91-108.

Hesse, C. H. (1995). Deconvolving a density from partially contaminated observations. *Journal of Multivariate Analysis*, 55(2), 246-260.

Hesse, C. H. (1996). How many "good"observations do you need for "fast" density deconvolution from supersmooth errors. *Sankhyā: The Indian Journal of Statistics, Series A*, 58, 491-506.

Hesse, C. H. (1999). Data-driven deconvolution. *Journal of Nonparametric Statistics*, 10(4), 343-373.

Holzmann, H., Bissantz, N., and Munk, A. (2007). Density testing in a contaminated sample. *Journal of Multivariate Analysis*, 98(1), 57-75.

Holzmann, H. and Boysen, L. (2006). Integrated square error asymptotics for supersmooth deconvolution. *Scandinavian Journal of Statistics*, 33(4), 849-860.

Kang, Y. and Qiu, P. (2021). Nonparametric deconvolution by fourier transformation and other related approaches. In G. Y. Yi, A. Delaigle, and P. Gustafson (Eds.), *Handbook of Measurement Error Models*, CRC, Chapter 11.

Kneip, A., Simar, L., and Van Keilegom, I. (2015). Frontier estimation in the presence of measurement error with unknown variance. *Journal of Econometrics*, 184(2), 379-393.

Kulik, R. (2008). Nonparametric deconvolution problem for dependent sequences. *Electronic Journal of Statistics*, 2, 722-740.

Liu, M. C. and Taylor, R. L. (1989). A consistent nonparametric density estimator for the deconvolution problem. *Canadian Journal of Statistics*, 17(4), 427-438.

Liu, M. C. and Taylor, R. L. (1990). Simulations and computations of nonparametric density estimates for the deconvolution problem. *Journal of Statistical Computation and Simulation*, 35, 145-167.

Lütkenöner, B. (2015). A family of kernels and their associated deconvolving kernels for normally distributed measurement errors. *Journal of Statistical Computation and Simulation*, 85(12), 2347-2363.

Masry, E. (1991). Multivariate probability density deconvolution for stationary random processes. *IEEE Transactions on Information Theory*, 37(4), 1105-1115.

Masry, E. (1993a). Asymptotic normality for deconvolution estimators of multivariate densities of stationary processes. *Journal of Multivariate Analysis*, 44(1), 47-68.

Masry, E. (1993b). Strong consistency and rates for deconvolution of multivariate densities of stationary processes. *Stochastic Processes and their Applications*, 47(1), 53-74.

Masry, E. (2003). Deconvolving multivariate kernel density estimates from contaminated associated observations. *IEEE Transactions on Information Theory*, 49(11), 2941-2952.

McIntyre, J. and Stefanski, L. (2011). Density estimation with replicate heteroscedastic measurements. *Annals of the Institute of Statistical Mathematics*, 63(1), 81-99.

Meister, A. (2006). Support estimation via moment estimation in presence of noise. *Statistics*, 40(3), 259-275.

Meister, A. (2007). Deconvolution from Fourier-oscillating error densities under decay and smoothness restrictions. *Inverse Problems*, 24(1), 015003.

Meister, A. (2009a). *Deconvolution Problems in Nonparametric Statistics.* Springer.

Meister, A. (2009b). On testing for local monotonicity in deconvolution problems. *Statistics & Probability Letters*, 79(3), 312-319.

Meister, A. and Neumann, M. H. (2010). Deconvolution from non-standard error densities under replicated measurements. *Statistica Sinica*, 20, 1609-1636.

Neumann, M. H. (1997). On the effect of estimating the error density in nonparametric deconvolution. *Journal of Nonparametric Statistics*, 7, 307-330.

Pensky, M. and Vidakovic, B. (1999). Adaptive wavelet estimator for nonparametric density deconvolution. *The Annals of Statistics*, 27(6), 2033-2053.

Potgieter, C. J. (2020). Density deconvolution for generalized skew-symmetric distributions. *Journal of Statistical Distributions and Applications*, 7(1), 1-20.

Rachdi, M. and Sabre, R. (2000). Consistent estimates of the mode of the probability density function in nonparametric deconvolution problems. *Statistics & Probability Letters*, 47(2), 105-114.

Song, W. (2010). Moderate deviations for deconvolution kernel density estimators with ordinary smooth measurement errors. *Statistics & Probability Letters*, 80, 169-176.

Stefanski, L. (1990). Rates of convergence of some estimators in a class of deconvolution problems. *Statistics & Probability Letters*, 9(3), 229-235.

Stefanski, L. and Carroll, R. J. (1990). Deconvolving kernel density estimators. *Statistics*, 21(2), 169-184.

Stefanski, L. and Cook, J. R. (1995). Simulation-extrapolation: The measurement error jackknife. *Journal of the American Statistical Association*, 90(432), 1247-1256.

Van Es, A. and Kok, A. (1998). Simple kernel estimators for certain nonparametric deconvolution problems. *Statistics & Probability Letters*, 39(2), 151-160.

Van Es, A. and Uh, H.-W. (2004). Asymptotic normality of nonparametric kernel type deconvolution density estimators: crossing the cauchy boundary. *Nonparametric Statistics*, 16, 261-277.

Van Es, A. and Uh, H.-W. (2005). Asymptotic normality of kernel-type deconvolution estimators. *Scandinavian Journal of Statistics*, 32(3), 467-483.

Van Es, B. and Gugushvili, S. (2010). Asymptotic normality of the deconvolution kernel density estimator under the vanishing error variance. *Journal of the Korean Statistical Society*, 39, 103-115.

Youndjé, É. and Wells, M. T. (2002). Least squares cross-validation for the kernel deconvolution density estimator. *Comptes Rendus Mathematique*, 334(6), 509-513.

Youndjé, É. and Wells, M. T. (2008). Optimal bandwidth selection for multivariate kernel deconvolution density estimation. *Test*, 17(1), 138-162.

Zhang, C.-H. (1990). Fourier methods for estimating mixing densities and distributions. *The Annals of Statistics*, 18, 806-831.

Zhang, S. and Karunamuni, R. J. (2000). Boundary bias correction for nonparametric deconvolution. *Annals of the Institute of Statistical Mathematics*, 52(4), 612-629.

Zhang, S. and Karunamuni, R. J. (2009). Deconvolution boundary kernel method in nonparametric density estimation. *Journal of Statistical Planning and Inference*, 139(7), 2269-2283.

Zu, Y. (2015). A note on the asymptotic normality of the kernel deconvolution density estimator with logarithmic chi-square noise. *Econometrics*, 3(3), 561-576.

# 11

# *Nonparametric Deconvolution by Fourier Transformation and Other Related Approaches*

**Yicheng Kang and Peihua Qiu**

**CONTENTS**



Nonparametric deconvolution in density estimation and its companion in regression (i.e., nonparametric regression with measurement errors) have broad applications. Many nonparametric deconvolution methods in the literature are based on kernel estimation. There are also some nonparametric deconvolution methods constructed based on the Fourier transformation, splines, wavelet, and other function expansions in specific basis function spaces. In this paper, some representative methods in the latter type are introduced. Some recent methods in the related image deblurring area are also described.

## 11.1 Introduction

Assume that we are interested in estimating the distribution of a random variable $X$, but it cannot be observed directly. What is observed is its

DOI: 10.1201/9781315101279-11

contaminated version $X^*$ defined by

$$X^* = X + U, \tag{11.1}$$

where $U$ is the measurement error, and $X$ and $U$ are assumed to be independent with probability density functions $f_X$ and $f_U$, respectively. From (11.1), it is obvious that

$$f_{X^*}(x^*) = \int f_U(x^* - x) f_X(x)\, dx, \tag{11.2}$$

where $f_{X^*}$ denotes the density of $X^*$. Namely, the density of $X^*$ is a convolution of the densities of $X$ and $U$. In the literature, it is often assumed that $f_U$ is known and we will make that assumption throughout this chapter; for the case where $f_U$ is unknown, see Delaigle and Van Keilegom (2021). Then, our major goal is to estimate $f_X$ from a set of observations of $X^*$ through (11.2), which is a *deconvolution* problem.

Let $\{X_1^*, X_2^*, \ldots, X_n^*\}$ be a set of independent and identically distributed (i.i.d.) observations of $X^*$. To obtain a nonparametric estimator of $f_X$, denoted as $\hat{f}_X$, we wish to "invert" (11.2), since $f_{X^*}$ can be estimated from the observations of $X^*$. Thus, the deconvolution problem is an *inverse* problem. More specifically, let $\mathcal{F}\{f\}(\omega)$ or $\tilde{f}(\omega)$ denote the Fourier transformation $\int_{-\infty}^{\infty} \exp(i\omega x) f(x) dx$ of a function $f(x)$, and $\mathcal{F}^{-1}\{\tilde{f}\}(x)$ denote the inverse Fourier transformation of $\tilde{f}(\omega)$. Then, by the property of the Fourier transformation that the Fourier transformation of the convolution of two functions equals the product of the Fourier transformations of the two individual functions, we have

$$\mathcal{F}\{f_{X^*}\}(\omega) = \mathcal{F}\{f_U\}(\omega)\mathcal{F}\{f_X\}(\omega).$$

Therefore, a reasonable estimator of $\mathcal{F}\{f_X\}(\omega)$, denoted as $\widehat{\mathcal{F}}\{f_X\}(\omega)$, can be defined as

$$\widehat{\mathcal{F}}\{f_X\}(\omega) = \frac{\widehat{\mathcal{F}}\{f_{X^*}\}(\omega)}{\mathcal{F}\{f_U\}(\omega)},$$

where $\widehat{\mathcal{F}}\{f_{X^*}\}(\omega)$ is an estimator of $\mathcal{F}\{f_{X^*}\}(\omega)$ that can be obtained from the observations of $X^*$ and $\mathcal{F}\{f_U\}(\omega)$ can be computed from the known function $f_U$. In the above expression, $\mathcal{F}\{f_U\}(\omega)$ generally approaches zero rapidly when $|\omega|$ increases, but for $|\omega|$ large, $\widehat{\mathcal{F}}\{f_{X^*}\}(\omega)$ is a poor estimator that oscillates. Therefore, the ratio $\widehat{\mathcal{F}}\{f_{X^*}\}(\omega)/\mathcal{F}\{f_U\}(\omega)$ is numerically unstable, which makes the deconvolution problem challenging to solve. Therefore, the deconvolution problem is a so-called "ill-posed" problem in the literature (Tikhonov and Arsenin, 1977).

The deconvolution problem has a vigorous history, including considerable work on kernel-based methods that involve estimating $f_{X^*}$ by a kernel estimator and then solving equation (11.2) using a Fourier transformation. See, for example, the contribution of Carroll and Hall (1988), Devroye (1989), Diggle and Hall (1993), Efromovich (1997), Fan (1991a), Fan (1991b), Liu and Taylor (1989), Masry (1991), Masry (1993), Stefanski (1990), Stefanski and Carroll (1990), Taylor and Zhang (1990), and Zhang (1990). In addition to the kernel-based methods, several alternative approaches using series expansions have been suggested over the years. For instance, a Fourier series (cosine-sine) method was proposed by Hall and Qiu (2005) and Delaigle et al. (2006). Spline-based methods were discussed by Mendelsohn and Rice (1982) and Koo and Park (1996). Wavelet methods were addressed by Pensky and Vidakovic (1999), Walter (1999), Fan and Koo (2002) and Pensky (2002). Taylor series low order approximation methods were explored by Carroll and Hall (2004).

Kernel-based methods for density and regression estimation are introduced in Chapters 10 (Delaigle, 2021) and 14 (Apanasovich and Liang, 2021). This chapter aims to introduce some of the alternative methods. Our introduction will focus on the main ideas of some fundamental methodologies, their major strengths and limitations, their potential applications in other areas (e.g., image analysis), and certain important open problems for future research. The remaining part of the chapter is organized as follows. Methods based on the Fourier series expansion are discussed in Section 11.2. Spline-based methods are described in Section 11.3. Wavelet methods are introduced in Section 11.4. Methods using low order approximations are discussed in Section 11.5. Then, in Section 11.6, we discuss the image deblurring problem which is essentially a deconvolution problem in image analysis. Some concluding remarks are given in Section 11.7.

## 11.2 Deconvolution by the Fourier Series Expansion

The deconvolution method suggested by Hall and Qiu (2005) is based on the Fourier series expansion. Its major idea is to use the property of trigonometric-series expansions that the effect of the random error $U$ in (11.1) can be factorized out and becomes separate from the effect of $X$. More specifically, assume that the support of the distribution of $X$ is contained in a known compact interval $\mathcal{I}$. This requires only knowledge of an upper bound for the support of $f_X$, although methodologies have been developed for estimating the actual support (e.g., Delaigle and Gijbels, 2006) when $\mathcal{I}$ is unknown. Without loss of generality, let $\mathcal{I} = [0, \pi]$. Then, we consider the cosine-series expansion of $f_X$ on $\mathcal{I}$ (the reason for choosing the cosine series, rather than the full cosine and sine series, will be explained later):

$$f_X(x) = a + \sum_{j\geq 1} a_{1j} \cos(jx),$$

where $a = \pi^{-1}$, $a_{kj} = (2/\pi)\int_{\mathcal{I}} f_X(x) cs_{kj}(x)\, dx$, and

$$cs_{kj}(x) = \begin{cases} \cos(jx), & k = 1, \\ \sin(jx), & k = 2. \end{cases}$$

The case where $k = 2$ is considered above because the related quantities will be used below. Then, $f_X$ can be estimated by $\overline{f}_X(x) = \pi^{-1} + \sum_{j\geq 1} \overline{a}_{1j}\cos(jx)$, where $\overline{a}_{kj}$ denotes an estimator of $a_{kj}$, for $k = 1, 2$ and $j \geq 1$. To obtain $\overline{a}_{kj}$, recall that $\alpha_{kj} = E[cs_{kj}(U)]$ is known for all $j$ and $k$. By the basic properties of trigonometric functions, we have

$$b_{kj} \equiv \frac{2}{\pi}E[cs_{kj}(X^*)] = \frac{2}{\pi}E[cs_{kj}(X+U)] = \begin{cases} a_{1j}\alpha_{1j} - a_{2j}\alpha_{2j}, & \text{if } k = 1, \\ a_{2j}\alpha_{1j} + a_{1j}\alpha_{2j}, & \text{if } k = 2. \end{cases} \tag{11.3}$$

Therefore, $b_j = (b_{1j}, b_{2j})^T$ can be expressed as $b_j = M_j a_j$, where $a_j = (a_{1j}, a_{2j})^T$ and $M_j$ is the $2 \times 2$ matrix with $(M_j)_{11} = (M_j)_{22} = \alpha_{1j}$ and $(M_j)_{21} = -(M_j)_{12} = \alpha_{2j}$. If

$$|\alpha_{1j}| + |\alpha_{2j}| \neq 0 \quad (j \geq 1), \tag{11.4}$$

then $a_j$ can be expressed as

$$\begin{pmatrix} a_{1j} \\ a_{2j} \end{pmatrix} = \frac{1}{\alpha_{1j}^2 + \alpha_{2j}^2}\begin{pmatrix} \alpha_{1j} & \alpha_{2j} \\ -\alpha_{2j} & \alpha_{1j} \end{pmatrix}\begin{pmatrix} b_{1j} \\ b_{2j} \end{pmatrix}. \tag{11.5}$$

So, $a_{1j}$ and $a_{2j}$ can be estimated by replacing $b_{1j}$ and $b_{2j}$ by their estimators on the right-hand side of (11.5). Now, $\hat{b}_{kj} = (2/\pi)n^{-1}\sum_i cs_{kj}(X_i^*)$ are the moment estimators of $b_{kj}$, for all $k$ and $j$, which are unbiased. Therefore, $a_{kj}$ can be estimated by

$$\begin{pmatrix} \hat{a}_{1j} \\ \hat{a}_{2j} \end{pmatrix} = \frac{1}{\alpha_{1j}^2 + \alpha_{2j}^2}\begin{pmatrix} \alpha_{1j} & \alpha_{2j} \\ -\alpha_{2j} & \alpha_{1j} \end{pmatrix}\begin{pmatrix} \hat{b}_{1j} \\ \hat{b}_{2j} \end{pmatrix}. \tag{11.6}$$

Thus, the following estimator of $a_{1j}$ is obtained:

$$\hat{a}_{1j} = \frac{\alpha_{1j}\hat{b}_{1j} + \alpha_{2j}\hat{b}_{2j}}{\alpha_{1j}^2 + \alpha_{2j}^2}. \tag{11.7}$$

In the literature, it is often assumed that the distribution of $U$ is known and symmetric about its mean. In such cases, without loss of generality, we can further assume that the mean of $U$ equals zero. Then, $\alpha_{2j} = 0$ and the assumption (11.4) reduces to $\alpha_{1j} \neq 0$, for each $j$. Then, (11.7) becomes $\hat{a}_{1j} = \alpha_{1j}^{-1}\hat{b}_{1j}$, and the corresponding estimator of $f_X(x)$ can be defined as

$$\overline{f}_X(x) = \pi^{-1} + \sum_{j=1}^{\infty} \alpha_{1j}\overline{b}_{1j}\cos(jx), \tag{11.8}$$

where $\bar{b}_{1j} = \hat{b}_{1j}$ for $j \leq m$ and 0 otherwise, and $m$ is a parameter. Here, $m$ works as a smoothing parameter and it can be chosen by a smoothing parameter selection procedure, such as the cross-validation procedure.

In (11.8), the cosine-series is used, instead of the sine-series or the full cosine/sine-series, because the corresponding estimator of $f_X(x)$ is robust against edge effects on $[0, \pi]$, as explained below. If $f_1(x)$ and $f_2(x)$ have a smooth derivative on $[0, \pi]$ and $[-\pi, \pi]$, respectively, then (by integration by parts)

$$\begin{aligned}\int_0^\pi f_1(x)\cos(jx)\,dx &= -\frac{1}{j}\int_0^\pi f_1'(x)\sin(jx)\,dx \\ &= \frac{1}{j^2}\left[(-1)^j f_1'(\pi) - f_1'(0)\right] - \frac{1}{j^2}\int_0^\pi f_1''(x)\cos(jx)\,dx \\ &= j^{-2}\left[(-1)^j f_1'(\pi) - f_1'(0)\right] + o\left(j^{-2}\right), \end{aligned} \tag{11.9}$$

Similarly, we have

$$\int_{-\pi}^\pi f_2(x)\sin(jx)\,dx = j^{-1}(-1)^{j+1}\left[f_2(\pi) - f_2(-\pi)\right] + o\left(j^{-1}\right). \tag{11.10}$$

Formula (11.10) implies that, unless $f_X(x)$ satisfies the periodic-continuity condition $f_X(\pi) = f_X(-\pi)$, coefficients in the full cosine/sine-series on $[-\pi, \pi]$ converge only at rate of $j^{-1}$. On the other hand, (11.9) implies that, without such a condition, the cosine-series on $[0, \pi]$ converges at rate of $j^{-2}$. This faster rate entails a smaller order of bias, and hence a faster rate of convergence in mean squares, of the estimator $\overline{f}_X$ in (11.10).

A counterpart of the deconvolution problem in regression is the errors-in-variables problem described below. Let $Y$ be a response variable, and $X$ be a predictor. We are interested in the functional relationship between $X$ and $Y$. However, $X$ cannot be observed directly. Instead, we can observe $X^*$. Then, a statistical model for describing this errors-in-variables problem can be the following one:

$$\begin{cases} Y = g(X) + V, \\ X^* = X + U, \end{cases} \tag{11.11}$$

where $U$ and $V$ are random errors, and $X$, $U$ and $V$ are independent of each other. Let $(X_1^*, Y_1)$, $(X_2^*, Y_2)$, ..., $(X_n^*, Y_n)$ be i.i.d. observations of $(X^*, Y)$. Then, the major goal of the errors-in-variables problem is to estimate the regression function $g$ from the observations $\{(X_i^*, Y_i), i = 1, 2, \ldots, n\}$. To this end, the method based on the cosine-series expansion discussed above can be modified for solving the errors-in-variables problem, as described below. Let $\psi(x) = g(x)f_X(x)$. We again assume that the support of $f_X$ is included in $[0, \pi]$. Then the support of $\psi$ is included in $[0, \pi]$ as well. In the case where we do not have knowledge of an upper bound for the support of $f_X$, we can estimate the support using the methodology proposed in Delaigle and Gijbels (2006).

Next, the cosine-series expansion of $\psi$ is

$$\psi(x) = \beta_0 + \sum_{j\geq 1} \beta_j \cos(jx), \qquad \text{for } x \in [0, \pi],$$

where $\beta_0 = \pi^{-1}$, and $\beta_j = (2/\pi)\int_0^\pi \psi(x)\cos(jx)\, dx$, for all $j$. Note that $\beta_j$ can be written as

$$\beta_j = \frac{2}{\pi} E\left[\cos(jX)g(X)\right].$$

By the elementary properties of the trigonometric functions, we have

$$\begin{aligned}\cos(jX^*)g(X) &= \cos(jX + jU)g(X) \\ &= \cos(jX)g(X)\cos(jU) - \sin(jX)g(X)\sin(jU). \end{aligned} \tag{11.12}$$

By the assumptions that the distribution of $U$ is symmetric about zero and $\alpha_{1j} \neq 0$, we have

$$E\left[\cos(jX)g(X)\right] = \alpha_{1j}^{-1} E\left[\cos(jX^*)g(X)\right].$$

Now, $E\left[\cos(jX^*)g(X)\right] = E\left[\cos(jX^*)Y\right]$ and $n^{-1}\sum_i \cos(jX_i^*)Y_i$ is an unbiased estimator of $E\left[\cos(jX^*)Y\right]$. So, $\psi(x)$ can be estimated by

$$\hat{\psi}(x) = \beta_0 + \sum_{j\geq 1} \hat{\beta}_j \cos(jx),$$

where $\hat{\beta}_j = (2/\pi)\alpha_{1j}^{-1}n^{-1}\sum_i \cos(jX_i^*)Y_i$ for $j \leq m$, and 0 otherwise. As below (11.8), $m$ is a smoothing parameter in the above expression. Next, one can construct the estimator of $g(x)$ by $\hat{g}(x) = \hat{\psi}(x)/\hat{f}_X(x)$, where $\hat{f}_X(x)$ can be $\overline{f}_X(x)$ defined in (11.8). A similar estimator of $g(x)$ in the special case when $X$ is uniformly distributed on an interval and $U$ has a normal distribution was considered in Efromovich (1994) and Efromovich (1999).

One advantage to use the Fourier series expansions as the basis for inference in the deconvolution problems is that the effect of the random errors can be factorized out in a way that is easy to handle empirically (i.e., (11.3) and (11.12)). This property is from the elementary addition formulae for sine and cosine functions, and it is not readily available when one is using methods based on the continuous Fourier transformation. It allows to construct relatively simple estimators, which are based on additions of finite series, rather than integrations. These methods are particularly effective when edge effects are involved, and they are easy to code too. However, there is room for improvement. For instance, the estimator defined by (11.8) can produce density estimates that take negative values when the true density is close to zero at certain places. Thus, when the method is used to estimate smooth densities it will suffer from the same vulnerability to negativity as kernel-based methods.

In comparison with kernel-based methods theoretically, the convergence rate achieved by the estimator (11.8) is governed by the rate of convergence of the cosine-series expansion, which is not a natural property for kernel estimators. In other words, it is possible to construct densities where the Fourier series approach gives much faster convergence rates than the kernel methods. We refer readers to the numerical examples provided in Section 3 in Hall and Qiu (2005) for more details.

Delaigle et al. (2006) modified the Fourier series approach described above for solving the so-called Berkson errors-in-variables problem which is the same as the problem described by (11.11), except that the positions of $X$ and $X^*$ are switched and $X^*$, $U$ and $V$ are assumed independent in this case. Interested readers can read the paper Delaigle et al. (2006) for more details.

## 11.3 Deconvolution by Splines

**Deconvolution by B-splines and least squares estimation.** Motivated by the analysis of DNA-content data obtained by microfluorimetry, Mendelsohn and Rice (1982) proposed to approximate $f_X$ by a function in a finite dimensional family of densities $\mathscr{L}_p$ of dimension $p$, where $p$ is a tuning parameter. Because of computational convenience of the B-splines, $\mathscr{L}_p$ can be chosen to be the space spanned by the B-spline basis functions with fixed knot locations. Then, the estimate of $f_X$, $\hat{f}_X$, can be defined as a linear combination of the B-spline basis functions

$$\hat{f}_X(x) = \sum_{j=1}^{p} \hat{\gamma}_j B_j(x), \tag{11.13}$$

where $B_j(x)$ is the $j$th B-spline basis function of degree $k-1$ with knots $t_1$, $t_2$, ..., $t_{p+k}$, the coefficients $\{\hat{\gamma}_j\}$ are the solution of the following least squares problem:

$$\min_{\gamma_j, 1\leq j\leq p} \sum_{i=1}^{m} \left( \hat{f}_{X^*}(s_i) - \sum_{j=1}^{p} \gamma_j f_U * B_j(s_i) \right)^2, \tag{11.14}$$

$\{\hat{f}_{X^*}(s_i), i = 1, 2, \ldots, m\}$ is a histogram estimate of $f_{X^*}$, and $f_U * B_j$ denotes the convolution product and can be numerically evaluated using the Simpson's rule.

One advantage to use the estimator (11.13) is that it is convenient to make $\hat{f}_X$ a legitimate probability density (i.e., a nonnegative function with a unit integration) as follows. By the properties of the B-splines that $\int B_j(x)\,dx = (t_{j+k} - t_k)/k$ and $B_j(x) \geq 0$, we can solve the least squares problem (11.14) by restricting the coefficients $\boldsymbol{\gamma} = (\gamma_1, \ldots, \gamma_p)^T$ to be $\boldsymbol{\gamma} \geq 0$ and $\mathbf{c}^T\boldsymbol{\gamma} = 1$, where $\mathbf{c} = (c_1, \ldots, c_p)^T$ and $c_j = (t_{j+k} - t_k)/k$, for $j = 1, 2, \ldots, p$. Then, it follows immediately that $\hat{f}_X$ is a probability density. On the other hand, there are several potential limitations with the above procedure. First, Mendelsohn and Rice (1982) suggested that the knots were chosen equally spaced and $p$ was determined by increasing its value until the occurrence of high frequency oscillations. This is similar to the eyeball method when choosing a bandwidth parameter for kernel smoothing methods. Thus, it is subjective and could be labor intensive as well. Second, in the application to the DNA-content data in Mendelsohn and Rice (1982), the data were used in the form of histograms, which might be less efficient compared to the likelihood-based approach to estimate the coefficients in (11.14). This latter approach was studied in Koo and Park (1996) and will be discussed in more details in the next part.

**Logspline deconvolution with the EM algorithm.** Koo and Park (1996) considered the deconvolution problem in the following complete-incomplete data specification. The complete unobserved data were $(X_1, X_1^*)$, $(X_2, X_2^*)$, ..., $(X_n, X_n^*)$, which was a random sample of size $n$ from the joint distribution of $(X, X^*)$ whose probability density was given by $f_{(X,X^*)}(x, x^*) = f_U(x^* - x)f_X(x)$. The incomplete observed data were $X_1^*$, $X_2^*$, ..., $X_n^*$. They considered how to estimate $f_X$ from the observed data alone. Let $L$ and $R$ be numbers such that $-\infty \leq L \leq R \leq \infty$, $L < t_1 < t_2 < \cdots < t_K < R$ be $K$ knots. Define $S$ to be the space of all twice continuously differentiable functions $s$ on $(L, R)$ such that $s$ is a cubic polynomial on each of the intervals $[t_1, t_2]$, $[t_2, t_3]$, ..., $[t_{K-1}, t_K]$, and is a linear function on each of the intervals $(L, t_1])$ and $[t_K, R)$. Then, all functions in $S$ are called natural cubic splines, and $S$ has a basis $B_1$, $B_2$, ..., $B_K$ that can be generated from the conventional B-splines (Stone and Koo, 1986). Now, we assume that the support of $f_X$ is $[L, R]$ and consider the following logspline model:

$$f_{X|\boldsymbol{\theta}}(x) = \exp(s(x; \boldsymbol{\theta}) - C(\boldsymbol{\theta})), \quad L < x < R,$$

where

$$s(x; \boldsymbol{\theta}) = \sum_{j=1}^{K-1} \theta_j B_j(x) \quad \text{and} \quad C(\boldsymbol{\theta}) = \log\left(\int_L^R \exp(s(x; \boldsymbol{\theta}))\, dx\right) < \infty.$$

Then $f_{X|\boldsymbol{\theta}}(\cdot)$ is a positive density function on $(L, R)$. Clearly, the logspline model assumes that $f_X$ is twice continuously differentiable. Also, by the property of B-splines that $\sum_{j=1}^{K} B_j(x) = 1$ for all $x \in (L, R)$, the last basis function will not be used in the above expression to make the logspline model identifiable (Stone and Koo, 1986). Now, the log likelihood function of the incomplete observed data $X_1^*, X_2^*, \ldots, X_n^*$ is

$$\begin{aligned} l_{X^*}(\boldsymbol{\theta}) &= \sum_{i=1}^{n} \log\left(\int_L^R f_U(X_i^* - x) f_{X|\boldsymbol{\theta}}(x)\, dx\right) \\ &= \sum_{i=1}^{n} \log\left(\int_L^R f_U(X_i^* - x) \exp\left(s(x;\boldsymbol{\theta}) - C(\boldsymbol{\theta})\right)\, dx\right) \\ &= \sum_{i=1}^{n} \log\left(\int_L^R f_U(X_i^* - x) \exp(s(x;\boldsymbol{\theta}))\, dx\right) - nC(\boldsymbol{\theta}). \end{aligned}$$

The usual maximum likelihood estimate $\hat{\boldsymbol{\theta}}$ is the maximizer of $l_{X^*}(\boldsymbol{\theta})$. Direct maximization of $l_{X^*}(\boldsymbol{\theta})$ is difficult numerically, because of the integrals inside the logarithms. The EM algorithm, which is briefly described below, provides a simpler approach. Let $f_{X|X^*,\boldsymbol{\theta}}(x|x^*)$ denote the conditional density of $X$ given $X^*$. We have

$$f_{X|X^*,\boldsymbol{\theta}}(x|x^*) = \frac{f_{(X,X^*)|\boldsymbol{\theta}}(x, x^*)}{f_{X^*|\boldsymbol{\theta}}(x^*)}.$$

In terms of log-likelihoods, we have

$$l_{X^*}(\boldsymbol{\theta}) = l_{(X,X^*)}(\boldsymbol{\theta}) - l_{X|X^*}(\boldsymbol{\theta}).$$

Taking conditional expectations with respect to the distribution of $X|X^*$ governed by the parameter $\boldsymbol{\theta}_0$ gives

$$\begin{aligned} l_{X^*}(\boldsymbol{\theta}) &= \mathrm{E}\left[l_{(X,X^*)}(\boldsymbol{\theta})|X^*, \boldsymbol{\theta}_0\right] - \mathrm{E}\left[l_{X|X^*}(\boldsymbol{\theta})|X^*, \boldsymbol{\theta}_0\right] \\ &\equiv G(\boldsymbol{\theta}|\boldsymbol{\theta}_0) - R(\boldsymbol{\theta}|\boldsymbol{\theta}_0). \end{aligned}$$

In each iteration of the EM algorithm, we first compute $G(\boldsymbol{\theta}|\boldsymbol{\theta}_0)$ (i.e., the expectation step) and then maximize $G(\boldsymbol{\theta}|\boldsymbol{\theta}_0)$ over $\boldsymbol{\theta}$ (i.e., the maximization step). Thus, a key quantity in the EM algorithm is the following conditional expectation:

$$\begin{aligned} G(\boldsymbol{\theta}|\boldsymbol{\theta}_0) &= E_{X|\boldsymbol{\theta}_0,X^*}\left[\log\left(f_{(X,X^*)|\boldsymbol{\theta}}(X_i, X_i^*)\right)\right] \\ &= \int_L^R f_{X|X^*,\boldsymbol{\theta}_0}(x|X_i^*) \log\left(f_U(X_i^* - x) f_{X|\boldsymbol{\theta}}(x)\right)\, dx \\ &= \int_L^R f_{X|X^*,\boldsymbol{\theta}_0}(x|X_i^*) s(x;\boldsymbol{\theta})\, dx - C(\boldsymbol{\theta}) + \text{terms not involving } \boldsymbol{\theta} \\ &= \sum_{j=1}^{K-1} \theta_j \int_L^R B_j(x) f_{X|X^*,\boldsymbol{\theta}_0}(x|X_i^*)\, dx - C(\boldsymbol{\theta}) \\ &\quad + \text{terms not involving } \boldsymbol{\theta}, \end{aligned}$$

where

$$f_{X|X^*,\boldsymbol{\theta}}(x|x^*) = f_U(x^* - x)\exp(s(x;\boldsymbol{\theta}) - C(\boldsymbol{\theta}|x^*)),$$
$$C(\boldsymbol{\theta}|x^*) = \log\left(\int_L^R f_U(x^* - x)\exp(s(x;\boldsymbol{\theta}))\,dx\right).$$

In the maximization step, if $\boldsymbol{\theta}_1$ maximizes $G(\boldsymbol{\theta}|\boldsymbol{\theta}_0)$, then we have $l_{X^*}(\boldsymbol{\theta}_1) \geq l_{X^*}(\boldsymbol{\theta}_0)$. To see this, note that $R(\boldsymbol{\theta}|\boldsymbol{\theta}_0)$ is the expectation of a log-likelihood of a density (indexed by $\boldsymbol{\theta}$), with respect to the same density indexed by $\boldsymbol{\theta}_0$. Hence, by Jensen's inequality, $R(\boldsymbol{\theta}|\boldsymbol{\theta}_0) \leq R(\boldsymbol{\theta}_0|\boldsymbol{\theta}_0)$ and it follows that

$$l_{X^*}(\boldsymbol{\theta}_1) - l_{X^*}(\boldsymbol{\theta}_0) = [G(\boldsymbol{\theta}_1|\boldsymbol{\theta}_0) - G(\boldsymbol{\theta}_0|\boldsymbol{\theta}_0)] - [R(\boldsymbol{\theta}_1|\boldsymbol{\theta}_0) - R(\boldsymbol{\theta}_0|\boldsymbol{\theta}_0)] \geq 0.$$

We now state the EM algorithm for computing $\hat{\boldsymbol{\theta}}$ in the complete-incomplete data specification. It starts with an initial estimate $\hat{\boldsymbol{\theta}}^0$ and iteratively updates the estimate as follows.

**Expectation-Step:** Given the current estimate $\hat{\boldsymbol{\theta}}^{(k)}$ of $\boldsymbol{\theta}$, calculate

$$b_j\left(\hat{\boldsymbol{\theta}}^{(k)}\right) = \sum_{i=1}^{n}\int_L^R B_j(x) f_{X|X^*,\hat{\boldsymbol{\theta}}^{(k)}}(x|X_i^*)\,dx, \quad 1 \leq j \leq K-1.$$

**Maximization-Step:** Determine the updated estimate $\hat{\boldsymbol{\theta}}^{(k+1)}$ by maximizing

$$Q\left(\boldsymbol{\theta}|\hat{\boldsymbol{\theta}}^{(k)}\right) = \sum_{j=1}^{K-1}\theta_j b_j\left(\hat{\boldsymbol{\theta}}^{(k)}\right) - nC(\boldsymbol{\theta}).$$

The EM algorithm stops when $l_{X^*}(\hat{\boldsymbol{\theta}}^{(k+1)}) - l_{X^*}(\hat{\boldsymbol{\theta}}^{(k)}) < 10^{-6}$. In the Maximization-step, the Newton-Raphson algorithm with step-halving can be employed for the maximization. More specifically, let $\mathbf{S}(\boldsymbol{\theta})$ be the score function at $\boldsymbol{\theta}$ with elements $b_j(\hat{\boldsymbol{\theta}}^{(k)}) - \partial C(\boldsymbol{\theta})/\partial\theta_j$ and let $\mathbf{H}(\boldsymbol{\theta})$ be the Hessian matrix of $C(\boldsymbol{\theta})$ at $\boldsymbol{\theta}$ with elements

$$\int_L^R B_{j_1}(x)B_{j_2}(x) f_{\mathbf{X}|\boldsymbol{\theta}}(x)\,dx - \int_L^R B_{j_1}(x) f_{\mathbf{X}|\boldsymbol{\theta}}(x)\,dx \int_L^R B_{j_2} f_{\mathbf{X}|\boldsymbol{\theta}}(x)\,dx.$$

Now, the computation of $\hat{\boldsymbol{\theta}}^{(k+1)}$ starts with $\tilde{\boldsymbol{\theta}}^{(0)} = \hat{\boldsymbol{\theta}}^{(k)}$ and iteratively determines $\tilde{\boldsymbol{\theta}}^{(m+1)}$ according to the expression

$$\tilde{\boldsymbol{\theta}}^{(m+1)} = \tilde{\boldsymbol{\theta}}^{(m)} + 2^{-q}\left[\mathbf{H}\left(\tilde{\boldsymbol{\theta}}^{(m)}\right)\right]^{-1}\mathbf{S}\left(\tilde{\boldsymbol{\theta}}^{(m)}\right),$$

where $q$ is the smallest nonnegative integer such that

$$l_{X^*}\left(\tilde{\boldsymbol{\theta}}^{(m)} + 2^{-q}\left[\mathbf{H}\left(\tilde{\boldsymbol{\theta}}^{(m)}\right)\right]^{-1}\mathbf{S}\left(\tilde{\boldsymbol{\theta}}^{(m)}\right)\right) \geq l_{X^*}\left(\tilde{\boldsymbol{\theta}}^{(m)}\right).$$

The Newton-Raphson algorithm stops when $l_{X^*}(\tilde{\boldsymbol{\theta}}^{(m+1)}) - l_{X^*}(\tilde{\boldsymbol{\theta}}^{(m)}) < 10^{-6}$.

To make the entire estimation procedure fully automatic, a data-driven rule for determining the final number and locations of knots is needed. Choosing the number of knots is similar to choosing a bandwidth in kernel smoothing. Too many knots would lead to a noisy estimate, and too few knots would give an estimate that is overly smoothed. The knot locations are also important, since more knots are needed in a region where the curvature of $f_X$ is larger. To this end, Koo and Park (1996) suggested the following stepwise knot deletion strategy. Let $K^*$ be an initial number of knots, and the knot locations are determined by an initial knot placement rule. Koo and Park (1996) suggested that $K^*$ can be chosen to be the integer closest to $3(\log n)^{1/2}$, and the knots can initially be placed at equally spaced percentiles of $X_i^*$ once the initial number of knots is given. Then, at each stage of the stepwise knot deletion process, the EM algorithm is used to obtain the estimate $\hat{\boldsymbol{\theta}}_K$ with $K$ being the number of remaining knots at that stage. The Bayesian information criterion (BIC) is calculated as:

$$\text{BIC} = -2l_{X^*}\left(\hat{\boldsymbol{\theta}}_K\right) + (K-1)\log n.$$

Delete the knote that results in the biggest drop in BIC and repeat this deletion process until BIC stops to decrease.

The logspline deconvolution method has advantages similar to those of logspline density estimates in the usual density estimation problem (cf., Kooperberg and Stone, 1991). It gives density estimates that are positive with unit integrations. However, that method also has some limitations. First, it is known that under fairly general conditions the EM algorithm could converge to a local maximum of $l_{X^*}(\boldsymbol{\theta})$. When this function is not concave, there is no guarantee that such a local maximum has unique maximizer, or that it is a global maximum. Second, the numerical studies in Koo and Park (1996) showed that the logspline deconvolution estimates may require a large sample size to perform well when the true density function has a complex (e.g., bimodal) structure. Third, the above procedure for determining $K^*$ is ad hoc in nature.

## 11.4 Deconvolution by Wavelets

Wavelet methods are well received in the literature of density estimation (e.g., Walter, 1981; Penskaya, 1985; Kerkyacharian and Picard, 1992; Masry, 1994; Hall and Patil, 1995) and curve estimation (e.g., Antoniadis et al., 1994; Abramovich and Silverman, 1998; Donoho and Johnstone, 1995; Hall et al.,

1998; Hall et al., 1997; Walter, 1994). Pensky and Vidakovic (1999) proposed several wavelet estimators of the density function $f_X$ in the deconvolution problem (11.1). The underlying idea is to represent $f_X$ via a wavelet expansion and estimate the coefficients using a deconvolution algorithm. Their estimators are based on the Meyer-type wavelets, which are band-limited and their Fourier transforms would have bounded supports (Hernández and Weiss, 1996). These wavelet estimators are constructed as follows.

Assume that $f_X$ is square integrable and the Fourier transform of $f_{X^*}$, denoted as $\tilde{f}_{X^*}(\omega)$, does not vanish for real $\omega$. Let $\varphi(x)$ and $\psi(x)$ be a scaling function and a wavelet for an orthonormal multi-resolution decomposition of $L^2(-\infty,\infty)$, respectively. Then, for any integer $m$, $f_X$ has the following expansion:

$$f_X(x) = \sum_{k\in\mathbb{Z}} a_{m,k}\varphi_{m,k}(x) + \sum_{k\in\mathbb{Z}}\sum_{j=m}^{\infty} b_{j,k}\psi_{j,k}(x), \tag{11.15}$$

where $\varphi_{m,k}(x) = 2^{m/2}\varphi(2^m x - k)$ and $\psi_{j,k}(x) = 2^{j/2}\psi(2^j x - k)$, and the coefficients $a_{m,k}$ and $b_{j,k}$ have the forms

$$a_{m,k} = \int_{-\infty}^{\infty} \varphi_{m,k}(x) f_X(x)\,dx, \quad b_{j,k} = \int_{-\infty}^{\infty} \psi_{j,k}(x) f_X(x)\,dx. \tag{11.16}$$

The scaling function $\varphi(x)$ and the wavelet function $\psi(x)$ can be defined as the functions whose Fourier transforms are (Walter, 1994; Zayed and Walter, 1996)

$$\tilde{\varphi}(\omega) = \left[\int_{\omega-\pi}^{\omega+\pi} dP\right]^{1/2}, \quad \tilde{\psi}(\omega) = \exp(-i\omega/2)\left[\int_{|\omega|/2-\pi}^{|\omega|-\pi} dP\right]^{1/2},$$

where $P$ is a probability measure that satisfies the following conditions: (i) support of $P$ is included in $[-\pi/3,\pi/3]$, and (ii) $\tilde{\varphi}(\omega)$ and $\tilde{\psi}(\omega)$ are $s \geq 2$ times continuously differentiable on $(-\infty,\infty)$. This ensures that $\varphi(x)$ and $\psi(x)$ have sufficient rates of descent as $|x| \to \infty$. Then, both $\tilde{\varphi}(\omega)$ and $\tilde{\psi}(\omega)$ would have bounded supports: supp $\tilde{\varphi} \subset [-4\pi/3, 4\pi/3]$ and supp $\tilde{\psi} \subset [-8\pi/3, -2\pi/3] \cup [2\pi/2, 8\pi/3]$. Moreover, we have

$$C_\varphi = \sup_x [|\varphi(x)|(|x|^s + 1)] < \infty, \quad C_\psi = \sup_x [|\psi(x)|(|x|^s + 1)] < \infty.$$

Let $u_{m,k}$ and $v_{j,k}$ be the solutions of the following equations:

$$\int_{-\infty}^{\infty} f_U(z-x) u_{m,k}(z)\,dz = \varphi_{m,k}(x), \quad \int_{-\infty}^{\infty} f_U(z-x) v_{j,k}(z)\,dz = \psi_{j,k}(x). \tag{11.17}$$

Then, the coefficients $a_{m,k}$ and $b_{j,k}$ can be viewed as mathematical expectations of the functions $u_{m,k}$ and $v_{j,k}$ (by (11.16)):

$$\begin{aligned} a_{m,k} &= \int_{-\infty}^{\infty}\int_{-\infty}^{\infty} f_U(z-x) f_X(x) u_{m,k}(z)\, dxdz \\ &= \int_{-\infty}^{\infty} f_{X^*}(z) u_{m,k}(z)\, dz = E\left[u_{m,k}(X^*)\right]; \qquad (11.18) \\ b_{j,k} &= \int_{-\infty}^{\infty}\int_{-\infty}^{\infty} f_U(z-x) f_X(x) v_{j,k}(z)\, dxdz \\ &= \int_{-\infty}^{\infty} f_{X^*}(z) v_{j,k}(z)\, dz. = E\left[v_{j,k}(X^*)\right]. \qquad (11.19) \end{aligned}$$

It is worth mentioning that (11.18) and (11.19) are much more convenient to work with, compared to (11.16), since the $X_i^*$'s are observable whereas the $X_i$'s are not. Before the wavelet estimators of $f_X$ can be formally defined, we still need to obtain the expressions for $u_{m,k}$ and $v_{j,k}$. To this end, after taking the Fourier transform on both sides of (11.17), we have $u_{m,k}(x) = 2^{m/2}U_m(2^m x - k)$, and $v_{j,k}(x) = 2^{j/2}V_j(2^j x - k)$, where $U_m(\cdot)$ and $V_j(\cdot)$ are the inverse Fourier transforms of the functions:

$$\tilde{U}_m(\omega) = \frac{\tilde{\varphi}(\omega)}{\tilde{f}_U(-2^m\omega)}, \quad \tilde{V}_j(\omega) = \frac{\tilde{\psi}(\omega)}{\tilde{f}_U(-2^j\omega)},$$

respectively. Thus, we can estimate $a_{m,k}$ and $b_{j,k}$ by

$$\hat{a}_{m,k} = \frac{1}{n}\sum_{i=1}^{n} 2^{m/2}U_m(2^m X_i^* - k), \quad \hat{b}_{j,k} = \frac{1}{n}\sum_{i=1}^{n} 2^{j/2}V_j(2^j X_i^* - k).$$

Then, from (11.15), we can define a linear wavelet estimator of $f_X$ as

$$\hat{f}_{X,n}^{(L)}(x) = \sum_{k\in\mathbb{Z}} \hat{a}_{m,k}\varphi_{m,k}(x),$$

and a nonlinear wavelet estimator of $f_X(x)$ as

$$\hat{f}_{X,n}^{(N)} = \sum_{k\in\mathbb{Z}} \hat{a}_{m,k}\varphi_{m,k}(x) + \sum_{j=m}^{m+r}\left[\sum_{k\in\mathbb{Z}} \hat{b}_{j,k}\psi_{j,k}(x)\right] I\left(\sum_{k\in\mathbb{Z}} \hat{b}_{j,k}^2 > \delta_{j,n}^2\right),$$

where $\delta_{j,n}$ are thresholding parameters. Note that $\hat{f}_{X,n}^{(L)}(x)$ and $\hat{f}_{X,n}^{(N)}(x)$ both seem computationally intractable since their definitions involve the calculation of infinite series. Under some minor conditions, we can modify the infinite series estimators $\hat{f}_{X,n}^{(L)}(x)$ and $\hat{f}_{X,n}^{(N)}(x)$ to be finite series estimators as follows

$$\hat{f}_{X,n}^{(LF)}(x) = \sum_{|k|\le K_n} \hat{a}_{m,k}\varphi_{m,k}(x),$$

$$\hat{f}_{X,n}^{(NF)} = \sum_{|k|\le M_n} \hat{a}_{m,k}\varphi_{m,k}(x) + \sum_{j=m}^{m+r}\left[\sum_{|k|\le L_n} \hat{b}_{j,k}\psi_{j,k}(x)\right] I\left(\sum_{|k|\le L_n} \hat{b}_{j,k}^2 > \delta_{j,n}^2\right),$$

without any loss in the convergence rates. Here, $K_n$, $M_n$, and $L_n$ are smoothing parameters.

Pensky and Vidakovic (1999) showed that $\hat{f}_{X,n}^{(L)}(x)$, $\hat{f}_{X,n}^{(LF)}(x)$, $\hat{f}_{X,n}^{(N)}(x)$, and $\hat{f}_{X,n}^{(NF)}(x)$ all achieve the optimal rates of convergence established in Fan (1993). Furthermore, in the case when $f_U$ is super smooth (i.e., $\tilde{f}_U(\omega)$ exponentially decreases as $\omega$ increases), the linear wavelet estimators $\hat{f}_{X,n}^{(L)}(x)$ and $\hat{f}_{X,n}^{(LF)}(x)$ are adaptive in the sense that the choice of $m$, which yields the optimal rate of convergence, does not depend on the unknown smoothness of the density $f_X$. Similarly, the nonlinear wavelet estimators $\hat{f}_{X,n}^{(N)}(x)$ and $\hat{f}_{X,n}^{(NF)}(x)$ are adaptive in the case when $\tilde{f}_U$ has a polynomial descent. Therefore, all these wavelet estimators have nice theoretical properties. However, the above construction of these estimators cannot guarantee that they are nonnegative with unit integrations. More recent work (e.g., Bigot and Van Bellegem, 2009) has lifted this limitation by proposing new wavelet-based methods that guarantee the related estimators to be legitimate density functions.

## 11.5 Deconvolution by Low Order Approximations

The deconvolution methods discussed in the previous sections all assume that the distribution of $U$ is known. This is a common assumption in the deconvolution literature because the related problem is difficult to solve otherwise. However, little information is generally available in practice about the distribution of $U$. Even under the assumption of a known $f_U$, Carroll and Hall (1988) have showed that the fastest possible convergence rate of a density estimator in the deconvolution problem is in the reciprocal of the logarithmic of the sample size when $U$ has a normal distribution. Fan (1991b) discussed settings in which the optimal convergence rate could be in the reciprocal of a polynomial of the sample size. Even in such settings, the optimal convergence rate is often slow, unless $f_U$ is very unsmooth (e.g., it has a discontinuity). The implication of these results is that consistent estimation of $f_X$ is difficult in practical terms. An alternative approach would be to estimate a function that approximates $f_X$ and is relatively easy to estimate. Carroll and Hall (2004) suggested an approach based on this idea. It requires knowledge of only low order moments of $f_U$. This information is often available either from a sample drawn from the distribution of $U$ or from a small number of repeated observations of $X^*$ for the same $X$. This approach is introduced below in two parts.

**Density estimation by low order approximations.** Conventional kernel estimators of $f_{X^*}$ and $f_X$ are given by

$$\hat{f}_{X^*}(x^*) = \frac{1}{nh}\sum_{i=1}^{n} K\left(\frac{x^* - X_i^*}{h}\right);$$
$$\hat{f}_X(x) = \frac{1}{nh}\sum_{i=1}^{n} K\left(\frac{x - X_i}{h}\right);$$

where $K(\cdot)$ is a kernel function and $h$ is a bandwidth. Because we do not observe the $X_i$'s in practice, $\hat{f}_X$ cannot be computed directly from the observed data. Nevertheless we can try to find a good approximation to $\hat{f}_X$ or its mean. To this end, let $K^{(j)}$ be the $j$th derivative of $K$. Define

$$\lambda_j(x) = E\left[K^{(j)}\left(\frac{x - X}{h}\right)\right];$$
$$\kappa_j(x) = E\left[K^{(j)}\left(\frac{x - X^*}{h}\right)\right];$$
$$u_j = E\left(U^j\right);$$

Assume that $U$ has finite moments and $K$ is an analytic function in the sense that all its derivatives are well defined on the entire real line. Obviously, the analyticity condition is satisfied for the commonly used Gaussian kernel function. Now, by the Taylor expansion of $K^{(j)}(\cdot)$ at $(x - X)/h$, we have

$$\begin{aligned}
\lambda_j(x) &= \kappa_j(x) - \sum_{k_1\geq 1} \frac{(-1)^{k_1} u_{k_1}}{k_1! h^{k_1}} \lambda_{j+k_1}(x) \\
&= \kappa_j(x) - \sum_{k_1\geq 1} \frac{(-1)^{k_1} u_{k_1}}{k_1! h^{k_1}} \left[\kappa_{j+k_1}(x) - \sum_{k_2\geq 1} \frac{(-1)^{k_2} u_{k_2}}{k_2! h^{k_2}} \lambda_{j+k_1+k_2}(x)\right] \\
&= \kappa_j(x) - \sum_{k_1\geq 1} \frac{(-1)^{k_1} u_{k_1}}{k_1! h^{k_1}} \kappa_{j+k_1}(x) + \sum_{k_1\geq 1}\sum_{k_2\geq 1} \frac{(-1)^{k_1+k_2} u_{k_1} u_{k_2}}{k_1! k_2! h^{k_1+k_2}} \lambda_{j+k_1+k_2}(x) \\
&\vdots \\
&= \kappa_j(x) + \sum_{r=1}^{\infty}\sum_{k_1=1}^{\infty}\cdots\sum_{k_r=1}^{\infty} \frac{(-1)^{k_1+\ldots+k_r+r}}{k_1!\ldots k_r! h^{k_1+\ldots+k_r}} u_{k_1}\cdots u_{k_r} \kappa_{k_1+\ldots+k_r+j}(x).
\end{aligned} \tag{11.20}$$

From (11.20), we have

$$\begin{aligned}
E[\hat{f}_X^{(j)}(x)] &= E[\hat{f}_{X^*}^{(j)}(x)] \\
&+ \sum_{r=1}^{\infty}\sum_{k_1=1}^{\infty}\cdots\sum_{k_r=1}^{\infty} \frac{(-1)^{k_1+\ldots+k_r+r}}{k_1!\ldots k_r!} u_{k_1}\cdots u_{k_r} E[\hat{f}_{X^*}^{(k_1+\ldots+k_r+j)}(x)].
\end{aligned}$$

Therefore, if $\hat{u}_j$ is a consistent estimator of $u_j$ and $\text{Var}(U) \to 0$, then a reasonable estimator of the $\nu$th-order approximation to $E[\hat{f}_X^{(j)}(x)]$ is

$$\hat{f}_{X,\nu}^{(j)}(x) = \hat{f}_{X^*}^{(j)}(x) + \sum_{r\geq 1, k_1\geq 1,\cdots,k_r\geq 1: k_1+\ldots+k_r\leq\nu} \cdots \sum \frac{(-1)^{k_1+\ldots+k_r+r}}{k_1!\ldots k_r!}\hat{u}_{k_1}\cdots\hat{u}_{k_r}\hat{f}_{X^*}^{(k_1+\ldots+k_r+j)}(x).$$

In particular, the estimators of the second-, fourth- and sixth-order approximations are given by

$$\hat{f}_{X,2}^{(j)}(x) = \hat{f}_{X^*}^{(j)}(x) + \hat{u}_1\hat{f}_Y^{(j+1)}(x) + \frac{1}{2}(2\hat{u}_1^2 - \hat{u}_2)\hat{f}_{X^*}^{(j+2)}(x); \tag{11.21}$$

$$\begin{aligned}\hat{f}_{X,4}^{(j)}(x) &= \hat{f}_{X,2}^{(j)}(x) + \frac{1}{6}(6\hat{u}_1^3 - 6\hat{u}_1\hat{u}_2 + \hat{u}_3)\hat{f}_{X^*}^{(j+3)}(x)\\ &+ \frac{1}{24}(24\hat{u}_1{}^4 - 36\hat{u}_1^2\hat{u}_2 + 8\hat{u}_1\hat{u}_3 + 6\hat{u}_2^2 - \hat{u}_4)\hat{f}_{X^*}^{(j+4)}(x);\end{aligned} \tag{11.22}$$

$$\begin{aligned}\hat{f}_{X,6}^{(j)}(x) &= \hat{f}_{X,4}^{(j)}(x) + \frac{1}{120}(120\hat{u}_1^5 - 240\hat{u}_1^3\hat{u}_2 + 60\hat{u}_1^2\hat{u}_3\\ &+ 180\hat{u}_1\hat{u}_2^2 + 10\hat{u}_1\hat{u}_4 - 20\hat{u}_2\hat{u}_3 + \hat{u}_5)\hat{f}_{X^*}^{(j+5)}(x)\\ &+ \frac{1}{720}(720\hat{u}_1^6 - 1800\hat{u}_1^4\hat{u}_2 + 480\hat{u}_1^3\hat{u}_3 + 1080\hat{u}_1^2\hat{u}_2^2 - 90\hat{u}_1^2\hat{u}_4\\ &+ 12\hat{u}_1\hat{u}_5 - 360\hat{u}_1\hat{u}_2\hat{u}_3 - 90\hat{u}_2^3 + 20\hat{u}_3^2 + 30\hat{u}_2\hat{u}_4 - \hat{u}_6)\hat{f}_{X^*}^{(j+6)}(x).\end{aligned} \tag{11.23}$$

In the literature, it is common to assume that the distribution of $U$ is symmetric. In such cases, we can let $\hat{u}_k = 0$, for odd $k$, and only use approximations of even orders. Then, the estimator of the $2\nu$-th order approximation to $E[\hat{f}_X^{(j)}(x)]$ can be simplified to

$$\hat{f}_{X,2\nu}^{(j)}(x) = \hat{f}_{X^*}^{(j)}(x) + \sum_{r\geq 1, k_1\geq 1,\cdots,k_r\geq 1: k_1+\ldots+k_r\leq\nu} \cdots \sum \frac{(-1)^r}{(2k_1)!\ldots(2k_r)!}\hat{u}_{2k_1}\cdots\hat{u}_{2k_r}\hat{f}_{X^*}^{(2k_1+\ldots+2k_r+j)}(x),$$

and the equations (11.21) – (11.23) would have simpler forms as well.

**Errors-in-variables regression by low order approximations.** It is worth mentioning that the above approximation procedure can also be applied to the errors-in-variables regression (cf., (11.11)). Let us consider the Nadaraya-Watson (NW) estimator of the regression function $g(x) = E(Y|X = x)$, defined by

$$\bar{g}_{NW}(x) = \frac{\sum_{i=1}^n Y_i K\left(\frac{x-X_i}{h}\right)}{\sum_{i=1}^n K\left(\frac{x-X_i}{h}\right)},$$

where $h$ is a bandwidth and $K$ is a kernel function. Again, because the $X_i$'s are unobservable, $\bar{g}_{NW}$ cannot be obtained from the observed data. Nonetheless we can obtain estimators of the low order approximations to its mean using results similar to (11.20). To this end, we have

$$E\left[YK\left(\frac{x-X}{h}\right)\right] = E\left[YK\left(\frac{x-X^*}{h}\right)\right] + \tag{11.24}$$
$$\sum_{r\geq 1}\sum_{k_1\geq 1}\cdots\sum_{k_r\geq 1}\frac{(-1)^{k_1+\ldots+k_r+r}}{k_1!\ldots k_r!h^{k_1+\ldots+k_r}}u_{k_1}\ldots u_{k_2}E\left[YK^{(k_1+\ldots+k_r)}\left(\frac{x-X^*}{h}\right)\right].$$

Then, by (11.20) and (11.24), an estimator of the second order (i.e., $\nu = 2$) approximation to $E(\bar{g}_{NW})$ is

$$\hat{g}_{NW}(x) = \frac{\sum_{i=1}^{n} Y_i L\left(\frac{x-X_i^*}{h}\right)}{\sum_{i=1}^{n} L\left(\frac{x-X_i^*}{h}\right)},$$

where $L(v) = K(v) - (\hat{u}_2/(2h^2))K^{(2)}(v)$. Of course, estimators of higher orders approximations can be constructed similarly.

## 11.6 Deconvolution Problems in Image Analysis

As discussed in Section 1, the deconvolution problem is an ill-posed inverse problem. There are similar ill-posed inverse problems in different disciplines and areas. In image processing, the image deblurring problem is a such inverse problem, which will be discussed below. In image deblurring, we aim to recover a true image $f$ from its blurred and noisy version $Z$, where the relationship between $Z$ and $f$ can be described by the following model:

$$Z(x,y) = (h*f)(x,y) + \varepsilon(x,y), \text{ for } (x,y)\in\Omega, \tag{11.25}$$

where $\varepsilon(x,y)$ denotes pointwise noise at $(x,y)$, $\Omega$ is the design space of the image, and $(h*f)(x,y) = \int\int f(x-u,y-v)h(u,v)\,dudv$ is a spatially blurred version of $f$. Obviously, the blurred image $(h*f)$ is the convolution between a *point spread function* (psf) $h$ and the true image $f$, and the blurring mechanism is described by the psf $h$. Similar to the density deconvolution problem (11.1), the image deblurring problem (11.25) is ill-posed in the following sense. In the case when $h$ is unknown, there could be many different sets of $h$ and $f$ that correspond to the same observed image. Even in cases when $h$ is completely known, an estimated true image is often numerically unstable, as discussed in Section 1 about the inverse problem (11.1). Thus, image deblurring is a challenging problem and has attracted much attention in the image processing community (cf., Campisi and Egiazarian, 2016; Hansen et al., 2006; Qiu, 2007).

Image deblurring methods that assume a known $h$ are often called *non-blind image deblurring* methods. The assumption that $h$ is known might be reasonable in certain applications. For instance, the linear psf $h$ is appropriate for describing the image blur caused by relative location move between the image acquisition device and the object. The Gaussian blur is often used for describing image blur caused by atmospheric turbulence in remote sensing and aerial imaging. After $h$ is specified, $f$ can be estimated based on the relationship that

$$\mathcal{F}\{Z\}(u,v) = \mathcal{F}\{h\}(u,v)\mathcal{F}\{f\}(u,v) + \mathcal{F}\{\varepsilon\}(u,v), \text{ for } (u,v) \in \mathbb{R}^2,$$

where $\mathcal{F}\{g\}$ denotes the Fourier transform of function $g$. Many estimators of $f$, called inverse filters in the image processing literature, have been proposed. A popular one is the Wiener filter (Gonzalez and Woods, 2008), defined by

$$\hat{f}(x,y) = \frac{1}{(2\pi)^2}\mathcal{R}\left\{\int\int \frac{\overline{\mathcal{F}\{h\}(u,v)}\mathcal{F}\{Z\}(u,v)}{|\mathcal{F}\{h\}(u,v)|^2 + \alpha(u^2+v^2)^{\beta/2}} \exp\{-i(ux+vy)\}\, dudv\right\}, \tag{11.26}$$

where $\overline{\mathcal{F}\{h\}(u,v)}$ denotes the complex conjugate of $\mathcal{F}\{h\}(u,v)$, $\mathcal{R}\{C\}$ denotes the real part of the complex number $C$, and $\alpha, \beta > 0$ are two parameters. It can be seen that $\hat{f}(x,y)$ in (11.26) bears some resemblance with the deconvolution kernel density estimator in Stefanski and Carroll (1990). In (11.26), inclusion of the term $\alpha(u^2+v^2)^{\beta/2}$ is mainly for handling the noise effect. If the pointwise noise in the observed image can be ignored, then we actually do not need this term. In cases where the pointwise noise is substantial, the noise effect would dominate the image estimator, because $\mathcal{F}\{f\}(u,v)$ and $\mathcal{F}\{h\}(u,v)$ usually converge to zero rapidly, as $u^2+v^2$ approaches infinity, but $\mathcal{F}\{\varepsilon\}(u,v)$ goes to zero much more slowly.

In many applications, however, it is difficult to specify the psf $h$ completely based on our prior knowledge about the image acquisition device. Image deblurring when $h$ is unknown is often referred to as *blind image deblurring.* A popular blind image deblurring approach in the literature is based on the total variation (TV) minimization. Based on the work by You and Kaveh (1996), Chan and Wong (1998) introduced the TV blind deblurring procedure as

$$\min_{f,h\in BV}\left\{||h*f-Z||_{L^2}^2 + \lambda_f\int_\Omega |\nabla h(x,y)|dxdy + \lambda_h\int_\Omega |\nabla f(x,y)|dxdy\right\}, \tag{11.27}$$

where $\lambda_f$ and $\lambda_h$ are two positive parameters, $\nabla$ is the gradient operator, and the space of all functions with bounded variation (BV) is defined as $BV = \{s \in L^1(\Omega) : \int_\Omega |\nabla s(x,y)|dxdy < \infty\}$. Clearly, in (11.27), the first term measures the goodness-of-fit of the estimators, and the second and third terms regularize their total variations. Chan and Wong (1998) solved the minimization problem by an iterative algorithm, after $\lambda_f$ and $\lambda_h$ are properly selected. More recently, Hall and Qiu (2007b) suggested estimating the psf $h$ from an observed test image of an imaging device. The true test image considered in the paper has a square block in the middle with a uniform background. The idea in the paper, however, can also be applied to cases when the test image has step edges at known locations with uniform background. In a follow-up research, Hall and Qiu (2007a) suggested a two-step image deblurring procedure. In the first step, the psf $h$ was estimated from an observed test image. Then, in the second step, any observed image $Z(x, y)$ taken by the same camera could be deblurred using the estimated psf obtained in the first step. The psf $h$ in this method was assumed to have a parametric form. This assumption was later removed in the paper Qiu (2008). A more flexible blind image deblurring method without restrictive assumptions on both $h$ and $f$ was proposed in Qiu and Kang (2015), based on the hierarchical nature of image blurring that the image structure was altered most significantly around step edges, less significantly around roof/valley edges, and least significantly at places where the true image intensity function was straight. For related discussions, see papers Kang (2020), Kang et al. (2018), and Kang and Qiu (2014).

## 11.7 Some Concluding Remarks

In the previous sections, we introduced some nonparametric deconvolution methods based on the discrete Fourier transformation and other series expansion approaches. These methods have their own strengths and limitations. For instance, the methods based on the Fourier series expansion are computationally convenient, but they cannot guarantee the estimators to be legitimate probability densities. The methods based on low order approximations are flexible to use in practice, because they only require information about the low order moments of the error distribution. However, they may not be statistically consistent. Therefore, the deconvolution problem is far away from being solved satisfactorily and much more future research is required. In addition, the deconvolution problem and its variants have broad applications in econometrics, signal processing, image restoration and many other areas. The related inverse problems in these applications often have similar structures (e.g., they are usually ill-posed), but with their own features and special properties. It should be helpful if the related research in different areas are better connected.

## Acknowledgments

The authors thank Professor Aurore Delaigle for her invitation and many helpful suggestions. This research is supported in part by an NSF grant.

## Bibliography

Abramovich, F. and Silverman, B. (1998). Wavelet decomposition approaches to statistical inverse problems. *Biometrika*, 85(1), 115-129.

Antoniadis, A., Gregoire, G. and McKeague, I. (1994). Wavelet methods for curve estimation. *Journal of the American Statistical Association*, 89(428), 1340-1353.

Apanasovich, T. and Liang, H. (2021). Nonparametric measurement errors models for regression. In *Handbook of Measurement Error Models*, G. Y. Yi, A. Delaigle, and P. Gustafson (Eds.), CRC, Chapter 14.

Bigot, J. and Van Bellegem, S. (2009). Log-density deconvolution by wavelet thresholding. *Scandinavian Journal of Statistics*, 36(4), 749-763.

Campisi, P. and Egiazarian, K. (2016). *Blind image deconvolution: theory and applications*. CRC press.

Carroll, R. J. and Hall, P. (1988). Optimal rates of convergence for deconvolving a density. *Journal of the American Statistical Association*, 83(404), 1184-1186.

Carroll, R. J. and Hall, P. (2004). Low order approximations in deconvolution and regression with errors in variables. *Journal of the Royal Statistical Society, Series B*, 66(1), 31-46.

Chan, T. F. and Wong, C.-K. (1998). Total variation blind deconvolution. *IEEE transactions on Image Processing*, 7(3), 370-375.

Delaigle, A. (2021). Deconvolution kernel density estimation. In *Handbook of Measurement Error Models*, G. Y. Yi, A. Delaigle, and P. Gustafson (Eds.), CRC, Chapter 10.

Delaigle, A. and Gijbels, I. (2006). Estimation of boundary and discontinuity points in deconvolution problems. *Statistica Sinica*, 16(3):773-788.

Delaigle, A., Hall, P. and Qiu, P. (2006). Nonparametric methods for solving the Berkson error-in-variables problem. *Journal of the Royal Statistical Society, Series B*, 68(2), 201-220.

Delaigle, A. and Van Keilegom, I. (2021). Deconvolution with unknown error distribution. In *Handbook of Measurement Error Models*, G. Y. Yi, A. Delaigle, and P. Gustafson (Eds.), CRC, Chapter 12.

Devroye, L. (1989). Consistent deconvolution in density estimation. *Canadian Journal of Statistics*, 17(2), 235-239.

Diggle, P. J. and Hall, P. (1993). A Fourier approach to nonparametric deconvolution of a density estimate. *Journal of the Royal Statistical Society, Series B*, 55(2):523-531.

Donoho, D. L. and Johnstone, I. M. (1995). Adapting to unknown smoothness via wavelet shrinkage. *Journal of the American Statistical Association*, 90(432), 1200-1224.

Efromovich, S. (1994). Nonparametric curve estimation from indirect observations. *Computing Science and Statistics*, 26, 196-200.

Efromovich, S. (1997). Density estimation for the case of supersmooth measurement error. *Journal of the American Statistical Association*, 92(438), 526-535.

Efromovich, S. (1999). *Nonparametric Curve Estimation: Methods, Theory, and Applications*. Springer, New York.

Fan, J. (1991a). Global behavior of deconvolution kernel estimates. *Statistica Sinica*, 1(2):541-551.

Fan, J. (1991b). On the optimal rates of convergence for nonparametric deconvolution problems. *The Annals of Statistics*, 19(3):1257-1272.

Fan, J. (1993). Adaptively local one-dimensional subproblems with application to a deconvolution problem. *The Annals of Statistics*, 600-610.

Fan, J. and Koo, J.-Y. (2002). Wavelet deconvolution. *IEEE Transactions on Information Theory*, 48(3), 734-747.

Gonzalez, R. C. and Woods, R. E. (2008). *Digital Image Processing*. Pearson Prentice Hall.

Hall, P., Kerkyacharian, G., Picard, D. (1998). Block threshold rules for curve estimation using kernel and wavelet methods. *The Annals of Statistics*, 26(3), 922-942.

Hall, P. and Patil, P. (1995). Formulae for mean integrated squared error of nonlinear wavelet-based density estimators. *The Annals of Statistics*, 23(3):905-928.

Hall, P., Penev, S., Kerkyacharian, G., and Picard, D. (1997). Numerical performance of block thresholded wavelet estimators. *Statistics and Computing*, 7(2), 115-124.

Hall, P. and Qiu, P. (2005). Discrete-transform approach to deconvolution problems. *Biometrika*, 92(1), 135-148.

Hall, P. and Qiu, P. (2007a). Blind deconvolution and deblurring in image analysis. *Statistica Sinica*, 17(4):1483-1509.

Hall, P. and Qiu, P. (2007b). Nonparametric estimation of a point-spread function in multivariate problems. *The Annals of Statistics*, 35(4):1512-1534.

Hansen, P. C., Nagy, J. G., and O'leary, D. P. (2006). *Deblurring Images: Matrices, Spectra, and Filtering*. SIAM.

Hernández, E. and Weiss, G. (1996). *A First Course on Wavelets*. CRC press.

Kang, Y. (2020). Consistent blind image deblurring using jump-preserving extrapolation. *Journal of Computational and Graphical Statistics*, 29(2), 372-382.

Kang, Y., Mukherjee, P., and Qiu, P. (2018). Efficient blind image deblurring using nonparametric regression and local pixel clustering. *Technometrics*, 60(4):522-531.

Kang, Y. and Qiu, P. (2014). Jump detection in blurred regression surfaces. *Technometrics*, 56, 539-550.

Kerkyacharian, G. and Picard, D. (1992). Density estimation in besov spaces. *Statistics & Probability Letters*, 13(1), 15-24.

Koo, J.-Y. and Park, B. U. (1996). B-spline deconvolution based on the em algorithm. *Journal of Statistical Computation and Simulation*, 54(4), 275-288.

Kooperberg, C. and Stone, C. J. (1991). A study of logspline density estimation. *Computational Statistics & Data Analysis*, 12(3), 327-347.

Liu, M. C. and Taylor, R. L. (1989). A consistent nonparametric density estimator for the deconvolution problem. *Canadian Journal of Statistics*, 17(4), 427-438.

Masry, E. (1991). Multivariate probability density deconvolution for stationary random processes. *IEEE Transactions on Information Theory*, 37(4), 1105-1115.

Masry, E. (1993). Strong consistency and rates for deconvolution of multivariate densities of stationary processes. *Stochastic Processes and Their Applications*, 47(1), 53-74.

Masry, E. (1994). Probability density estimation from dependent observations using wavelets orthonormal bases. *Statistics & Probability Letters*, 21(3), 181-194.

Mendelsohn, J. and Rice, J. (1982). Deconvolution of microfluorometric histograms with b splines. *Journal of the American Statistical Association*, 77(380), 748-753.

Penskaya, M. (1985). Projection estimators of the density of an a prior distribution and of functionals of it. *Theory of Probability and Mathematical Statistics*, 31, 113-124.

Pensky, M. (2002). Density deconvolution based on wavelets with bounded supports. *Statistics & Probability Letters*, 56(3), 261-269.

Pensky, M. and Vidakovic, B. (1999). Adaptive wavelet estimator for nonparametric density deconvolution. *The Annals of Statistics*, 27(6), 2033-2053.

Qiu, P. (2007). Jump surface estimation, edge detection, and image restoration. *Journal of the American Statistical Association*, 102, 745-756.

Qiu, P. (2008). A nonparametric procedure for blind image deblurring. *Computational Statistics and Data Analysis*, 52, 4828-4841.

Qiu, P. and Kang, Y. (2015). Blind image deblurring using jump regression analysis. *Statistica Sinica*, 25, 879-899.

Stefanski, L. A. (1990). Rates of convergence of some estimators in a class of deconvolution problems. *Statistics & Probability Letters*, 9(3), 229-235.

Stefanski, L. A. and Carroll, R. J. (1990). Deconvolving kernel density estimators. *Statistics*, 21(2), 169-184.

Stone, C. J. and Koo, C.-Y. (1986). Logspline density estimation. *Contemp. Math*, 59(1), 15.

Taylor, R. and Zhang, H. (1990). On a strongly consistent nonparametric density estimator for the deconvolution problem. *Communications in Statistics-Theory and Methods*, 19(9), 3325-3342.

Tikhonov, A. N. and Arsenin, V. Y. (1977). *Solutions of Ill-posed Problems.* John Wiley, New York.

Walter, G. (1981). Orthogonal series estimators of the prior distribution. *Sankhyā: The Indian Journal of Statistics, Series A*, 43(2):228-245.

Walter, G. G. (1994). *Wavelets and Other Orthogonal Systems with Applications.* CRC Press, Boca Raton, FL.

Walter, G. G. (1999). Density estimation in the presence of noise. *Statistics & Probability Letters*, 41(3), 237-246.

You, Y.-L. and Kaveh, M. (1996). A regularization approach to joint blur identification and image restoration. *IEEE Transactions on Image Processing*, 5(3), 416-428.

Zayed, A. I. and Walter, G. G. (1996). Characterization of analytic functions in terms of their wavelet coefficients. *Complex Variables and Elliptic Equations*, 29(3), 265-276.

Zhang, C.-H. (1990). Fourier methods for estimating mixing densities and distributions. *The Annals of Statistics*, 18(2):806-831.

# 12

# *Deconvolution with Unknown Error Distribution*

**Aurore Delaigle and Ingrid Van Keilegom**

## CONTENTS



## 12.1 Introduction

In the nonparametric literature on the classical measurement error problem, where the goal is to do inference on the distribution of a variable $X$ observed with independent additive error $U$, it is often assumed that the error density $f_U$ is perfectly known. In applications this is often too restrictive, since in many cases one does not know much about the complexity and imperfect nature of the underlying data. In this chapter we present approaches for non- and semiparametric inference on the distribution of $X$ developed in papers that do not assume the density $f_U$ to be (fully) known. Unless otherwise specified, we assume throughout that all the variables are continuous and the data follow the classical additive measurement error model (see (12.1) on the following pages) or a heteroscedastic variant of it (see model (12.15)). Apart

DOI: 10.1201/9781315101279-12

from some qualitative or parametric assumptions on $f_U$, we do not use other models. In particular, we do not consider the case where the variable $X$ is a covariate in a regression model, that one wishes to estimate by taking the measurement error on $X$ into account.

There are basically two ways to avoid assuming that $f_U$ is known: either we observe additional data (in the form of repeated contaminated measurements, longitudinal data, validation data, auxiliary variables, instrumental variables, etc.) that can be used to estimate $f_U$, or we make assumptions on the laws of $X$ and $U$ that allow to identify and estimate $f_U$ without the need to collect additional data. In Section 12.2 we show how to estimate $f_X$ nonparametrically when additional data are available; the case without additional observations is the topic of Section 12.3. In Section 12.4 we discuss the related challenging problem of estimating the boundary of the support of $X$ in the case without additional data. Finally, in Section 12.5, we consider the case where one has neither enough data nor enough information about the underlying densities to be able to estimate $f_U$ consistently; we discuss how nonparametric estimators of $f_X$ are impacted by misspecification of $f_U$.

## 12.2 Estimation of $f_X$ when Additional Data Are Available

In this section we discuss techniques for estimating the density $f_X$ nonparametrically from data coming from the classical measurement error model, in the case where the error density is unknown but it can be estimated from additional observations. For example, we may have access to a sample from the error distribution or may be able to measure the data repeatedly. There are other situations where some type of additional data are available, which can be used for identifying and constructing an estimator of $f_U$ and $f_X$. They include the case when validation data are available (i.e. when some of the data points are measured without error), when panel or longitudinal data are observed, or when auxiliary variables or instrumental variables are available. In each of these cases it is possible to identify the distribution of the signal $X$ under certain assumptions.

In this section we consider three different scenarios. In Section 12.2.1, we discuss the simplest case where we observe a direct sample from the errors, which are assumed to be homoscedastic. Section 12.2.2 introduces techniques that can be applied in the more common situation where the contaminated observations are observed repeatedly and the errors are homoscedastic. We extend those technique to the more general heteroscedastic case in Section 12.2.3.

### 12.2.1 Sample from $f_U$ in the Classical Error Model

Suppose we observe an i.i.d. sample of contaminated data $X_1^*, \ldots, X_n^*$ distributed like a random variable $X^*$ coming from the classical error model

$$X^* = X + U,\ X \text{ and } U \text{ independent, } X \sim f_X \text{ and } U \sim f_U\,. \tag{12.1}$$

As usual in the deconvolution literature, we assume that

$$f_U \text{ is symmetric and } \varphi_U(t) \neq 0 \text{ for all } t \in \mathbb{R}\,, \tag{12.2}$$

where here and throughout, $\varphi_A(t)$ denotes the characteristic function of $A$ if $A$ is a random variable, or the Fourier transform of $A$ if $A$ is a function. (Note that since $f_U$ is symmetric, $\varphi_U$ is real and thus $\varphi_U(t) \neq 0$ is equivalent to $\varphi_U(t) > 0$.)

In the basic setting where $f_U$ is known, a popular nonparametric estimator of $f_X$ is the deconvolution kernel estimator (Carroll and Hall, 1988; Stefanski and Carroll, 1990). See also Apanasovich and Liang (2021) for more details regarding kernel deconvolution methods for regression with classical errors, and Kang and Qiu (2021) for other deconvolution approaches. For all $x \in \mathbb{R}$, it is defined by

$$\hat{f}_X(x) = \frac{1}{nh} \sum_{j=1}^{n} K_U\Big(\frac{x - X_j^*}{h}\Big)\,, \tag{12.3}$$

where $h > 0$ is a bandwidth and, letting $K$ be a kernel function,

$$K_U(x) = \frac{1}{2\pi} \int e^{-itx} \frac{\varphi_K(t)}{\varphi_U(t/h)}\, dt\,, \tag{12.4}$$

where $i$ denotes the complex number such that $i^2 = -1$; see Delaigle (2021).

When $f_U$ is unknown, we cannot compute the estimator at (12.3). In Diggle and Hall (1993), the authors considered the case where, in addition to the $X_i^*$'s, an i.i.d. sample $\widetilde{U}_1, \ldots, \widetilde{U}_m$ from the error density $f_U$ is observed. There, they suggested to replace the unknown $\varphi_U(t)$ at (12.4) by the empirical characteristic function $\hat{\varphi}_U(t) = m^{-1} \sum_{j=1}^{m} e^{it\widetilde{U}_j}$ to obtain

$$\hat{K}_U(x) = \frac{1}{2\pi} \int e^{-itx} \frac{\varphi_K(t)}{\hat{\varphi}_U(t/h)}\, dt\,, \tag{12.5}$$

and they proposed to estimate $f_X(x)$ by

$$\hat{f}_X(x) = \frac{1}{nh} \sum_{j=1}^{n} \hat{K}_U\Big(\frac{x - X_j^*}{h}\Big)\,. \tag{12.6}$$

Under certain regularity conditions, they showed that as long as $n = O(m)$, estimating $\varphi_U$ has no first order asymptotic impact on the integrated squared error of the estimator at (12.3). However, in practice $\hat{\varphi}_U(t)$ is a poor estimator of $\varphi_U(t)$ for large $|t|$ (i.e. where $\varphi_U(t)$ takes small values). Indeed, since $\hat{\varphi}_U$ is unbiased and has a variance of order $m^{-1}$, then values of $|\hat{\varphi}_U|$ much smaller than $m^{-1/2}$ are essentially noise and can create numerical instability of the integral at (12.6). These difficulties can be avoided by regularising $\hat{\varphi}_U$ in its tails, using for example the estimator $\tilde{f}_X(x) = (nh)^{-1} \sum_{j=1}^n \tilde{K}_U\{(x - X_j^*)/h\}$ suggested by Neumann (1997), where

$$\tilde{K}_U(x) = \frac{1}{2\pi} \int e^{-itx} \frac{\varphi_K(t)}{\hat{\varphi}_U(t/h)} 1\{|\hat{\varphi}_U(t/h)| \geq m^{-1/2}\}\, dt. \tag{12.7}$$

In practice, $h$ needs to be chosen from the data; Neumann (1997) briefly mentions the possibility of using cross-validation of the type as in Stefanski and Carroll (1990), but without giving any detail. Perhaps this could be done by replacing, in each term of the cross-validation criterion used by Stefanski and Carroll (1990), $\varphi_U$ by $\hat{\varphi}_U$, using as well $1\{|\hat{\varphi}_U(t/h)| \geq m^{-1/2}\}$ as above, but this approach is studied neither in theory nor in practice.

### 12.2.2 Replicated Measurements with Homoscedatisc Errors

Observing a sample from $f_U$, like in Section 12.2.1, is only possible in some particular applications. Instead, what is often more realistic is to assume that we can observe replicated contaminated measurements

$$X_{jk}^* = X_j + U_{jk}, \text{ for } k = 1, \ldots, m_j \text{ and } j = 1, \ldots, n, \tag{12.8}$$

where $m_j \geq 1$ is the number of replicates available for the $j$th individual, at least a fraction of the $m_j$'s are greater or equal to 2, $X_j \sim f_X$, $U_{jk} \sim f_U$ and the $X_j$'s and the $U_{jk}$'s are totally independent.

For example, in nutrition studies, the long term nutrient intake $X$ of a patient is often measured through several 24 hour recalls. At each 24 hour recall, the $j$th patient reports their food intake over the last 24 hours, which is only a rough approximation to their long term intake $X_j$. After a transformation (typically the log transform), the data from the 24 hour recalls are often assumed to behave like $X_{jk}^*$ at (12.8).

To understand why replicates can be used to make progress when $f_U$ is unknown, note that if we subtract two replicates, say $X_{j1}^*$ and $X_{j2}^*$, for a given individual, then we have $X_{j1}^* - X_{j2}^* = U_{j1} - U_{j2}$. Since the $U_{jk}$'s are i.i.d., this can be exploited to estimate quantities related to $f_U$. In the simplest version of this problem, a parametric model is assumed for $f_U$. Often, the errors are assumed to be of zero mean, and the only unknown in $f_U$ is the variance $\sigma_U^2$, which can be estimated by

$$\hat{\sigma}_U^2 = \sum_{j=1}^n \sum_{k=1}^{m_j} (X_{jk}^* - \bar{X}_j^*)^2 / \sum_{j=1}^n (m_j - 1). \tag{12.9}$$

This approach is commonly used in the parametric literature on measurement errors. See for example Madansky (1959), Carroll and Stefanski (1990), Gleser (1990), Carroll et al. (1993) and Carroll et al. (2006, p.71). It can be combined with either a parametric estimator of $f_X$ or with the deconvolution estimator at (12.3), replacing there all instances of $\varphi_U$ by the corresponding parametric estimator.

However, if we assume that (12.2) holds, the distribution of $U$ can be estimated consistently without such parametric assumptions, as we show now. Under (12.2), since the $U_{jk}$'s are i.i.d., we have

$$X_{j1}^* - X_{j2}^* = U_{j1} - U_{j2} \sim f_U * f_U\,,$$

where, for two functions $f$ and $g$, $f * g(x) = \int f(x-u)g(u)\,du$ denotes the convolution of $f$ and $g$. Therefore, the characteristic function of $X_{j1}^* - X_{j2}^*$ is equal to $\varphi_U^2$ and we can estimate $\varphi_U^2$ by the empirical characteristic function of all the possible differences $X_{jk}^* - X_{j\ell}^*$, $k \neq \ell$,

$$\hat{\varphi}_U^2(t) = \frac{1}{N}\sum_j \sum_{k<\ell} e^{it(X_{jk}^* - X_{j\ell}^*)} = \frac{1}{N}\sum_j \sum_{k<\ell} e^{it(U_{jk} - U_{j\ell})}\,, \tag{12.10}$$

where $\sum_j$ refers to the sum over the individuals for which $m_j \geq 2$, and $N$ denotes the number of terms in the triple sum $\sum_j \sum_{k<\ell}$. See Delaigle et al. (2007) and Delaigle et al. (2008).

Under (12.2), for all $t \in \mathbb{R}$ we can write $\varphi_U(t) = \{\varphi_U^2(t)\}^{1/2}$. Since $\hat{\varphi}_U^2$ is an empirical characteristic function, it is not guaranteed to be real nor positive, unlike $\varphi_U^2(t)$. However, these two properties can be enforced by replacing $\hat{\varphi}_U^2(t)$ by $|\Re\{\hat{\varphi}_U^2(t)\}|$, where $\Re$ denotes the real part (the imaginary part is of no interest in practice, and ignoring it makes no asymptotic difference since it vanishes asymptotically). Motivated by these arguments and noting that, for all $x \in \mathbb{R}$ we have $\Re(e^{ix}) = \cos x$, Delaigle et al. (2008) proposed to estimate $\varphi_U(t)$ by

$$\hat{\varphi}_U(t) = \left|\Re\{\hat{\varphi}_U^2(t)\}\right|^{1/2} = \left|\frac{1}{N}\sum_j \sum_{k<\ell} \cos\{t(X_{jk}^* - X_{j\ell}^*)\}\right|^{1/2}, \tag{12.11}$$

where $N$ and the sums are as at (12.10). Then, they estimate $f_X(x)$ by

$$\hat{f}_X(x) = \frac{1}{nh}\sum_{j=1}^n \hat{K}_U\Big(\frac{x - X_j^*}{h}\Big), \tag{12.12}$$

with

$$\hat{K}_U(x) = \frac{1}{2\pi}\int e^{-itx}\frac{\varphi_K(t)}{\hat{\varphi}_U(t/h)+\rho}\,dt, \tag{12.13}$$

where $\rho > 0$ is a ridge parameter (usually a small number) introduced to avoid problems with the denominator getting too close to zero. Under sufficient regularity conditions, Delaigle et al. (2008) show that, if $n = O(N)$ and the distribution of $X$ is sufficiently smooth compared to that of $U$, $\hat{f}_X$ at (12.12) has the same first order asymptotic properties as $\hat{f}_X$ at (12.3).

In practice it is difficult to choose an appropriate $\rho$ from the data, and other techniques can be employed to reduce the impact of the unreliability of $\hat{\varphi}_U$ in its tails. For example, one could use Neumann's (2007) truncation approach introduced in Section 12.2.1. Delaigle et al.'s (2008) alternative suggestion is to replace $\hat{\varphi}_U(t) + \rho$ by

$$\tilde{\varphi}_U(t) = \hat{\varphi}_U(t)\, 1\{t \in A\} + \hat{\varphi}_{U,P}(t)\, 1\{t \notin A\}, \tag{12.14}$$

where $A$ denotes an interval on which $\hat{\varphi}_U$ is not too unreliable, and $\hat{\varphi}_{U,P}$ denotes a parametric estimator of $\varphi_U$. For example, $A$ could be taken to be the truncation interval used by Neumann (2007), or the largest interval around 0 on which the estimator $\hat{\varphi}_U(t)$ does not oscillate. For the parametric model $\varphi_{U,P}$, arguments from Meister (2004) and Delaigle (2008) suggest that a good choice is to use a Laplace distribution. Delaigle et al. (2008) follow this approach, and take $\hat{\varphi}_{U,P}(t) = (1 + \hat{\sigma}_P^2 t^2)^{-1}$, where $\hat{\sigma}_P^2$ is half the empirical variance of $U$ computed as at (12.9). Delaigle (2008) suggest using the plug-in method bandwidth of Delaigle and Gijbels (2002, 2004), replacing there each occurrence of $\varphi_U$ by $\tilde{\varphi}_U$.

Li and Vuong (1998) suggested a more complex approach which, in principle, could be used regardless of symmetry properties of the error density $f_U$. Their technique is based on properties of the characteristic function of pairs of replicates, but it suffers from at least two drawbacks. First, it is not clear how it could be implemented in practice. Second, the authors established consistency of their estimator under the assumption that the density and the characteristic function of $U$ and $X$ are both compactly supported. As noted by Delaigle et al. (2008), it seems difficult to satisfy those conditions simultaneously.

### 12.2.3 Replicated Measurements with Heteroscedastic Errors

The estimator at (12.12) introduced in Section 12.2.2 can be extended to the setting where the $U_{jk}$'s at (12.8) are not identically distributed. In practice, heteroscedastic errors arise when individuals are not observed under similar conditions. For example, the observations may have been collected in several laboratories or from different studies, and groups of individuals (e.g. smoker/non smoker, male/female) may be contaminated by different types of errors. There are several ways to model heteroscedasticity of the errors. One possibility is to assume that instead of coming from the model at (12.8), the replicated contaminated observations are generated from the model

$$X^*_{jk} = X_j + U_{jk},\ X_j \sim f_X,\ U_{jk} \sim f_{U_j},\ \text{for } k = 1, \ldots, m_j \text{ and } j = 1, \ldots, n, \tag{12.15}$$

where $m_j > 1$ is the number of replicates available for the $j$th individual, the $X_j$'s and the $U_{jk}$'s are totally independent and, letting $n_j = m_j(m_j - 1)/2$,

$$f_{U_j} \text{ is symmetric for } j = 1, \ldots, n \text{ and } \sum_{j=1}^{n} n_j |\varphi_{U_j}(t)|^2 > 0 \text{ for all } t \in \mathbb{R}\,, \tag{12.16}$$

where $\varphi_{U_j}$ denote the characteristic function of $U_{jk}$, for $k = 1, \ldots, m$. Note that unlike the homoscedastic case from Section 12.2.2, the measurements need to be replicated at least once ($m_j > 1$) for all individuals.

Under these conditions, Delaigle and Meister (2008) proposed an alternative to (12.12) that can be computed from the data at (12.15). To understand their technique, note that using (12.16), since $(X_{jk}^* + X_{j\ell}^*)/2 = X_j + (U_{jk} + U_{j\ell})/2$, we have

$$E\Big(\sum_{j=1}^{n} \sum_{k<\ell} e^{it\frac{X_{jk}^* + X_{j\ell}^*}{2}}\Big) = \varphi_X(t) \sum_{j=1}^{n} n_j |\varphi_{U_j}(t/2)|^2 \,.$$

Likewise, since $(X_{jk}^* - X_{j\ell}^*)/2 = (U_{jk} - U_{j\ell})/2$, we have

$$E\Big(\sum_{j=1}^{n} \sum_{k<\ell} e^{it\frac{X_{jk}^* - X_{j\ell}^*}{2}}\Big) = \sum_{j=1}^{n} n_j |\varphi_{U_j}(t/2)|^2 \,.$$

These calculations suggest estimating $\varphi_X(t)$ by

$$\hat\varphi_X(t) = \sum_{j=1}^{n} \sum_{k<\ell} e^{it(X_{jk}^* + X_{j\ell}^*)/2} \Big/ \sum_{j=1}^{n} \sum_{k<\ell} e^{it(X_{jk}^* - X_{j\ell}^*)/2} \,.$$

However, as in Section 12.2.2, since the denominator is an empirical characteristic function, it can get close to zero, especially for large $|t|$, even if (12.16) holds. To overcome this difficulty, Delaigle and Meister (2008) use a ridge parameter $\rho > 0$, and propose to estimate $f_X(x)$ by

$$\hat f_X(x) = \frac{1}{2\pi} \int e^{-itx} \frac{\sum_{j=1}^{n} \sum_{k<\ell} e^{it(X_{jk}^* + X_{j\ell}^*)/2}}{\sum_{j=1}^{n} \sum_{k<\ell} e^{it(X_{jk}^* - X_{j\ell}^*)/2} + \rho} \varphi_K(ht)\, dt \,.$$

To choose $(\rho, h)$ in practice, we can use the SIMEX bandwidth of Delaigle and Hall (2008). Alternatives such as the one discussed at (12.14) could also be used to avoid having to use $\rho$. In this case, the only parameter to choose is $h$. While for this we could also use the SIMEX bandwidth of Delaigle and Hall (2008), inspired by Delaigle et al. (2008), another approach that seems reasonable and which we prefer is to use a plug-in procedure of the type in Delaigle and Gijbels (2002, 2004). This approach consists in choosing $h$ by minimising an estimator of the asymptotic mean squared error of version of the estimator $\hat f_X$ that assumes that the $\varphi_{U_j}$'s are known, i.e., of

$$\tilde f_X(x) = \frac{1}{2\pi} \int e^{-itx} \sum_{j=1}^{n} \sum_{k<\ell} e^{it(X_{jk}^* + X_{j\ell}^*)/2} \varphi_K(ht) \Big/ \sum_{j=1}^{n} n_j |\varphi_{U_j}(t/2)|^2 \, dt \,.$$

### 12.2.4 Related Literature

In the case where replicated data are available and the errors $U_i$ are normally distributed, McIntyre and Stefanski (2011) suggested an alternative kernel density estimator in the heteroscedastic context. In the regression context, Delaigle and Meister (2007) also suggested an alternative SIMEX procedure, which can be easily adapted to the density estimation setting. Meister and Neumann (2010) considered the replication model in cases where $\varphi_U$ has zeros, and Horowitz and Markatou (1996) and Neumann (2007) considered a related problem using panel data. See also Schennach (2004).

## 12.3 Estimation of $f_U$ and $f_X$ without Additional Data

In the previous section we assumed that we had additional data that could be used to estimate the error density $f_U$. However, additional data are not always available, a situation that has received increasing attention in the recent literature. Although this problem is much harder than the previous ones, fortunately one can still correct for the measurement error in certain cases. In this section we present some settings where we can identify and estimate the densities $f_U$ and $f_X$ without the additional data from Section 12.2. This will be done first for the case where $f_U$ is partially known (e.g., normal distribution with unknown variance), and then for the case where only some qualitative information about $f_U$ is available (like symmetry). The former model is referred to as the semiparametric model (as $f_X$ is nonparametric and $f_U$ is parametric), whereas the latter is nonparametric.

We will assume throughout this section that the classical additive error model is valid, i.e. we have a sample $X_1^*, \ldots, X_n^*$ of i.i.d. copies of $X^*$, where $X^*$ comes from the model at (12.1).

### 12.3.1 Semiparametric Estimation without Additional Data

In the literature on this estimation problem, two quite different main streams of ideas are developed. The first one makes assumptions on the behavior of the characteristic function of $X$; in the second approach, the identifiability of the model is obtained by making assumptions on the support of $X$. We refer also to Wang (2021), which goes deeper into the important issue of identifiability of measurement error models.

The first line of research is initiated by Matias (2002), and later extended to more general densities $f_X$ and $f_U$ by Butucea and Matias (2005), Meister (2006) and Butucea et al. (2008). It focuses on the supersmooth class of error distributions introduced in Delaigle (2021). Below we explain in detail the method developed by Butucea and Matias (2005). Then we briefly explain the different contributions of the other three papers.

Suppose that the error $U$ is supersmooth of a known order, i.e. the error is such that its characteristic function $\varphi_U$ satisfies

$$d_0 \exp(-|t\sigma|^\beta) \le |\varphi_U(t)| \le d_1 \exp(-|t\sigma|^\beta) \quad \text{for all } |t| > M \qquad (12.17)$$

for some constants $0 < d_0, d_1, M < \infty$, where $\beta > 0$ is a known constant and $\sigma > 0$ is an unknown scale parameter. This includes the case of normal errors with unknown variance, in which case $\beta = 2$ and $\sigma^2 = \sigma_U^2/2$, where $\sigma_U^2$ is the variance of $U$. It also includes the case where $U$ has a stable distribution with unknown scale parameter $\sigma$, and with all other parameters known.

The density of $U$ then only depends on the unknown parameter $\sigma$, and we will therefore focus in what follows on the identifiability and estimation of $\sigma$. Once the density of $U$ is estimated, classical deconvolution methods, like the one at (12.6), can be used to estimate the density $f_X$.

Suppose that the characteristic function $\varphi_X$ of $X$ satisfies either

$$|\varphi_X(t)| \ge c_0 |t|^{-\alpha} \quad \text{for } |t| \text{ large enough,} \qquad (12.18)$$

for some unknown constant $c_0 > 0$ and a known constant $\alpha > 1$ (which is e.g. the case for the exponential density) or

$$|\varphi_X(t)| \ge c_0 \exp(-c_1 |t|^\alpha) \quad \text{for } |t| \text{ large enough,} \qquad (12.19)$$

for some known constants $0 < \alpha < \beta$ and $c_1 > 0$, and an unknown constant $c_0 > 0$, which is satisfied for the normal density, among many others. Under (12.17), since $\varphi_{X^*} = \varphi_X \varphi_U$ by (12.1), we have, for $|t|$ large enough,

$$\log\{|\varphi_X(t)|\}/|t|^\beta + \log(d_0)/|t|^\beta - \sigma^\beta \le \log\{|\varphi_{X^*}(t)|\}/|t|^\beta \le 0\,,$$

where we used the fact that $\varphi_{X^*}(t) \le 1$ for all $t$. Under either of (12.18) or (12.19), $\log\{|\varphi_X(t)|\}$ tends to infinity more slowly than $|t|^\beta$. Therefore, we have

$$\lim_{|t|\to\infty} \log\{|\varphi_{X^*}(t)|\}/|t|^\beta = -\sigma^\beta.$$

This shows that $\sigma$ can be identified from the distribution of $X^*$ alone.

To derive an estimator of $\sigma$, define $\Psi(s,t) = \varphi_{X^*}(t)\exp(s^\beta t^\beta)$, and note that for $s > \sigma$,

$$\lim_{t\to+\infty} |\Psi(s,t)| = \lim_{t\to\infty} |\varphi_X(t)|\,|\varphi_U(t)| \exp(s^\beta t^\beta) = \infty,$$

whereas for $s \le \sigma$, $\lim_{t\to+\infty} |\Psi(s,t)| = 0$, since $|\varphi_U(t)|\exp(s^\beta t^\beta)$ tends to a positive constant when $s = \sigma$, to 0 when $s < \sigma$ and to infinity faster than $|\varphi_X(t)|$ tends to zero when $s > \sigma$. Motivated by this, Butucea and Matias (2005) proposed to estimate $\sigma$ by

$$\hat\sigma = \inf\{s : s > 0 \text{ and } |\hat\Psi(s, t_n)| \ge 1\},$$

where $\hat{\Psi}(s,t) = \hat{\varphi}_{X^*}(t)\exp(s^\beta t^\beta)$, with $\hat{\varphi}_{X^*} = n^{-1}\sum_{j=1}^n e^{itX_j^*}$ the empirical characteristic function of $X^*$, and where $t_n$ is a smoothing parameter satisfying $t_n \to +\infty$ as $n \to \infty$.

Butucea and Matias' (2005) work shows that it is possible to estimate the unknown parameter $\sigma$ of a parametric supersmooth error distribution, but their method requires strong assumptions on the target density $f_X$, since we need to know that the characteristic function $\varphi_X$ decreases to zero in the tails more slowly than the characteristic function of the errors, $\varphi_U$, and this information is often not available in practice. Moreover, their estimator depends in a sensitive way on the smoothing parameter $t_n$, as they explain at the end of their Section 2.

In Butucea et al. (2008) the above method was adapted to the case where $U$ has a stable symmetric distribution, that is has characteristic function

$$\varphi_U(t) = \exp(-|\sigma t|^\beta)$$

for all $t$, where the scale parameter $\sigma > 0$ is supposed to be known and the self-similarity index $\beta > 0$ is unknown. So in this case instead of assuming that $\sigma$ is unknown and $\beta$ is known (which is a special case of the model in Butucea and Matias, 2005), they make the reverse assumption. They show that the parameter $\beta$ is identified, and they propose an estimator which is (as in Butucea and Matias, 2005) based on the idea of selecting the smallest value of $\beta$ that satisfies a certain property. As before, the estimator depends on a tuning parameter $t_n$ that needs to go to infinity as $n \to \infty$ and that depends on parameters that are unknown in practice.

The work of Butucea and Matias (2005) is also related to the papers by Matias (2002) and Meister (2006), who considered the special case of a normal error $U \sim N(0, \sigma_U^2)$. We focus here on the method proposed by Meister (2006); the one by Matias (2002) is rather similar. Meister (2006) assumed that for a constant $M > 0$,

$$c_0|t|^{-\alpha} \le |\varphi_X(t)| \le c_1|t|^{-\alpha} \quad \text{for all } |t| > M,$$

where $c_0$ and $c_1$ are positive finite constants and $\alpha > 1$ (not necessarily known). Under these conditions, since $\varphi_{X^*} = \varphi_X\varphi_U$, by (12.1), for all $\gamma > 1$ and $c_2 > 0$, we have

$$\lim_{|t|\to\infty} t^{-2}\log\left\{\frac{|\varphi_{X^*}(t)|}{c_2|t|^{-\gamma}}\right\} \le \lim_{|t|\to\infty} \frac{\log(c_1/c_2) + \log\left(|t|^{\gamma-\alpha}\right)}{t^2} - \frac{\sigma_U^2}{2} = -\frac{\sigma_U^2}{2},$$

since $\varphi_U(t) = \exp(-\sigma_U^2 t^2/2)$.

Using these ideas, Meister (2006) proposed to estimate $\sigma_U^2$ by

$$\hat{\sigma}_U^2 = \min\left\{\max\left(0, -2\log\left\{|\hat{\varphi}_{X^*}(t_n)|/(c_2 t_n^{-\gamma})\right\}/t_n^2\right), \sigma_n^2\right\}, \tag{12.20}$$

with $\sigma_n^2$ and $t_n$ two sequences tending to infinity as $n \to \infty$ (see Meister, 2006), and where $c_2 = c_0$ and $\gamma = \alpha$ if $c_0$ and $\alpha$ are known. If they are unknown, $c_2$ and $\gamma$ are chosen arbitrarily.

Let us now turn to the second stream of techniques mentioned at the start of this subsection, namely the idea of identifying the measurement error model by making assumptions on the support of $X$. Schwarz and Van Bellegem (2010) assumed that $U \sim N(0, \sigma_U^2)$ with $\sigma_U^2 > 0$ unknown, and that the density $f_X$ vanishes on a set of positive measure. They show that under this model, $\sigma_U^2$ and $f_X$ are identified. The proof of this result relies on the fact that for any probability distributions $P_1$ and $P_2$ and for any $0 < \sigma_1 < \sigma_2$, we have that $P_1 = P_2 * N(0, \sigma_2^2 - \sigma_1^2)$ whenever $P_1 * N(0, \sigma_1^2) = P_2 * N(0, \sigma_2^2)$.

Based on this identification result, Schwarz and Van Bellegem (2010) proposed to estimate $\sigma_U^2$ and $\varphi_X$ by minimizing a weighted $L_1$ distance between the characteristic function $\hat{\varphi}_{X^*}$ of the data, and the characteristic function $\varphi_{X^*} = \varphi_X \varphi_{\sigma_U}$ under the model, with $\varphi_{\sigma_U}$ the characteristic function of a normal with variance $\sigma_U^2$. More precisely, they defined their estimators by any pair $(\hat{\sigma}_U^2, \hat{\varphi}_X)$ that satisfies

$$\rho(\hat{\sigma}_U^2, \hat{\varphi}_X) \le \inf_{\tilde{\sigma}_U^2 > 0, \tilde{\varphi}_X \in \Phi_{\mathcal{C}}} \rho(\tilde{\sigma}_U^2, \tilde{\varphi}_X) + \delta_n,$$

where $\delta_n$ is some sequence tending to zero, $\Phi_{\mathcal{C}}$ is the set of all characteristic functions corresponding to some class of distributions $\mathcal{C}$, and

$$\rho(\tilde{\sigma}_U^2, \tilde{\varphi}_X) = \int_{\mathbb{R}} |\tilde{\varphi}_X(t) \varphi_{\tilde{\sigma}_U}(t) - \hat{\varphi}_{X^*}(t)| w(t)\, dt,$$

for some strictly positive and continuous weight function $w$. While they established consistency of their estimator under some conditions, they did not propose a way to compute their estimator in practice (e.g., how to choose $\delta_n$, $\mathcal{C}$ and $w$ nor how to solved the optimisation problem).

The approaches in the preceding paragraphs are important in that they come up with theoretical ways to identify the model without the need to collect additional data. However, those estimators all suffer from one or more of the following problems: they depend on one or several tuning parameters for which no clear guidelines are given, no (or limited) practical implementation is discussed, and they might lead to practical identifiability issues.

To overcome these problems, Bertrand et al. (2019) proposed a new method for the case where the error $U$ is normal with unknown variance $\sigma_U^2$, and the support of $X$ is compact. The identifiability of this model is guaranteed by Schwarz and Van Bellegem (2010). Assume that the support of $X$ is equal to $[b, a+b]$, with $a > 0$ and $b \in \mathbb{R}$ two unknown constants, and write

$$X = aS + b\,,$$

where $S = (X - b)/a$ is a continuous random variable taking values on $[0, 1]$.

The advantage of formulating the problem through $S$ is that Bernstein (1912) showed that any continuous function $f(s)$ defined on $[0,1]$ can be approximated uniformly by the limit, as $m$ tends to infinity, of a Bernstein polynomial of degree $m$, defined as follows:

$$B_m(s) = \sum_{k=0}^{m} \alpha_{k,m} b_{k,m}(s), \qquad s \in [0,1]\,,$$

where $b_{k,m}(s) = \binom{m}{k} s^k (1-s)^{m-k}$, for $k = 0, \ldots, m$ and $\alpha_{k,m} = f(k/m)$. Thus, for $m$ large enough, the density $f_S(s)$ of $S$ can be approximated by

$$\tilde{f}_{S,m}(s;\boldsymbol{\theta}_m) = \sum_{k=0}^{m} f_S(k/m) b_{k,m}(s) = \sum_{k=0}^{m} \theta_{k,m} f_{B_{k+1,m-k+1}}(s), \quad s \in [0,1],$$

where $\boldsymbol{\theta}_m = (\theta_{0,m}, \ldots, \theta_{m,m})$, with $\theta_{k,m} = (m+1)^{-1} f_S(k/m)$ some unknown positive parameters, and where $f_{B_{k+1,m-k+1}}$ denotes the Beta density with parameters $k+1$ and $m-k+1$.

We deduce, using (12.1), that $f_{X^*}(t) = f_X * f_U(t) = a^{-1} \int f_S\{(x - b)/a\} \phi_{\sigma_U}(t-x)\,dx$, where $\phi_{\sigma_U}$ is the density of a $N(0,\sigma_U^2)$. Thus, we can approximate $f_{X^*}(t)$ by

$$\tilde{f}_{X^*,m}(t;\sigma_U,a,b,\boldsymbol{\theta}_m) = \sum_{k=0}^{m} \theta_{k,m} \int f_{a,B_{k+1,m-k+1}}(x-b)\phi_{\sigma_U}(t-x)\,dx\,,$$

where $f_{a,B_{k+1,m-k+1}}(x) = a^{-1} f_{B_{k+1,m-k+1}}(x/a)$. It can be shown that if $f_S$ is continuous, we have $\lim_{m\to\infty} \sup_t \left|\tilde{f}_{X^*,m}(t;\sigma_U,a,b,\boldsymbol{\theta}_m) - f_{X^*}(t)\right| = 0$.

The unknown parameters $\sigma_U, a, b$ and $\boldsymbol{\theta}_m$ of this approximation are estimated by maximum likelihood, under the constraint that the $\theta_{k,m}$'s are non negative and sum to 1, which ensures that the estimator of $\tilde{f}_{S,m}(\cdot\,;\boldsymbol{\theta}_m)$ is a density. Letting $\hat{\sigma}_U, \hat{a}, \hat{b}$ and $\hat{\boldsymbol{\theta}}_m$ denote the resulting maximum likelihood estimators, the estimator of $f_X(x)$ is then given by

$$\hat{f}_X(x) = \sum_{k=0}^{m} \hat{\theta}_{k,m} f_{\hat{a},B_{k+1,m-k+1}}(x-\hat{b})\,.$$

Bertrand et al. (2019) suggested choosing $m$ using the Bayesian Information Criterion (BIC).

### 12.3.2 Nonparametric Estimation without Additional Data

In the previous section we made some parametric assumptions on the error density $f_U$, assuming for example that $U$ is normal with unknown variance or that $U$ has a stable distribution with either scale or self-similarity index unknown and estimated from the data. In this section we go one step further and make only qualitative assumptions on the density $f_U$, from which we can still identify and estimate $f_X$.

A first paper on this topic is by Meister (2007), who assumed that the characteristic function $\varphi_U$ is known on a compact interval around zero. Based on this assumption, he shows that the density $f_X$ is identifiable. To estimate $f_X$ in practice, he decomposes its characteristic function $\varphi_X$ in a Legendre polynomial basis, estimates the unknown coefficients of the decomposition, and then deduces an estimator of $f_X$ by an inverse Fourier transform smoothed by some kernel. While this work constitutes a first step in this difficult estimation problem, assuming that $\varphi_U$ is known on a compact interval around zero is only slightly less strong than assuming that $f_U$ is completely known; for example it implies that all moments of $U$ are known (if they exist).

Delaigle and Hall (2016) relaxed the conditions on $f_U$, assuming only that $f_U$ satisfies the standard deconvolution assumption at (12.2). They introduced their technique for both continuous and discrete distributions but here we discuss only the continuous case. Under (12.2), if we do not impose any constraint on $f_X$ then it is impossible to distinguish $f_X$ from $f_U$ based on data on $X^*$. For example, if $X$ has a symmetric density $f_X$ and we observe $X^* = X + U$ whereas all we know about $X$ and $U$ is that they are independent and $f_U$ is symmetric, then $f_{X^*}$, $f_X$ and $f_U$ could each play the role of $f_U$ since these three densities are symmetric (here and below we let $f_T$ denote the density of any variable $T$).

Thus, under (12.2), $f_X$ cannot be identified from data on $X^*$ if it is not asymmetric, but asymmetry does not suffice to ensure identifiability. Indeed, suppose that $X$ can be expressed as

$$X = Y + Z\,, \tag{12.21}$$

where $Y$ and $Z$ are independent and have a non degenerate distribution, $f_Z$ is symmetric and $f_Y$ is asymmetric. Then $f_X$ is asymmetric, but since $X^* = X + U = Y + Z + U$, and each of $f_U$, $f_Z$ and $f_{Z+U}$ are symmetric, then each of these three densities can play the role of the symmetric error density $f_U$, which shows that we cannot identify $f_U$ from data on $X^*$. Motivated by these considerations, Delaigle and Hall (2016) assumed that

$$f_X \text{ is asymmetric and } X \text{ cannot be decomposed as at (12.21).} \tag{12.22}$$

The condition at (12.22) may appear very restrictive as it excludes many distributions commonly used in statistics. However, Delaigle and Hall (2016) argued that in real life, data can come from such a diverse, infinite set of distributions, that we can rarely expect that $f_X$ will be so nice and regular that it exactly satisfies (12.21). By contrast, the errors tend to be more structured (for example they are often averages of several random variables) and can often reasonably be assumed to have a nice and symmetric distribution.

The distributions for which (12.21) does not hold are known in the probability literature as non-decomposable distributions, and are notoriously difficult to characterise. However, some results suggest that "in general, a distribution is indecomposable"; see Parthasarathy et al. (1962). See also Delaigle and Hall (2016), who proved that (12.21) often does not hold in the discrete case.

Under (12.2) and (12.22), Delaigle and Hall (2016) developed a methodology based on the phase function, which, for a random variable $T$, is defined by $\rho_T(t) = \varphi_T(t)/|\varphi_T(t)|$, for all $t \in \mathbb{R}$. In this notation, since (12.2) implies that $\varphi_U = |\varphi_U|$ and recalling that $X^* = X + U$, we have

$$\rho_{X^*} = \varphi_{X^*}/|\varphi_{X^*}| = \varphi_X \varphi_U/|\varphi_X \varphi_U| = \rho_X \,. \tag{12.23}$$

Now, we can easily estimate $\rho_X$ from data on $X^*$ (it suffices to replace $\varphi_{X^*}$ in (12.26) by its empirical estimator). Thus, if we could uniquely identify a distribution from its phase function, we could deduce an estimator of $f_X$.

However, a phase function does not uniquely identify a distribution. To see why, let

$$T = X + V \,, \tag{12.24}$$

where $V$ and $X$ are independent and $V$ has a non degenerate distribution. If $V$ has a symmetric density $f_V$, then $\rho_T = \rho_X$ (this is shown in the same way as the proof of (12.26)). Likewise, if we could express $X$ as at (12.21), then we would have $\rho_X = \rho_Y$. Note too that, in these notations, we have $\text{var}(Y) < \text{var}(X) < \text{var}(T)$. Now, as argued above, in many cases, (12.21) will not hold. Since, for $T$ at (12.24), we have $\text{var}(X) < \text{var}(T)$, this motivated Delaigle and Hall (2016) to assume that, in addition to (12.22), the distribution $F_X$ of $X$ is such that

$F_X$ is the unique distribution with smallest variance among all distributions with phase function $\rho_X$. (12.25)

Note that (12.25) does not follow from (12.22). Indeed, even though, under (12.22), (12.21) cannot hold, where $\rho_Y = \rho_X$ and $\text{var}(Y) < \text{var}(X)$, this does not ensure that there is no random variable $V$ which has neither the form at (12.24) nor that of $Y$ at (12.21), but which is such that $\rho_V = \rho_X$ and $\text{var}(V) < \text{var}(X)$. As mentioned above, too little is known about properties of non-decomposable distributions for it to be possible to characterise the distributions that satisfy (12.22) and (12.25). However, Delaigle and Hall (2016) argued that, in many real applications, it is reasonable to assume that these conditions hold.

Thus, in theory, their goal is to find the distribution $F_X$ with phase function $\rho_X$ such that $\rho_X = \rho_{X^*}$, or equivalently, such that

$$\varphi_{X^*}(t) - \rho_X(t)|\varphi_{X^*}(t)| = 0 \quad \text{for all } t \,, \tag{12.26}$$

which has the smallest possible variance. In practice, to estimate $F_X$ under assumptions (12.2), (12.22) and (12.25), they start by estimating the phase function of $X$ by $\hat{\rho}_X = \hat{\rho}_{X_*} = \hat{\varphi}_{X^*}/|\hat{\varphi}_{X^*}|$, where $\hat{\varphi}_{X^*}(t) = n^{-1} \sum_{j=1}^n e^{itX_j^*}$

is the empirical characteristic function of $X^*$. Then, to make the optimisation problem tractable in practice, they approximate $F_X(x)$ by a discrete distribution $F(x|p) = \sum_{j=1}^m p_j I(x_j \le x)$ which puts mass $0 \le p_j \le 1$ at $x_j$, for $j = 1, \ldots, m$, where $\sum_{j=1}^m p_j = 1$; they take $m = 5\sqrt{n}$ and choose the $x_j$'s at random, uniformly over $[\min_i X_i^*, \max_i X_i^*]$. Let $\rho(t|p) = \varphi(t|p)/|\varphi(t|p)|$ denote the phase function of the distribution $F(x|p)$, where $\varphi(t|p) = \sum_{j=1}^m p_j \exp(itx_j)$. Motivated by (12.26), and noting that the quality of $\hat{\varphi}_{X^*}(t)$ degrades as $|t|$ increases, Delaigle and Hall (2016) propose to search for $\hat{p} = (\hat{p}_1, \ldots, \hat{p}_m)$ that minimises

$$T(p) = \int \Big|\varphi_{X^*}(t) - \rho(t|p)|\hat{\varphi}_{X^*}(t)|\Big|^2 w(t)\, dt\,,$$

where $w$ is a weight function, and minimises, at the same time, the variance of the distribution $F(x|p)$. See Delaigle and Hall (2016) for details of implementation. Then they estimate $\varphi_U(t)$ by $\hat{\varphi}_U(t) = \hat{\varphi}_{X^*}(t)/\varphi(t|\hat{p})$. In the continuous case, they deduce a density estimator of $f_X(x)$ by taking $\hat{f}_X(x) = (2\pi)^{-1} \int e^{-itx} \varphi(t|\hat{p}) \varphi_K(ht)/\tilde{\varphi}_U(t)\, dt$, where $\tilde{\varphi}_U$ is obtained from $\hat{\varphi}_U$ as at (12.14), $K$ is a kernel function, and $h$ is the plug-in bandwidth of Delaigle and Gijbels (2002, 2004), replacing there each occurrence of $\varphi_U$ by $\tilde{\varphi}_U$.

It is worth mentioning that typically, in practice, when minimising $T(p)$ most of the $\hat{p}_j$'s are equal to zero and a more recent suggestion is to take $m$ small and minimise over both the $x_j$'s and the $p_j$'s; see the R package `deconvolve` by Delaigle et al. (2021).

### 12.3.3 Related Literature

So far, we focused on the case where the only available model equation is the measurement error model. In some case, we also know that $X$ is the covariate of a regression model of the form $Y = g(X) + \epsilon$, where $X$, $\epsilon$ and $U$ are mutually independent, $E(\epsilon) = 0$, and we have an i.i.d. sample $(X_i^*, Y_i)$, $i = 1, \ldots, n$ with the same distribution as $(X^*, Y)$. In such cases, this regression model can be used in an attempt to identify and estimate $f_U$ (in addition to the other model components). This approach has been followed by Reiersøl (1950) in a seminal paper that assumes that $g$ is linear, and by Schennach and Hu (2013), who showed conditions under which this model is identified in a fully nonparametric setting. As it turns out, there are three mutually exclusive cases, and for each case Schennach and Hu (2013) established conditions under which the model components are identified. The result establishes when the knowledge of the joint distribution of the observable variables $Y$ and $X^*$ uniquely determines the unobservable quantities of interest, namely the function $g$ and the distributions of $X$, $U$ and $\epsilon$. We also refer to Schennach and Hu (2013) for related papers regarding identification in this type of models, and to the review paper by Schennach (2016) (Section 5) for papers that deal with partial identification in these models.

## 12.4 Boundary Estimation with Measurement Error

We now turn to the estimation of the endpoints of the support of $X$, when we observe $X^*$ at (12.1), where the distribution of $U$ is (partially) unknown and no additional data are available. We suppose that $X$ is not supported on the whole real line and our goal is to estimate the endpoints of its support. Without loss of generality, we suppose that it is the right endpoint $\tau$ of the support of $X$ that is finite. Our goal in this section is to estimate $\tau$. The case of a left endpoint is dealt with similarly. Note that most of the methods presented in the previous sections implicitly assumed that $f_X$ was either supported on the whole real line or vanished at the endpoints of its support. For example, it is well known that kernel density estimators are not consistent near the boundary of their domain unless they vanish at the boundary.

The problem of estimating the frontier or boundary of a variable has received a lot of attention in the literature, in particular in economics where the efficiency of a firm is often measured by the distance between the output (production) of the firm and the maximal possible output. This output variable is often measured with some noise, and often not much information is available about the distribution of this noise. In that example, $\tau$ above corresponds to the largest possible output.

If $X$ is assumed to be supported on a bounded interval, and if $U \sim N(0, \sigma_U^2)$ with unknown $\sigma_U^2$, then the method proposed by Bertrand et al. (2019) (see Section 12.3.1) can be applied since it provides estimators of each of $\sigma_U^2$,$f_X$ and the support $[b, a+b]$ of $X$.

If $X$ is not assumed to be supported on a compact interval, a number of other approaches exist in the literature. When the error $U$ has an unknown compact support $[-c, c]$ and is unimodal with unique mode at zero (and is otherwise unknown), Hall and Simar (2002) proposed to estimate $\tau$ by:

$$\hat{\tau} = \text{argmax}_{t \in \mathcal{J}} |\hat{f}'_{X^*}(t)|, \tag{12.27}$$

where $\mathcal{J}$ is an interval in the right tail of $X^*$ including $\tau$, and $\hat{f}'_{X^*}$ denotes the derivative of a standard kernel density estimator based on the data $X_1^*, \ldots, X_n^*$.

Note that in the error-free case, that is if $X^* = X$, this is a standard procedure for estimating an endpoint of the support of a distribution. In the error case, a natural approach that leads to a consistent estimator of $\tau$ consists in replacing $\hat{f}'_{X^*}$ at (12.27) by a deconvolution kernel density estimator of $f'_X$ (see Delaigle and Gijbels, 2006). However, Hall and Simar (2002) show that, under some conditions, the naive approach at (12.27) provides a consistent estimator of $\tau$ too (recall that in the error setting, a naive estimator is an estimator that applies to contaminated data, a technique that is consistent in the error-free case).

To understand why, they considered the toy example where the density $f_X$ is constant (say equal to $K > 0$) on some (small) interval $[a, \tau]$. Then, if $\tau > a + 2c$ (which is the case for small $c$), it can be easily seen that

$$f'_{X^*}(t) = \begin{cases} 0 & \text{if } a + c < t < \tau - c \\ -K f_U(t - \tau) & \text{if } \tau - c < t < \tau + c \\ 0 & \text{if } t > \tau + c. \end{cases}$$

Hence, the maximizer of $|f'_{X^*}(t)|$ for $t$ in the right tail equals the maximizer of $f_U(t - \tau)$, which is $\tau$ thanks to the unimodality of $f_U$. They showed that when the density $f_X$ is not flat to the left of $\tau$ but satisfies certain regularity conditions, and $\sigma_U$ (and hence $c$) is small, then $\text{argmax}_t |f'_{X^*}(t)| = \tau + O(\sigma_U^2)$. Exploiting the fact that $\sigma_U^2 = o(1)$, they proposed a refined estimator, obtained by adding a bias correction term to $\hat{\tau}$. The improved estimator has a bias term of order $O(\sigma_U^3)$ if $f_U$ has a symmetric density around zero.

Another approach was considered by Schwarz et al. (2012), under the assumption that the error $U \sim N(0, \sigma_U^2)$ with $\sigma_U^2$ unknown. Their work considered a general problem of frontier estimation, but here we discuss only the part of their technique that can be used to estimate the right endpoint $\tau$ of the distribution of $X$. To ensure that the model is identifiable, the authors followed Schwarz and Van Bellegem (2010) (see Section 12.3.1) and assumed that the probability distribution of $X$ vanishes on a set of positive measure. Without loss of generality, suppose that $\tau > 0$ (can be satisfied by pre-transforming the data to the positive real line).

Their approach for estimating $\tau$ is based on the observation that for any $A > \tau$, we have $\int_0^A \lim_{m\to\infty} \{F_X(x)\}^m \, dx = \int_0^A 1\{x \geq \tau\} \, dx = A - \tau$, which suggests that, for $m$ large enough, we can estimate $\tau$ by $A - \int_0^A \lim_{m\to\infty} \{\hat{F}_X(x)\}^m \, dx$, where $\hat{F}_X$ denotes a consistent estimator of $F_X$. To construct $\hat{F}_X$, the authors use a sieve estimator. Specifically, they approximate the distribution of $X$ by a discrete distribution with atoms $0 \leq \delta_1 \leq \ldots \leq \delta_{K_n}$ where $K_n \to \infty$ as $n \to \infty$; that is, they take $F_{X,\delta}(x) = K_n^{-1} \sum_{k=1}^{K_n} I(\delta_k \leq x)$. Let $\hat{F}_{X^*}(t) = n^{-1} \sum_{j=1}^{n} I(X_j^* \leq t)$ denote the empirical distribution function and $F_{\delta,\sigma_U} = F_{X,\delta} * \phi_{\sigma_U}$. To estimate the $\delta_k$'s and $\sigma_U^2$, they propose to minimise the following weighted $L_1$-distance:

$$\int_{\mathbb{R}} \left|F_{\delta,\sigma_U}(t) - \hat{F}_{X^*}(t)\right| w(t) \, dt \,,$$

under the constraint that the $\delta_k$'s and $\sigma_U$ are less than a constant $D_n$, which is such that $D_n \to \infty$ as $n \to \infty$. Finally they estimate $\tau$ by the order-$m_n$ frontier estimator, defined by

$$\hat{\tau} = A - \int_0^A \{F_{X,\hat{\delta}}(x)\}^{m_n} \, dx, \tag{12.28}$$

where $m_n \to \infty$ as $n \to \infty$, but they didn't propose a practical choice of $m_n$.

Next, we consider the method proposed by Kneip et al. (2015), which also assumes that $U \sim N(0, \sigma_U^2)$ with $\sigma_U^2$ unknown. Their approach relies on transforming the error model at (12.1) to the exponential scale by taking $\tilde{X}^* = \tilde{X} \cdot \tilde{U}$, where for a random variable $T$, $\tilde{T} = \exp(T)$. This has the advantage that the support of $\tilde{X}$ is compact since it is included in $[0, \tilde{\tau}]$, where $\tilde{\tau} = \exp(\tau)$ (by contrast, all we know of $X$ is that is its support is included in $(-\infty, \tau]$).

Then they estimate $\tilde{\tau}$ by maximum likelihood under this multiplicative model. To do this, for any $\check{\tau} > 0$, $\sigma > 0$ and density $h$ with support included in $[0, 1]$, let

$$f_{\check{\tau},\sigma,h}(t) = t^{-1} \int_0^1 \phi_\sigma \big[ \log\{t/(z\check{\tau})\} \big] h(z) \, dz \, . \tag{12.29}$$

We have $f_{\tilde{X}^*}(t) = \int_0^{\tilde{\tau}} f_{\tilde{U}}(t/x) f_{\tilde{X}}(x)/x \, dx$, where $f_{\tilde{U}}(u) = \phi_{\sigma_U}(\log u)/u$ with $\phi_{\sigma_U}$ the density of a $N(0, \sigma_U^2)$. By a change of variable, we deduce that $f_{\tilde{X}^*}(t) = f_{\tilde{\tau},\sigma_U,h^*}(t)$, with $h^*(z) = \tilde{\tau} f_{\tilde{X}}(z\tilde{\tau})$.

Since $h^*$, $\tilde{\tau}$ and $\sigma_U^2$ are unknown, to estimate $\tau$ by maximum likelihood, we need to maximise $\sum_{i=1}^n \log f_{\check{\tau},\sigma,h}(\tilde{X}_i^*)$ with respect to the parameters $\check{\tau} > 0$ and $\sigma > 0$, and the density $h$ whose support is included in $[0, 1]$. Since minimising over the set of such densities $h$ is not possible in practice, Kneip et al. (2015) approximate $h(z)$ by a histogram of the type

$$h_\gamma(z) = \gamma_1 I(z = 0) + \sum_{k=1}^{M_n} \gamma_k I(q_{k-1} < z \le q_k) \, ,$$

for $0 \le z \le 1$, where $q_k = k/M_n$, $M_n \to \infty$ and $n \to \infty$ and $\gamma = (\gamma_1, \ldots, \gamma_{M_n}) \in \Gamma_n$, defined by

$$\Gamma_n = \big\{ \gamma = (\gamma_1, \ldots, \gamma_{M_n}) : \gamma_k > 0 \text{ for all } k \text{ and } \sum_{k=1}^{M_n} \gamma_k = M_n \big\} \, .$$

Finally, estimators $\hat{\tilde{\tau}}$, $\hat{\sigma}_U$ and $\hat{h} = h_{\hat{\gamma}}$ are obtained by maximizing the following penalized likelihood :

$$(\hat{\tilde{\tau}}, \hat{\sigma}_U, \hat{\gamma}) = \text{argmax}_{\tilde{\tau}>0,\sigma_U>0,\gamma\in\Gamma_n} \Big\{ n^{-1} \sum_{i=1}^n \log f_{\tilde{\tau},\sigma_U,h_\gamma}(\tilde{X}_i^*) - \lambda \, \text{pen}(f_{\tilde{\tau},\sigma_U,h_\gamma}) \Big\},$$

where $\lambda \ge 0$ is a fixed constant independent of $n$, and $\text{pen}(f_{\tilde{\tau},\sigma_U,h_\gamma}) = \max_{3 \le j \le M_n} |\gamma_j - 2\gamma_{j-1} + \gamma_{j-2}|$ is a smoothness penalty.

Under regularity conditions, Kneip et al. (2015) showed that, as long as the density $f_{\tilde{X}}$ has a jump at the boundary $\tilde{\tau}$, the estimators $\hat{\tilde{\tau}}$ and $\hat{\sigma}_U$ are consistent and converge at a logarithmic rate. In practice they recommended using $M_n = \max\{3, 2\,[n^{1/5}]\}$, with $[a]$ the nearest integer to $a$; for $\lambda$ they selected the value of $\lambda$ by minimizing, over the grid $\log_{10} \lambda = -2, -1, 0, 1, 2$, a bootstrap estimator of the relative root mean squared error of $\hat{\tilde{\tau}}$.

Recently, Florens et al. (2020) proposed an estimator of $\tau$ that makes minimal assumptions on the error density $f_U$. For $X^*$ at (12.1), write $X^* = \tau - Z + U$, where $Z = \tau - X$ is an unobservable random variable independent of $U$, supported on $[0, \infty)$ and with density $f_Z$. Suppose that $f_U$ is symmetric around zero.

Their approach is based on the identifiability of the cumulants of $Z$. Denote the $\ell$-th cumulant of $Z$ and $X^*$ by $\kappa_Z(\ell)$ and $\kappa_{X^*}(\ell)$, respectively. Using standard properties of cumulants, it can be proved that

$$\kappa_{X^*}(1) = E(X^*) = \tau - \kappa_Z(1), \qquad \kappa_{X^*}(2p+1) = -\kappa_Z(2p+1), \quad p \geq 1,$$
$$\kappa_{X^*}(2p) = \kappa_Z(2p) + \kappa_U(2p) \quad \text{for } p \geq 1.$$

Thus, the odd cumulants of $Z$ of order 3 and higher are identifiable since they can be expressed in terms of the observable $X^*$. On the other hand, since the even cumulants of $f_U$ do not vanish in general, the even cumulants of $Z$ are not identifiable from the distribution of $X^*$. This shows that to make the distribution of $Z$ identifiable, we have to restrict $f_Z$ to a class of densities that are determined by the odd cumulants of order 3 and higher.

The above formulation can also be expressed through characteristic functions, as follows. For any random variable $V$, let $\eta_V(t) = \frac{\partial}{\partial t}\{\text{Im} \log \varphi_V(t)\}$, where Im denotes the imaginary part, and let

$$T_V(t) = \eta_V(t) - \eta_V(0) = \sum_{p=1}^{\infty} \frac{(-1)^p t^{2p}}{(2p)!} \kappa_V(2p+1) . \tag{12.30}$$

Then the class of densities $f_V$ that are determined by their odd cumulants of order 3 and higher is equivalent to the class of densities that are determined by $T_V(t)$ for all $t$. Thus, if $f_Z$ belongs to a class of densities $f_V$ that are determined by $T_V(t)$ for all $t$, it is identifiable from the distribution of $X^*$.

In practice Florens et al. (2020) suppose that $f_Z$ belongs to a flexible parametric family $\{f_Z(\cdot|\lambda) : \lambda \in \Lambda\}$, where $\Lambda$ is a compact subset of $\mathbb{R}^m$; thus, $f_Z(\cdot) = f_Z(\cdot|\lambda_0)$ for some $\lambda_0 \in \Lambda$. Let $T_\lambda(t) = \eta_V(t) - \eta_V(0)$, where $V \sim f_Z(\cdot|\lambda)$. The results above show that $\lambda$ (and hence $f_Z$) is identified if the parametric class is such that

$$T_\lambda \equiv T_{\lambda_0} \Longrightarrow \lambda = \lambda_0 . \tag{12.31}$$

Note in particular that we have $T_{\lambda_0} = -T_{X^*}$. Once $f_Z$ is identified, we can identify $\tau$ and $\sigma_U^2 = \text{var}(U)$ from the distribution of $X^*$ since

$$\tau = E(X^*) + E(Z) \quad \text{and} \quad \sigma_U^2 = \text{var}(X^*) - \text{var}(Z) . \tag{12.32}$$

For a parametric family satisfying (12.31), to estimate $\lambda$, Florens et al. (2020) minimise a penalised weighted $L_2$-distance

$$\hat{\lambda}_\alpha = \text{argmin}_{\lambda \in \Lambda} \Big\{ \int_{\mathbb{R}} \{\hat{T}_{X^*}(t) - T_\lambda(t)\}^2 w(t)\, dt + \alpha \|\lambda\|^2 \Big\},$$

where $\alpha > 0$ is a regularization parameter, $w$ is a weight function, $\|\lambda\|$ is the Euclidean norm of $\lambda$ and $\widehat{T}_{X^*}(t) = \hat{\eta}_{X^*}(t) - \hat{\eta}_{X^*}(0)$, with $\hat{\eta}_{X^*}(t) = \frac{\partial}{\partial t}\{\text{Im} \log \hat{\varphi}_{X^*}(t)\}$ and $\hat{\varphi}_{X^*}(t) = n^{-1}\sum_{j=1}^{n} \exp(itX_j^*)$. Then, using (12.32), they estimate $\tau$ and $\sigma_U^2$ by $\hat{\tau}_\alpha = \overline{X^*} + E_{\hat{\lambda}_\alpha}(Z)$ and $\hat{\sigma}_{U,\alpha}^2 = \hat{\sigma}_{X^*}^2 - \text{var}_{\hat{\lambda}_\alpha}(Z)$, where $\overline{X^*}$ and $\hat{\sigma}_{X^*}^2$ are the sample mean and variance of the $X_i^*$'s, and $E_{\hat{\lambda}_\alpha}(Z)$ and $\text{var}_{\hat{\lambda}_\alpha}(Z)$ are the mean and variance corresponding to the density $f_Z(z|\hat{\lambda}_\alpha)$.

In practice, Florens et al. (2020) suggest the following flexible parametric family $\{f_Z(z|\lambda) : \lambda \in \Lambda\}$:

$$f_Z(z|\lambda) = \frac{e^{-z}}{\|\lambda\|^2}\Big\{\sum_{k=0}^{m} \lambda_k v_k(z)\Big\}^2,$$

where $\lambda_0 = 1$, $\lambda = (\lambda_1, \ldots, \lambda_m) \in \mathbb{R}^m$, and $v_k$ are Laguerre polynomials, i.e. polynomials that are orthonormal with respect to the exponential density $e^{-z}$. It can be shown that as the number $m$ of parameters tends to infinity, the Hellinger distance (restricted to an interval $A$) between any continuous density $f_Z$ defined on $\mathbb{R}^+$ and its Laguerre approximation $f_Z(\cdot|\lambda)$ tends to zero. In practice Florens et al. (2020) recommended to choose the regularization parameters $\alpha$ and the number of polynomials $m$ by minimizing the bootstrap estimate of the root mean squared error of the estimator $\hat{\tau}_\alpha$.

## 12.5 Effect of Misspecifying the Error Distribution

Consistent estimation of the error density is not always possible and it is important to understand the effect that misspecifying the error distribution can have on the nonparametric deconvolution estimators of $f_X$ such as those introduced in the previous sections. Clearly, in standard asymptotic terms, where properties of an estimator are analyzed for $n \to \infty$, misspecifying the error distribution implies non consistency of deconvolution estimators.

Indeed, if we assume that the error density is, say, $f_\xi$ instead of the true $f_U$, then estimators such as the one at (12.3) will consistently estimate

$$(2\pi)^{-1} \int e^{-itx} \varphi_{X^*}(t)/\varphi_\xi(t)\, dt = (2\pi)^{-1} \int e^{-itx} \varphi_X(t)\varphi_U(t)/\varphi_\xi(t)\, dt,$$

which in general is different from $f_X$ if $\varphi_U \neq \varphi_\xi$. Further this integral is not even guaranteed to exist, nor to be equal to a density. In particular, if $\varphi_\xi(t)$ tends to zero faster than $\varphi_U(t)$ as $|t| \to \infty$, i.e. if we misspecify the error density in such a way that we assume it is smoother than it really is, then not only is the resulting estimator of $f_X$ not consistent, but it also does not converge to a well defined quantity. (Here, as usual in the deconvolution literature, we qualify the smoothness of a distribution through the speed of decay of its characteristic function in the tails, where a faster decay corresponds to a smoother distribution). A thorough theoretical study of this error misspecification problem has been studied in Meister (2004).

These considerations suggest that the consequences of assuming that the error distribution is smoother than it really is are so severe that, when in doubt, we should rather assume that the error density is not very smooth. In particular, recalling the distinction between ordinary smooth and supersmooth errors introduced in Delaigle (2021), we should preferably assume that the error is ordinary smooth with a low level of smoothness, rather than supersmooth. For example, in many cases we could assume that the errors have a Laplace distribution, since this distribution is ordinary smooth with $\beta = 2$ (and thus not very smooth).

Using a completely different approach, arguments in favor of a Laplace distribution were also provided by Delaigle (2008). There, the author suggested that, in measurement error problems, if it reasonable to derive asymptotic properties of estimators (in particular of the deconvolution kernel density estimator) taking $n \to \infty$ and $\sigma_U^2 = \text{var}(U) \to 0$. The rationale behind this approach is that, in the conventional error-free case, asymptotics where $n \to \infty$ usually describe properties of an estimator in situations where the sample becomes ideal (i.e. of increasingly better quality). In the context with errors, the quality of a sample does not depend only on its size, but also on the value of $\sigma_U^2$, and an ideal sample is a sample that has both a large sample size and a small error variance. This approach was also used by Fan (1992) in the supersmooth error case, by Hall and Simar (2002) in the context of boundary estimation, and by Staudenmayer and Ruppert (2004) to justify their SIMEX procedure. Delaigle (2008) shows that the deconvolution kernel estimator is relatively robust to error misspecification, as long as the error variance $\sigma_U^2$ is reasonably well estimated. Further, as in the standard asymptotic approach, the effect of error misspecification is more serious if we assume that the error distribution is smoother than it is, compared to assuming that the error distribution is less smooth than it is. In particular, in this context too, it is preferable to assume that the error is ordinary smooth, and assuming that the error is Laplace seems to guarantee relative robustness of the estimator.

This double asymptotic approach is useful to understand several issues that are encountered in practice, but which are not accessible via classical theory. For example, this work explains why, in practice, assuming Laplace errors often results in estimators that perform well, even if the error distribution is not Laplace. In particular it provides some theoretical underpinning to the low-order estimator of Carroll and Hall (2004), which can work really well in practice when $\sigma_U^2$ is not too large (the advantage of the low-order approach is that it only requires to estimate low-order moments of the error, whereas the deconvolution estimator requires knowledge of the entire error distribution). These double asymptotics also justify theoretically the fact that, when the error variance is not too large, the rate of convergence of the deconvolution kernel estimator with Gaussian errors can be much faster than logarithmic (it can be as fast as algebraic). Intuitively this is clear: if there is little noise in the data, then even if this noise is Gaussian, deconvolving should not be too difficult. However, the classical theory does not take into account the magnitude of the error variance. For example, even though, in finite samples, deconvolving Laplace errors with $\text{var}(U) = 2\text{var}(X)$ is much more difficult than deconvolving normal errors with $\text{var}(U) = 0.2\text{var}(X)$, the classical asymptotic theory only states that rates in the latter case are logarithmic, whereas rates in the former case are algebraic, thus considerably faster.

## Acknowledgments

Delaigle acknowledges support from the Australian Research Council (DP170102434); Van Keilegom acknowledges support from the European Research Council (2016-2021, Horizon 2020/ ERC grant agreement No. 694409).

## Bibliography

Apanasovich, T. and Liang, H. (2021). Nonparametric measurement errors models for regression. In *Handbook of Measurement Error Models*, G. Y. Yi, A. Delaigle, and P. Gustafson (Eds.), CRC, Chapter 14.

Bernstein, S. (1912). Démonstration du théorème de Weierstrass fondée sur le calcul des probabilités. *Communications de la Société mathématique de Kharkow*, 13, 1–2.

Bertrand, A., Van Keilegom, I. and Legrand, C. (2019). Flexible parametric approach to classical measurement error variance estimation without auxiliary data. *Biometrics*, 75(1), 297–307.

Butucea, C. and Matias, C. (2005). Minimax estimation of the noise level and of the signal density in a semiparametric convolution model. *Bernoulli*, 11, 309–340.

Butucea, C., Matias, C. and Pouet, C. (2008). Adaptivity in convolution models with partially known noise distribution. *Electronic Journal of Statistics*, 2, 897–915.

Carroll, R., Eltinge, J., and Ruppert, D. (1993). Robust linear regression in replicated measurement error models. *Statistics & probability letters*, 16(3), 169–175.

Carroll, R. and Hall, P. (1988). Optimal rates of convergence for deconvolving a density. *Journal of the American Statistical Association*, 83(404), 1184–1186.

Carroll, R. and Hall, P. (2004). Low order approximations in deconvolution and regression with errors in variables. *Journal of the Royal Statistical Society, Series B*, 66(1), 31–46.

Carroll, R., Ruppert, D., Stefanski, L., and Crainiceanu, C. (2006). *Measurement Error in Nonlinear Models: A Modern Perspective.* CRC Press.

Carroll, R. and Stefanski, L. (1990). Approximate quasi-likelihood estimation in models with surrogate predictors. *Journal of the American Statistical Association*, 85(411), 652–663.

Delaigle, A. (2008). An alternative view of the deconvolution problem. *Statistica Sinica*, 18, 1025–1045.

Delaigle, A. (2021). Deconvolution kernel density estimator. In *Handbook of Measurement Error Models*, G. Y. Yi, A. Delaigle, and P. Gustafson (Eds.), CRC, Chapter 10.

Delaigle, A. and Gijbels, I. (2002). Estimation of integrated squared density derivatives from a contaminated sample. *Journal of the Royal Statistical Society: Series B*, 64(4), 869–886.

Delaigle, A. and Gijbels, I. (2004). Practical bandwidth selection in deconvolution kernel density estimation. *Computational Statistics & Data Analysis*, 45(2), 249–267.

Delaigle, A. and Gijbels, I. (2006). Estimation of boundary and discontinuity points in deconvolution problems. *Statistica Sinica*, 773–788.

Delaigle, A. and Hall, P. (2008). Using SIMEX for smoothing-parameter choice in errors-in-variables problems. *Journal of the American Statistical Association*, 103(481), 280–287.

Delaigle, A. and Hall, P. (2016). Methodology for non-parametric deconvolution when the error distribution is unknown. *Journal of the Royal Statistical Society, Series B*, 78, 231–252.

Delaigle, A., Hall, P., and Meister, A. (2008). On deconvolution with repeated measurements. *The Annals of Statistics*, 36(2), 665–685.

Delaigle, A., Hall, P., and Müller, H. (2007). Accelerated convergence for nonparametric regression with coarsened predictors. *The Annals of Statistics*, 35(6), 2639–2653.

Delaigle, A., Hyndman, T. and Wang, T. (2021). deconvolve: Deconvolution tools for measurement error problems. R package version 0.1.0.

Delaigle, A. and Meister, A. (2007). Nonparametric regression estimation in the heteroscedastic errors-in-variables problem. *Journal of the American Statistical Association*, 102, 1416–1426.

Delaigle, A. and Meister, A. (2008). Density estimation with heteroscedastic error. *Bernoulli*, 14, 562–579.

Diggle, P. and Hall, P. (1993). A Fourier approach to nonparametric deconvolution of a density estimate. *Journal of the Royal statistical society: series B*, 55(2), 523–531.

Fan, J. (1992). Deconvolution with supersmooth distributions. *Canadian Journal of Statistics*, 20(2), 155–169.

Florens, J.-P., Simar, L. and Van Keilegom, I. (2020). Estimation of the boundary of a variable observed with symmetric error. *Journal of the American Statistical Association*, 115(529), 425–441.

Gleser, L. (1990). Improvements of the naive approach to estimation in nonlinear errors-in-variables regression models. *Contemp. Math*, 112, 99–114.

Hall, P. and Simar, L. (2002). Estimating a changepoint, boundary, or frontier in the presence of observation error. *Journal of the American Statistical Association*, 97, 523–534.

Horowitz, J. and Markatou, M. (1996). Semiparametric estimation of regression models for panel data. *The Review of Economic Studies*, 63(1), 145–168.

Kang, Y. and Qiu, P. (2021). Nonparametric deconvolution by Fourier transformation and other related approaches. In *Handbook of Measurement Error Models*, G. Y. Yi, A. Delaigle, and P. Gustafson (Eds.), CRC, Chapter 11.

Kneip, L., Simar, L. and Van Keilegom, I. (2015). Frontier estimation in the presence of measurement error with unknown variance. *Journal of Econometrics*, 184, 379–393.

Li, T. and Vuong, Q. (1998). Semiparametric deconvolution with unknown noise variance. *Journal of Multivariate Analysis*, 65, 139–165.

Madansky, A. (1959). The fitting of straight lines when both variables are subject to error. *Journal of the American Statistical Association*, 54, 173–205.

Matias, C. (2002). Semiparametric deconvolution with unknown noise variance. *ESAIM, Probability and Statistics*, 6, 271–292.

McIntyre, J. and Stefanski, L. (2011). Density estimation with replicate heteroscedastic measurements. *Annals of the Institute of Statistical Mathematics*, 63(1), 81–99.

Meister, A. (2004). On the effect of misspecifying the error density in a deconvolution problem. *Canadian Journal of Statistics*, 32(4), 439–449.

Meister, A. (2006). Density estimation with normal measurement error with unknown variance. *Statistica Sinica*, 16, 195–211.

Meister, A. (2007). Deconvolving compactly supported densities. *Mathematical Methods of Statistics*, 16, 63–76.

Meister, A. and Neumann, M. H. (2010). Deconvolution from non-standard error densities under replicated measurements. *Statistica Sinica*, 1609–1636.

Neumann, M. (1997). On the effect of estimating the error density in nonparametric deconvolution. *Journal of Nonparametric Statistics*, 7, 307–330.

Neumann, M. H. (2007). Deconvolution from panel data with unknown error distribution. *Journal of Multivariate Analysis*, 98(10), 1955–1968.

Parthasarathy, K., Rao, R. and Varadhan, S. (1962). On the category of indecomposable distributions on topological groups. *Transactions of the American Mathematical Society*, 102, 200–217.

Reiersøl, O. (1950). Identifiability of a linear relation between variables which are subject to error. *Econometrika*, 18, 375–389.

Schennach, S. M. (2004). Nonparametric regression in the presence of measurement error. *Econometric Theory*, 20(6), 1046–1093.

Schennach, S. M. (2016). Recent advances in the measurement error literature. *Annual Review of Economics*, 8, 341–377.

Schennach, S. M. and Hu, Y. (2013). Nonparametric identification and semiparametric estimation of classical measurement error models without side information. *Journal of the American Statistical Association*, 108, 177–186.

Schwarz, M. and Van Bellegem, S. (2010). Consistent density deconvolution under partially known error distribution. *Statistics and Probability Letters*, 80, 236–241.

Schwarz, M., Van Bellegem, S., and Florens, J.-P. (2012). Nonparametric frontier estimation from noisy data. In *Exploring research frontiers in contemporary statistics and econometrics* - Festschrift in Honor of L. Simar, Van Keilegom, I. and Wilson, P.W. (eds.), 45–64. Springer.

Staudenmayer, J. and Ruppert, D. (2004). Local polynomial regression and simulation-extrapolation. *Journal of the Royal Statistical Society, Series B*, 66, 17–30.

Stefanski, L. and Carroll, R. (1990). Deconvolving kernel density estimators. *Statistics*, 21(2), 169–184.

Wang, L. (2021). Identifiability in measurement error models. In *Handbook of Measurement Error Models*, G. Y. Yi, A. Delaigle, and P. Gustafson (Eds.), CRC, Chapter 5.

# 13

# *Nonparametric Inference Methods for Berkson Errors*

**Weixing Song**

## CONTENTS



Due to the nature of error structures, statistical inference related to Berkson measurement error have not received much attention from statisticians and practitioners. The reasons are mixed, the main reason may be that, from a theoretically point of view, dealing with Berkson measurement error in parametric models may not be as challenging as in classical measurement error setups. For example, in linear regression models, unlike the classical error case, the naive estimation procedures do provide a consistent estimator for the regression coefficient. Although this pleasant phenomenon is not shared in nonlinear regression models, the bias can be easily corrected by regressing the response variable on the noisy variables, which has a tractable form if the distribution of the measurement error is known, a common assumption in measurement error modeling literature.

DOI: 10.1201/9781315101279-13

The necessity of calling more attention to the statistical inference related to Berkson measurement errors comes from the interesting fact that, compared to parametric inference, nonparametric inference related to Berkson measurement errors appears much more difficult. Although many inference procedures have already been developed for estimating the density and regression functions, there are still many theoretical voids waiting to be filled out.

This chapter will briefly introduce some nonparametric techniques for estimating density and the regression functions when only Berkson errors are present in the model. Hopefully it can help graduate students and researchers to gain some familiarity with these interesting topics and develop more advanced statistical inference tools for more complicated models related to Berkson measurement errors.

## 13.1 Introduction

To facilitate our discussion, assume that $X$, possibly multidimensional, is the random variable of interest. Due to some uncontrollable reasons, $X$ cannot be directly measured. Instead, a proxy variable $X^*$ is observed. In the classical measurement error modeling, it is often assumed that

$$X^* = X + U, \tag{13.1}$$

while in the Berkson measurement error modeling, we assume thtat

$$X = X^* + U. \tag{13.2}$$

In both structures (13.1) and (13.2), the random variable $U$ is the measurement error. What separates these two structures is not the displacement of $X$ and $X^*$, but the stochastic relationships among these variables. In the classical measurement error model (13.1), $X$ and $U$ are independent, but in the Berkson measurement error model (13.2), $X^*$ and $U$ are independent. It is commonly believed that the first research on Berkson measurement errors was done by Berkson (1950) in the regression context. The Berkson measurement error structure is widely practiced in designed experiments in which there are some target values that an experimenter wants to apply to experimental units, but the actual delivered values may differ from the target values. For example, a nominal amount of nitrogen ($X^*$) is applied to a crop, but the actual amount of nitrogen ($X$) absorbed by the crop could be different from the nominal one and is difficult to measure. In this scenario, the relationship between the actual amount of nitrogen and the nominal one is better explained by a Berkson measurement error structure. Many other examples of real data applications with Berkson measurement errors can be found in many areas including agriculture experiments, bioassay studies, and epidemiology, among others, as described in the monograph Carroll et al. (2006), journal papers, Carroll et al. (2007), Delaigle (2007), and Long et al. (2016), and the references therein.

Compared to the research done on classical measurement error, relatively little interest has been shown on research involving Berkson measurement errors. One reason why the Berkson measurement error is less popular among statisticians is the ease of dealing with the parametric model. It is well known that in the linear regression model where instead of observing the covariate $X$, we observe $X^*$ in (13.2), the naive estimator, that is, simply replacing $X$ with $X^*$ in the least squares estimation procedure, is still consistent. In nonlinear regression models $Y = g(X;\theta) + \varepsilon$, for $X^*$ in (13.2),

$$E(Y|X^*) = \int g(X^* + u;\theta) f_U(u)du$$

often possesses a known and tractable parametric form, and the least squares estimation procedure based on data $(X_1^*, Y_1), \ldots, (X_n^*, Y_n)$ from $(X^*, Y)$,

$$\hat{\theta}_n = \operatorname*{argmin}_{\theta} \sum_{j=1}^{n} \left\{ Y_j - \int g(Z_j + u;\theta) f_U(u)du \right\}^2$$

generally provides a consistent estimator for $\theta$. Here the integral is understood as a $p$-fold integral, and $p$ is the dimension of $X$. Similar ideas based on methods-of-moments have been used in Huwang and Huang (2000) and Wang (2003, 2004, 2007) for estimation in polynomial, general nonlinear and mixed Berkson measurement error models.

Recent years have seen increased interest in developing nonparametric inference procedures related to Berkson measurement errors. Compared to classical measurement error, nonparametric inference with Berkson measurement errors faces many unique challenges, and some seemingly simple questions present nontrivial challenges. In this chapter, we will focus on modeling the relationship between a scalar response variable $Y$ and a scalar covariate $X$ which is contaminated with Berkson measurement error. In particular, we will try to fit the following regression model

$$Y = g(X) + \varepsilon, \quad X = X^* + U \tag{13.3}$$

based on an i.i.d. sample $\{(Y_i, X_i^*)\}_{i=1}^n$ from (13.3). To ensure the identifiability of $g$, we will assume that the density function $f_U$ of $U$ is known.

As an application of model (13.3), Delaigle et al. (2006) considers data collected from a survey conducted by the US Department of Agriculture. To estimate areas growing specific crops, three methods are discussed: aerial photography, satellite imagery and personal statements of the farmers. The goal is to detect the link between the data gained by aerial photography and by satellite imagery. However, when aerial photography data $X$ are not available, the data from personal interviews are considered as the proxy $X^*$, with the satellite imagery data used as the response variable $Y$. The unobserved random variables $X = X^* + U$ represent the aerial photography data. Carroll et al. (2007) discusses a data set from a Nevada test side thyroid disease study. The goal of the study is to investigate the link between radiation exposure and thyroid disease outcomes. The predictor data $X^*$ denote the observed log radiation exposure, which represent only a part of the true log radiation exposure $X$ of an individual. $X$ is unobserved and may be interpreted as $X^* + U$. The response variable $Y$ is the absence or presence of thyroid disease, coded as 0 and 1, respectively.

In this chapter, we will discuss two topics: the estimation of the density function of $X$ and of the regression function $g$ in model (13.3). These topics are the most classical research areas in nonparametric statistics, and have been fully developed for error-free cases and for the classical measurement error setup. In classical measurement error cases, the deconvolution technique can be viewed as one of the most representative achievements in nonparametric smoothing.

For the sake of brevity, we will assume throughout the observed variable $X$ to be one dimensional.

## 13.2 Density Estimation

In classical measurement error, estimating the distribution of $X$ is a very important research topic, and the deconvolution kernel estimation procedure provides a viable way to estimate the density function of $X$. Kang and Qiu (2021) in Chapter 11 has explored some alternative methods to estimate the density function of $X$ other than the Fourier transformation. In the context of Berkson measurement error, Delaigle (2007) is the first paper to investigate the density estimation problem. Note that Delaigle (2007) studies a more comprehensive setting including both Berkson and classical errors. Later, Long et al. (2016) discusses the bandwidth selection issues in kernel based estimation procedures. The main results in this section are adapted from Delaigle (2007) and Long et al. (2016).

Clearly, if the density function of $U$ is unknown, then the density function of $X$ will be unidentifiable. Hereafter, we shall assume that the density function of $U$ is known.

Assume a random sample, $X_1^*, X_2^*, \ldots, X_n^*$, of size $n$, obeys the Berkson model (13.2). In the following discussion, for a generic random variable $X$, $f_X$ and $\varphi_X$ will be used to denote its density function and characteristic function, respectively.

### 13.2.1 A Simple $\sqrt{n}$-Consistent Estimator

The relationship $X = X^* + U$ and the independence between $X^*$ and $U$ implies that $f_X$ is the convolution of $f_{X^*}$ and $U$. That is

$$f_X(x) = f_{X^*} * f_U(x) = \int f_U(x - x^*) f_{X^*}(x^*) dx^*,$$

which immediately leads to the following simple estimator of $f_X$ given in Delaigle (2007),

$$\hat{f}_X(x) = \frac{1}{n} \sum_{i=1}^{n} f_U(x - X_i^*). \tag{13.4}$$

If $f_U$ is square integrable and $f_{X^*}$ is bounded, then $\hat{f}_X(x)$ is unbiased with a MISE that converges to 0 at rate $n^{-1}$.

The estimator proposed in (13.4) is very simple to calculate and does not need any specification of smoothing parameters, unlike the standard kernel density estimator in the error-free case or the deconvolution kernel estimator in the classical measurement error case. However, as noted by Long et al. (2016), a disadvantage of (13.4) is that in cases where $U$ is concentrated around 0, the estimator will have large spikes at the sample points $X_i^*$ and thus have high variance.

### 13.2.2 Kernel Based Estimator

From $X = X^* + U$ and the independence of $X^*$ and $U$, we have

$$\varphi_X(t) = \varphi_{X^*}(t) \varphi_U(t). \tag{13.5}$$

Let $K$ be a univariate unimodal density function, and $h = h_n$ be a sequence of positive real numbers. Using the classical kernel density estimator of $X^*$, the characteristic function of $X^*$ can be smoothly estimated by

$$\hat{\varphi}_{X^*}(t) = \int e^{itx^*} \frac{1}{nh} \sum_{j=1}^{n} K\left\{h^{-1}(x^* - X_j^*)\right\} dx^* = \tilde{\varphi}_{X^*}(t) \int e^{ithx^*} K(x^*) \, dx^*,$$

where $\tilde{\varphi}_{X^*}(t) = n^{-1} \sum_{j=1}^{n} \exp(itX_j^*)$ is the empirical characteristic function of $X^*$. Then $\hat{\varphi}_{X^*}(t) = \tilde{\varphi}_{X^*}(t) \varphi_K(ht)$. Hence, using (13.5), $\varphi_X(t)$ can be estimated by

$$\hat{\varphi}_X(t) = \tilde{\varphi}_{X^*}(t) \varphi_K(ht) \varphi_U(t).$$

Let $L_1$ be the class of absolutely integrable functions with respect to Lebesgue measure. Assuming that $\varphi_U \in L_1$, which implies that $\hat{\varphi}_X(t) \in L_1$, then by Fourier inversion, an estimator of $f_X(x)$ can be defined as

$$\hat{f}_{X,h}(x) = \frac{1}{2\pi} \int e^{-itx} \hat{\varphi}_X(t) dt = \frac{1}{2\pi} \int e^{-itx} \tilde{\varphi}_{X^*}(t) \varphi_K(ht) \varphi_U(t) dt. \tag{13.6}$$

In fact, the estimator defined in (13.6) has another more tractable form. To see this, substituting the empirical characteristic function $\tilde{\varphi}_{X^*}(t)$ into the definition of $\hat{f}_{X,h}(x)$, we have

$$\begin{aligned} \hat{f}_{X,h}(x) &= \frac{1}{2\pi}\int e^{-itx}\frac{1}{n}\sum_{j=1}^{n}\exp(itX_j^*)\varphi_K(ht)\varphi_U(t)dt \\ &= \frac{1}{n}\sum_{j=1}^{n}\frac{1}{2\pi}\int e^{-it(x-X_j^*)}\varphi_K(ht)\varphi_U(t)dt. \end{aligned}$$

Note that $\varphi_K(ht) = \int e^{ihtx}K(x)dx = \int e^{itx}K_h(x)dx$, where $K_h(x) = h^{-1}K(x/h)$, thus $\varphi_K(ht)\varphi_U(t) = \varphi_{K_h}(t)\varphi_U(t) = \varphi_{K_h * f_U}(t)$. Since for two functions $f$ and $g$, the Fourier transform of the convolution $f * g(x) = \int f(x-u)g(u)du$ is $\varphi_{f*g} = \varphi_f\varphi_g$, we deduce that

$$\hat{f}_{X,h}(x) = \frac{1}{n}\sum_{j=1}^{n}\int K_h(x-u-X_j^*)f_U(u)du = \int \hat{f}_{X^*,h}(x-u)f_U(u)du, \quad (13.7)$$

where $\hat{f}_{X^*,h}(x^*)$ is simply the standard kernel density estimator of $f_{X^*}(x^*)$. In fact, the above estimator can be directly obtained by replacing $f_{X^*}(x^*)$ with its kernel density estimator in the convolution relationship $f_X(x) = \int f_{X^*}(x-u)f_U(u)du$.

In particular, letting $h = 0$ allows us to recover the kernel-free estimator (13.4) defined in Delaigle (2007).

### 13.2.3 Mean Integrated Squared Error

The following theorem summarizes the mean integrated squared error (MISE) for the estimator $\hat{f}_{X,h}(x)$ defined in (13.6).

**Theorem 13.1 (Long et al., 2016)** *Assume* $\varphi_X(t), \hat{\varphi}_{X^*}(t) \in L_1$. *Then*

$$\text{MISE}(h) = \frac{1}{2\pi}\int |1-\varphi_K(ht)|^2 d\mu(t) + \frac{1}{2\pi n}\int |\varphi_K(ht)|^2 dv(t), \quad (13.8)$$

*where*

$$d\mu(t) = |\varphi_U(t)\varphi_{X^*}(t)|^2 dt, \quad dv(t) = |\varphi_U(t)|^2\{1-|\varphi_{X^*}(t)|^2\}dt.$$

Requiring $\varphi_X$ and $\hat{\varphi}_X$ to be $L_1$ integrable guarantees that the estimator $\hat{f}_X(x)$ is a bounded density. The condition $\hat{\varphi}_X$ can be replaced by assuming that $\varphi_U \in L_1$. The proof of Theorem 13.1 can be found in Long et al. (2016).

The first term on the right hand side of (13.8) is the integrated squared bias and the second term is the integrated variance. Applying the Parseval identity, equation (13.8) can be written as:

$$\begin{aligned}\text{MISE}(h) &= \frac{1}{2\pi}\int |1-\varphi_K(ht)|^2 d\mu(t) + \frac{1}{2\pi n}\int |\varphi_K(ht)|^2 dv(t) \\ &= \frac{1}{2\pi nh}\int \varphi_K^2(t)|\varphi_U(t/h)|^2 dt + (1-n^{-1})\int \{K_h * f_X(x)\}^2 dx \\ &\quad + \int f_X^2(x)dx - 2\int \{K_h * f_X(x)\} f_X(x)dx,\end{aligned}$$

which coincides with the result of Theorem 2 in Delaigle (2007) when only Berkson measurement errors are present. In particular, letting $h = 0$ gives

$$\begin{aligned}\text{MISE}(0) &= \frac{1}{2\pi n}\int |\varphi_U(t)|^2[1-|\varphi_Z(t)|^2]dt \\ &= \frac{1}{n}\int f_U^2(u)du - \frac{1}{n}\int f_X^2(x)dx \qquad (13.9)\end{aligned}$$

which is the MISE of the estimator (13.4), and corresponds to the result of Theorem 1 in Delaigle (2007) when only Berkson measurement errors are present. Note that the right hand side of (13.9) is positive by the Cauchy-Schwarz inequality.

It is well known that the bandwidth plays a crucial role in kernel density estimation. Smaller bandwidths generally introduce more variability and larger bandwidths lead to more bias. Therefore, any bandwidth selection procedure tries to balance the bias and variance.

Define $\sigma_K^2 = \int x^2 K(x)dx$. Then based on Theorem 13.1, we have the following corollary.

**Corollary 13.1** (Long et al., 2016) *Assume that*

- *$K$ is a symmetric density, four times differentiable;*
- $\int t^8|\varphi_U(t)|^8 dt < \infty$, $\int |\varphi_U(t)|dt < \infty$.

*Then* MISE$(h)$ *has the following expansion*

$$\begin{aligned}&\text{MISE}(h) \qquad (13.10)\\ &= \frac{1}{2\pi n}\int dv(t) + \frac{1}{2\pi}\left\{\frac{h^4\sigma_K^4}{4}\int t^4 d\mu(t) - \frac{h^2\sigma_K^2}{n}\int t^2 dv(t)\right\}\{1+O(h^2)\}.\end{aligned}$$

The first term of the right hand side of (13.10) is free of $h$. Therefore, a theoretical optimal bandwidth $h$ is the one that minimizes the leading term in the second term of the right hand side of (13.10), or

$$\operatorname*{argmin}_h \left\{\frac{h^4\sigma_K^4}{4}\int t^4 d\mu(t) - \frac{h^2\sigma_K^2}{n}\int t^2 dv(t)\right\} = \sqrt{\frac{2\int t^2 dv(t)}{n\sigma_K^2 \int t^4 d\mu(t)}}.$$

Denote the right hand side of the above expression as $h_{\text{opt}}$. Accordingly, the MISE at $h_{\text{opt}}$ is

$$\text{MISE}(h_{\text{opt}}) = \frac{1}{2\pi n}\int dv(t) - \frac{1}{n^2}\frac{\left\{\int t^2 dv(t)\right\}^2}{\int t^4 d\mu(t)} + O\left(\frac{1}{n^3}\right).$$

This asymptotically optimal bandwidth depends on unknown quantities such as the characteristic function $\varphi_X$. Long et al. (2016) provide a rule-of-thumb bandwidth selector by choosing $\sigma_K^2 = 1$ and pretending $f_{X^*}$ to be normal with variance $\sigma_{X^*}^2$ which is estimated by the sample variance $\hat{\sigma}_{X^*}^2$. Thus one can use the following simple practical bandwidth to implement the kernel density estimation procedure

$$\hat{h}_{\text{opt}} = \sqrt{\frac{2\int t^2|\varphi_U(t)|^2(1 - e^{-\hat{\sigma}_{X^*}^2 t^2})dt}{n\int t^4 e^{-\hat{\sigma}_{X^*}^2 t^2}|\varphi_U(t)|^2 dt}}.$$

However, in general, this bandwidth is too large and the resulting estimator tends to oversmooth the data.

Based on the relationship between the kernel estimators $\hat{f}_X$ and $\hat{f}_{X^*}$, Long et al. (2016) also discusses the possibility of using the asymptotically optimal bandwidth for $\hat{f}_{X^*}$ to smooth $\hat{f}_X$, however, this strategy is not recommended since it leads to suboptimal rate of MISE convergence.

## 13.3 Regression with Berkson Measurement Error

In some medical and agricultural studies, the proxy variable $X^*$ in the Berkson measurement error model is treated as a fixed quantity. For example, to study how the yield of a certain crop is affected by a fertilizer, the dial on the fertilizing device is set at various pre-specified levels $X^*$, but the actual amount absorbed by the crop $X$ depends on many random factors such as soil types, wind directions and precipitation among other things. This is the reason why $X^*$ sometimes is also called a "controlled" variable, see Section 13.6 in Cheng and John (1999) for more explanation. However, theoretical research on this subject often treats $X^*$ as a random variable. Indeed, the methodology and theoretical results developed for the random cases continue to hold for some fixed cases where the values of $X^*$ are chosen from an equally spaced design, resulting in estimators with properties that are similar to those for random designs with uniform distributions. Also, there are many applications where $X^*$ should be viewed as random variables. See Delaigle et al. (2006) for more discussion on this issue. In this section, we assume that $X^*$ is random. The discussion on nonparametric regression in the classical measurement error setup can be found in Apanasovich and Liang (2021).

In the measurement error-free cases, a commonly used nonparametric estimator of the regression function $E(Y|X = x)$ is the so-called Nadaraya-Watson estimator, which takes the form of

$$\hat{E}(Y|X = x) = \frac{\sum_{j=1}^{n} K_h(x - X_j)Y_j}{\sum_{j=1}^{n} K_h(x - X_j)},$$

where $(Y_j, X_j)$, $j = 1, 2, \ldots, n$ is an i.i.d. sample from the population $(Y, X)$, $K_h(x) = h^{-1}K(x/h)$ with $K$ being a kernel density function and $h$ is a bandwidth. The readers are referred to Wand and Jones (1995) for more introduction on the kernel smoothing techniques. Note that $n^{-1}\sum_{j=1}^{n} K_h(x-X_j)$ is an estimator of the density function of $X$. Since we have developed some density estimators of $X$ in Section 13.2, it might be tempting to try the Nadaraya-Watson protocol. For example, using the estimator (13.4), we may think

$$\tilde{g}_n(x) = \frac{\sum_{j=1}^{n} f_U(x - X_j^*)Y_j}{\sum_{j=1}^{n} f_U(x - X_j^*)}$$

is a natural estimator of $g(x)$. However, Koul and Song (2009) and Delaigle (2014) have shown that as $n \to \infty$, $\tilde{g}_n(x)$ converges to $E\{E(g(X)|X^*)|X = x\}$ in probability. That is, $\tilde{g}_n$ is not a consistent estimator of $g$.

In fact, constructing a nonparametric estimator for $g$ in model (13.3) is far more complicated. Delaigle et al. (2006) points out that under the assumptions that $E|\varepsilon| < \infty$, $E\varepsilon = 0$, and $g$ is bounded and continuous, only quantities which can be expressed as functionals of $\gamma(x^*) = Eg(x^* + U)$ can be consistently estimated using nonparametric methods. This implies that $g$ can be consistently estimated if and only if $g$ is uniquely determined by knowing $\gamma(x^*)$ for all $x^*$ in the support of the distribution of $X^*$. Indeed, noting that $\gamma(x^*) = E(Y|X^* = x^*)$, a consistent estimator of $\gamma(x^*)$ can be easily constructed by applying some nonparametric smoothing technique on a sample from $(X^*, Y)$, such as a kernel estimator, which implies that if $g$ is a functional of $\gamma$, then a consistent estimator of $g$ can be obtained by simply plugging the consistent estimator of $\gamma$ in the functional.

### 13.3.1 Methods Based on Trigonometric Functions

In this section, we will introduce the discrete transform method developed in Delaigle et al. (2006). Their approach is more appealing for the Berkson measurement error model, since it is relatively unaffected by the difficulties that are caused by distributions of $U$ for which the characteristic function has infinitely many 0's, which pose a big challenge when applying the deconvolution kernel method. Kang and Qiu (2021) applied the same approach in the classical measurement error cases.

For model (13.3), we assume that $\varepsilon$ satisfies $E|\varepsilon| < \infty$, $E\varepsilon = 0$ and $g$ is bounded and continuous. Both $g$ and $f_U$ are compactly supported, and, without loss of generality, both support intervals are rescaled to be contained in $\mathcal{I} = [-\pi, \pi]$.

On $\mathcal{I}$, $g$ has a trigonometric expansion

$$g(x) = g_0 + \sum_{j=1}^{\infty} \{g_{1j} \cos(jx) + g_{2j} \sin(jx)\},$$

where $g_0 = (2\pi)^{-1} \int_{\mathcal{I}} g(x)dx$,

$$g_{1j} = \pi^{-1} \int_{\mathcal{I}} g(x) \cos(jx)dx, \quad g_{2j} = \pi^{-1} \int_{\mathcal{I}} g(x) \sin(jx)dx.$$

Then accordingly, $\gamma(x^*) = Eg(x^* + U)$ has the following trigonometric expansion,

$$\gamma(x^*) = g_0 + \sum_{j=1}^{\infty} \{\gamma_{1j} \cos(jx^*) + \gamma_{2j} \sin(jx^*)\},$$

where

$$\begin{aligned} \gamma_{1j} &= \pi^{-1} \int_{\mathcal{I}} \gamma(x^*) \cos(jx^*)dx^* = g_{1j}\alpha_{1j} + g_{2j}\alpha_{2j}, \\ \gamma_{2j} &= \pi^{-1} \int_{\mathcal{I}} \gamma(x^*) \sin(jx^*)dx^* = -g_{1j}\alpha_{2j} + g_{2j}\alpha_{1j}, \end{aligned}$$

$\alpha_{1j} = E\cos(jU)$, and $\alpha_{2j} = E\sin(jU)$. So, provided $|\alpha_{1j}| + |\alpha_{2j}| \neq 0$ for $j \geq 1$,

$$\begin{pmatrix} g_{1j} \\ g_{2j} \end{pmatrix} = \frac{1}{\alpha_{1j}^2 + \alpha_{2j}^2} \begin{pmatrix} \alpha_{1j} & -\alpha_{2j} \\ \alpha_{2j} & \alpha_{1j} \end{pmatrix} \begin{pmatrix} \gamma_{1j} \\ \gamma_{2j} \end{pmatrix}. \tag{13.11}$$

Note that $E(Y|X^* = x^*) = \gamma(x^*)$. Based on data $\{(X_j^*, Y_j)\}_{j=1}^n$, we can estimate $\gamma$ consistently using popular nonparametric smoothing techniques, such as a local linear smoother as discussed in Fan and Gijbels (1996). Then the coefficients $\gamma_{kj}$ can be estimated by

$$\hat{\gamma}_{kj} = \pi^{-1} \int_{\mathcal{J}} \hat{\gamma}(x^*) \mathrm{cs}_{kj}(x^*)dx^*,$$

where $\mathcal{J} \subseteq \mathcal{I}$ contains the support of $\gamma$, and $\mathrm{cs}_{kj}(x^*)$ denotes $\cos(jx^*)$ or $\sin(jx^*)$ according to $k = 1$ or 2.

Since $(2\pi)^{-1} \int_{\mathcal{I}} g(x^*)dx^* = (2\pi)^{-1} \int_{\mathcal{I}} \gamma(x^*)dx^*$, $g_0$ can be estimated by

$$\hat{g}_0 = (2\pi)^{-1} \int_{\mathcal{J}} \hat{\gamma}(x^*)dx^*,$$

and based on (13.11), the coefficients $g_{kj}$ can be estimated by

$$\begin{pmatrix} \hat{g}_{1j} \\ \hat{g}_{2j} \end{pmatrix} = \frac{1}{\alpha_{1j}^2 + \alpha_{2j}^2} \begin{pmatrix} \alpha_{1j} & -\alpha_{2j} \\ \alpha_{2j} & \alpha_{1j} \end{pmatrix} \begin{pmatrix} \hat{\gamma}_{1j} \\ \hat{\gamma}_{2j} \end{pmatrix}.$$

Thus the resulting estimator of $g$ can be defined as

$$\hat{g}(x) = \hat{g}_0 + \sum_{j=1}^{m}\{\hat{g}_{1j}\cos(jx) + \hat{g}_{2j}\sin(jx)\}, \tag{13.12}$$

where the threshold value $m$ denotes the number of Fourier frequencies that are included in the estimator. Delaigle (2007, p.209) proposes a modified cross validation criterion to choose $m$ in practice which will be shown later. Also in Delaigle et al. (2006), the local linear smoother is used to estimate $\gamma(x^*)$. To prevent aberrant behavior by the local linear smoother $\hat{\gamma}(x^*)$, some modifications are made on $\hat{\gamma}(x^*)$ in their theoretical study: set $\hat{\gamma}(x^*)$ to 0 if it is not well defined, or its absolute value exceeds $B_1 n^{B_2}$, or $|x^*|$ lies outside a compact interval that is known to contain the support of $\gamma$. Here $B_1$ and $B_2$ are some fixed positive constants.

To state the theoretical properties of the proposed estimator defined in (13.12), the following technical conditions are assumed.

(D1). The supports of $f_Z$ and $f_U$ are contained within $\mathcal{I}$, and $f_Z$ is bounded away from zero on an interval $\mathcal{J}$.

(D2). $f_U$ is symmetric, in which case each $\alpha_{2j} = 0$, and each $\alpha_{1j}$ does not vanish, being bounded above and below by strictly positive constant multiples of $j^{-a}$, $a > 0$.

(D3). $f_\varepsilon$ has finite variance and zero mean.

(D4). $h$ is chosen to be $B_3 n^{-B_4} \le h \le B_5 n^{-1/4}$, where $B_3, B_5 > 0$ and $1/4 < B_4 < 1$.

Also, given $b > 2, B > 0$, we define the following family of functions

$$\mathcal{C}_{\text{regr}}(b) = \{g : \text{Supp}(\gamma) \subseteq \mathcal{J}, g_0, g_{kj} \text{ are such that } |g_0| \le B, |g_{kj}| \le Bj^{-b}\}.$$

The following theorem provides the uniform convergence rate for the MISE of the proposed estimator (13.12) and also a theoretical optimal bound of the convergence rate when the regression error $\varepsilon$ has a normal distribution.

**Theorem 13.2** (Delaigle, 2007) *Suppose the conditions (D1)-(D4) hold. Then*

$$\sup_{g\in\mathcal{C}_{\text{regr}}(b)} \left\{\int_{\mathcal{I}} E_g(\hat{g} - g)^2\right\} = O(n^{-(2b-1)/\{2(a+b)\}}).$$

*Further, if we assume that $\varepsilon$ is normal, then*

$$\liminf_{n\to\infty} n^{(2b-1)/\{2(a+b)\}} \inf_{g_n} \sup_{g\in\mathcal{C}_{\text{regr}}(b)} \left\{\int_{\mathcal{I}} E_g(g_n - g)^2\right\} > 0,$$

*where $g_n$ denotes any arbitrary nonparametric estimators of $g$.*

From Theorem 13.2, we can see that when $g \in \mathcal{C}_{\text{regr}}(b)$, no nonparametric estimator can achieve a faster convergence rate than $n^{-(2b-1)/\{2(a+b)\}}$ in the mean square sense, and the proposed estimator (13.12) attains this optimal convergence rate.

According to Delaigle (2006), if the $X_i^*$'s are obtained by placing $k \geq 2$ replicates at each of $v$ points that are equally spaced within $\mathcal{I}$, with $n = kv$, then the conclusion in Theorem 13.2 still holds after some minor modifications. Provided that $k$ is fixed and $v$ increases, the conclusions in Theorem 13.2 are identical to those that would be obtained if $f_{X^*}$ were uniform on $\mathcal{I}$.

The implementation of the estimation procedure (13.12) requires two smoothing parameters: the bandwidth $h$ when constructing the local linear smoother for $\gamma(x^*)$, and the threshold value $m$ in the trigonometric expansion. Delaigle et al. (2006) recommends using $h = h_{\text{PI}} n^{1/5-c}$ with $1/4 \leq c < 1$, where $h_{\text{PI}}$ is the plug-in bandwidth selector of Ruppert et al. (1995). To select $m$, the following cross-validation criterion is used

$$\hat{m}_{CV} = \text{argmin}_m \left( \sum_{i=1}^{n} [Y_i - E\{\hat{g}^{-1}(X_i; m) | X_1^*, \ldots, X_n^*\}]^2 \right),$$

where $\hat{g}^{-i}(\cdot; m)$ denotes the version of $\hat{g}$ that is constructed by omitting $(X_i^*, Y_i)$ from the sample, using $m$ terms in the Fourier series, and where the conditional expectation $E\{\hat{g}^{-1}(X_i; m) | X_1^*, \ldots, X_n^*\}$ can be estimated by

$$\int \frac{\sum_k S_k(z) Y_k - S_i(z) Y_i}{1 - S_i(z)} \left\{ \frac{1}{2\pi} + \frac{1}{\pi} \sum_{j=1}^{m} \cos[j(z - Z_i)] \right\} dz.$$

The detailed derivation of the above expression can be found in Delaigle et al. (2006).

### 13.3.2 Kernel Methods

The second method provided in Delaigle et al. (2006) is a kernel method. However, its theoretical properties, such as convergence rates, have not been discussed.

The proposed estimator is motivated by the following observation. Note that

$$\begin{aligned} \gamma(x^*) &= E(Y|X^* = x^*) = Eg(x^* + U) = \int g(x^* + u) f_U(u) du \\ &= \int g(x^* - u) f_{U^-}(u) du = g * f_{U^-}(x^*), \end{aligned}$$

where $f_{U^-}(u) = f_U(-u)$. Thus we have $\varphi_\gamma(t) = \varphi_g(t)\varphi_U(-t)$. If $\varphi_U(-t) \neq 0$ for all $t$, by Fourier inversion, we could write $g(x) = (2\pi)^{-1} \int e^{-itx} \varphi_\gamma(t)/\varphi_U(-t) dt$. Since $f_U$ is compactly supported, $\varphi_U(t)$ can equal zero for some $t$. To avoid dividing by 0, Delaigle et al. (2006) suggest estimating $g(x)$ by

$$\tilde{g}(x) = \frac{1}{2\pi} \int \exp(-itx)\varphi_{\hat{\gamma}}(t)\varphi_U^{-1}(-t)I\{|\varphi_U(-t)| > \eta\}dt, \qquad (13.13)$$

where $\varphi_{\hat{\gamma}}$ is the Fourier transform of $\hat{\gamma}$, an estimator of $\gamma$, and $\eta$ denotes a small positive threshold which plays the role of a smoothing parameter. Then the estimator of $g(x)$ is defined as

$$\hat{g}(x) = \Re\{\tilde{g}(x)\},$$

the real part of $\tilde{g}(x)$.

Delaigle et al. (2006) state that the Trigonometric method performs better than the kernel method, which is a direct consequence of imposing the truncation $I\{|\varphi_U(-t)| > \eta\}$ on the inverse Fourier transformation. However, more numerical studies are needed to illustrate the superiority of the former over the latter.

As we mentioned before, if $f_U$ is unknown, then the distribution of $X$ is not identifiable, hence $g$ is also not identifiable. Moreover, assuming a parametric form for the density function of $U$ does not help the identifiability issue.

Just like in the classical measurement error case, the assumption of a known $f_U$ is strict. In the case where $f_U$ is unknown, one has to explore other resources to identify it. These resources or data include possible observations from $f_U$, internal or external validation data on $(X, X^*)$, or repeated measurements $X_{kl} = X_k^* + U_{kl}, k \geq 2$. As Delaigle et al. (2006) point out, these resources might not be easy to acquire, but the chances are increasing due to advancement of new technology producing data of many kinds. See Delaigle and Van Keilegom (2021) in Chapter 12 for a review of the unknown error case in the classical error setting.

### 13.3.3 Estimators for Some Special Measurement Errors

In this section, we introduce two nonparametric regression estimators for the regression function $g$ in model (13.3) when the measurement error $U$ follows a normal distribution or a Laplace distribution. Generally speaking, the more information we can use, the better estimator we can construct.

#### 13.3.3.1 Berkson Regression: Normal Measurement Error

The estimation procedures introduced in the last two sections require some strong conditions on the relationships between the supports of $f_U$, $g$ and $f_{X^*}$. These conditions might be reasonable in some cases but seem to be rather stringent in many real data applications. Meister (2010) argues that such strong assumptions on the supports can be omitted when the error density $f_U$ is normal. In particular, under normal measurement error, this estimation procedure can estimate $g$ consistently on the whole real line, although the design variables $X_i^*$'s all fall into a fixed compact interval $\mathcal{I}$. Meister (2010) further argues that the identifiability of $g$ over the whole real line when $f_U$ is normal is due to the fact that the function $E[g(X)|X^* = x^*]$ is analytic if $f_U$ is normal even if only finitely many derivatives of $g$ exist.

The claim made by Meister (2010) seems contradictory to the relevant statement made by Delaigle et al. (2006) that only quantities of functionals of $\gamma(x^*) = Eg(x^* + U)$ can be consistently estimated. This seemingly contradiction can be resolved by noting that the condition imposed in Delaigle et al. (2006) is that the regression function $g$ is bounded and continuous, whereas in Meister (2010), the regression functions are assumed to be differentiable to certain order (the parameter $K$ defined in (13.15) on the following page).

In the following, we will assume that $f_U$ is normal with mean 0 and variance $\sigma^2 > 0$, and $|g(x)| \leq C\exp(D|x|)$, $x \in \mathbb{R}$ for some constants $C, D > 0$. Due to the complexity of the estimation procedure, the main steps to construct the estimator of $g$ in Meister (2010) are summarized below.

*Step 1: Approximating $\gamma(x^*)$ by a Taylor expansion of $\gamma(x^*)$.*

By a Taylor expansion of order $K - 1$ for some positive integer $K > 1$ which will be specified later, we have

$$\gamma(x^*) = \sum_{k=1}^{K-1} \frac{\gamma^{(k)}(0)}{k!} x^{*k} + R_K(x^*), \tag{13.14}$$

where $\gamma^{(k)}(0)$ is the $k$-th derivative of $\gamma$ evaluated at 0. Note that $U$ has a normal distribution with mean 0 and variance $\sigma^2$, so by changing variable, $\gamma(x^*) = Eg(x^* + U)$ can be written as

$$\gamma(x^*) = \frac{1}{\sqrt{2\pi}\sigma} \int g(y) \exp\{-(x^* - y)^2/(2\sigma^2)\} dy.$$

Therefore, for any integer $k \geq 0$, the $k$-th order derivative of $\gamma(x^*) = E(Y|X^* = x^*)$ can be written as

$$\begin{aligned} \gamma^{(k)}(x^*) &= \frac{1}{\sqrt{2\pi}\sigma} \int g(y) \frac{d^k}{dx^{*k}} \exp\{-(x^* - y)^2/(2\sigma^2)\} dy \\ &= \frac{(-1)^k}{\sqrt{2\pi}\sigma^k} \int g(x^* - \sigma y) \exp(-y^2/2) H_k(y) dy, \end{aligned}$$

where $H_k$ denotes the $k$-th Hermite polynomial. Then by (13.14), we have

$$\gamma(x^*) = \sum_{k=0}^{K-1} \frac{(-1)^k}{\sqrt{2\pi}\sigma^k k!} \int g(-\sigma y) \exp(-y^2/2) H_k(y) dy \cdot x^{*k} + R_K(x^*),$$

with the remainder term $|R_K(x^*)| \le c(K!)^{-1/2}|x^*/\sigma|^K \exp(D|x^*|)$. Thus, we can use

$$\gamma_{K,1}(x^*) = \sum_{k=0}^{K-1} \frac{(-1)^k}{\sqrt{2\pi}\sigma^k k!} \int g(-\sigma y) \exp(-y^2/2) H_k(y) dy \cdot x^{*k} \tag{13.15}$$

to approximate $\gamma(x^*)$.

*Step 2: Approximating $\gamma(x^*)$ by a Legendre polynomial.*

For any positive integer $k \ge 0$, let

$$\tilde{L}_k(x^*) = \frac{1}{2^k k!} \frac{d^k}{dz^{*k}} \{(x^{*2} - 1)^k\}$$

be the $k$-th Legendre polynomial. Define

$$L_k(x^*) = \sqrt{\frac{2k+1}{X^*_{(n)} - X^*_{(1)}}} \cdot \tilde{L}_k \left\{ \frac{2x^* - (X^*_{(n)} + X^*_{(1)})}{X^*_{(n)} - X^*_{(1)}} \right\},$$

where $X^*_{(i)}$, $i = 1, 2, \ldots, n$ are the order statistics of $X^*_i$, $i = 1, 2, \ldots, n$. Then the sequence $L_k, k \ge 0$ forms an orthonormal basis for the Hilbert space consisting of all square-integrable functions on the domain $[X^*_{(1)}, X^*_{(n)}]$. So for all $x^* \in [X^*_{(1)}, X^*_{(n)}]$, $\gamma(x^*) = E(Y|X^* = x^*)$ can be estimated by

$$\hat{\gamma}_{K,2}(x^*) = \sum_{k=1}^{K-1} \hat{c}_k L_k(x^*),$$

where $\hat{c}_k$ is defined as

$$\hat{c}_k = \sum_{j=1}^{n-1} Y_{[j]} \int_{X^*_{(j)}}^{X^*_{j+1}} L_k(x^*) dx^*,$$

and $Y_{[j]}$ is the response variable corresponding to $X^*_{(j)}$. Note that although the polynomials $L_k$ are defined in $[X^*_{(1)}, X^*_{(n)}]$, they can uniquely be continued to $\mathbb{R}$ in a natural way. The parameter $K$ can be viewed as the smoothing parameter, and a guideline for choosing $K$ is provided later in Theorem 13.3 .

*Step 3: Estimating the coefficients of $x^{*k}$ in (13.15).*

Rewrite $L_k(x^*)$ as $L_k(x^*) = \sum_{j=0}^{k} \lambda_{k,j} x^{*j}$. Then

$$\hat{\gamma}_{K,2}(x^*) = \sum_{k=0}^{K-1} \hat{c}_k L_k(x^*) = \sum_{k=0}^{K-1} \sum_{j=0}^{k} \hat{c}_k \lambda_{k,j} x^{*j} = \sum_{j=0}^{K-1} \left( \sum_{k=j}^{K-1} \hat{c}_k \lambda_{k,j} \right) x^{*j}. \tag{13.16}$$

Therefore, by comparing the coefficients of $x^{*j}$, $j = 1, 2, \ldots, K-1$, in (13.15) and (13.16), $\hat{d}_j = \sum_{k=j}^{K-1} \hat{c}_k \lambda_{k,j}$ can be used to estimate

$$\frac{(-1)^j}{\sqrt{2\pi}\sigma^j j!} \int g(-\sigma y) \exp(-y^2/2) H_j(y) dy \tag{13.17}$$

based on (13.15).

*Step 4: Constructing the estimator of g.*

For any two functions $f, g$, we use $\langle f, g \rangle = \int f(x) g(x) \exp(-x^2/2) dx$ to denote their inner product in the Hilbert space

$$\mathcal{H} = \{f : \|f\|^2 = \langle f, f \rangle < \infty\}.$$

It is well known that Hermite polynomials form an orthogonal basis of the Hilbert space $\mathcal{H}$. Denote $g_\sigma(x^*) = g(-\sigma x^*)$. Then we have

$$g(-\sigma x^*) = \sum_{k=0}^{\infty} \frac{1}{\sqrt{2\pi} k!} < g_\sigma, H_k > H_k(x^*).$$

From Step 3, we know that $\langle g_\sigma, H_k \rangle$ can be estimated by $(-1)^k \hat{d}_k \sigma^k k! \sqrt{2\pi}$. This implies that, after changing the variable $-\sigma x^*$ to $x^*$, $g(x^*)$ can be estimated by

$$\hat{g}(x^*) = \sum_{k=0}^{\lfloor c_K (K-1) \rfloor} (-1)^k \sigma^k \hat{d}_k H_k(-x^*/\sigma), \tag{13.18}$$

where $c_K$ is some number chosen from $(0, 1)$, and the cut-off value $\lfloor c_K(K-1) \rfloor$, the largest integer less than $c_K(K-1)$, plays a similar role as the bandwidth in kernel regression. Meister (2010) claims that the choice of $c_K$ is not critical.

To state the asymptotic properties of $\hat{g}(x)$ defined in (13.18), the following condition is needed.

> **D**: The design variables are either fixed with $c_1 n^{-1} \leq X^*_{(j+1)} - X^*_{(j)} < c_2 (\log n)/n$ for all $n$ and $j$, where $c_1, c_2$ are two positive constants; all $X_j^*$'s fall into some fixed closed interval; or the $X_j^*$'s are random and located in some fixed closed interval and have a density function $f_{X^*}$ bounded below from zero by a constant and bounded above by a positive constant.

We further define a family of functions $\mathcal{G}$ to be

$$\left\{ g : g \text{ is } \beta\text{-fold differentiable on } \mathbb{R}, \int |x^{*k} g^{(j)}(x^*)|^2 \exp\{-x^{*2}/(2\sigma^2)\} dx^* < C_G \right\}$$

for some constant $C_G$. The following theorem provides a uniform convergence rate for a weighted MISE of $\hat{g}$.

**Theorem 13.3** (Meister, 2010) *Assume that Condition* **D** *holds. Choose* $K = K_n = c\lfloor \log n / \log\log n \rfloor$ *for some constant* $c$, *and* $c_K \in (0,1)$ *such that*

$$\lim_{n\to\infty} \frac{c_K K \log\log n}{\log n} \in (0,1).$$

*Then,*

$$\sup_{g\in\mathcal{G}} E\int |\hat{g}(x^*) - g(x^*)|^2 \exp\{-x^{*2}/(2\sigma^2)\}dx^* = O\left\{(\log n/\log\log n)^{-\beta}\right\}.$$

Unfortunately, no data-driven procedures for selecting the smoothing parameters $K$ and $c_K$ are provided in Meister (2010).

From Theorem 13.3, we also have

$$\sup_{g\in\mathcal{G}} E\int_a^b |\hat{g}(x^*) - g(x^*)|^2 dx^* = O\left\{(\log n/\log\log n)^{-\beta}\right\}.$$

For the optimal convergence rate in the mean square sense, we have the following result.

**Theorem 13.4** (Meister, 2010) *Assume that Condition* **D** *holds, and* $T_n(x^*)$ *is an arbitrary estimator of* $g$ *based on* $\{(X_j^*, Y_j)\}_{j=1}^n$. *Assume that* $\beta > 2$ *and* $C_G$ *is sufficiently large; and suppose* $\varepsilon$ *has a standard normal distribution. Then for any* $a < b$, *we have*

$$\sup_{g\in\mathcal{G}} E\int |\hat{T}_n(x^*) - g(x^*)|^2 dx^* \geq c\left\{(\log n)^{-\beta}\right\}$$

*for* $n$ *sufficiently large.*

Combing the above two theorems, we can see that the estimator $\hat{g}$ achieves nearly optimal convergence rates up to an iterated logarithmic factor under smoothness constraints.

#### 13.3.3.2 Berkson Regression: Special Ordinary Smooth Cases

From Apanasovich and Liang (2021) and Delaigle (2021), we know that in classical measurement error setups, the nonparametric estimation procedures associated with ordinary smooth measurement error are much easier than in the super smooth case. In particular, the convergence rates of the deconvolution kernel density estimator and regression estimator in the former case are much faster than in the latter scenario. In this section, we will see that when the measurement error $U$ has a characteristic function $\varphi_U$ of the form

$$1/\varphi_U(t) = \sum_{j=0}^{J} a_j \sigma^j t^j, \tag{13.19}$$

for some positive integer $J$, where $a_0 = 1, a_1, \ldots, a_J$ are real-valued constants, $a_J > 0$, $\sigma^2$ is the variance of $U$, it is possible to construct a simple estimator of regression function $g$. More technical details can be found in Delaigle and Meister (2011).

Recall that $\gamma(x^*) = E(g(X)|X^* = x^*) = Eg(x^* + U)$ implies that $\varphi_\gamma(t) = \varphi_g(t)\varphi_U(-t)$. Then by the Fourier inversion, as well as (13.19), we have

$$\begin{aligned} g(x^*) &= \frac{1}{2\pi}\int \exp(-itx^*)\varphi_\gamma(t)/\varphi_U(-t)dt \\ &= \sum_{j=0}^{J} a_j\sigma^j \frac{1}{2\pi}\int (-t)^j \exp(-itx^*)\varphi_\gamma(t)dt \qquad (13.20) \\ &= \sum_{j=0}^{J}(-i)^j a_j \sigma^j \gamma^{(j)}(x^*) \end{aligned}$$

for almost all $x^* \in \mathbb{R}$. Therefore, an estimator of $g$ can be constructed by plugging any estimators of $\gamma^{(j)}$, $j = 1, 2, \ldots, J$, using the observed data $X^*$ in (13.20). This relationship also echoes Delaigle et al. (2006)'s statement on the identifiability of $g$ in model (13.3) that only quantities that can be expressed as functionals of $\gamma(x^*)$ can be consistently estimated using nonparametric methods.

As an example, suppose $U$ has a Laplace distribution with mean 0 and variance $\sigma^2$ and its characteristic function $\varphi_U^{-1}(t) = 1 + \sigma^2 t^2/2$, which has the form of (13.19) with $J = 2$, $a_0 = 1, a_1 = 0$ and $a_2 = 1/2$. Therefore, from (13.20), $g(x^*) = \gamma(x^*) - \sigma^2\gamma''(x^*)/2$. By choosing a proper nonparametric estimator $\hat{\gamma}(x^*)$ for $\gamma(x^*)$, e.g., the local linear smoother, $g(x^*)$ can be estimated by

$$\hat{g}(x^*) = \hat{\gamma}(x^*) - \frac{\sigma^2}{2}\hat{\gamma}''(x^*). \qquad (13.21)$$

In fact, (13.21) can be also obtained from the kernel methods discussed in Delaigle et al. (2006) by letting $\eta = 0$ in (13.13).

Similar to classical nonparametric smoothers, for a particular kernel estimate of $\gamma(x^*)$, a theoretically optimal bandwidth can be found by deriving an asymptotic expansion of the MISE of $\hat{g}$ defined in (13.21). The consistency, as well as the asymptotic normality, can be easily established in a standard manner.

As a partial extension, Shi et al. (2020) discusses the estimation of $g$ for multivariate $X$ by assuming the measurement error follows a multivariate Laplace distribution.

## 13.4 Final Remarks

The research on nonparametric statistical inferences related to Berkson measurement error has gained much momentum in recent years, as evidenced by many real data applications and theoretical developments. By assuming an instrument variable can be obtained, Schennach (2013) claims that the regression function, as well as all other unknown quantities, are all identified, and consistent estimators are constructed. In the presence of certain mixtures of classical and Berkson errors, estimation of the regression function has been investigated in Carroll et al. (2007), Delaigle (2007), Delaigle and Meister (2011), and Yin et al. (2013). It is noted that the estimators constructed in the last four references can be used to derive the nonparametric density and the regression function estimators in the case of only Berkson measurement error by nullifying the classical measurement error.

Literature has seen less research on hypothesis testing involving Berkson measurement errors. A series of work done by Koul and Song (2008, 2009, 2010, 2016) develops some lack-of-fit test procedures for checking the adequacy of certain parametric forms for the regression functions based on empirical processes and nonparametric smoothing techniques.

Compared to classical measurement errors, nonparametric inference procedures related to Berkson measurement errors are not full-fledged. However, given the rapid accumulation of various types of data and the advancement of technology, the opportunities for estimating statistical models with Berkson measurement error structure are growing.

## Bibliography

Apanasovich, T. and Liang, H. (2021). Nonparametric measurement errors models for regression. In *Handbook of Measurement Error Models*, G. Y. Yi, A. Delaigle, and P. Gustafson (Eds), CRC, Chapter 14.

Berkson, J. (1950). Are there two regressions? *Journal of the American Statistical Association*, 45(250), 164–180.

Carroll, R. J., Delaigle, A., and Hall, P. (2007). Non-parametric regression estimation from data contaminated by a mixture of Berkson and classical errors. *Journal of the Royal Statistical Society, Series B*, 69, 859-878.

Carroll, R., Rupper, D., Crainiceanu, C., and Stefanski, L. (2006). *Measurement Error in Nonlinear Models: A Modern Perspective* 2nd ed. Chapman and Hall/CRC.

Cheng, C. L. and John, W. V. N. (1999). *Statistical Regression with Measurement Error.* John Wiley & Sons, Ltd.

Delaigle, A. (2007). Nonparametric density estimation from data with a mixture of Berkson and classical errors. *Canadian Journal of Statistics*, 35(1), 89-104.

Delaigle, A. (2014). Nonparametric kernel methods with errors-in-variables: Constructing estimators, computing them, and avoiding common mistakes. *Australian & New Zealand Journal of Statistics*, 56(2), 105-124.

Delaigle, A. (2021). Deconvolution kernel density estimator. In *Handbook of Measurement Error Models*, G. Y. Yi, A. Delaigle, and P. Gustafson (Eds). CRC, Chapter 10.

Delaigle, A., Hall, P., and Qiu, P. H. (2006). Nonparametric methods for solving the Berkson errors-in-variables problem. *Journal of the Royal Statistical Society, Series B*, 68, 201-220.

Delaigle, A. and Meister, A. (2011). Rate-optimal nonparametric estimation in classical and Berkson errors-in-variables problems. *Journal of Statistical Planning and Inference*, 141(1), 102-114.

Delaigle, A. and Van Keilegom, I. (2021). Deconvolution with unknown error distribution. In *Handbook of Measurement Error Models*, G. Y. Yi, A. Delaigle, and P. Gustafson (Eds). CRC, Chapter 12.

Fan, J. and Gijbels, I. (1996). *Local Polynomial Modelling and its Applications*. Chapman and Hall/CRC.

Huwang, L. and Huang, Y. H. S. (2000). On errors-in-variables in polynomial regression-Berkson case. *Statistica Sinica*, 10(3), 923-936.

Kang, Y. and Qiu, P. (2021). Nonparametric deconvolution by Fourier transformation and other related approaches. In *Handbook of Measurement Error Models*, G. Y. Yi, A. Delaigle, and P. Gustafson (Eds). CRC, Chapter 11.

Koul, H. L. and Song, W. X. (2008). Regression model checking with Berkson measurement errors. *Journal of Statistical Planning and Inference*, 138(6), 1615-1628.

Koul, H. L. and Song, W. X. (2009). Minimum distance regression model checking with Berkson measurement errors. *Annals of Statistics*, 37(1), 132-156.

Koul, H. L. and Song, W. X. (2010). Model checking in partial linear regression models with Berkson measurement errors. *Statistica Sinica*, 20(4), 1551-1579.

Koul, H. L. and Song, W. X. (2016). Minimum distance partial linear regression model checking with Berkson measurement errors. *Journal of Statistical Planning and Inference*, 174, 129-152.

Long, J. P., E. Karoui, N., and Rice, J. A. (2016). Kernel density estimation with Berkson error. *Canadian Journal of Statistics*, 44(2), 142-160.

Meister, A. (2010). Nonparametric Berkson regression under normal measurement error and bounded design. *Journal of Multivariate Analysis*, 101(5), 1179-1189.

Ruppert, D., Sheather, S. J., and Wand, M. P. (1995). An effective bandwidth selector for local least squares regression. *Journal of the American Statistical Association*, 90(432), 1257-1270.

Schennach, S. M. (2013). Regressions with Berkson errors in covariates-a nonparametric approach. *Annals of Statistics*, 41(3), 1642-1668.

Shi, J. H., Bai, X. Q., and Song, W. X. (2020). Nonparametric regression estimate with Berkson laplace measurement error. *Statistics & Probability Letters*, 166(7). doi: 10.1016/j.spl.2020.108864

Wand, M.P. and Jones, M.C. (1995). *Kernel Smoothing.* Chapman and Hall, Ltd., London.

Wang, L. Q. (2003). Estimation of nonlinear Berkson-type measurement error models. *Statistica Sinica*, 13(4), 1201-1210.

Wang, L. Q. (2004). Estimation of nonlinear models with Berkson measurement errors. *Annals of Statistics*, 32(6), 2559-2579.

Wang, L. Q. (2007). A unified approach to estimation of nonlinear mixed effects and Berkson measurement error models. *Canadian Journal of Statistics*, 35(2), 233-248.

Yin, Z. H., Gao, W., Tang, M. L., and Tian, G. L. (2013). Estimation of nonparametric regression models with a mixture of Berkson and classical errors. *Statistics & Probability Letters*, 83(4), 1151-1162.

# 14

# *Nonparametric Measurement Errors Models for Regression*

**Tatiyana Apanasovich and Hua Liang**

## CONTENTS



DOI: 10.1201/9781315101279-14

## 14.1 Introduction

Measurement error models have been extensively studied in statistical literature and widely applied in different scientific areas like nutrition and epidemiology. Comprehensive literature reviews can be found in monographs by Carroll et al. (2006) and Fuller (1987). Broadly, the types of models studied in the literature can be divided into (i) linear measurement error models; (ii) nonlinear measurement error models; (iii) nonparametric and semiparametric measurement errors models. Reviews of earlier results on linear models can be found in Fuller (1987), while Schennach (2016) gave a comprehensive survey on estimation and inference methods for nonlinear measurement errors models. Carroll et al. (2006) surveyed nonparametric models and thorough analysis of theory of nonparametric deconvolution techniques can be found in the monographs by Meister (2009). In this chapter, we review selective published results on nonparametric measurement errors models with emphases on two major methods: deconvolution based methods and unbiased score based methods. We aim at introducing main methodological advances and briefly discuss their implementation and inference. Hence instead of stating technical conditions rigorously, we describe key ideas and refer readers to the original papers for details.

Consider nonparametric estimation of a regression function $m(x) = \mathrm{E}(Y|X = x)$ when $X$ is measured with some error and is not directly observable. Let $(Y_1, W_1), \cdots, (Y_n, W_n)$ denote a random sample assumed to follow the classical error model

$$Y_i = m(X_i) + \epsilon_i, \quad W_i = X_i + U_i, \quad i = 1, \cdots, n, \tag{14.1}$$

where the regression errors $\epsilon_i$ are independent, have an unknown density such that $\mathrm{E}(\epsilon_i|X_i = x) = 0$, $\mathrm{Var}(\epsilon_i|X_i = x) < \infty$. The measurement errors $U_i$ are independent and identically distributed, and independent of the $(X_i, \epsilon_i)$s. Denote the densities of $W$, $X$ and $U$ by $f_W(\cdot)$, $f_X(\cdot)$ and $f_U(\cdot)$, respectively. In the most general setting, neither of $f_W(\cdot)$, $f_X(\cdot)$ are known. While $f_W(\cdot)$ can be estimated from data, estimating $f_X(\cdot)$ requires either a sample of $X_j$s or at least an estimate of an error density, $f_U(\cdot)$, which is generally assumed to be known in most of the early studies.

In Section 14.2.3.2 we will discuss the line of research when $f_U(\cdot)$ is partially or completely unknown. For a comprehensive discussion on these topics, one may refer to Delaigle and Van Keilegom (2021). In Section 14.2.3.3 we will discuss the case when the $U_i$s are independent, but not identically distributed, so that $U_i \sim f_{U_i}$, but the $f_{U_i}(\cdot)$s are known or estimated from additional data.

If the $X_i$s are observable, the kernel estimator of the regression function (also called Nadaraya-Watson estimator) has the following form (Fan and Gijbels, 2003):

$$\widehat{m}(x) = \frac{(nh)^{-1}\sum_{i=1}^{n} Y_i K\left(\frac{x-X_i}{h}\right)}{(nh)^{-1}\sum_{i=1}^{n} K\left(\frac{x-X_i}{h}\right)}, \tag{14.2}$$

where $K(\cdot)$ is a kernel function and $h > 0$ is a smoothing parameter also known as a bandwidth.

More generally, the local polynomial estimator of $m(x)$ of order $p$ is defined as $\widehat{m}(x) = \widehat{\beta}_{0,x}$, where $\widehat{\beta}_{0,x}$ is obtained through the following minimization problem:

$$\text{argmin}_{\beta_{0,x},\cdots,\beta_{p,x}} \sum_{i=1}^{n} \left\{ Y_i - \sum_{j=0}^{p} \beta_{i,x}(X_i - x)^i \right\}^2 K\left(\frac{x - X_i}{h}\right). \tag{14.3}$$

In this review we focus on the case where the $X_i$s not observable so (14.2) and (14.3) have to be modified accordingly. For the review of the nonparametric methods for the Berkson error see Song (2021).

If we simply use $W_i$ instead of $X_i$ in (14.2) and (14.3), we will arrive at biased estimators (Fan and Truong, 1993). The most popular solutions to modification of (14.2) follow the theme of deconvolution kernel pioneered in the density estimation problem (Carroll and Hall, 1988). The chapter is organized as follows. We discuss deconvolution methods in Section 14.2. The methods proposed to construct local polynomial estimators based on unbiased scores are reviewed in Section 14.3. In Section 14.4, we discuss issues related to implementation of reviewed methods in practice. Section 14.5 contains multiple miscellaneous topics.

## 14.2 Deconvolution Methods

The general problem of deconvolution in statistics is to estimate a function $f(\cdot)$ which is related to an empirically estimable quantity $g(\cdot)$ through a convolution with a probability distribution $G$ (Meister, 2009),

$$g(x) = \int f(x-y)dG(y).$$

Hence $f(\cdot)$ can be estimated indirectly by inverting a convolution operator after $g$ is estimated from data. Fourier methods are very popular in deconvolution as they change the convolution into a simple multiplication. Therefore the construction of deconvolution estimators as well as understanding their properties requires rigorous results from Fourier analysis, functional analysis and probability theory. See also Kang and Qiu (2021) for other approaches to density deconvolution, and Delaigle (2021) for a review of deconvolution-based kernel estimators for the density.

### 14.2.1 General Form of the Estimator

Note that the kernel estimator of $m(\cdot)$, (14.2), in error free case can be written as

$$\widehat{m}(x) = \frac{(nh)^{-1}\sum_{i=1}^{n} Y_i K\left(\frac{x-X_i}{h}\right)}{\widehat{f}_X(x)},$$

where $\widehat{f}_X(x) = (nh)^{-1}\sum_{i=1}^{n} K\left(\frac{x-X_i}{h}\right)$ is a kernel estimator of the density of covariate $X$. Hence the problems of estimating the regression function $m(\cdot)$ and the density $f_X(\cdot)$ are related. That relationship has been explored in the case of mismeasured $X$ by Fan and Truong (1993) in the following way. In the classical measurement error model (14.1), the errors are additive, $W = X+U$, and it is easy to see that $f_W(w) = \int_{-\infty}^{\infty} f_X(w-x)f_U(x)dx$ and $\phi_W(t) = \phi_X(t)\phi_U(t)$, where $\phi_A(t)$ denotes a characteristic function of a random variable $A$. Hence we can deconvolve the first equation using its Fourier version to get an expression for $f_X(\cdot)$, assuming that conditions of Fourier inversion theorems apply and $\inf_{t\in\mathbb{R}} |\phi_U(t)| > 0$, which is

$$f_X(x) = \frac{1}{2\pi}\int_{-\infty}^{+\infty} \exp(-\imath tx)\phi_W(t)/\phi_U(t)dt.$$

If we estimate $\phi_W(t)$ by the empirical characteristic function $\widehat{\phi}_W(t) = n^{-1}\sum_{i=1}^{n} \exp(\imath tW_i)$ and assuming that $\phi_U(\cdot)$ is known, we may estimate $f_X(x)$ by

$$\widehat{f}_X(x) = \frac{1}{2\pi}\int_{-\infty}^{+\infty} \exp(-\imath tx)\widehat{\phi}_W(t)/\phi_U(t)dt. \tag{14.4}$$

However $\widehat{\phi}_W(t)$ has large fluctuations at its tails and $1/\phi_U(t) \to \infty$ as $|t| \to \infty$ making $\widehat{f}_X(\cdot)$ highly unstable. Several modifications have been proposed. One approach is to add a damping factor inside the integral (14.4). Carroll and Hall (1988) and Stefanski and Carroll (1990) suggested the deconvolution kernel density estimator of $f_X(\cdot)$ defined by

$$\widehat{f}_X(x) = \frac{1}{2\pi}\int_{-\infty}^{+\infty} \exp(-\imath tx)\phi_K(th)\frac{\widehat{\phi}_W(t)}{\phi_U(t)}dt, \tag{14.5}$$

where $h > 0$ and $\phi_K(\cdot)$ is the Fourier transformation of a kernel function $K(\cdot)$. Here, $\phi_K(\cdot)$ is used to dampen effect of the unreliability of $\widehat{\phi}_W(t)$ for large $|t|$ as $K(\cdot)$ is chosen such that $\phi_K(\cdot)$ is compactly supported.

Alternatively one can interpret (14.5) as using an adjustment to $\widehat{f}_X(\cdot)$ in (14.4) to have an empirical characteristic function of $W_i$s estimated as

$$\widehat{\phi}_W(t) = \frac{1}{n}\sum_{i=1}^{n}\phi_K(th)\exp(\imath tW_i). \tag{14.6}$$

Note that if $\phi_K(\cdot)$ is compactly supported, then (14.6) is compactly supported, which in turn guarantees that the numerator vanishes well before the denominator causes the ratio in (14.4) to diverge.

One can present (14.5) as

$$\widehat{f}_X(x) = \frac{1}{nh}\sum_{i=1}^{n} K_U\left(\frac{x-W_i}{h}\right), \tag{14.7}$$

where

$$K_U(u) = \frac{1}{2\pi}\int_{-\infty}^{+\infty}\frac{\exp(-\imath tu)\phi_K(t)}{\phi_U(t/h)}dt. \tag{14.8}$$

$K_U(\cdot)$ is also called a deconvolution kernel. As one can see the deconvolution kernel is constructed from the original kernel $K(\cdot)$ for assumed distribution of errors through $\phi_U(\cdot)$. For example, take the following second order kernel

$$K(x) = \frac{48\cos x}{\pi x^4}\left(1-\frac{15}{x^2}\right) - \frac{144\sin x}{\pi x^5}\left(2-\frac{5}{x^2}\right),$$

whose characteristic function has a compact support:

$$\phi_K(t) = (1-t^2)^3 I(|t|\leq 1).$$

Suppose that $U$ is a normal error with mean 0 and variance $\sigma^2$. Then, we get the following deconvolution kernel

$$K_U(u) = \frac{1}{\pi}\int_0^1 \cos(tu)(1-t^2)^3\exp(\sigma^2t^2/2)dt.$$

Using (14.7) and (14.8), Fan and Truong (1993) proposed the following nonparametric estimator of $m(\cdot)$:

$$\widehat{m}(x) = \frac{(nh)^{-1}\sum_{i=1}^{n} Y_i K_U\left(\frac{x-W_i}{h}\right)}{(nh)^{-1}\sum_{i=1}^{n} K_U\left(\frac{x-W_i}{h}\right)}. \tag{14.9}$$

Note that unlike the error free case, the convolution kernel $K_U(\cdot)$ does not have to be positive everywhere and is not compactly supported. Hence in practice, the denominator can be close to 0 or even vanish. Therefore, Hall and Meister (2007) suggested to replace (14.9) by

$$\widehat{m}(x) = \frac{\sum_{i=1}^{n} Y_i K_U\left(\frac{x-W_i}{h}\right)}{\max\left\{\sum_{i=1}^{n} K_U\left(\frac{x-W_i}{h}\right), \rho\right\}},$$

where $\rho > 0$ is referred as a ridge parameter. More ridge techniques will be discussed in Section 14.2.3.1.

### 14.2.2 Asymptotic Properties

In this section we discuss the asymptotic behavior of the deconvolution kernel regression estimator (14.9) as the number of observations $n$ tends to infinity. Meister (2009) formulated strong consistency results, $\widehat{m}(x) \to m(x)$ *a.s.*, at some value $x \in \mathbb{R}$. He discussed the assumptions needed to ensure the participating Fourier transforms well defined, e.g. boundedness of $f_X(\cdot)$, $m(\cdot)$ and $\phi_U(\cdot) \neq 0$ as well as the rates at which $h := h_n$ converges to 0 as $n \to \infty$. We outline some of these assumptions in Section 14.2.2.1.

The other relevant question is how fast $\widehat{m}(x)$ converges to $m(x)$. The rates of convergence for (14.9) were first established in Fan and Truong (1993). They provided optimal weak convergence rates for types of noises ($U$) they defined. The authors claimed that the traditional arguments for establishing lower bounds in kernel estimators cannot be generalized to the context of error-in-variables. Fan and Truong (1993) developed a new approach for establishing the bounds by connecting the regression problem with the density estimation problem, which was considered in Carroll and Hall (1988) and Fan (1991). They showed that the rates not only depend on the number of bounded derivatives the regression function $m(\cdot)$ has, but also on the smoothness of the error density, $f_U(\cdot)$, and the density of $X$, $f_X(\cdot)$. We briefly discuss the convergence rates and their optimality in Section 14.2.2.2. To establish asymptotic normality of the estimator, regularity conditions were presented in Fan (1991). The assumptions are stronger than those needed to define the estimator and surveyed in Section 14.2.2.3. Liang (2000) applied the approach of Fan and Truong (1993) to partially linear models for establishing asymptotically normal estimators of the linear parameter.

#### 14.2.2.1 Consistency

Next we outline the approach Meister (2009) proposed to prove weak and strong consistency. Observing the numerator and denominator of (14.9), it is easy to see that the denominator is a kernel estimator of $f_X(\cdot)$ discussed in Carroll and Hall (1988) and the numerator is

$$\widehat{p}(x) := \frac{1}{2\pi n} \sum_j Y_j \int_{-\infty}^{+\infty} \exp(-\imath tx)\phi_K(th)\exp(\imath tW_j)/\phi_U(t)dt.$$

By taking the expectation of the numerator, Meister (2009) showed that it is dominated by $p(x) := m(x)f_X(x)$. Meister (2009) established consistency by using the argument that $\widehat{m}(x)$ is a reasonable estimator of $p(x)/f_X(x)$. He assumed that $\phi_U(t) \neq 0$ for all $t \in \mathbb{R}$, $K(\cdot) \in L(\mathbb{R}) \cap L_2(\mathbb{R})$ and $\phi_K(\cdot)$ supported on $[-1, 1]$. It was assumed that $p(\cdot)$ is a Lebesgue integrable function so that its Fourier transform, $\phi_p(\cdot)$, is well defined. That is satisfied when $f_X(\cdot)$ and $m(\cdot)$ are bounded, continuous and $\phi_p(\cdot), \phi_X(\cdot) \in L_1(\mathbb{R})$. The rates at which $h := h_n$ converges to 0 as $n \to \infty$ were also discussed (Meister, 2009).

#### 14.2.2.2 Optimal Convergence Rates

In their theoretical statements, Fan and Truong (1993) described the smoothness of a density in terms of the asymptotic rate of decay of its Fourier transform as $t \to \infty$. It is known that the number of derivatives of a continuous density is directly related to the asymptotic behavior of its Fourier transform as $t \to \infty$. Carroll and Hall (1988) discussed how the tail behavior of $\phi_U(\cdot)$ affects the convergence in the context of density estimation. Fan (1991) introduced a notion of ordinary smooth and supersmooth functions. Ordinary smooth functions admit a finite number of continuous derivatives and their Fourier transform decays as $|t|^{-\alpha}$ for some $\alpha > 0$,

$$d_1|t|^{-\alpha} \leq |\phi_U(t)| \leq d_2|t|^{-\alpha}, \text{ for all } t \in \mathbb{R}, \text{ with } d_1, d_2 > 0. \tag{14.10}$$

Supersmooth functions admit an infinite number of derivatives and their Fourier transform decays as $\exp(-|t|^{\alpha})$ for some $\alpha > 0$,

$$d_1|t|^{\gamma}\exp(-d_3|t|^{\alpha}) \leq |\phi_U(t)| \leq d_2|t|^{\gamma}\exp(-d_3|t|^{\alpha}), \quad \text{for all } t \in \mathbb{R}, \text{ with } d_1, d_2, d_3 > 0.$$

Examples of ordinary smooth functions are gamma, uniform and double exponential; examples of supersmooth functions are normal and Cauchy. If the density of $U$ is ordinary smooth, the kernel deconvolution exhibits a convergence rate of the form of $n^{-c}$ for some $c > 0$. When the density of $U$ is supersmooth, the convergence rate is $(\ln n)^{-c}$ for some $c > 0$, which is slower than any negative power of $n$ suggesting that essentially there is no hope to recover $m(\cdot)$ with a reasonably small error for reasonable sample sizes. This conclusion is often interpreted as a general pessimistic message about the Gaussian deconvolution problem (Meister, 2009).

To determine the precise behavior of the estimator, some additional assumptions are needed to quantify the smoothness degree of $m(\cdot)$ and $f_X(\cdot)$. More conditions are imposed on $m(\cdot)$, $f_X(\cdot)$ and $K(\cdot)$ to guarantee the optimality in minimax sense as discussed in Meister (2009). $f_X(\cdot)$ is uniformly bounded and Hölder continuous for $\beta \geq 1$. $p(\cdot)$ is uniformly bounded, continuous integrable and Hölder continuous for $\beta \geq 1$. $K(\cdot) \in L_1(\mathbb{R}) \cap L_2(\mathbb{R})$ and is a $\beta$-order kernel, that is

$$\int_{-\infty}^{+\infty} K(y)dy = 1, \quad \int_{-\infty}^{+\infty} y^j K(y)dy = 0, j = 1, \cdots, \lfloor\beta\rfloor,$$
$$\int_{-\infty}^{+\infty} |y|^{\beta}|K(y)|dy < \infty.$$

Moreover, $\phi_K(\cdot)$ is supported on $[-1, 1]$. With respect to regression errors, it is assumed that $||\mathrm{var}(Y_j|X_j = \cdot)||_{\infty} \leq C < \infty$.

Under these conditions Fan and Truong (1993) showed that the local and global rates of convergence of the defined kernel estimators are optimal. Specifically, the authors established the lower bounds for these rates and showed that they match the lower bounds for all possible estimators for the same class of problems. However, their framework requires assumptions which are difficult to check in practice. For example the theoretical selection of the kernel and bandwidth parameter requires knowledge of the joint smoothness degree $\beta$ of $p(\cdot)$ and $f_X(\cdot)$.

#### 14.2.2.3 Asymptotic Normality

The difference between the estimator $\widehat{m}(x)$ and $m(x)$ can be decomposed into the bias term and a centered random variable. The bias term is deterministic and the random deviation of the estimator and its expectation should converge to the degenerated random variable in distribution, which follows from consistency. It was proved in Fan and Masry (1992) that the expectation of the limiting distribution of $\widehat{m}(x) - m(x)$ is the same as in the error-free case. Therefore, as in the error-free case, the bias depends on the smoothness of $m(\cdot)$ and $f_X(\cdot)$, the number of finite moments of $Y$ and the order of kernel $K(\cdot)$. Most conditions are fairly standard to error-free context. For example, $f_X(\cdot)$ is twice differentiable such that $||f_X^{(j)}(\cdot)||_\infty < \infty$ for $j = 0, 1, 2$; $m(\cdot)$ is three times differentiable, $||m^{(j)}(\cdot)||_\infty < \infty$ for $j = 0, \cdots, 3$. Stronger moment conditions on $Y$ are common in measurement error contexts, e.g. for some $\eta > 0$, $\mathrm{E}\{|Y - m(X)|^{2+\eta}|X = x\}$ is bounded for all $x$. See Fan and Masry (1992) and Fan and Truong (1993).

The asymptotic variance of the estimator differs from the error-free case since it depends strongly on the type of measurement errors (Fan and Masry, 1992). Different conditions on kernel $K(\cdot)$ are needed for ordinary smooth and supersmooth errors. These conditions are also standard in deconvolution problems, see for example Fan and Truong (1993).

Asymptotic normality in the ordinary smooth error case is pretty straightforward to establish. The expressions are given in Delaigle et al. (2009). The optimal bandwidth is found by the usual trade-off between the squared bias and the variance. For example the rate of that bandwidth is $n^{-2/(2\alpha+5)}$ when $f_X(\cdot)$ is twice differentiable and $U$ is ordinary smooth of order $\alpha$ as in (14.10).

In the case of supersmooth error, a technical condition, which is a refined version of the Lyapounov condition is needed. A lower bound on the bandwidth is essential and the rate of that lower bound is logarithmic in $n$. Note that the variance of the estimator is negligible compared to the squared bias and the estimator converges at a logarithmic rate.

### 14.2.3 Modifications of the Classical Estimator

Kernel methods for deconvolution based on (14.9) have many attractive features. However, they also have disadvantages, which include assumptions that seem unrealistic in many situations. In the next sections we will discuss the attempts made to relax some of them.

#### 14.2.3.1 $\phi_U(\cdot)$ Vanishes on the Real Line

Kernel methods discussed above require the characteristic function of the error distribution $\phi_U(\cdot)$ to be positive on the entire real line, for example, the characteristic functions correspond to error distributions that cannot be compactly supported. Some of the infinitely supported distributions are also excluded. One approach to deal with zeros in $\phi_U(\cdot)$ is to replace $\phi_U(\cdot)$ by an approximation of $\phi_U(\cdot)$ that does not have any zeros but usually depends on the number of parameters in addition to a bandwidth. Hall and Meister (2007) suggested methods based on ridging as they proposed to replace a kernel in (14.7) by

$$K_U(t) = \begin{cases} h^{-(r+2)}(t)\phi_U(-t)|\phi_U(t)|^r, & \text{if } |\phi_U(t)| \leq h(t), \\ \{\phi_U(t)\}^{-1}, & \text{if } |\phi_U(t)| > h(t), \end{cases}$$

where $r \geq 0$ is a tuning parameter, $h(t)$ is a positive ridge function, generally depending on $n$, e.g. $h(t) = n^{-\xi}|t|^\rho$, where $\xi > 0$ and $\rho > 0$. Hence the estimator of $m(\cdot)$ becomes the real part of

$$\frac{\int \phi_U(-t)|\phi_U(t)|^r\widehat{v}(t)/\{|\phi_U(t)| \vee h(t)\}^{r+2}\exp(-\imath tx)dt}{\int \phi_U(-t)|\phi_U(t)|^r\widehat{\phi}_W(t)/\{|\phi_U(t)| \vee h(t)\}^{r+2}\exp(-\imath tx)dt},$$

where $\widehat{v}(t) = n^{-1}\sum_j Y_j \exp(\imath tW_j)$ and $x \vee y = \max(x, y)$. See Hall and Meister (2007) for the results about theoretical properties of their estimators in a wide variety of settings. Note that the authors generalized the ordinary smooth and supersmooth errors into, respectively

$$|\phi_U(t)| \geq c_1|\sin\{(\pi t)/\lambda\}|^\nu(1 + |t|)^{-\alpha},$$

for all $t \in \mathbb{R}$ with $c_1 > 0$, and

$$|\phi_U(t)| \geq c_1|\sin\{(\pi t)/\lambda\}|^\nu|t|^\gamma \exp(-d|t|^\alpha),$$

for all $t \in \mathbb{R}$ with $c_1 > 0$, $d > 0$, and $\gamma \geq 0$ some constants, and for both generalizations $\nu \in \mathbb{Z}$, $\nu, \lambda > 0$. One can see that for errors in both classes, $\phi_U(\cdot)$ can have isolated zeros at non-zero integer multiples of $\lambda$.

Methods outlined in Hall and Meister (2007) require a selection of a functional smoothing parameter, $h(t)$, which can be reduced to the selection of two parameters. The authors suggested a way to choose them.

The ridge-based method enjoys optimal convergence rates, both in standard (or nonoscillatory) cases where characteristic functions do not vanish, and in oscillatory cases where those functions have infinitely many zeros. However, for oscillatory cases the optimal rates are slower. In some cases, the rates depend only on the smoothness of the error distribution, but in others, the convergence rates of such estimators depend on the number of zeros. For example, the estimators cannot achieve a better convergence rate than $n^{-1/(2\nu)}$, as pointed out by Hall and Meister (2007), where $\nu$ describes the order of the isolated zeros of $\phi_U(\cdot)$.

Delaigle and Meister (2007) proposed an estimator, which attains the standard deconvolution rate and has only the bandwidth as a tuning parameter. They assumed, however, that $m(\cdot)$ and $f_X(\cdot)$ are supported on $I \subset [a,b]$, where $a, b$ are finite constants. The authors used a clever idea instead of trying to estimate $f_X(\cdot)$ directly, they estimate another function which related to $\phi_X(\cdot)$ and is well defined for all $t$, and reconstruct $f_X(\cdot)$ from it.

Specifically, Delaigle and Meister (2007) estimated $m(\cdot)$ by

$$\widehat{m}(x) = \frac{\sum_{i=1}^{n} Y_i K_U\left(\frac{x-W_i}{h}\right) I_{[a,b](x)}}{\max\left\{\sum_{i=1}^{n} K_U\left(\frac{x-W_i}{h}\right) I_{[a,b]}(x), \rho\right\}},$$

where $\rho > 0$ is referred to as a ridge parameter, and

$$K_U(x) = \frac{1}{2\pi}\int \exp(-\imath t x)\frac{\phi_K(t)}{\phi_U(t/h)}\left\{\sum_{k=0}^{J}\eta_k \exp\left(\frac{2\imath t k\pi}{\lambda h}\right)\right\}$$
$$\times\left\{\exp\left(\frac{2\imath t\pi}{\lambda h}\right) - 1\right\}^{\nu} dt,$$

where $J + 1 > (x-a)\lambda/(2\pi)$ and $(\eta_0, \cdots, \eta_J) = (1, 0, \cdots, 0)\Gamma^{-1}$ and $\Gamma_{jk} = \gamma_{\nu,k-j}$

$$\gamma_{\nu,k} = \begin{cases} \binom{\nu}{k}(-1)^{\nu-k} & \text{if } k \in \{0, \cdots, \nu\}, \\ 0 & \text{otherwise.} \end{cases}$$

The authors advise to choose $J = \lceil (x-a)\lambda/(2\pi)\rceil$, and claim that their estimator reaches the optimal rates when $a$ is finite, which hints that large $J$ should work. In practice the estimator of $f_X(\cdot)$ would suffer from numerical instability if $J$ is large.

#### 14.2.3.2 Error Distribution is Unknown or Partially Known

In practical work, the assumption of a perfectly known error density $f_U(\cdot)$ is not always realistic. Moreover, Meister (2004) showed that misspecification of the error density in the standard deconvolution kernel estimator may have a critical influence on the asymptotic behavior of the estimator.

Most of authors addressing this issue assume that the error density can be estimated directly from additional data and the measurement system can be calibrated (Carroll et al., 2006). For example, for some units both $W$ and $X$ can be observed, then $U = W - X$. Hence one assumes that there is a sample $U_1, \cdots, U_m$ with $U_i \sim f_U$, then an unknown $\phi_U$ can be estimated by (Delaigle et al., 2008)

$$\widehat{\phi}_U(t) = \frac{1}{m}\sum_{k=1}^{m}\exp(\imath t U_k).$$

Johannes (2009) stated the conditions to ensure that the estimator of $\phi_U$ is asymptotically negligible.

Another approach is based on replicated measurements where the random variable $X$ is independently measured several times but each measurement is affected by error, hence we observe data

$$W_{jk} = X_j + U_{jk}, \quad j = 1, \cdots, n, \quad k = 1, \cdots, N_j.$$

If the real valued $\phi_U(\cdot)$ does not vanish at any point on the real line, a consistent estimator of $\phi_U(\cdot)$ is (Delaigle et al., 2008)

$$\widehat{\phi}_U(t) = \left| \frac{1}{N} \sum_{j=1}^{n} \sum_{k_1, k_2 \in S_j} \exp\{\imath t(W_{jk_1} - W_{jk_2})\} \right|^{1/2},$$

where $S_j$ denotes the set of $N_j(N_j - 1)/2$ distinct pairs $(k_1, k_2)$ with $k_1 < k_2 \leq N_j$, $N = N(n) = \sum_{j \leq n} N_j(N_j - 1)/2$ ignoring the case when $N_j = 1$. The deconvolution kernel is then given by

$$K_U(x) = \frac{1}{2\pi} \int \exp(-\imath tu) \frac{\phi_K(t)}{\widehat{\phi}_U(t/h) + \rho} dt,$$

where the ridge parameter $\rho \geq 0$ is used for compensating the fluctuations of the denominator. Delaigle et al. (2008) showed that even if the number of repeated observations is small, it is possible for the proposed modified kernel estimator to achieve the same level of performance they would have if the error distributions were known.

Some authors used semiparametric approaches to the deconvolution with partly known noise density (Butucea and Matias, 2005; Meister, 2006). They showed that if there is a parametric model for the error density $f_U(\cdot)$ and additional constraints on the density $f_X(\cdot)$, it is possible to estimate an unknown parameter of $f_U(\cdot)$ without any additional observations. Specifically, these authors assumed

$$W_j = X_j + \sigma U_j, \quad j = 1, \cdots, n,$$

where the error variables $U_j$ have a known density $f_U(\cdot)$ (e.g., normal as in Meister (2006)) and $\sigma > 0$ denotes a scaling parameter. This model is considered under the assumption that $\phi_X(\cdot)$ has a specific known positive lower bound, so that $\sigma$ can be estimated consistently. Under additional assumptions, some of these semiparametric estimators achieve nearly optimal rates (Meister, 2006).

Carroll and Hall (2004) suggested new methods, which are based on defining a low order approximation of an estimating equation, and proceed by constructing relatively accurate estimators of it. They argued that their framework can result in consistent estimators, but in many contexts consistency is impossible to achieve unless the number of replications grows with the sample size. The general form of error-in-variables distribution is assumed to be unknown but its low order moments either known or can be estimated from repeated measurements.

Delaigle and Hall (2016) assumed $\phi_U(\cdot)$ is completely unknown, but placed a number of assumptions on $f_U(\cdot)$ and $f_X(\cdot)$. For example, they assumed that $\phi_U(\cdot)$ is real valued and non-negative; in the discrete case it vanishes at most a countable number of points, and in the continuous case it is strictly positive on the real line. Note that these are standard assumptions in deconvolution problems, most of the time the distribution of $U$ is symmetric. The density function $f_X(\cdot)$ is assumed to be asymmetric. Moreover, it is assumed that the random variable $X$ does not have a symmetric component. Hence, there is a special type of asymmetric distribution for $X$ that cannot be recovered by their method, when $f_X(\cdot)$ is itself a convolution of a skew distribution and a symmetric distribution. As discussed in Delaigle and Hall (2016) if one were to assume that the density function $f_X(\cdot)$ were sampled from a random universe of distributions, this critical assumption is satisfied with probability 1.

Next we provide a brief overview of how the method of Delaigle and Hall (2016) can be implemented. Define the phase function of a random variable $V$ as $\rho_V(t) = \phi_V(t)/|\phi_V(t)|$. Note that the symmetry of $f_U(\cdot)$ implies that $\phi_U(t) = |\phi_U(t)|$ and one can deduce that $\rho_X(t) = \rho_W(t) = \phi_W(t)/|\phi_W(t)|$ for $\phi_U(t) \neq 0$.

They suggested to estimate $\rho_W(t)$ by $\widehat{\rho}_W(t) = \widehat{\phi}_W(t)/|\widehat{\psi}_W(t)|^{1/2}$, where $\widehat{\phi}_W(t) = \sum_j \exp(\imath t W_j)$ is a root $n$ consistent estimators of $\phi_W(t)$ and

$$\widehat{\psi}_W(t) = \frac{1}{n(n-1)} \sum\sum_{j \neq k} \exp\{\imath t(W_j - W_k)\}$$

is a root $n$ consistent estimator of $|\phi_W(t)|^2$.

Let $w(t)$ denote a non-negative weight function chosen to avoid numerical difficulties that can arise when dividing by very small numbers. Also let $x_i$ denote a set of arbitrary values with respective probability masses $p_i$ to be estimated. Specifically, Delaigle and Hall (2016) suggested sampling the $x_i$ uniformly on the interval $[\min(W_j), \max(W_j)]$, with $i = 1, \cdots, m$, $m = 5\sqrt{n}$, so that $\phi_X(t|\mathbf{p}) := \sum_j p_j \exp(\imath t x_j)$. The goal is then to find the set $\mathbf{p} = \{p_i\}_{i=1}^m$ that minimizes

$$T(\rho) = \int_{-\infty}^{+\infty} \left| \widehat{\rho}_W(t) - \frac{\phi_X(t|\mathbf{p})}{|\phi_X(t|\mathbf{p})|} \right|^2 w(t)dt$$

and also minimizes the variance of the corresponding (discrete) distribution, $\sum_{i=1}^m p_i x_i^2 - (\sum_{i=1}^m p_i x_i)^2$. This non-convex optimization problem of finding the solution $\{\widehat{p}_i\}_{i=1}^m$ can be solved using various methods. Details were given in Delaigle and Hall (2016). Hence, the proposed estimator of $m(x)$ is

$$\widetilde{m}(x) = \frac{(2\pi)^{-1} \int \exp(-\imath tx)\{\widehat{\phi}_{YW}(t)/\widehat{\phi}_U(t)\}\phi_K(ht)dt}{\max[(2\pi)^{-1} \int \exp(-\imath tx)\{\widehat{\phi}_W(t)/\widehat{\phi}_U(t)\}\phi_K(ht)dt, \rho]},$$

where

$$\widehat{\phi}_{YW}(t) = \sum_{j=1}^{n} Y_j \exp(\imath t W_j), \quad \widehat{\phi}_U(t) = \widehat{\phi}_W(t)/\widehat{\phi}_X(t),$$

and $\rho$ is a ridge parameter. The authors also offered a ridging for $\widehat{\phi}_X(\cdot)$ which we will not discuss here.

Delaigle and Hall (2016) showed that the performance of the resulting estimators is excellent, as it is often equal or even better than the estimators that are based on the additional data through extensive numerical studies.

#### 14.2.3.3 Heteroscedastic Errors-in-Variables

Delaigle and Meister (2007) proposed methods that relax the assumption that the measurement errors are identically distributed. They considered the heteroscedastic error-in-variable problem where $X_i \sim f_X(\cdot)$ (still) but $U_i \sim f_{U_i}(\cdot)$ and therefore $W_i \sim f_{W_i}(\cdot)$, $i = 1, \cdots, n$. If the $f_{U_i}(\cdot)$s are known, then the authors proposed to use

$$\widehat{m}(x) = \frac{(h)^{-1} \sum_{i=1}^{n} Y_i K_{U_i}\left(\frac{x-W_i}{h}\right)}{(h)^{-1} \sum_{i=1}^{n} K_{U_i}\left(\frac{x-W_i}{h}\right)}$$

with convolution kernels defined by

$$K_{U_i}(u) = \frac{1}{2\pi} \int \exp(-\imath t u) \phi_K(t) \Psi_i(t/h) dt,$$

where $\Psi_i(t) = \frac{\phi_{U_i}(-t)}{\sum_{k=1}^{n} |\phi_{U_k}(t)|^2}$ replaces the term $\{n\phi_U(t)\}^{-1}$ used in the homoscedastic settings. Note, if we just replace $\phi_U(\cdot)$ with $\phi_{U_i}(\cdot)$ in (14.8) so that now $K_U(\cdot)$ becomes $K_{U_i}(\cdot)$ in (14.9) we still have consistent estimates. However, one can easily see that its rates of convergence are dictated by the least favorable $U_i$s, which makes that approach less desirable than the proposed one. In fact, Delaigle and Meister (2007) showed that their estimator is the optimal one in a minimax sense with respect to any nonparametric regression estimator.

The authors also considered the case when the error density is unknown. Delaigle and Meister (2007) studied the general case when each observation is replicated at least once, and the replications do not need to have the same error distribution. Specifically, suppose that we have replicated data in the form $(W_{jk}, Y_j)$, $j = 1, \cdots, n$, $k = 1, ..., r_j$, and

$$W_{jk} = X_j + U_{jk}, \quad U_{jk} \sim f_{U_{jk}}, \quad r_j \geq 2.$$

They showed that it is possible to define an estimator of $m(\cdot)$ even without accurate estimate of each component $f_{U_j}(\cdot)$ from a large number of replications. In fact, they only require at least two replications per individual. The only assumption needed for the identification is that at least one of the densities $f_{U_{jk}}(\cdot)$, $k = 1, \cdots, r_j$ is symmetric around 0 for each $j = 1, \cdots, n$. Without loss of generality, we assume that $f_{U_{jr_j}}(\cdot)$ has this property. Let

$$\widehat{\phi}_W(t) = n^{-1} \sum_{j=1}^{n} \sum_{k=1}^{r_j - 1} \exp\{\imath t(W_{jk} + W_{jr_j})/2\};$$

$$\widehat{\phi}_U(t) = n^{-1} \sum_{j=1}^{n} \sum_{k=1}^{r_j - 1} \exp\{\imath t(W_{jk} - W_{jr_j})/2\};$$

$$\widehat{\phi}_Y(t) = n^{-1} \sum_{j=1}^{n} Y_j \sum_{k=1}^{r_j - 1} \exp\{\imath t(W_{jk} + W_{jr_j})/2\}.$$

Let $\rho \geq 0$ be the ridge parameter introduced to prevent the denominator from getting too close to 0 and

$$\widetilde{\phi}_U(t) = \frac{|\widehat{\phi}_U(t)|^2 + \rho|\widehat{\phi}_U(t)|}{\widehat{\phi}_U(-t)}.$$

Then the proposed regression estimator is defined by

$$\widehat{m}(x) = \frac{\int \exp(-\imath tx)\phi_K(th)\widehat{\phi}_Y(t)/\widetilde{\phi}_U(t)dt}{\int \exp(-\imath tx)\phi_K(th)\widehat{\phi}_W(t)/\widetilde{\phi}_U(t)dt}.$$

The authors postulated that the convergence rates for this estimator are the same as those for the estimator for the case of known error densities. They did not provide proofs, instead stated that it would require much technical calculations and assumptions. They did not claim optimality, but stressed their estimator's simplicity.

### 14.2.4 Nonparametric Prediction

Nonparametric prediction of a random variable $Y$ conditional on the value of an explanatory variable $X$ is an important problem in many applications. Carroll et al. (2009) considered the problem of predicting the random variable $Y$ by estimating $\mathrm{E}(Y|T = x)$, where $T$ is an observed future explanatory variable generated by $T = X + U^F$, where the density of $U^F$, $f_{U^F}(\cdot)$, is known. Moreover, past observations $\{(Y_j, W_j)\}_{j=1}^n$ are such that $W_j = X_j + U_j$, the unobserved $X_j$ have a common unknown density $f_X(\cdot)$, but the measurement errors $U_j$ are heterogeneously distributed with known (or estimable) densities denoted by $f_{U_j}(\cdot)$. Let $f_{TY}(\cdot)$ denote the joint density of $T$ and $Y$, $f_T(\cdot)$ denote the marginal density of $T$. The task is to estimate

$$\mu(x) = \mathrm{E}(Y|T = x) = \frac{\int y f_{TY}(x, y)dy}{f_T(x)}.$$

The authors exploited the relationship between $T$ and each $W_j$ expressed in terms of their characteristic functions $\phi_T(t) = \phi_X(t)\phi_{U^F}(t)$, and $\phi_X(t) = \phi_{W_j}(t)/\phi_{U_j}(t)$.

Assuming that $f_{U_j}(t) > 0$ and $\phi_T(t)$ is integrable, one can write

$$\phi_T(t) = \phi_{U_F}(t)\sum_j\{\phi_{W_j}(t)/\phi_{U_j}(t)\} = \phi_{U_F}(t)\sum_j\{\phi_{W_j}(t)\Psi_j(t)\},$$

where

$$\Psi_j(t) = \frac{\phi_{U_j}(-t)}{\sum_{k=1}^{n}|\phi_{U_k}(t)|^2}.$$

Let

$$K_{T,j,h}(x) = \frac{1}{2\pi}\int_{-\infty}^{\infty}\exp(-\imath tx)\phi_K(t)\phi_{U^F}(t/h)\Psi_j(t/h)dt.$$

Carroll et al. (2009) proposed to estimate $m(x)$ by

$$\widetilde{m}(x) = \frac{\sum_j Y_j K_{T,j}\{(x-W_j)/h\}}{\sum_j K_{T,j}\{(x-W_j)/h\}}.$$

They showed that the estimator enjoys optimal accuracy, in the sense that the rates of weak convergence are the best possible. It is worth nothing that those rates can vary from parametric rates ($n^{-1/2}$) to much slower rates. The authors remarked that the results regarding the parametric rates do not suggest that it might be beneficial to artificially add noises to some of the data.

## 14.3 Unbiased Score Method

Unbiased scores approach is a method used to derive an estimator for the error-in case from the error-free one. See Stefanski and Carroll (1987) and Stefanski (1989) for an introduction to the methods. Briefly, suppose in an error-free case an unknown true parameter is denoted by $\theta_0$ and there exists $\Phi(\cdot)$ such that $\mathrm{E}\{\Phi(Y, X, \theta_0)\} = 0$. Then $\theta_0$ can be estimated by $\widehat{\theta}$ satisfying

$$\frac{1}{n}\sum_{i=1}^{n}\Phi(Y_i, X_i, \widehat{\theta}) = 0.$$

Under general regularity conditions, the asymptotic normality and consistency of $\widehat{\theta}$ can be easily proved. Assume there is a function $\Psi(\cdot)$, such that

$E\{\Psi(Y,W,\theta_0)|Y,X\} = \Phi(Y,X,\theta_0)$. Then an estimator defined as a solution of

$$\frac{1}{n}\sum_{i=1}^{n}\Psi(Y_i,W_i,\widehat{\theta}) = 0$$

would be consistent and asymptotically normal and is known as an unbiased score estimator.

One can show that an estimator of the form (14.9) is an unbiased score estimator. Since $\widehat{m}(x)$ in (14.2) is a solution of

$$\frac{1}{nh}\sum_{i=1}^{n}\left\{m(x)K\left(\frac{x-X_i}{h}\right) - Y_iK\left(\frac{x-X_i}{h}\right)\right\} = 0,$$

an estimator

$$\frac{(nh)^{-1}\sum_{i=1}^{n}Y_iL\left(\frac{x-W_i}{h}\right)}{(nh)^{-1}\sum_{i=1}^{n}L\left(\frac{x-W_i}{h}\right)},$$

is an estimator of $m(x)$ based on unbiased score when $X_i$s are mismeasured, where $L(\cdot)$ is such that

$$E\{L(x-W_i)/h|X_i\} = K\{(x-X_i)/h\}.$$

Delaigle et al. (2009) showed that $L(x) = K_U(x)$, where $K_U(x)$ is a deconvolution kernel (14.8).

In general it is really hard to solve the equation above in its original form and simulations based methods are warranted (see Section 14.3.1 for details). However, an unbiased score equation is turned out to be much simpler if it is formulated in the Fourier domain. See Section 14.3.2 for details on how this observation led to a solution to the general problem of local polynomial estimators in the errors-in-variable case.

### 14.3.1 Monte Carlo Methods

McIntyre et al. (2018) and McIntyre and Stefanski (2011) proposed a simulation based kernel estimator inspired by the unbiased scoring method. Specifically, they considered the problem with replicated measurements for the $r$th subject, $(Y_{rj}, W_{rj})$, $r = 1,\cdots,n$, $j = 1,\cdots,m_r$ and measurement errors $U_{rj}$ to follow the normal distribution with means zero and unknown variances $\sigma_r^2$. Let $\bar{Y}_r$ be a sample mean of $Y_{rj}$, $\bar{W}_r$ and $\widehat{\sigma}_r^2$ be the sample mean and the sample variance of the $W_{rj}$s. Define $T_r = Z_{r1}(Z_{r1}^2+\cdots+Z_{rm_r-1}^2)^{-1/2}$, where the $Z_{rj}$s are a random sample of standard normal variables. Then the proposed estimator is

$$\widehat{m}(x) = \frac{\sum_{r=1}^{n}\bar{Y}_rK_r^*(x,\bar{W}_r,\widehat{\sigma}_r^2,m_r,\lambda,T_r)}{\sum_{r=1}^{n}K_r^*(x,\bar{W}_r,\widehat{\sigma}_r^2,m_r,\lambda,T_r)}, \tag{14.11}$$

where

$$K_r^*(x, \bar{W}_r, \widehat{\sigma}_r^2, m_r, \lambda, T_r) = \mathrm{E}\left\{K\left(\Lambda(x, \bar{W}_r, \widehat{\sigma}_r^2, m_r, T_r)/\lambda\right) \Big| \bar{W}_r, \widehat{\sigma}_r^2\right\}$$

with $\Lambda(x, \bar{W}_r, \widehat{\sigma}_r^2, m_r, T_r) = x - [\bar{W}_r + \imath\{(m_r - 1)/m_r\}^{1/2}\widehat{\sigma}_r T_r]$. Here, $K(\cdot)$ is a probability density that is entire on a complex plane, $\lambda > 0$ is a bandwidth parameter. McIntyre and Stefanski (2011) showed that the estimator $K_r^*(\cdot)$ is unbiased estimator of the deconvolution kernel of Stefanski and Carroll (1990) for the case of normal measurement error with variance $\sigma_r^2/m_r$

$$\mathrm{E}\{K_r^*(x, \bar{W}_r, \widehat{\sigma}_r^2, m_r, \lambda, T_r)|X_r\} = K\left(\frac{x - X_r}{\lambda}\right).$$

Note that even though $K(\cdot)$ is complex-valued, its expectation, $K^*(\cdot)$ is real-valued. In most cases, $K_r^*(\cdot)$ does not have a simple closed-form expression. Monte Carlo approximations to the conditional expectations can be used to compute $K_r^*(\cdot)$ and (14.11), respectively. For $b = 1, \cdots, B$, let $T_{r1}, \cdots, T_{rb}$ be independent replicates of $T_r$. Then Monte Carlo approximation of (14.11) is

$$\widehat{m}(x) = \frac{\sum_{r=1}^n \bar{Y}_r \sum_{b=1}^B \mathrm{Re}\left\{K\left(\Lambda(x, \bar{W}_r, \widehat{\sigma}_r^2, m_r, T_{rb})/\lambda\right)\right\}}{\sum_{r=1}^n \sum_{b=1}^B \mathrm{Re}\left\{K\left(\Lambda(x, \bar{W}_r, \widehat{\sigma}_r^2, m_r, T_{rb})/\lambda\right)\right\}}.$$

When $m_r = 2$ for all $r$, the estimator simplifies and may be computed without Monte Carlo simulation (McIntyre and Stefanski, 2011). McIntyre et al. (2018) provided arguments establishing the pointwise consistency of their estimators.

### 14.3.2 Local Polynomial Estimators

Recall that in the error-free case (Fan and Gijbels, 2003), the local polynomial estimator of order $p$ of $m(x)$ can be written as

$$\widehat{m}(x) = e_1^\top \widehat{\mathbf{S}}_n^{-1} \widehat{\mathbf{T}}_n,$$

where $e_1 = (1, 0, \cdots, 0)^\top$, $\widehat{\mathbf{S}}_n = (\widehat{S}_{n,k,k'})_{0 \le k,k' \le p}$ is a $(p+1) \times (p+1)$ matrix, with

$$\widehat{S}_{n,k,k'} = \frac{1}{nh^{k+k'+1}} \sum_{j=1}^n K\left(\frac{X_j - x}{h}\right)(X_j - x)^{k+k'}, \quad k, k' = 0, \cdots, p, \quad (14.12)$$

and $\widehat{\mathbf{T}}_n = (\widehat{T}_{n,0}, \cdots, \widehat{T}_{n,p})^\top$, with

$$\widehat{T}_{n,k} = \frac{1}{nh^{k+1}} \sum_{j=1}^n Y_j K\left(\frac{X_j - x}{h}\right)(X_j - x)^k. \quad (14.13)$$

To construct a consistent estimator of $m(\cdot)$ that can be computed from errors-in data $(Y_i, W_i)$, Delaigle et al. (2009) suggested replacing $\widehat{\mathbf{S}}_n$ and $\widehat{\mathbf{T}}_n$ by unbiased scores. Specifically, they offered functions $L_l$ that satisfy

$$\mathrm{E}\left\{L_l\left(\frac{W_j - x}{h}\right)(W_j - x)^l | X_j\right\} = K\left(\frac{X_j - x}{h}\right)(X_j - x)^l, \quad l = 0, \cdots, 2p.$$

The key to finding such functions is to solve Fourier version of the above equality. The details and conditions for interchangeability of integration and expectation, and derivative and integration can be found in Delaigle et al. (2009). The following is deduced from the Fourier inversion theorem, given that the conditions for expressions to be well defined are met:

$$L_l(x) = \imath^{-l} x^{-l} \frac{1}{2\pi} \int \exp(-\imath t x) \phi_K^{(l)}(t) / \phi_U(t/h) dt,$$

where $(l)$ denotes the $l$th derivative. Then,

$$\begin{aligned} \widehat{S}_{n,k,k'} &= \frac{1}{nh^{k+k'+1}} \sum_{j=1}^{n} L_{k+k'}\left(\frac{X_j - x}{h}\right)(X_j - x)^{k+k'}; \\ \widehat{T}_{n,k} &= \frac{1}{nh^{k+1}} \sum_{j=1}^{n} Y_j L_k \left(\frac{X_j - x}{h}\right)(X_j - x)^k; \end{aligned}$$

$k, k' = 0, \cdots, p$. Note that the estimator of Fan and Truong (1993) is a special case with $p = 0$.

The authors showed asymptotic normality of their estimators and derived their asymptotic bias and variance. Delaigle et al. (2009) showed that the bias of their estimator is exactly the same as the bias of the local polynomial estimator in the error-free case. As in the case of Nadaraya-Watson estimators (Fan and Truong, 1993), the measurement errors only affect the variance of the estimator. The optimal bandwidth is found by the usual trade-off between the squared bias and the variance.

The authors mentioned the fact that their estimator enjoys the design-adaptive property similar to error- free case discussed in Fan and Gijbels (2003). Moreover these estimators provide a natural and elegant solution to the problem of derivative estimation.

Delaigle et al. (2009) showed that, for $p = 1$, the proposed estimator is different from that of Fan and Truong (1993), but it converges at the same rate. For $p > 1$, the local polynomial estimator converges at faster rates, which is the main advantages of local polynomial estimators over the Nadaraya Watson one which corresponds to $p = 0$. In theory, a higher order of polynomial should lead to theoretical improvements. However, in practice, the order of $p > 1$ is not noticeable in finite samples. The authors discussed various generalizations of their estimators e.g. the case of unknown error distribution and heteroscedastic measurement errors.

Huang and Zhou (2017) proposed a new estimator, which is a clever spin of the following equality

$$m^{nv}(w)f_W(w) = (mf_X) * f_U(w),$$

where $m^{nv}(w) := \mathrm{E}(Y|W = w)$ and $(mf_X) * f_U(w)$ is a convolution given by $\int_{-\infty}^{+\infty} m(x)f_X(x)f_U(w - x)dx$. So the local polynomial of order $p$ from Huang and Zhou (2017), assuming all the relevant Fourier transforms are well defined and $\phi_U(\cdot)$ never vanish, is

$$\widehat{m}_{HZ}(x) = \frac{1}{2\pi}\frac{\int_{-\infty}^{+\infty} \exp(-\imath tx)\phi_{\widehat{m}^{nv}\widehat{f}_W}(t)/\phi_U(t)dt}{\widehat{f}_X(x)},$$

where $\widehat{f}_X(\cdot)$ is the deconvolution kernel density estimator of $f_X(\cdot)$ in Stefanski and Carroll (1990), and $\phi_{\widehat{m}^{nv}\widehat{f}_W}(\cdot)$ is the Fourier transform of $\widehat{m}^{nv}\widehat{f}_W$. $\widehat{m}^{nv}(\cdot)$ is the $p$-th order local polynomial estimator of $m^{nv}(\cdot)$, which results from replacing $X_j$s by $W_j$s in (14.12) and (14.13). $\widehat{f}_W(\cdot)$ is the regular kernel density estimator of $f_W(\cdot)$ (Fan and Gijbels, 2003).

It can be shown that, when $p = 0$, this new estimator is the same as the estimator given by Delaigle et al. (2009), both reducing to the local constant estimator in Fan and Truong (1993). Other than this special case, these two estimators differ in general. Huang and Zhou (2017) studied asymptotic properties of the proposed estimators. They proved asymptotic normality and derived the asymptotic bias and variance of the proposed estimators. Huang and Zhou (2017) used similar regularity conditions as in Delaigle et al. (2009). Through numerical studies the authors showed that their estimators are comparable in performance to Delaigle et al. (2009).

## 14.4 Implementation

One can encounter significant difficulties when computing estimators in practice. In Section 14.4.1 we discuss common problems related to numerical integration and divisions associated with (14.9). However, the biggest challenge in implementation of nonparametric estimators is their reliance on the bandwidth. We introduce one of the most prominent methods for bandwidth selection (Section 14.4.2).

There is an R package called `decon` developed by Wang and Wang (2011) aims to implement the deconvolution estimator. However, the latest available version 1.2 − 4 of this package has been criticized by Delaigle (2014) as it suffers from a number of problems with bandwidth selection. Specifically, the default bandwidth option for the errors-in-variables local constant estimator is a bandwidth from the density estimation part whose initial guess does not have the correct theoretical order of magnitude.

There is another R package on GitHub called `deconvolve` developed by Delaigle et al. (2021), which offers solutions to deconvolution problems with homoscedastic and heteroscedastic errors. The bandwidth selection methods include plug-in estimators, SIMEX and cross-validation for homoscedastic errors only.

### 14.4.1 Numerical Instability of the Estimators

While the choice of the kernel is usually not that important in error-free estimation, one needs to be careful when choosing kernel in (14.9) so that the integral in (14.8) exists. This is not trivial, as for example Gaussian kernel with normal measurement errors would result in a deconvolution kernel valid only for large $h$. Delaigle and Gijbels (2007) discussed some issues related to numerical integration when computing valid deconvolution kernel $K_U(\cdot)$ as in most cases there is no closed form analytical expression for it. Moreover, in practice estimators can be numerically unstable when either numerator or denominator or both take unusual values. Delaigle et al. (2008) suggested ridge estimator when the denominator takes unusually small values. See Section 14.2.3.1. When the numerator is too large at certain values, Delaigle (2014) suggested a following practical strategy. Under the regularity conditions, $m(x)$ should lie close to most of points $Y_i$s for which the $X_i$s are close to $x$. In particular, as $n$ increases, $m(x)$ is expected to lie inside $[q_{0.05,x}, q_{0.95,x}]$, where $q_{\alpha,x}$ denotes the $\alpha$-level quantile of the $Y_i$s whose $X_i$s are in a small neighborhood of $x$. Since the $X_i$s are not observed, it is suggested to calculate quantiles for $Y_i$s for which the $W_i$s $\in [x - \sigma_U, x + \sigma_U]$, where $\sigma_U^2 = \text{Var}(U)$. Hence the corrected estimator would be

$$\begin{aligned}\widetilde{m}(x) = {} & \widehat{m}(x) I\{\widehat{m}(x) \in [q_{0.05,x}, q_{0.95,x}]\} \\ & + q_{0.05,x} I\{\widehat{m}(x) < q_{0.05,x}) + q_{0.95,x} I\{\widehat{m}(x) > q_{0.95,x}\}.\end{aligned}$$

### 14.4.2 Bandwidth Selection

Recall that the criterion for the bandwidth selection is the mean integrated squared error (MISE), defined by

$$\text{MISE}(h) = \text{E}\left[\int_{-\infty}^{+\infty} \{\widehat{m}(x) - m(x)\}^2 f_X(x) dx\right].$$

Plug-in methods minimize the approximated MISE and work well for error free cases. However, they are difficult to implement in the case of measurement errors because such bandwidths depend not only on smoothness of $m(\cdot)$, but on a tail behavior of $\phi_U(\cdot)$ (see Section 14.2.2.1).

The conventional cross-validation (CV) bandwidth $h_0$ is

$$h_0 = \text{argmin}_{h>0} \frac{1}{n} \sum_{j=1}^{n} \{Y_j - \widehat{m}_{-j}(X_j; h)\}^2 \omega(X_j),$$

where $\widehat{m}_{-j}(\cdot)$ denotes the version of $\widehat{m}(\cdot)$, computed from a reduced sample with the omitted $j$th observation. The nonnegative function $\omega(\cdot)$ represents a weight, used to reduce the effects of greater variability when attempting to estimate $m(x)$ for values of $x$ that lie in the tails of the distribution of $X$. But the $X_j$s are not observable, and so the straightforward implementation of cross-validation is infeasible.

The best solution to this problem was offered by Delaigle and Hall (2008). They adopted the simulation-extrapolation algorithm (SIMEX, Cook and Stefanski, 1994) into a bandwidth selector. Delaigle et al. (2008) advocated adding whole measurement errors in two steps as follows.

The method entails using Monte Carlo simulation to add additional multiples of measurement errors to the observed data. Specifically, let $U_1^*, \cdots, U_n^*$ and $U_1^{**}, \cdots, U_n^{**}$ denote independent and identically distributed random variables, also independent of the $(Y_i, W_i)$s and having the distribution of $U$. Let $W_j^* = W_j + U_j$ and $W_j^{**} = W_j + U_j^* + U_j^{**}$. Consider the problem of estimating $m^*(\cdot) = \text{E}(Y|W = x)$ from the contaminated data $(Y_j, W_j^*)$ and of estimating $m^{**}(\cdot) = \text{E}(Y|W^* = x)$ from values of $(Y_j, W_j^{**})$. Since the $W_i$s and $W_i^*$s are known, the standard cross-validation can be calculated over a grid of candidate bandwidths. To reduce the effects of individual $(W^*, W^{**})$, the cross-validation scores are averaged over a number of Monte Carlo replicates, and this average is then used to identify the bandwidths $h_1$ and $h_2$ that minimize the scores based on the $(Y_j, W_j^*)$s and the $(Y_j, W_j^{**})$s, respectively. Note that $W^{**}$ relates to $W^*$ in the same way as $W^*$ to $W$, and $W$ to $X$. Thus we expect the relationship between $h_0$ and $h_1$ to be similar to that between $h_1$ and $h_2$. The linear back extrapolation step in the SIMEX leads to $h_0 = h_l^2/h_2$. A more general approach that leads to a 'composite bandwidth' was also discussed.

## 14.5 Contemporary Topics

There is a number of topics which are considered as active research in the area of nonparametric measurement errors models. Below we discuss a few of the directions for which some work has been done recently but there are open problems associated with them.

### 14.5.1 Confidence Interval and Bands

Confidence intervals and bands are an informative way of quantifying the reliability of estimators. Delaigle et al. (2015) offered methodologies for constructing pointwise confidence intervals and confidence bands. The authors showed that the problem is more complex than in the standard error-free settings. Specifically, they argued that the asymptotic variance of the deconvolution kernel estimator of $m(\cdot)$ is non-trivial to estimate and thus inference based on limiting distributions is difficult to implement. Delaigle et al. (2015) focused on bootstrap based percentile methods, which estimate variance implicitly. However, it is not straightforward to devise a way to implement bootstrap for inference on $m(\cdot)$ due to the unobservability of $X$ in data. The authors proposed novel techniques for bootstrap sampling and tuning parameter choice aimed at minimizing the coverage error of confidence bands we briefly discuss next.

Let $U^* = \{U_i^*\}_{i=1}^n$, $X^* = \{X^*\}_{i=1}^n$ and $\epsilon^* = \{\epsilon^*\}_{i=1}^n$ denote samples drawn by sampling randomly from the distributions with distribution functions $F_U(\cdot)$, $\widehat{F}_X(\cdot)$, and $\widehat{F}_\epsilon(\cdot)$, respectively. It is assumed that the distribution of $U$ is known. The case when it has to be estimated from the data was discussed without formal theoretical results provided. $\widehat{F}_X(\cdot)$ is the estimator of $F_X(\cdot)$ with bandwidth as in Hall and Lahiri (2008). $\widehat{F}_\epsilon(\cdot)$ is constructed by moment matching because the proposed methods require the knowledge of first three moments only and not the entire $F_\epsilon(\cdot)$. The samples are drawn such that conditionally on the original data set, they are comprised of independent data which are independent of one another. Using the bootstrap data in place of the original data, the authors proposed to compute the bootstrap analogue $\widehat{m}^*(\cdot)$ of $\widehat{m}(\cdot)$. Delaigle et al. (2015) showed that with carefully chosen bandwidths, the distribution of $\widehat{m}(\cdot) - m(\cdot)$ resembles the distribution of $\widehat{m}^*(\cdot) - \widehat{m}(\cdot)$.

For the nominal coverage of the confidence band to be $1-\alpha$, where $0 < \alpha < 1$, the authors defined a nominal $1 - \alpha/2$ level percentile pointwise confidence band for $m(\cdot)$, constructed over the compact interval $I$, by

$$\{(x, y) : x \in I \text{ and } \widehat{m}(x) - \widehat{t}_{1-\alpha/2}(x) \leq y \leq \widehat{m}(x) - \widehat{t}_{\alpha/2}(x)\},$$

where, $\widehat{t}_{1-\alpha/2}(x)$ and $\widehat{t}_{\alpha/2}(x)$ are quantities to ensure that

$$\begin{aligned} &P\{\widehat{m}^*(x) - \widehat{m}(x) \leq \widehat{t}_{1-\alpha/2}(x)|(Y_i, W_i)_{i=1}^n\} \\ &\qquad = P\{\widehat{m}^*(x) - \widehat{m}(x) > \widehat{t}_{\alpha/2}(x)|(Y_i, W_i)_{i=1}^n\} = \alpha/2. \end{aligned}$$

The quantiles $\widehat{t}_{\alpha/2}$ and $\widehat{t}_{1-\alpha/2}$ are computed as the empirical quantiles obtained from $B$ bootstrap samples. Hence due to additional variability associated with the bootstrap distribution and the Monte Carlo approximation algorithm, the desired coverage can be achieved only approximately. To improve coverage accuracy, the authors suggested to calibrate the intervals through a standard double bootstrap method.

Delaigle et al. (2015) mentioned that their bootstrap methodology would be largely unchanged if the bands were simultaneous and the main alteration would be to the critical point determining interval width. However, their theoretical results do not formally cover that case.

### 14.5.2 Multivariate Regression

A number of authors, e.g., Fan and Masry (1992); Guo and Liu (2017); Han and Park (2018), considered the case when $X$, $W$ and $U$ are $d$-dimensional. Denote $\mathbf{X}_i = (X_{i1}, \cdots, X_{id})$, $\mathbf{W}_i = (W_{i1}, \cdots, W_{id})$ and $\mathbf{U}_i = (U_{i1}, \cdots, U_{id})$, respectively, so that the model becomes

$$Y_i = m(\mathbf{X}_i) + \epsilon_i, \quad \mathbf{W}_i = \mathbf{X}_i + \mathbf{U}_i, \quad i = 1, \cdots, n.$$

The authors assumed that $\mathbf{U}_i$ are independent of $\mathbf{X}_i$ and have known densities. Fan and Masry (1992) and Guo and Liu (2017) utilized the multivariate kernel defined as a tensor product of one-dimensional ones

$$\mathbf{K}(\mathbf{x}) = \prod_{l=1}^{d} K(x_l), \quad \mathbf{x} \in \mathbb{R}^d, \quad x_l \in \mathbb{R}.$$

The multivariate Fourier transform is $\phi_{\mathbf{A}}(\mathbf{t}) = \int_{R^d} \exp(\imath \mathbf{t}^\top \mathbf{x}) f_{\mathbf{A}}(d\mathbf{x})$ and the multivariate deconvolution kernel becomes

$$\mathbf{K_U}(\mathbf{u}) = \frac{1}{(2\pi)^d} \int_{\mathbb{R}^d} \exp(-\imath \mathbf{t}^\top \mathbf{u}) \phi_{\mathbf{K}}(\mathbf{t}) / \phi_{\mathbf{U}}(\mathbf{t}/h) d\mathbf{t},$$

where $h > 0$ is a scalar bandwidth. Analogously to (14.9) the estimator of $m(\mathbf{x})$ becomes

$$\widehat{m}(\mathbf{x}) = \frac{(nh)^{-1} \sum_{i=1}^{n} Y_i \mathbf{K_U}\left(\frac{\mathbf{x} - \mathbf{W}_i}{h}\right)}{(nh)^{-1} \sum_{i=1}^{n} \mathbf{K_U}\left(\frac{\mathbf{x} - \mathbf{W}_i}{h}\right)}.$$

Fan and Masry (1992) introduced more general settings than mentioned above where they let $\{X_j\}_{j=-\infty}^{\infty}$ and $\{Y_j\}_{j=-\infty}^{\infty}$ be jointly stationary processes. The authors established asymptotic normality for both strongly mixing and $\rho$-mixing processes, when the error distribution function is either ordinarily smooth or super smooth.

Guo and Liu (2017) extended consistency theorems (Fan and Truong, 1993; Meister, 2009) from one to multidimensional settings, when a noise density has no zeros in the Fourier domain. Moreover they extended Delaigle and Meister (2011), and showed the desired convergence rate.

Han and Park (2018) assumed $m(\mathbf{X}) = m_1(X_{i1}) + \cdots + m_d(X_{di})$ and studied estimation of the additive regression model

$$Y_i = m_1(X_{i1}) + \cdots + m_d(X_{di}) + \epsilon_i.$$

The authors developed a new smooth backfitting method and theory for it. Specifically, they proposed a new kernel function that suitably deconvolves the measurement error density while keeping its integral along the line of local smoothing equal to one. The normalization property of the kernel function is required for a projection interpretation of the smooth backfitting method estimator, which is a key element in the theoretical development of the method.

The estimator can handle the cases of ordinary smooth errors while it cannot be easily adapted to the case of supersmooth measurement errors.

Han and Park (2018) proved that their method achieves the optimal rates of convergence in one-dimensional deconvolution problems when the smoothness of measurement error distribution is less than a threshold value; when it is above the threshold, convergence is slower than the univariate rate but still much faster than the optimal rate in multivariate deconvolution problem discussed above.

Lee et al. (2018) considered partially linear additive models where both parametric and nonparametric predictors are contaminated by errors. The authors utilized the smoothed normalized deconvolution kernel of Han and Park (2018) and only considered the case of ordinary smooth $f_U(\cdot)$, so that its characteristic function, $\phi_U(t)$ decays at a rate $|t|^{-\beta}$ as $|t| \to \infty$ for some $\beta > 0$. The proposed estimator of a parametric part achieves $\sqrt{n}$-consistency when $\beta < 1/2$. In the case $\beta \geq 1/2$, the estimator has the rate $O_p(n^{-1/(1+2\beta)})$. Furthermore, they suggested an estimator of the additive function in the nonparametric part that achieves the optimal one-dimensional convergence rates in nonparametric deconvolution problems similar to Han and Park (2018).

## Bibliography

Butucea, C. and Matias, C. (2005). Minimax estimation of the noise level and of the deconvolution density in a semiparametric convolution model. *Bernoulli*, 11(2), 309-340.

Carroll, R. J., Delaigle, A., and Hall, P. (2009). Nonparametric prediction in measurement error models. *Journal of the American Statistical Association*, 104(487), 993-1003.

Carroll, R. J. and Hall, P. (1988). Optimal rates of convergence for deconvolving a density. *Journal of the American Statistical Association*, 83(404), 1184-1186.

Carroll, R. J. and Hall, P. (2004). Low-order approximations in deconvolution and regression with errors in variables. *Journal of the Royal Statistical Society, Series B*, 66, 31-46.

Carroll, R. J., Ruppert, D., Stefanski, L. A., and Crainiceanu, C. M. (2006). *Measurement Error in Nonlinear Models: A Modern Perspective*, 2nd ed. Chapman and Hall, New York.

Cook, J. R. and Stefanski, L. A. (1994). Simulation-extrapolation estimation in parametric measurement error models. *Journal of the American Statistical Association*, 86, 1314-1328.

Delaigle, A. (2014). Nonparametric kernel methods with errors-in-variables: Constructing estimators, computing them, and avoiding common mistakes. *Australian & New Zealand Journal of Statistics*, 56, 105-124.

Delaigle, A. (2021). Deconvolution kernel density estimator. In *Handbook of Measurement Error Models*, G. Y. Yi, A. Delaigle, and P. Gustafson (Eds), CRC, Chapter 10.

Delaigle, A. and Gijbels, I. (2007). Frequent problems in calculating integrals and optimizing objective functions: A case study in density deconvolution. *Statistics and Computing*, 17, 349-355.

Delaigle, A. and Hall, P. (2008). Using SIMEX for smoothing-parameter choice in errors-in-variables problems. *Journal of the American Statistical Association*, 103(481), 280-287.

Delaigle, A. and Hall, P. (2016). Methodology for non-parametric deconvolution when the error distribution is unknown. *Journal of the Royal Statistical Society, Series B*, 78(1), 231-252.

Delaigle, A., Hall, P., and Jamshidi, F. (2015). Confidence bands in nonparametric errors-invariables regression. *Journal of the Royal Statistical Society, Series B*, 77(1), 149-169.

Delaigle, A., Hall, P., and Meister, A. (2008). On deconvolution with repeated measurements. *The Annals of Statistics*, 36(2), 665-685.

Delaigle, A., Hyndman, T., and Wang, T. (2021). Deconvolve: Deconvolution tools for measurement error problems. R package version 0.1.0.

Delaigle, A. and Meister, A. (2007). Nonparametric regression estimation in the heteroscedastic errors-in-variables problem. *Journal of the American Statistical Association*, 102(480), 1416-1426.

Delaigle, A. and Meister, A. (2011). Rate-optimal nonparametric estimation in classical and Berkson errors-in-variables problems. *Journal of Statistical Planning and Inference*, 141(1), 102-114.

Delaigle, A. and Van Keilegom, I. (2021). Deconvolution with unknown error distribution. In *Handbook of Measurement Error Models*, G. Y. Yi, A. Delaigle, and P. Gustafson (Eds), Chapter 12.

Fan, J. (1991). On the optimal rates of convergence for nonparametric deconvolution problems. *The Annals of Statistics*, 19(3), 1257-1272.

Fan, J. and Gijbels, I. (2003). *Local Polynomial Modelling and its Applications.* CRC Press, Boca Raton.

Fan, J. and Masry, E. (1992). Multivariate regression estimation with errors-invariables: asymptotic normality for mixing processes. *Journal of Multivariate Analysis*, 43, 237-271.

Fan, J. and Truong, Y. K. (1993). Nonparametric regression with errors in variables. *The Annals of Statistics*, 21, 1900-1925.

Fuller, W. A. (1987). *Measurement Error Models.* New York: John Wiley and Sons.

Guo, H. J. and Liu, Y. M. (2017). Convergence rates of multivariate regression estimators with errors-in-variables. *Numerical Functional Analysis and Optimization*, 38(12), 1564-1584.

Hall, P. and Lahiri, S. (2008). Estimation of distributions, moments and quantiles in deconvolution problems. *Annals of Statistics*, 36(5), 2110-2134.

Hall, P. and Meister, A. (2007). A ridge-parameter approach to deconvolution. *The Annals of Statistics*, 35(4), 1535-1558.

Han, K. and Park, B. U. (2018). Smooth backfitting for errors-in-variables additive models. *The Annals of Statistics*, 46, 2216-2250.

Huang, X. and Zhou, H. (2017). An alternative local polynomial estimator for the error-in-variables problem. *Journal of Nonparametric Statistics*, 29(2), 301-325.

Johannes, J. (2009). Deconvolution with unknown error distribution. *The Annals of Statistics*, 37(5A), 2301-2323.

Kang, Y. and Qiu, P. (2021). Nonparametric deconvolution by Fourier transformation and other related approaches. In *Handbook of Measurement Error Models*, G. Y. Yi, A. Delaigle, and P. Gustafson (Eds), CRC, Chapter 11.

Lee, E. R., Han, K., and Park, B. (2018). Estimation of errors-in-variables partially linear additive models. *Statistica Sinica*, 28, 2353-2373.

Liang, H. (2000). Asymptotic normality of parametric part in partially linear models with measurement error in the nonparametric part. *Journal of Statistical Planning and Inference*, 86(1), 51-62.

McIntyre, J., Johnson, B., and Rappaport, S. (2018). Monte Carlo methods for nonparametric regression with heteroscedastic measurement error. *Biometrics*, 74(2), 498-505.

McIntyre, J. and Stefanski, L. (2011). Regression-assisted deconvolution. *Statistics in Medicine*, 30(14), 1722-1734.

Meister, A. (2004). On the effect of misspecifying the error density in a deconvolution problem. *Canadian Journal of Statistics*, 32(4), 439-449.

Meister, A. (2006). Density estimation with normal measurement error with unknown variance. *Statistica Sinica*, 16, 195-211.

Meister, A. (2009). *Deconvolution Problems in Nonparametric Statistics.* Springer-Verlag, Berlin/Heidelberg.

Schennach, S. M. (2016). Recent advances in the measurement error literature. *Annual Review of Economics*, 8, 341-377.

Song, W. (2021). Nonparametric inference methods for Berkson errors. In *Handbook of Measurement Error Models*, G. Y. Yi, A. Delaigle, and P. Gustafson (Eds), CRC, Chapter 13.

Stefanski, L. (1989). Unbiased estimation of a nonlinear function of a normal mean with application to measurement error models. *Communications in Statistics. Theory and Methods*, 18(12), 4335-4358.

Stefanski, L. and Carroll, R. J. (1987). Conditional scores and optimal scores for generalized linear measurement-error models. *Biometrika*, 74(4), 703-716.

Stefanski, L. and Carroll, R. J. (1990). Deconvolving kernel density estimators. *Statistics*, 21(2), 169-184.

Wang, X. and Wang, B. (2011). Deconvolution estimation in measurement error models: The R packages. *Journal of Statistical Software*, 39(10), 1-24.

# Part V

# Applications

# 15

# *Covariate Measurement Error in Survival Data*

**Jeffrey S. Buzas**

## CONTENTS



## 15.1 Introduction

In the absence of covariate measurement error, the analysis of time to event data presents challenges beyond those in ordinary regression modeling. Survival data are typically skewed, have some form of censoring or truncation and

DOI: 10.1201/9781315101279-15

may have time dependent covariates. Semi-parametric regression models are also widely used for modeling survival data. Modeling and estimation methods for survival data must account for these features.

Adjusting for covariate measurement error adds to the above challenges, and many approaches that have been developed for general measurement error problems either do not directly apply to survival models, or need significant modification.

The measurement error literature on survival models developed rapidly in the years after Prentice (1982) published his seminal article. The voluminous literature on measurement error methods for survival data can easily overwhelm an analyst or researcher new to the field. The purpose of this chapter is to describe the effects of covariate measurement error in survival analysis models, and to provide a broad overview of the field, including an introduction to several approaches that correct for covariate measurement error induced bias. The chapter is not a step-by-step guide to analyzing data, nor does it delve too deeply into technical details. It is also not comprehensive–there are too many flavors of survival models, measurement error models and proposals for adjustment to consider here.

Other excellent overviews of adjusting for covariate measurement error in survival models include Prentice (2005), and the relevant chapters in Carroll et al. (2006) and Yi (2017).

This chapter is organized as follows. The first section reviews features of survival models and data in the absence of measurement error. Models for covariate measurement error are then considered, followed by a discussion of the effects of measurement error on parameter estimation. Several approaches to correcting for the effects of covariate measurement error are then described, including regression calibration, SIMEX (Simulation-extrapolation), likelihood methods and Bayesian methods. The chapter closes with a discussion and conclusions.

## 15.2 Overview of Survival Models

The purpose of this section is to review the fundamental concepts in survival models, including hazard functions, regression models, censoring and likelihoods.

### 15.2.1 Hazard Function

The hazard function occupies a central place in the modeling and analysis of survival data. The hazard function is defined as

$$\lambda(t) = \lim_{\Delta t \to 0^+} \frac{P(t < T \leq t + \Delta t \mid T \geq t)}{\Delta t} \qquad \text{for} \quad t \geq 0,$$

and can be interpreted as the rate of change of the probability of surviving just beyond time $t$ conditional on surviving up to time $t$. Noting that $\lambda(t)\Delta t \approx P(t < T \leq t + \Delta t \mid T \geq t)$, the hazard can be also be interpreted as proportional to the probability of a death in the interval $(t, t + \Delta t)$ given survival up to time $t$. The ease of interpretation is why it is common to formulate models in terms of the hazard function.

A straightforward calculation shows that

$$\lambda(t) = \frac{f(t)}{1 - F(t)} = -\frac{d}{dt}\log(1 - F(t)),$$

where $f(t)$ and $F(t)$ are the density and distribution functions for $T$, respectively. Then $F(t) = 1 - \exp(-\Lambda(t))$ where $\Lambda(t) = \int_0^t \lambda(u)du$ is the cumulative hazard function, showing that the hazard determines $F(\cdot)$ and vice-versa. Therefore, to model and compare survival functions we can model hazard functions. The *survivor function*, $S(t) = 1 - F(t)$, is also commonly used in survival data modeling.

**Example:** (Exponential) For $t > 0$, the exponential distribution with mean $1/\eta$ has density and survivor functions $f(t) = \eta e^{-\eta t}$, $S(t) = e^{-\eta t}$ and hazard $\lambda(t) = f(t)/S(t) = \eta$. Note that the hazard is constant with respect to time $t$, a result of the memoryless property of the exponential distribution.

**Example** (Weibull): The Weibull is a generalization of the exponential, with density, survivor and hazard functions $f(t) = p(\eta t)^{p-1}\eta e^{-(\eta t)^p}$; $S(t) = e^{-(\eta t)^p}$ and $\lambda(t) = \eta p(\eta t)^{p-1}$, where $\eta$ and $p$ are positive constants. There is significant flexibility modeling the hazard function by varying $p$ and $\eta$, including constant hazard ($p = 1$), linear hazard ($p = 2$) and increasing hazard $p \geq 1$ and decreasing hazard ($0 < p < 1$). However, the Weibull hazard is necessarily monotonic, precluding its use in some applications.

**Example** (Piecewise constant): A piecewise constant hazard can adapt to most hazard shapes and is commonly used, perhaps most often to model the baseline hazard in proportional hazards models. It is straightforward to understand and estimate using likelihood or Bayesian methods. The idea is to a priori choose a sequence of constants $0 = a_0 < a_1 < \cdots < a_K = \infty$ where $a_{K-1}$ is chosen so that the probability that $T_i > a_{K-1}$ is essentially zero. Let $A_k = (a_{k-1}, a_k]$ for $k = 1, \ldots, K$ and let $\rho = (\rho_1, \rho_2, \ldots, \rho_K)^T$ be a vector of parameters. The piecewise constant hazard is defined as

$$\lambda(t) = \sum_{k=1}^{K} \rho_k I(t \in A_k), \tag{15.1}$$

where $I(\cdot)$ is the indicator function. The cumulative hazard is then $\Lambda(t) = \sum_{k=1}^{K} \rho_k u_k(t)$ where $u_k(t) = |A_k \cap (0, t]|$ is the length of intersection of $A_k$ with $(0, t]$. As noted in Yi (2017), $K$ in the range of 4 to 6 often works well, and the

$a_k$ are commonly chosen so that the intervals $(a_{k-1}, a_k]$ contain approximately equal numbers of observed failures. Using this prescription, the $a_k$ are not chosen a priori and the uncertainty in defining the $a_k$ could be accounted for in an analysis, though this is likely rarely done.

Note when $K = 1$, the piecewise constant model reduces to the exponential model with constant hazard over $[0, \infty)$.

### 15.2.2 Regression Models

There are two primary classes of regression models in use for survival data, namely accelerated failure time models (AFT) and proportional hazards models (PH). Let $\lambda_0(t)$ and $S_0(t)$ be baseline hazard and survivor functions corresponding to a random variable $T_0$ and $Z$ a vector of covariates.

AFT models are defined as follows. Let $T = e^{-Z^T\beta}T_0$ where $\beta$ is a vector of parameters. Then the survivor and hazard functions of $T$ are $S(t \mid Z) = S(te^{Z^T\beta}))$ and $\lambda(t \mid Z) = e^{Z^T\beta}\lambda_0(te^{Z^T\beta})$. AFT models are related to linear models as follows. Let $Y = \log T$. Then $Y = -Z^T\beta + \log T_0 = -Z^T\beta + \epsilon$ where $\epsilon = \log T_0$ is the random error term.

The PH models assume that $\lambda(t \mid Z) = e^{Z^T\beta}\lambda_0(t)$. Note that for covariate vectors $Z_1$ and $Z_2$,

$$\frac{\lambda(t \mid Z_1)}{\lambda(t \mid Z_2)} = e^{(Z_1 - Z_2)^T\beta},$$

which does not depend on $t$, i.e. the hazards are proportional.

To aid in understanding the effects of covariates on the AFT and PH models, consider two observations $T_1$ and $T_2$ for two subjects with covariate vectors $Z_1$ and $Z_2$ such that $e^{Z_1^T\beta} = 1$ and $e^{Z_2^T\beta} = 2$. Then for the PH model, $\lambda(t \mid Z_1) = \lambda_0(t)$ and $\lambda(t \mid Z_2) = 2\lambda_0(t)$. In other words, the *hazard* is twice as large for the subject with covariate vector $Z_2$.

For the AFT model, $\Pr(T_1 \geq t) = S(t)$ and $\Pr(T_2 \geq t) = S(2t)$, demonstrating that the covariates directly affect the survivor function. Furthermore, for the AFT model it can be shown that $E[T_2] = \frac{1}{2}E[T_1]$, providing a very straightforward interpretation; the subject with covariate vector $Z_1$ is expected to live twice as long as the subject with covariate $Z_2$. Analogous identities hold for relations between the median and any other percentile for the two subjects.

Additive hazards have also been considered for modeling survival data. However, they will not be considered in this chapter. See Yi (2017) for a summary of approaches to ameliorating the effects of covariate measurement error for additive hazards models.

### 15.2.3 Censoring

A distinctive and common feature of survival data is that the survival time is not always observed, but rather is censored. This is not a missing data problem. Right censoring is when we do not observe the survival time but know it is greater than some value $C_R$. Left censoring is when we only know the survival time is less than a value $C_L$. Interval censoring occurs when we only know that $C_L < T < C_R$ for known values $C_L$ and $C_R$ with $C_L < C_R$. Survival data can also be truncated. Only right censoring is considered in this chapter.

### 15.2.4 Likelihoods

We begin the subsection with a representation of the full likelihood for right censored data in the absence of measurement error, and follow with the definition of the partial likelihood used for estimation and inference in the semi-parametric proportional hazards model.

The construction of the likelihood in the absence of measurement error typically assumes the failure time and censoring time are independent conditional on the covariates, i.e. that $f(t, c \mid z) = f(t \mid z)f(c \mid z)$. Let $T_i$ denote the survival time, $C_i$ the censoring time, $\delta_i = I(T_i \leq C_i)$ and $t_i = \min(T_i, C_i)$. The likelihood for the observed data is then ( Kalbfleisch and Prentice, 2002)

$$L = \prod_{i=1}^{n} L_i = \prod_{i=1}^{n} (f(t_i \mid Z_i))^{\delta_i} (S(t_i \mid Z_i))^{1-\delta_i}$$
$$= \prod_{i=1}^{n} (\lambda(t_i \mid Z_i))^{\delta_i} S(t_i \mid Z_i). \tag{15.2}$$

For fully parametric models, parameter estimation can be achieved via maximum likelihood. For the semi-parametric PH models, the likelihood depends on the unspecified baseline hazard $\lambda_0(t)$, and typically partial likelihood, which is not dependent on $\lambda_0(t)$, is used for estimation. The partial likelihood function is given by

$$L_{P,i} = \prod_{i=1}^{n} \left\{ \frac{\lambda(t_i \mid Z_i)}{\sum_{j=1}^{n} R_j(t_i)\lambda(t_i \mid Z_j)} \right\}^{\delta_i}, \tag{15.3}$$

where $R_j(t_i) = I(t_j \geq t_i)$.

For the PH model $\lambda(t \mid X, Z) = \lambda_0(t)\exp\{\beta_x^T X + \beta_z^T Z\}$, the log-partial likelihood is then

$$l_{P,i} = \sum_{i=1}^{n} \delta_i \left( \{\beta_x^T X_i + \beta_z^T Z_i\} - \log \left[ \sum_{j=1}^{n} R_j(t_i) \exp\{\beta_x^T X_j + \beta_z^T Z_j\} \right] \right). \tag{15.4}$$

There are interesting connections between the full and partial likelihoods. For example, the partial likelihood score for the proportional hazards model can be obtained in the limit from the full likelihood score when the baseline hazard is modeled with the piecewise constant hazard (equation (15.1)) and the partition is such that $|A_k| \to 0$ as $K \to \infty$, and where $a_{K-1}$ is fixed at a large value beyond which there is no chance of observing events (Yi and Lawless, 2007). See Sinha et al. (2003) for a Bayesian justification of the partial likelihood.

## 15.3 Measurement Error Models and Identifiability

In the following discussion we retain $Z$ to represent error-free covariates and let $X$ represent error-prone covariates, where we use $X^*$ to be the observed version for $X$. The two primary considerations in formulating a covariate measurement error model are the stochastic and functional relations between the observed covariate $X^*$ and the unobserved true covariate $X$, and the joint distribution of $(T, C, X^*)$ conditional on $(X, Z)$. Additional modeling of the distribution of $(X^*, X, Z)$ often depends on parameters that are weakly identified, essentially necessitating the need for auxiliary data in addition to $(T, C, X^*, Z)$.

### 15.3.1 Measurement Error Models

The measurement error model considered here is the classical additive model where $X^* = X + U$ and where $X$ is possibly vector-valued. The random measurement error $U$ is such that $E[U] = 0$ and $\text{Var}(U) = \Sigma_u$, i.e. we assume $X^*$ is an unbiased measurement of $X$ and the measurement error is homoscedastic. It is assumed that $X^*$ provides no information about $(T, C)$ when $X$ is known, i.e. $f(t, c \mid x, z, x^*) = f(t, c \mid x, z)$. This assumption is the survival model analog of non-differential measurement error, and measurements satisfying this property are often called surrogates. Combined with the assumption of conditional independence between the survival and censoring times described in Section 15.2.4, it follows that $f(t, c, x^*, x, z) = f(t, c \mid x, z)f(x^*, x, z) = f(t \mid x, z)f(c \mid, x, z)f(x^*, x, z)$. The implication of these identities is that attention can be focused on the model for $T$ given $(X, Z)$ and the measurement error model $f(x^*, x, z)$.

There are many variations on the classical measurement error model that will not be addressed here, including heteroscedastic measurement error, multiplicative measurement error, differential measurement error, and the classic Berkson error model: $X = X^* + U$ with $U$ independent of $X^*$. The effect of measurement error in proportional hazards models with Berkson error was shown to be minimal, see Küchenhoff et al. (2007).

### 15.3.2 Identifiability and Auxiliary Data

A probability model $f(d \mid \theta)$ for data $d$ depending on a possibly vector-valued parameter $\theta$ is identified when distinct values of $\theta$ uniquely determine $f(d \mid \theta)$. Parameter identification is a necessary condition for the existence of consistent estimators for $\theta$. The practical import of identifiability, or lack thereof, is that there is very little information in the data for unidentified parameters.

Covariate measurement error does not generally render the regression coefficients of interest unidentified, see Schennach and Yu (2013). However, normal theory linear models are not identified (Reiersol, 1950), suggesting that the information in the data for parameters of interest may be weak for models that are approximately linear with approximately normal errors. Furthermore, many of the modeling strategies that have been proposed in the literature for linear and nonlinear measurement error models require additional data to allow estimation of parameters in the expanded models. Typically, additional data that enables consistent estimation of the measurement error variance (covariance matrix in the case of multiple covariates measured with error) is sufficient to construct estimators that reduce most of measurement error induced bias. Many of the methods described in this chapter can be implemented when there are auxiliary data that can identify the measurement error variance. Alternatively, the proposal in Betrand et al. (2019) can be used to estimate the measurement error variance without auxiliary data when the support of the distribution of $X$ is finite. In some situations, their method over-estimated the measurement error variance, and caution is recommended.

Sources of information that enable estimation of the measurement error variance can be internal or external to the study data, and include replicate measurements, instrumental variables, and validation data. Instrumental variables are additional measurements of $X$ that satisfy the surrogate assumption described above. Validation data, considered the gold standard, consist of precise measurements of $X$ on a subset of the study participants.

Carroll et al. (2006) strongly recommend designing studies to obtain internal validation data whenever possible, because "...it can be used with all known techniques, permits direct examination of the error structure, and typically leads to much greater precision of estimation and inference."

## 15.4 Effect of Measurement Error

The effect of measurement error on parameter estimation is often complex and can depend on other covariates in the model and the strength of their correlation with the mis-measured covariate. The *induced hazard*, first studied in Prentice (1982), is the first step toward understanding these effects.

### 15.4.1 Induced Hazard Function

When $X^*$ is observed instead of $X$, it is natural to inquire about the induced hazard function $\lambda^*(t \mid X^*, Z)$ and understand its relation to $\lambda(t \mid X, Z)$. The comparison serves two purposes: i) to understand the effects of measurement error on parameter estimation; ii) to suggest approaches for ameliorating the effect of measurement error. The induced hazard is defined as:

$$\lambda^*(t \mid X^*, Z) = \lim_{\Delta t \to 0} \frac{\Pr(t \leq T < t \mid T \geq t, X^*, Z)}{\Delta t}.$$

The superscript on $\lambda$ is to indicate that the functional form of the induced hazard may be quite different from the hazard in the absence of measurement error. It follows from a straightforward argument using iterated expectations and the assumption of non-differential measurement error that:

$$\lambda^*(t \mid X^*, Z) = E\left[\lambda(t \mid X, Z)\right] \mid T \geq t, X^*, Z].$$

Note that for most realistic models relating $X^*$ to $X$, $\lambda^*(t \mid X^*, Z) \neq \lambda(t \mid X = X^*, Z)$.

**Example:** Consider the proportional hazards model $\lambda(t \mid X, Z) = \lambda_0(t)e^{\beta_X^T X + \beta_Z^T Z}$. The induced hazard is then

$$\lambda^*(t \mid X^*, Z) = \lambda_0(t)e^{\beta_Z^T Z} E\left[e^{\beta_X^T X} \mid T \geq t, X^*, Z\right].$$

The example brings up several important points. First, the expectation defining the induced hazard is conditional on $T \geq t$, and therefore the induced hazard may depend on the unspecified baseline hazard $\lambda_0(t)$ in a way such that it is no longer in the class of proportional hazards. Second, as noted by Prentice (1982), uniqueness results for moment generating functions require full specification of the distribution for $X \mid T \geq t, X^*, Z$ in order to evaluate $E[e^{\beta_X^T X} \mid T \geq t, X^*, Z]$. Finally, non-linearity of $e^{\beta_X^T X}$ means that even in the special case where dependence on the conditioning event $T \geq t$ is minimal, $E[e^{\beta_X^T X} \mid T \geq t, X^*, Z] \neq e^{\beta_X^T X^*}$. In other words, a naive analysis replacing $X$ with $X^*$ will not recover the induced hazard, even under ideal circumstances.

### 15.4.2 Effect of Measurement Error in Proportional Hazards Model

To aid in understanding the effect of covariate measurement error on parameter estimation, we examine the induced hazard for the proportional hazards model under some simplifying assumptions. If failures are infrequent, then $\Pr(T \geq t \mid X, Z) \approx 1$, implying $E[e^{\beta_X^T X} \mid T \geq t, X^*, Z] \approx E[e^{\beta_X^T X} \mid X^*, Z]$. Under the normality assumption

$$\begin{pmatrix} X^* \\ X \\ Z \end{pmatrix} \sim \text{MVN} \begin{pmatrix} \mu_X & \Sigma_X + \Sigma_U & \Sigma_X & \Sigma_{XZ} \\ \mu_X, & \Sigma_X & \Sigma_X & \Sigma_{XZ} \\ \mu_Z & \Sigma_{ZX} & \Sigma_{ZX} & \Sigma_Z \end{pmatrix}$$

and using the properties of multivariate normal distributions, it follows that

$$\lambda^*(t \mid X^*, Z) \propto \lambda_0(t) \exp\left[\beta_X^T E[X \mid X^*, Z] + \beta_Z Z\right],$$

demonstrating that the induced hazard is, advantageously, in the class of proportional hazards models. The proportionality above is approximate owing to the assumption of infrequent failures.

Conveniently, the above analysis implies that the effect of measurement error in the proportional hazards model under normality and rare events can be understood using existing results for the effect of measurement error in the linear model. Let $\Sigma_{X|Z}$ denote the conditional variance of $X$ given $Z$, $\Omega = \Sigma_{X|Z}(\Sigma_{X|Z} + \Sigma_U)^{-1}$ and define $\Gamma_z$ through the conditional expectation $E[X \mid Z] = \Gamma_0 + \Gamma_z Z$; $(\Gamma_z = \Sigma_{XZ}\Sigma_Z^{-1})$. Using properties of multivariate normal distributions and under the infrequent failures assumption, it can be shown that

$$\lambda^*(t \mid X^*, Z) \propto \lambda_0(t) \exp\left[\beta_{x^*}^{*T} X^* + \beta_z^* Z\right],$$

where $\beta_x^* = \Omega^T \beta_x$ and $\beta_z^* = \beta_z + \Gamma_z^T(I - \Omega^T)\beta_x$. The effects of ignoring measurement error on parameter estimation is seen to be complex. In the case of a single covariate measured with error, $\Omega = \Sigma_{X|Z}^2/(\Sigma_{X|Z}^2 + \Sigma_U^2)$ where $\Sigma_{X|Z}$ and $\Sigma_U$ are scalars, implying that the magnitude of $\beta_x$ is underestimated, and that the attenuation increases with the strength of the correlation between $X$ and $Z$. Measurement error in $X$ is also seen to bias estimation of $\beta_z$ in a complex way, except in the case where $X$ and $Z$ are uncorrelated. As noted in Carroll (1989), if $Z$ represents whether a subject received treatment, then measurement error in $X$ can affect the ability to estimate the treatment effect.

The analytic results in the above analysis required simplifying assumptions. Quantifying the effects of measurement error on parameter estimation more generally is not possible, as it will depend on the type of regression model, the distributional relation between covariates and failure time, and potentially the censoring process. See Hughes (1993) for further analysis of the effect of measurement error in PH models.

## 15.5 Methods for Correcting for Measurement Error

As discussed in the last section, ignoring measurement error and proceeding with the usual analysis will result in biased, inconsistent estimators of regression coefficients. Many proposals have been developed in the measurement error literature that provide corrections for the effect of covariate measurement error for the analysis of survival data. The goal for the remainder of the chapter is to describe several general strategies for correcting for the effects covariate measurement error.

### 15.5.1 Regression Calibration

Regression calibration (RC) was described in detail as a general approach to correcting for covariate measurement error, see Chapter 7. Strengths of regression calibration are that it is easy to understand and implement, and it is applicable across a wide range of regression models. At a basic level, RC can be described as developing a regression model to impute values for the unobserved covariate $X$ using the observed covariates $(X^*, Z)$, and then using the imputed values in the regression of $Y$ on $(X, Z)$. Regression calibration estimation consists of three steps:

1. Model and estimate the regression of $X$ on $(X^*, Z)$ to obtain an imputed value $\widetilde{X}$ where $\widetilde{X} = E(X \mid X^*, Z)$.
2. Regress $Y$ on $(\widetilde{X}, Z)$ to obtain regression parameter estimates.
3. Adjust standard errors of regression parameter estimates to incorporate the uncertainty in imputing $\widetilde{X}$.

When $(X^*, X, Z)$ is approximately jointly normal, or when $X$ is strongly correlated with $(X^*, Z)$, the regression of $X$ on $(X^*, Z)$ is approximately linear:

$$E[X \mid X^*, Z] \approx \mu_X + \Sigma_{X|X^*Z}\Sigma_{X^*Z}^{-1} \begin{pmatrix} X^* - \mu_X \\ Z - \mu_Z \end{pmatrix},$$

where $\Sigma_{x|x^*z}$ is the covariance of $X$ with $(X^*, Z)$ and $\Sigma_{x^*z}$ is the variance matrix of $(X^*, Z)$. In general, auxiliary data are needed to estimate these parameters. The right hand side is also the best linear predictor of of $X$, see Carroll et al. (2006), providing additional justification for using the approximation.

Regression calibration is not immediately transportable to survival models owing to the fact that the calibration function generally is conditional on $T \geq t$ in addition to $(X^*, Z)$.

For example, a first order approximation to the induced hazard is

$$\lambda^*(t \mid X, Z) \approx \lambda(t \mid E[X \mid T \geq t, X^*, Z], Z),$$

and it is seen that the regression of $X$ on $(X^*, Z)$ is also conditional on $T \geq t$. Interestingly, starting with a survival model with time independent covariates, first order regression calibration results in a model with time dependent covariates. If we assume events are infrequent, then

$$\lambda^*(t \mid X, Z) \approx \lambda(t \mid E[X \mid X^*, Z], Z),$$

and the usual regression calibration algorithm can be applied. A word of caution–first order regression calibration can do a poor job removing bias when there is significant measurement error, when the effect of the mis-measured predictor $X$ is large or when the regression model for the response on covariates is highly nonlinear (Carroll et al., 2006); Buonaccorsi, 2010).

Modifications to the regression calibration algorithm have been developed for applications where the rare disease assumption is untenable, see Clayton (1991), Tsiatis et al. (1995), and Wang et al. (1997).

Xie et al. (2001) generalize the results of Clayton (1991). The following describes their approach. They assume a classical additive error model and the availability of replicate measurements for each study subject: $X_{ij}^* = X_i + U_{ij}$ for $i = 1, \ldots, n, j = 1, \ldots, k$, where the $U_{ij}$ are identically distributed and independent of all random variables. For notational simplicity, it is assumed that each subject has the same number of replicates ($k$) available. It is straightforward to relax this assumption. Let $\bar{X}_i^* = (1/k)\sum_{j=1}^k X_{ij}^*$. Ignoring additional covariates $Z$ for now, the main idea of the approach is to estimate the calibration function among subjects still at risk at time $t$:

$$E[X \mid T \geq t, \bar{X}^*] \approx \mu_X(t) + \Sigma_X(t)\Sigma_{\bar{X}^*}^{-1}(t)\left(\bar{X}^* - \mu_X(t)\right),$$

where $\mu_X(t) = E[X \mid T \geq t], \Sigma_X(t) = \text{Var}(X \mid T \geq t)$ and $\Sigma_{\bar{X}^*}(t) = \text{Var}(\bar{X}^* \mid T \geq t) = \text{Var}(X \mid T \geq t) + (1/k)\text{Var}(U) = \Sigma_X(t) + (1/k)\Sigma_U$.

Estimates for the parameters in the calibration function are obtained using a standard variance components approach applied to subjects still at risk at time $t$:

$$\widehat{\mu}_X(t) = \frac{\sum_{i=1}^n R_i(t)\bar{X}_i^*}{\sum_{i=1}^n R_i(t)};$$

$$\widehat{\Sigma}_U = \frac{1}{n(k-1)}\sum_{i=1}^n\sum_{j=1}^k \left(X_{ij}^* - \bar{X}_i^*\right)\left(X_{ij}^* - \bar{X}_i^*\right)^T;$$

$$\widehat{\Sigma}_X(t) = \frac{\sum_{i=1}^n R_i(t)\left(\bar{X}_i^* - \widehat{\mu}_X(t)\right)\left(\bar{X}_i^* - \widehat{\mu}_X(t)\right)^T}{\sum_{i=1}^n R_i(t)} - \frac{1}{k}\widehat{\Sigma}_U.$$

Imputed values for $X_i$ at time $t$ are then

$$\widetilde{X}_i(t) = \widehat{\mu}_X(t) + \widehat{\Sigma}_X(t)\widehat{\Sigma}_{\bar{X}^*}^{-1}(t)\left(\bar{X}_i^* - \widehat{\mu}_X(t)\right),$$

where $\widehat{\Sigma}_{\bar{X}^*}(t) = \widehat{\Sigma}_X(t) + (1/k)\widehat{\Sigma}_U$. The regression calibration partial likelihood estimator is defined as the value of $\beta_x$ that maximizes (15.4) with $\widetilde{X}_i(t)$ replacing $X_i$:

$$\widehat{\beta}_x = \underset{\beta_x}{\text{argmax}}\sum_{i=1}^n \delta_i\left(\{\beta_x^T\widetilde{X}_i(t_i)\} - \log\left[\sum_{j=1}^n R_j(t_i)\exp\{\beta_x^T\widetilde{X}_j(t_i)\}\right]\right).$$

The asymptotic distribution of $\widehat{\beta}_x$ can be used for inference, see Xie et al. (2001) for details on deriving and estimating the asymptotic covariance matrix. Additional covariates measured without error are handled by redefining $X = (X^T, Z^T)^T$ and $X_{ij}^* = \{(X_i + U_{ij})^T, Z_i^T\}^T$ and proceeding with the above analysis.

### 15.5.2 SIMEX

SIMEX (Simulation-Extrapolation) is an approach to correcting for the effects of covariate measurement error that is applicable to a very large class of regression models (Cook and Stefanski, 1995), including semi-parametric PH models and AFT models.

SIMEX is popular in applications because the bias correction process is straightforward and transparent, resulting in a visual display of the effect of measurement error on parameter estimation. Additionally, standard software can often be easily adapted to implement the method, and it is not necessary to model the distribution for the true covariate $X$. The idea is to incrementally increase the amount of measurement error in $X^*$ using simulated random errors (simulation step), and plot the resulting regression coefficients against the amount of measurement error, thereby establishing a relation between the bias in $\beta$ and the amount of measurement error in $X^*$. The SIMEX estimator extrapolates the relation to the case of no measurement error (extrapolation step). SIMEX requires an estimate of the measurement error variance. Recently, Bertrand et al. (2019) apply SIMEX in a PH model utilizing a novel method for estimating the measurement error variance that does not rely on auxiliary data. Details of the SIMEX method are given in Carroll et al. (2006), and the description there can be straightforwardly applied to the survival data regression models described in this chapter. Carroll et al. (2006) also provide a data application of SIMEX in the PH setting where the effect of the true covariate on the hazard is modeled with a spline.

SIMEX for survival data has been widely studied in the literature. Green and Cai (2004) derive asymptotic properties of SIMEX estimators for multivariate PH failure time models. SIMEX was successfully extended to AFT models, see He et al. (2007), and these authors also provide an R package to implement their methodology, see He et al. (2012). Yi and He (2012) describe and extend SIMEX estimation in proportional odds models. Oh et al. (2018) use SIMEX to address measurement error in the survival time outcome. Bertrand et al. (2017) study SIMEX for survival cure models. A word of caution, Yi and He (2012) noted that SIMEX can be sensitive to the assumption of normally distributed errors.

### 15.5.3 Likelihood Methods

There is a large literature studying likelihood approaches to covariate measurement error in survival data. The approaches can be categorized as a) constructing the full likelihood for the observed data; b) using the induced hazard to construct an induced likelihood or partial likelihood conditional on $(X^*, Z)$; c) constructing a "corrected" likelihood; and d) constructing an approximately unbiased likelihood (or partial likelihood) score.

Approach a) is considered first. Assuming non-differential measurement error, the conditional density for the observed data $(t, \delta, X^*, Z)$ is obtained through the identity $f_{T,\delta,X^*|Z}(t,\delta,x^* \mid z) = \int f_{T,\delta|X,Z}(t,\delta \mid x,z) f_{X^*|X,Z}(x^* \mid x,z) f_{X|Z}(x \mid z) dx = \int \lambda(t \mid X,Z)^{\delta} S(t \mid X,Z) f_{X^*|X,Z}(x^* \mid x,z) f_{X|Z}(x \mid z) dx$. In the case of the proportional hazards model, the resulting likelihood is

$$L = \prod_{i=1}^{n} \int \left\{\lambda_0(t_i)\exp\{\beta_x^T x + \beta_z^T Z_i\}\right\}^{\delta_i} \times \exp\left\{-\int_0^{t_i} \lambda_0(u) e^{(\beta_x^T x + \beta_z^T Z_i)} du\right\} f_{X^*|X,Z}(X_i^*; x, Z_i) f_{X|Z}(x; Z_i) dx. \tag{15.5}$$

An appealing feature of a full likelihood approach is asymptotic efficiency, assuming all of the many modeling choices are correct. There are several challenges with using the above likelihood for estimation of the regression parameters $(\beta_x^T, \beta_z^T)^T$. The likelihood

1. depends on the unknown baseline hazard $\lambda_0(t)$;
2. requires specifying distributions for $X^* \mid X, Z$ and $X \mid Z$, up to a set of unknown parameters;
3. requires numerical evaluation of an analytically intractable integral;
4. may not be straightforward to maximize.

Some common modeling choices are the following. The baseline hazard can be modeled with the piece-wise constant model, with knots taken to be the at the distinct observed failure times or chosen as described above (Section 15.2.1). Under the additive model $X^* = X + U$ with $U$ independent of all other variables, $f_{X^*|X,Z}(x^* \mid x,z) = f_{X^*|X}(x^* \mid x)$. Typically, the measurement error is modeled with a normal distribution, i.e. $X^* \mid X \sim N(X, \Sigma_U)$. For the unobserved covariate, a normal model $X \mid Z \sim N(E[X \mid Z], \Sigma_{X|Z})$ could also be employed, in which case the mean could be modeled using the observed data by noting $E[X \mid Z] = E[X^* \mid Z]$. Auxiliary data are typically needed to model/estimate the variances $\Sigma_U$ and $\Sigma_{X|Z}$, and these observations would need to be incorporated in the likelihood.

When there are no mis-measured covariates, Hu et al. (1998) investigate the use of semi-parametric and non-parametric densities for the distribution of $X$, and they discuss details for evaluating numerically the integral in equation (15.5) and estimation of standard errors for the resulting regression parameter estimates. Rigorous derivation of the asymptotic distributions for their estimation proposals are provided by Dupuy (2005). A significant constraint to their proposals is they do not allow for additional covariates measured without error.

Note that, in contrast to regression calibration and SIMEX, the full likelihood approach requires estimating the distribution of the unobserved $X$, a daunting task in the absence of validation data. While efficiency may be gained with a correct model, it may be accompanied by a lack of robustness to mis-specification.

Another route to likelihood analysis is to use the induced hazard defined in Section 15.4.1, along with an analogously defined induced survivor function. This approach results in the conditional distribution $f_{t,\delta|X^*,Z}(t,\delta \mid x^*,z)$, in contrast to the likelihood given above for $f_{t,\delta,X^*|Z}(t,\delta,x^* \mid z)$. The induced survivor function can be computed via

$$\begin{aligned} S^*(t \mid X^*, Z) &= P(T > t \mid X^*, Z) = E\left[P(T > t \mid X^*, Z) \mid X, X^*, Z)\right] \\ &= E\left[P(T > t \mid X, X^*, Z) \mid X^*, Z\right] \\ &= E\left[P(T > t \mid X, Z) \mid X^*, Z\right] \\ &= E\left[S(t \mid X, Z) \mid X^*, Z\right], \end{aligned}$$

where the fourth equality follows from the assumption $X^*$ is a surrogate for $X$. Similarly, $f^*(t \mid X^*, Z) = E\left[f(t \mid X, Z) \mid X^*, Z\right]$ where the expectation is with respect to the conditional distribution of $X \mid X^*, Z$. Finally, $\lambda^*(t \mid X^*, Z) = f^*(t \mid X^*, Z)/S^*(t \mid X^*, Z)$. Note that this approach for obtaining the induced hazard avoids having to specify the distribution for $X$ conditional on $(T \geq t, X^*, Z)$ as done in Section 15.4.1.

These quantities can be plugged into either the full or partial likelihoods given by equations (15.2) and (15.3), see Zucker (2005). Either approach necessitates modeling the baseline hazard with, essentially, the piece-wise constant hazard.

When validation data is available, Zhou and Pepe (1995) and Zhou and Wang (2000) provided estimates the induced hazard without having to specify the distribution for $X \mid X^*, Z$.

Plugging the induced hazard function into the partial likelihood does not seem compelling as the induced hazard may not be in the class of proportional hazards models, and therefore the induced partial likelihood will not be independent of the baseline hazard $\lambda_0(t)$. However, Zucker (2005) gives several reasons for preferring the induced partial likelihood approach, most notably that it seems more robust to estimation of $\lambda_0(t)$, and the resulting estimating equations were easier to solve than those defining the full induced likelihood. There is also the advantage that in the absence of measurement error the approach reduces to the usual partial likelihood estimator. Yi (2017) provides a thorough and clear exposition of the induced likelihood and partial likelihood approaches.

### 15.5.4 Corrected Likelihood

A general approach to estimation in the presence of covariate measurement error, termed the insertion correction strategy by Yi (2017, Ch. 2), is to derive a log-likelihood (or score function) that is unbiased for the log-likelihood or score used in the absence of measurement error. Suppose there exists $l_i^*(t_i, X_i^*, Z_i, \delta_i)$ such that $E[l_i^* \mid t_i, \delta_i, X_i, Z_i] = l_i$ where $l_i$ is defined as the logarithm of $L_i$, see equation (15.2). Then provided differentiation and expectation can be interchanged, the *corrected score*, obtained by taking the derivative of the corrected log-likelihood $l_i^*$, will have expectation zero and will result in consistent estimation of regression parameters under regularity conditions. Augustin (2004) and Yi and Lawless (2007) independently developed insertion correction strategies for the proportional hazard model. The following is cast after the latter reference.

For the proportional hazards model, the log of the likelihood in equation (15.2) is given by

$$l_i = \delta_i\{\log \lambda_0(t_i) + \beta_x^T X_i + \beta_z^T Z_i\} - \exp\{\beta_x^T X_i + \beta_z^T Z_i\}\Lambda_0(t_i).$$

With additive, non-differential measurement error, the score

$$l_i^* = \delta_i\{\log \lambda_0(t_i) + \beta_x^T X_i^* + \beta_z^T Z_i\} - \{M(\beta_x)\}^{-1} \exp\{\beta_x^T X_i^* + \beta_z^T Z_i\}\Lambda_0(t_i) \tag{15.6}$$

is easily seen to have the property $E[l_i^* \mid X_i, Z_i, T_i, C_i] = l_i$ where $M(\beta_x) = E[e^{\beta_x^T U} \mid X, Z]$ is the moment generating function for the measurement error $U$ evaluated at $\beta_x$. An independent normal model for the measurement error is typically used, resulting in $M(\beta_x) = \exp\{\beta_x^T \Sigma_U \beta_x/2\}$.

The corrected likelihood depends on the unknown baseline hazard $\lambda_0(t)$. The piece-wise constant model, see equation (15.1), is often used to model the baseline hazard. Then $l_i^*$ is a function of the parameter $\theta = (\beta^T, \rho^T)^T$ where $\beta^T = (\beta_x^T, \beta_z^T)^T$ and $\rho = (\rho_1, \rho_2, \ldots, \rho_K)^T$ are the parameters in the piece-wise hazard, again refer to (15.1). The measurement error corrected estimator $\widehat{\theta}$ is defined as the solution to the corrected likelihood score estimating equations given by

$$S(\widehat{\theta}) = \partial/\partial\theta \frac{1}{n}\sum_{i=1}^{n} l_i^* = \frac{1}{n}\sum_{i=1}^{n} S_i(\theta) = 0$$

where $S_i(\theta) = \partial l_i^*/\partial\theta$. The robust sandwich estimator for the asymptotic variance of $\widehat{\theta}$ can be used for inference:

$$\mathrm{Var}(\widehat{\theta}) \approx \frac{1}{n}\Gamma^{-1}(\widehat{\theta})\Sigma(\widehat{\theta})\Gamma^{-T}(\widehat{\theta})$$

where $\Sigma(\widehat{\theta}) = \frac{1}{n}\sum_{i=1}^{n} S_i(\widehat{\theta})S_i^T(\widehat{\theta})$, $\Gamma(\widehat{\theta}) = \frac{1}{n}\sum_{i=1}^{n} S_i'(\widehat{\theta})$ and $S_i'(\theta) = (\partial/\partial\theta^T)S_i(\theta)$.

The corrected full likelihood defined above depended on the baseline hazard $\lambda_0(t)$. A corrected partial likelihood would avoid this problem. Unfortunately, the existence result in Stefanski (1989) precludes the possibility of constructing a corrected score when the measurement error is normally distributed, prompting Nakamura (1992) to propose a first order corrected partial likelihood score that was originally thought to result in only approximately consistent estimators. Kong and Gu (1999) showed Nakamura's estimator was consistent. Interestingly, the first order score was later shown to be equivalent to the derivative of (15.6) when the Breslow estimation scheme for $\lambda_0(t)$ is employed, providing intuition for Kong and Gu's result, see Augustin (2004) and Yi and Lawless (2007).

Buzas (1998) derived an unbiased partial likelihood type score using an extended insertion approach, see Yi (2017) for a clear exposition of the method. Hu and Lin (2002) extended the approaches of Nakamura (1992) and Buzas (1998), and Yan and Yi (2015) unify several proposals using a corrected profile likelihood method.

### 15.5.5 Bayesian Methods

A Bayesian analysis of survival data with covariate measurement error is in principle straightforward. Starting with the likelihood and priors for the model without measurement error, the Bayesian approach simply requires adding prior probability models for the mis-measured covariates, measurement errors and the priors for the parameters of these models.

Gustafson (2004) notes that the Bayesian approach via MCMC may be the easiest approach to likelihood type analyzes, see page 89 middle paragraph.

Let $f_{T|X,Z,\beta}(t \mid x, z, \beta), f_{X^*|X,Z,\alpha}(x^* \mid x, z, \alpha)$ and $f_{X|Z,\gamma}(x \mid z, \gamma)$ denote the probability models for the survival time, measurement error and covariate where $\beta, \alpha$ and $\gamma$ are the parameters in the respective models. A Bayesian analysis requires specifying priors for $\theta = (\beta^T, \alpha^T, \gamma^T)$. Typically, independent priors are specified for $\theta$, i.e. $f_\theta(\theta) = f_\beta(\beta) f_\alpha(\alpha) f_\gamma(\gamma)$.

For example, suppose we model survival times with the proportional hazards model $\lambda(t \mid X, Z) = \lambda_0(t) \exp\{\beta_x X + \beta_z^T Z\}$, and employ a normal theory additive measurement error model $W = X + U$ for the scalar covariate $X$ where $X \sim N(\gamma_0, \sigma_x^2)$ and $U \sim N(0, \sigma_u^2)$. Kalbfleisch (1978) and Sinha et al. (2003) provide justification for using the partial likelihood for computing the posterior distribution. If we use the partial likelihood for estimation, no prior is required for the infinite dimensional baseline hazard $\lambda_0(t)$, as it factors out of the partial likelihood. A Bayesian analysis would then require prior specification for $\beta = (\beta_x, \beta_z^T)$, $\gamma = (\gamma_0, \sigma_x^2)$ and $\sigma_u^2$. Typical choices for priors for $\beta$ include improper flat priors, multivariate normal priors and Zellner's g-prior. These prior choices are also common for the regression parameters in linear models. Uninformative priors for $\gamma_0$ include a normal prior with large variance or an improper flat prior. Independent inverse gamma priors are often used for the variance parameters $\sigma_x^2$ and $\sigma_u^2$. The resulting posterior for $\beta$ is analytically intractable and Markov chain Monte Carlo (MCMC) methods must be employed to obtain a sample from the posterior. Alternatively, the posterior can be approximated using the integrated nested Laplace approximation (INLA), see Muff et al. (2017). Computational details for both approaches are beyond the scope of this chapter.

If the full likelihood is used for estimation in the PH model with $\lambda_0(t)$ unspecified, a common choice of prior for $\lambda_0(t)$ is the gamma process prior, see Ibrahim et al. (2001) for details. Alternatively, if the piecewise constant hazard is used, independent gamma priors are commonly used for $\rho$, i.e., $\rho_k \sim \text{gamma}(a_k, b_k)$. Taking $a_k = b_k = 0$ results in an uninformative improper prior for the $\rho_k$. As above, models for $X$ and $U$ are added to the models comprising the likelihood.

The models above may not be identified without additional data such as replicates, instrumental variables or validation data. While posterior distributions for unidentified parameters using proper priors can still result, the posterior will not converge to the true parameter values. Any additional identifying observations would need to be incorporated into the likelihood with priors specified for the corresponding model parameters.

The Bayesian approach described above requires specification of probability models for the survival time, unobserved covariate, measurement error, and auxiliary identifying observations. In addition, priors are required for all model parameters. As in any Bayesian analysis, it is important to understand the sensitivity to the choice of probability models for data and priors.

Bartlett and Keogh (2018) use simulation to compare regression calibration to a Bayesian analysis for a proportional hazards model, and conclude that the approaches provide similar results when the amount of measurement error is moderate, but the Bayesian approach is preferred when the magnitude of measurement error and covariate effect ($\beta_x$) are large. It is generally true that first order regression calibration can perform poorly when these conditions are present, see for example Buzas et al. (2014) and Hu et al. (1998). Cheng and Crainiceanu (2009) study Bayesian analysis for survival data using nonparametric models for the baseline hazard and event time/covariate model. Muff et al. (2017) develop a Bayesian analysis of the Weibull AFT model with two covariates measured with error.

### 15.5.6 Conclusions and Discussion

The effect of covariate measurement error on parameter estimation in survival models is complex. Under simplifying assumptions, the effect of classical additive measurement error is similar to that in linear models–namely the magnitude of the regression coefficient for the mis-measured covariate is shrunk toward zero. The effects on coefficients of covariates measured without error are difficult to parse, and depend in a complex way on the correlation between $X$ and $Z$. The Berkson error model was not considered here. As noted above, the effect of measurement error in proportional hazards models with Berkson error was shown to be minimal, see Küchenhoff et al. (2007).

The default methods for adjusting for covariate measurement error effects for general nonlinear models are regression calibration and SIMEX. The reasons for this is that they are easy to understand, do not require assumptions on the distribution of $X$, are widely applicable and can mostly be implemented with existing software. I consider these the default methods for survival models when the magnitude of the measurement error is modest relative to the variation in $X$, and with the caveat that regression calibration may need to be modified to account for dependence on survival time. Both methods generally require auxiliary data for successful implementation, and studies should be planned with this in mind. SIMEX has been implemented in the statistical software packages R and Stata. Regression calibration has been implemented in Stata, and SAS macros implementing variations of regression calibration for survival models are available at https://www.hsph.harvard.edu/donna-spiegelman/software/rrc-macro/ (accessed July 24, 2019).

Several other successful strategies for addressing covariate measurement error were discussed herein, including likelihood and Bayesian approaches. A strategy not discussed here is conditional scores, which retain efficiency properties similar to maximum likelihood estimators (Stefanski and Carroll, 1987). Tsiatis and Davidian (2001) derive a conditional score for covariate measurement error in the proportional hazards model with time dependent covariates, see also Song and Huang (2005).

There are many modeling variations for survival data and covariate measurement error, resulting in a large product space of models. For survival data, models not considered here include additive hazards, frailty models, proportional odds, survival cure, time dependent covariates, and multivariate survival data. Measurement error models not considered, except perhaps briefly, include multiplicative measurement error, mis-classification, heteroscedastic measurement error, instrumental variables, and measurement error in the outcome. Yi (2017) is an excellent reference for many of these topics. See also Li and Lin (2003) on the use of SIMEX in frailty measurement error models, Song and Wang (2008) and Liao et al. (2011) for time varying covariates, Huang and Wang (2000) for a nonparametric estimating score approach, and Chen (2019) for survival cure model methods.

## Bibliography

Augustin, T. (2004). An exact corrected log-likelihood function for Cox's proportional hazards model under measurement error and some extensions. *Scandinavian Journal of Statistics*, 31, 43-50.

Bartlett, J.W. and Keogh, R.H. (2018). Bayesian correction for covariate measurement error: A frequentist evaluation and comparison with regression calibration. *Statistical Methods in Medical Research*, 2018, 27(6), 1695-1708.

Bertrand, A., Legrand, C., Carroll, R.J., De Meester. C., and Van Keilegom, I. (2017). Inference in a survival cure model with mismeasured covariates using a simulation-extrapolation approach. *Biometrika*, 104(1), 31-50.

Bertrand, A., Van Keilegom, I., and Legrand, C. (2019). Flexible parametric approach to classical measurement error variance estimation without auxiliary data. *Biometrics*, 75(1), 297-307.

Buonaccorsi, J.P. (2010). *Measurement Error: Models, Methods, and Applications.* Chapman and Hall/CRC Press, London.

Buzas, J.S. (1998). Unbiased scores in proportional hazards regression with covariate measurement error. *Journal of Statistical Planning and Inference*, 67, 247-257.

Buzas, J.S., Stefanski, L.A., and Tosteson, T.D. (2014). In *Handbook of Epidemiology*, 2nd ed., Vol. 3, Ahrens, W. and Pigeot, I. (Eds), Springer-Verlag, 1241-1282.

Carroll, R.J. (1989). Covariance analysis in generalized linear measurement error models. *Statistics in Medicine*, 8, 1075-1093.

Carroll, R.J., Ruppert, D., Stefanski, L.A., and Crainiceanu, C.M. (2006). *Measurement Error in Nonlinear Models*, 2nd ed. Chapman & Hall, London.

Chen, L.P. (2019). Semiparametric estimation for cure survival model with left-truncated and right-censored data and covariate measurement error. *Statistics & Probability Letters*, 154, 108547.

Cheng, Y.J. and Crainiceanu, C.M. (2009). Cox models with smooth functional effect of covariates measured with error. *Journal of the American Statistical Association*, 104, 1144-1154.

Clayton, D.G. (1991). Models for the analysis of cohort and case-control studies with inaccurately measured exposures. In *Statistical Models for Longitudinal Studies of Health*, Dwyer, J.H., Feinleib, M., Lipsert, P. et al. (eds.) Oxford University Press, New York, 301-331.

Cook, J. and Stefanski, L.A. (1995). A simulation extrapolation method for parametric measurement error models. *Journal of the American Statistical Association*, 89, 1314-1328.

Dupuy, J.F. (2005) The proportional hazards model with covariatemeasurement error. *Journal of Statistical Planning and Inference*, 135, 260-275.

Greene, W.F. and Cai, J. (2004). Measurement error in covariates in the marginal hazards model for multivariate failure time data. *Biometrics*, 60, 987-996.

Gustafson, P. (2004). *Measurement Error and Misclassification in Statistics and Epidemiology: Impacts and Bayesian Adjustments.* Chapman and Hall/CRC Press, London.

He, W., Yi, G.Y., and Xiong, J. (2007). Accelerated failure time models with covariates subject to measurement error. *Statistics in Medicine*, 26, 4817-4832.

He, W., Xiong, J., and Yi, G.Y. (2012). SIMEX R package for accelerated failure time models with covariate measurement error. *Journal of Statistical Software*, 2012, (46), 1-14.

Hu, P., Tsiatis, A.A., and Davidian, M. (1998). Estimating the parameters in the Cox model when covariate variables are measured with error. *Biometrics*, 54, 1407-1419.

Hu, C. and Lin, D.Y. (2002). Cox regression with covariate measurement error. *Scandanavian Journal of Statistics*, 29, 637-655.

Huang, Y. and Wang, C.Y. (2000). Cox regression with accurate covariates unascertainable: a nonparametric-correction approach. *Journal of the American Statistical Association*, 95, 1209-1219.

Hughes, M.D. (1993) Regression dilution in the proportional hazards model. *Biometrics*, 49, 1056-1066.

Ibrahim, J.G., Chen, M., and Sinha, D. (2001). *Bayesian Survival Analysis.* Springer, New York.

Kalbfleisch, J.D. (1978). Non-parametric Bayesian analysis of survival time data. *Journal of the Royal Statistical Society, Series B*, 40, 214-221.

Kalbfleisch, J.D. and Prentice, R.L. (2002). *The Statistical Analysis of Failure Time Data*, 2nd Ed. John Wiley & Sons, Hoboken, New Jersey.

Kong, F.H. and Gu, M. (1999). Consistent estimation in Cox proportional hazards model with covariate measurement errors. *Statistica Sinica*, 9, 953-969.

Küchenhoff, H., Bender, R., and Langner I. (2007). Effect of Berkson measurement error on parameter estimates in Cox regression models. *Lifetime Data Analysis*, 13, 261-272.

Li, Y. and Lin, X. (2003). Functional inference in frailty measurement error models for clustered survival data using the SIMEX approach. *Journal of the American Statistical Association*, 98, 191-203.

Liao, X., Zucker, D.M., Li, Y. and Spiegelman, D. (2011). Survival analysis with error-prone time varying covariates: a risk set calibration approach. *Biometrics*, 67(1), 50-58.

Muff, S., Ott, M., Braun, J., and Held, L. (2017). Bayesian two-component measurement error modelling for survival analysis using INLAA case study on cardiovascular disease mortality in Switzerland. *Computational Statistics & Data Analysis*, 113, 177-193.

Nakamura, T. (1992). Proportional hazards models with covariates subject to measurement error. *Biometrics*, 48, 829-838.

Oh, E.J., Shepherd, B.E., Lumley, T., and Shaw, P.A. (2018). Considerations for analysis of time-to-event outcomes measured with error: Bias and correction with SIMEX. *Statistics in Medicine*, 37(8), 1276-1289.

Prentice. R.L. (1982). Covariate measurement errors and parameter estimation in a failure time regression model. *Biometrika*, 69, 331-342.

Prentice, R.L. (2005). *Measurement Error in Survival Analysis. Encyclopedia of Biostatistics*, John Wiley & Sons, Ltd.

Reiersol, O. (1950). Identifiability of a linear relation between variables which are subject to error. *Econometrica*, 18(4), 375-389.

Schennach, S.M., and Hu, Y. (2013). Nonparametric identification and semiparametric estimation of classical measurement error models without side information. *Journal of the American Statistical Association*, 108(501), 177-186.

Sinha, D., Ibrahim, J.G., and Chen, M. (2003). A Bayesian justification of Coxs partial likelihood. *Biometrika*, 90(3), 626-641.

Song, X. and Huang, Y. (2005). On corrected score approach for proportional hazards model with covariate measurement error, *Biometrics*, 61, 702-714.

Song, X. and Wang, C.Y. (2008). Semiparametric approaches for joint modeling of longitudinal and survival data with time-varying coefficients. *Biometrics*, 64, 557-566.

Stefanski, L.A. and Carroll, R.J. (1987). Conditional scores and optimal scores in generalized linear measurement error models. *Biometrika*, 74, 703-716.

Stefanski, L.A. (1989). Unbiased estimation of a nonlinear function of a normal mean with application to measurement error models. *Communications in Statistics — Theory and Methods*, 18, 4335-4358.

Tsiatis, A.A., DeGruttola, V., and Wulfsohn, M.S. (1995). Modeling the relationship of survival to longitudinal data measured with error: Applications to survival and CD4 counts in patients with AIDS. *Journal of the American Statistical Association*, 90, 27-37.

Tsiatis, A.A. and Davidian, M. (2001). A semiparametric estimator for the proportional hazards model with longitudinal covariates measured with error. *Biometrika*, 88, 447-458.

Wang, C.Y., Hsu, Z.D., Feng, Z.D., and Prentice, R.L. (1997). Regression calibration in failure time regression. *Biometrics*, 53, 131-145.

Xie, S.X., Wang, C.Y. and Prentice, R.L. (2001). A risk set calibration method for failure time regression by using a covariate reliability sample. *Journal of the Royal Statistical Society, Series B*, 63, 855-870.

Yi, G.Y. (2017). *Statistical Analysis with Measurement Error or Misclassification.* Springer, New York.

Yi, G.Y. and He, W. (2012). Bias analysis and the simulation-extrapolation method for survival data with covariate measurement error under parametric proportional odds models. *Biometrical Journal*, 54, 343-360.

Yi, G.Y. and Lawless, J.F. (2007). A corrected likelihood method for the proportional hazards model with covariates subject to measurement error. *Journal of Statistical Planning and Inference*, 137, 1816-1828.

Yan, Y. and Yi, G.Y. (2015). A corrected profile likelihood method for survival data with covariate measurement error under the Cox model. *The Canadian Journal of Statistics*, 43(3), 454-480.

Zhou, H. and Pepe, M.S. (1995). Auxiliary covariate data in failure time regression analysis. *Biometrika*, 82, 139-149.

Zhou, H. and Wang, C.Y. (2000). Failure time regression with continuous covariates measured with error. *Journal of the Royal Statistical Society, Series B*, 62, 657-665.

Zucker, D.M. (2005). A pseudo-partial likelihood method for semiparametric survival regression with covariate errors, *Journal of the American Statistical Association*, 100(472), 1264-1277.

# 16

# Mixed Effects Models with Measurement Errors in Time-Dependent Covariates

**Lang Wu, Wei Liu, and Hongbin Zhang**

## CONTENTS



## 16.1 Introduction

In a longitudinal study, data are collected on a sample of subjects repeatedly over time until the end of the study. For example, in an HIV/AIDS study, viral load and CD4 cell counts are often measured repeatedly over time. Figure 16.1 shows CD4 and viral load longitudinal data during an anti-HIV treatment. The observed values of CD4 and viral load change over time, and there seem large variations between the individuals. To model these data, mixed effects models

DOI: 10.1201/9781315101279-16

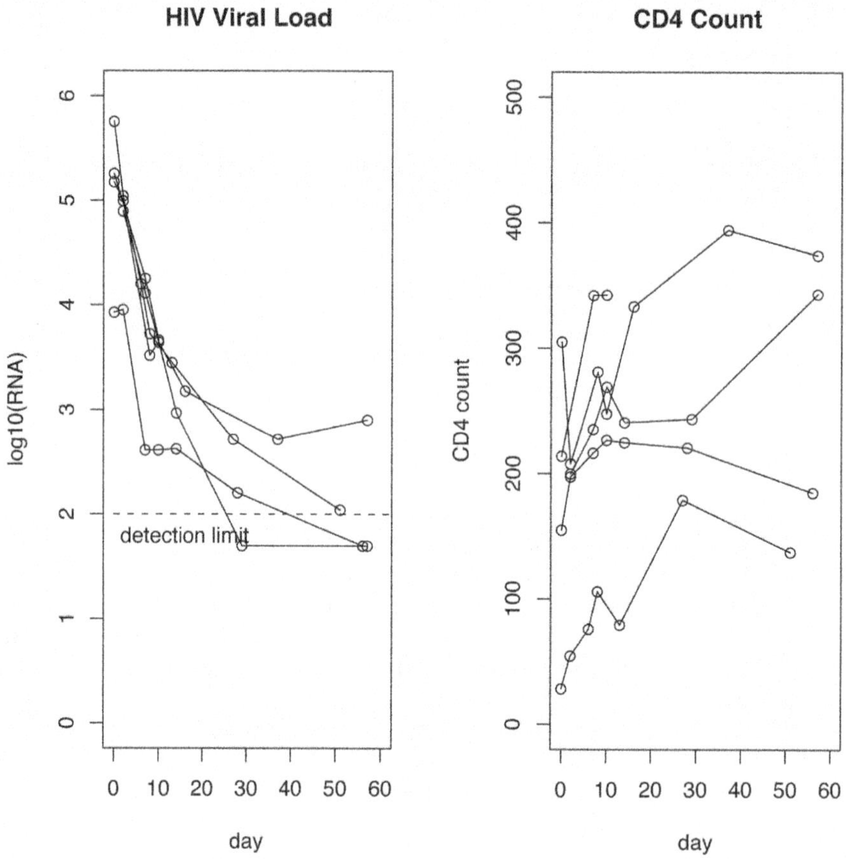


**FIGURE 16.1**
CD4 and viral load data for five randomly selected patients from an AIDS study.

are widely used since they allow for individual-specific inference. Often, one variable such as viral load is chosen as a response variable, and other variables such as CD4 are chosen as time-dependent covariates to partially explain the variations in the response variable. This leads to mixed effects models with time-dependent covariates.

For statistical inference of mixed effects models with time-dependent covariates, a common challenge is that some variables such as CD4 and viral load are usually measured with substantial errors. That is, the observed values of these variables may not be their true values but values with measurement errors. The large variations among the repeated measurements within each individual in Figure 16.1 indicate such measurement errors. Failing to address the measurement errors may lead to misleading statistical analyses and results (Carroll et al., 2006; Wu, 2009; Yi, 2017).

In the presence of covariate measurement errors, replicates of the covariate values can be required to estimate the magnitude of the measurement errors. For time-dependent covariates, repeated measurements over time of the covariates allow us to model the covariate process and thus allow us to estimate the magnitude of the measurement errors. In other words, repeated measurements may be viewed as replicates. In this chapter, we consider mixed effects models with error-prone time-dependent covariates. We discuss linear mixed effects (LME) models, nonlinear mixed effects (NLME) models, generalized linear mixed models (GLMMs), and survival mixed (frailty) models with error-prone time-dependent covariates.

## 16.2 Generalized Linear Mixed Models (GLMM) with Covariate Measurement Errors

Generalized linear mixed models (GLMM) are widely used to model longitudinal data. They may be viewed as extensions of generalized linear models (GLM) for cross-sectional data to longitudinal data by including random effects in some of the regression parameters. These random effects not only reflect the variation between individuals but also incorporate the association among the repeated measurements in longitudinal data. A linear mixed effects (LME) model is a special case of GLMMs. In this section, we consider GLMMs with time-dependent covariates which may be measured with errors.

### 16.2.1 Measurement Error Models for Time-Dependent Covariates

In linear mixed effects (LME) models, random effects may be viewed as "individual effects", reflecting the individual deviations from population averages. Since each individual shares the same random effects, the associations among the repeated measurements on an individual are partially incorporated through the shared random effects. A main advantage of a mixed effects model for longitudinal data is that it allows for both individual-specific inference and usual population-average inference.

For example, for the CD4 data shown in Figure 16.1, we see large variations between the longitudinal trajectories of the CD4 profiles. Suppose that a sample of $n$ individuals is obtained, with individual $i$ having $m_i$ repeated measurements. To incorporate the large between-individual variation, as well as the association among the repeated measurements on the same individuals, we may fit the following LME model

$$\begin{aligned} x_{ij}^* &= \beta_{0i} + \beta_{1i} t_{ij} + \beta_{2i} t_{ij}^2 + e_{ij}, \qquad (16.1) \\ \beta_{0i} &= \beta_0 + b_{0i}, \qquad \beta_{1i} = \beta_1 + b_{1i}, \qquad \beta_{2i} = \beta_2 + b_{2i}, \\ & (b_{0i}, b_{1i}, b_{2i})^T \sim N(0, B_{3\times 3}), \qquad e_{ij} \sim N(0, \sigma^2), \\ & i = 1, 2, \cdots, n, \qquad j = 1, 2, \cdots, m_i, \end{aligned}$$

where $x_{ij}^*$ is the observed CD4 value for individual $i$ at time $t_{ij}$, $\beta_k$'s are fixed effect parameters (or population parameters), $b_{ki}$'s are random effects, $B_{3\times 3}$ is a general $3 \times 3$ covariance matrix incorporating correlations between the 3 random effects, $\sigma^2$ is the variance parameter for the repeated measurements within an individual, and $e_{ij}$ is measurement error or random error for the repeated measurements. We assume that the random effects $(b_{0i}, b_{1i}, b_{2i})$ are independent of the random error $e_{ij}$, and we also assume that the random errors $\{e_{i1}, e_{i2}, \cdots, e_{im_i}\}$ of the within-individual repeated measurements are independent and identically distributed (i.i.d.). The variance parameter $\sigma^2$ measures the variations of the repeated measurements within an individual. The variances of the random effects, i.e., the diagonal elements of the covariance matrix $B_{3\times 3}$, measure the variations between individuals. In the following, we write $B_{3\times 3}$ as $B$ when the dimensions are clear, and we use similar notation for other matrices or vectors. Figure 16.2 shows the (individual-specific) fitted curves for four randomly selected individuals. We see that the quadratic polynomial fitted the observed longitudinal CD4 data reasonably well.

It is well known that CD4 values are usually measured with substantial errors. To address measurement errors in CD4, model (16.1) may be treated as a measurement error model, where the (unobserved) true CD4 values are assumed to change smoothly over time. To see this, we write model (16.1) as follows

$$x_{ij}^* = x_{ij} + e_{ij}, \qquad e_{ij} \sim N(0, \sigma^2),$$

where $x_{ij} = \beta_{0i} + \beta_{1i} t_{ij} + \beta_{2i} t_{ij}^2$ may be interpreted as the (unobserved) true value of CD4 for individual $i$ measured at time $t_{ij}$, $x_{ij}^*$ is the observed but contaminated CD4 value, and $e_{ij}$ represents measurement error. In this case, the value of $\sigma$ reflects the magnitude of measurement errors. Here we assume that the magnitude of measurement errors is the same for all individuals over time.

Let

$$\widehat{\beta}_{0i} = \widehat{\beta}_0 + \widehat{b}_{0i}, \qquad \widehat{\beta}_{1i} = \widehat{\beta}_1 + \widehat{b}_{1i}, \qquad \widehat{\beta}_{2i} = \widehat{\beta}_2 + \widehat{b}_{2i},$$

be the estimates of the individual-specific parameters in model (16.1), where $\widehat{\beta}_k$ is the maximum likelihood estimate (MLE) of $\beta_k$ and $\widehat{b}_{ki}$ is the empirical Bayes estimate of $b_{ki}$, $k = 0, 1, 2; i = 1, 2, \cdots, n$. The value on the fitted individual curves (displayed in Figure 16.2)

$$\widehat{x}_{ij}^* = \widehat{\beta}_{0i} + \widehat{\beta}_{1i} t_{ij} + \widehat{\beta}_{2i} t_{ij}^2$$

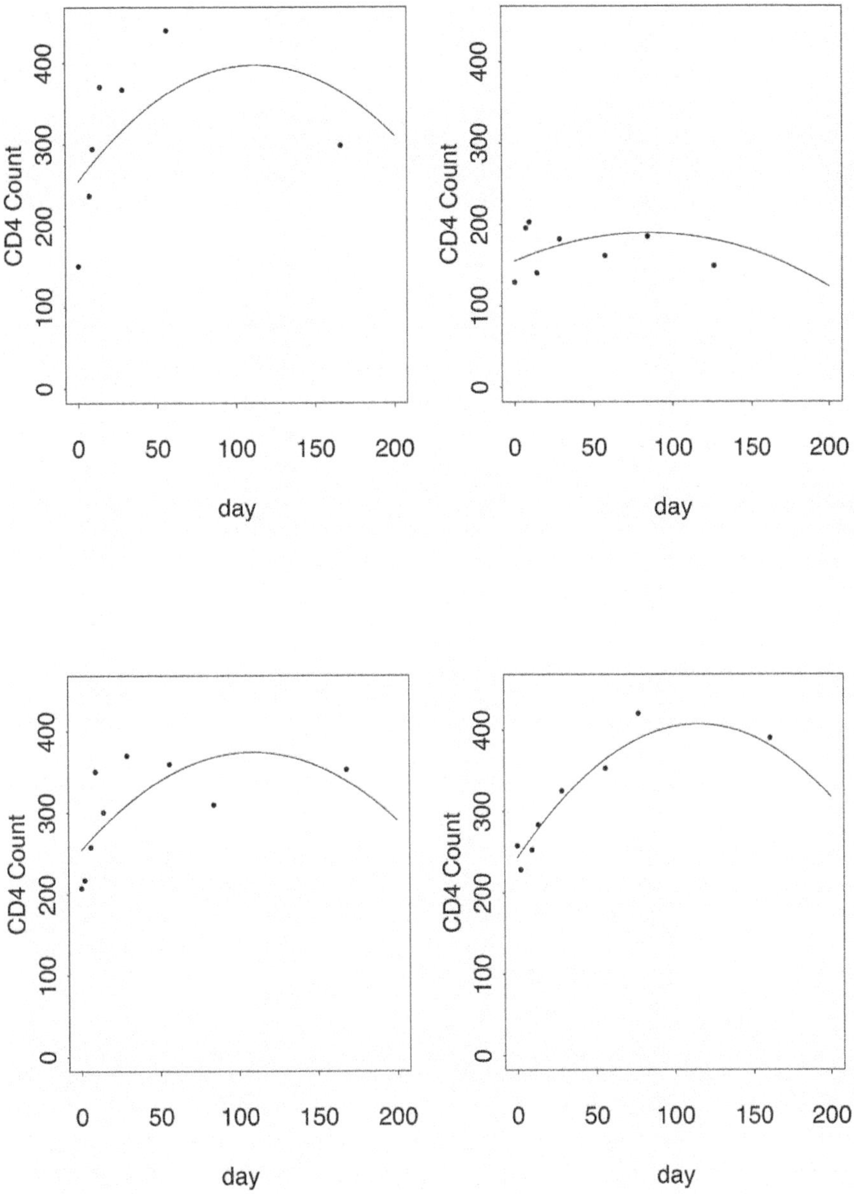


**FIGURE 16.2**
Individually fitted curves for the CD4 longitudinal data on four individuals.

may be viewed as an estimate of the true value $x_{ij}$. The above measurement error model is often called a *classical measurement error model.* In this approach, we have assumed that the true values of CD4 change smoothly over time. If the CD4 trajectories are too complicated for a parametric model to be appropriate, we may consider more flexible nonparametric mixed effects models, which may be approximated by LME models.

More generally, let the observed data of the time-dependent error-prone covariate be $\{x_i^*, \quad i = 1, 2, \cdots, n\}$, where $x_i^* = (x_{i1}^*, x_{i2}^*, \cdots, x_{im_i}^*)^T$. To address measurement errors in $x$, we may model the observed covariate data based on the following LME model

$$\begin{aligned} x_i &= U_i\beta + V_i b_i + e_i, \\ & \quad b_i \sim N(0, B), \qquad e_i \sim \sigma^2 I_{m_i}, \qquad i = 1, 2, \cdots, n, \end{aligned} \tag{16.2}$$

where $U_i$ and $V_i$ are $m_i \times p$ and $m_i \times d$ design matrices respectively, $\beta = (\beta_0, \beta_1, \cdots, \beta_p)^T$ is a $p \times 1$ vector of unknown fixed effect parameters, $b_i = (b_{0i}, b_{1i}, \cdots, b_{di})^T$ is a $d \times 1$ vector of random effects, $B$ is a $d \times d$ unknown covariance matrix of the random effects, $e_i = (e_{i1}, e_{i2}, \cdots, e_{im_i})^T$ is a vector of random errors, and $I_{m_i}$ is the $m_i \times m_i$ identity matrix. We assume that $b_i$ and $e_i$ are independent. The unknown parameter $\sigma$ reflects the magnitude of measurement errors of the observed covariate data, which may be estimated from the observed data.

### 16.2.2 GLMM with Covariates Measurement Errors

For the response longitudinal data, we consider GLMMs, which includes LME models as special cases. For simplicity, we focus on one time-dependent and error-prone covariate in the GLMM. Let $Y$ be a response random variable and $y$ be the observed value of $Y$. Let $y_{ij}$ be the value of the response variable for individual $i$ at time $t_{ij}$, $i = 1, 2, \cdots, n$; $j = 1, 2, \cdots, m_i$, and let $y_i = (y_{i1}, y_{i2}, \cdots, y_{im_i})^T$. Let $W_i$ be a $m_i \times q$ matrix of error-free covariates for individual $i$, which may contain both time-dependent and time-independent covariates, with the $j$-th column contains values of $j$-th covariate, $j = 1, 2, \cdots, q$. A general GLMM can be written as

$$h(E(y_i)) = W_i\alpha + Z_i a_i + \alpha_x x_i^*, \qquad i = 1, 2, \cdots, n, \tag{16.3}$$

where $h(\cdot)$ is a known link function, $\alpha = (\alpha_1, \cdots, \alpha_q)^T$ is a vector of unknown fixed effect parameters, $Z_i$ is a $m_i \times r$ design matrix which is usually a submatrix of $W_i$, $\mathbf{a}_i = (a_{0i}, a_{1i}, \cdots, a_{ri})^T$ is a vector of random effects in the response model, and $\alpha_x$ is an unknown parameter associated with the error-prone covariate $x_i^*$. We assume that $Y$ follows a distribution in the exponential family, such as a normal distribution and a binomial distribution. We also assume that the random effects $a_i \sim N(0, A)$, where $A$ is an $r \times r$ unknown covariance matrix. Note that, throughout this chapter, the random effects in the response model are denoted by vector $a_i$ while the random effects in the covariate model are denoted by vector $b_i$.

When the link function $h(y) = y$ and $Y$ follows a normal distribution, the GLMM (16.3) reduces to an LME model

$$E(y_i) = W_i\alpha + Z_i a_i + \alpha_x x_i^*.$$

When the link function is the logit link $h(y) = \log(y/(1-y))$ and $Y$ is binary taking values 0 and 1, the GLMM (16.3) is a logistic regression model with random effects

$$\log\left(\frac{P(y_{ij}=1)}{1-P(y_{ij}=1)}\right) = W_i\alpha + Z_i a_i + \alpha_x x_i,$$

where $Y$ is assumed to follow a Bernoulli distribution. The exponential family also contains other parametric distributions such as Poisson distributions and Negative binomial distributions. Thus, the GLMM (16.3) includes a wide variety of models useful for modelling various longitudinal data.

Since the time-dependent covariate $x^*$ is measured with error, we may replace model (16.3) by

$$h(E(y_i)) = W_i\alpha + Z_i a_i + \alpha_x x_i, \tag{16.4}$$

in which the observed covariate value $x_i^*$ is replaced by the unobserved true value $x_i$. In other words, the response $y$ depends on the true covariate value $x$ rather than the mis-measured value $x^*$. To estimate model parameters in GLMM (16.4), there are two commonly used methods: (i) two-step method; and (ii) joint likelihood method. These two methods are described below.

For the two-step method, we first fit the LME model (16.2) to the observed covariate data and obtain the predicted (fitted) covariate values $\widehat{x}_i$:

$$\widehat{x}_i = U_i\widehat{\beta} + V_i\widehat{b}_i, \qquad i = 1, 2, \cdots, n,$$

where $\widehat{b}_i$ is the empirical Bayes estimate of the random effects $b_i$. Then, in the second step, we fit the GLMM (16.4), with the unknown true covariate values $x_i$ in the model substituted by their estimates from the first step $\widehat{x}_i$:

$$h(E(y_i)) = W_i\alpha + Z_i a_i + \alpha_x\widehat{x}_i, \qquad i = 1, 2, \cdots, n.$$

To incorporate the estimation uncertainty in the first step, we may use a bootstrap method to obtain the standard errors of the parameter estimates in the GLMM. An advantage of this two-step method is that standard software can be used to fit the LME covariate model and the GLMM response model respectively.

For the joint likelihood method, we obtain MLEs of all parameters (denoted by $\theta$) in both the covariate model (16.2) and the response model (16.4) based on the likelihood

$$L(\theta|\text{data}) = \prod_{i=1}^{n}\int\int f(y_i|x_i, a_i, \theta)f(x_i^*|b_i, \theta)f(a_i|A)f(b_i|B)\; da_i db_i,$$

where $f(\cdot)$ denotes a generic density function. The resulting MLEs are consistent, asymptotically normal, and asymptotically most efficient under some regularity conditions.

A main challenge of the joint likelihood method is computational, since the likelihood involves a high-dimensional and intractable integration. A standard approach is to use the EM algorithm by treating the random effects $(a_i, b_i)$ as "missing data". At iteration $t$ ($t = 1, 2, 3, \cdots,$), the E-step computes the conditional expectation

$$Q(\theta; \theta^{(t)}) = E\Big[f(y_i|x_i, a_i, \theta)f(x_i^*|b_i, \theta)f(a_i|A)f(b_i|B) \mid y_i, x_i^*, \theta^{(t)}\Big],$$

where $\theta^{(t)}$ is the parameter estimate at iteration $t$, and the expectation is taken with respect to the conditional distribution of the "missing data" $(a_i, b_i)$ given the observed data $(y_i, x_i^*)$, evaluated at $\theta = \theta^{(t)}$. Monte-Carlo methods can be used to approximate this conditional expectation. The M-step then maximizes $Q(\theta; \theta^{(t)})$ using (say) the Newton-Raphson method. Beginning with some starting values and iterating the E-step and the M-step until convergence, we obtain a (possibly local) maxima. The EM algorithm can be slow to converge. Thus, computationally more efficient approximate methods, such as that based on Laplace approximations to the integral, are useful.

The above method addresses covariate measurement errors by modelling the longitudinal covariate data to estimate (unobserved) true covariate values and the magnitudes of measurement errors. The method may be most useful when the longitudinal covariate trajectories exhibit distinct patterns such as quadratic patterns.

## 16.3 Extensions

The basic ideas and approaches described in the previous section can be extended to other models with error-prone time-varying covariates. In the following, we briefly discuss four extensions: (i) nonlinear mixed effects response models; (ii) survival response models; (iii) mechanistic nonlinear covariate models; and (iv) nonparametric covariate models.

### 16.3.1 NLME Models with Measurement Errors in Time-Varying Covariates

Nonlinear mixed effects (NLME) models are extensions of LME models to allow the response variable to depend on parameters and random effects in nonlinear fashions. NLME models are usually mechanistic models in the sense that they are derived based on the underlying data-generation mechanisms, such as models for pharmacokinetics and HIV viral dynamics. Thus, NLME models are often called *mechanistic models* or *scientific models* (Wu, 2009). Since NLME models are based on the true data-generation mechanisms, they are more reliable for predictions than GLMMs. On the other hand, GLMM and LME models are usually empirical models in the sense that they only approximate the observed data without much understanding of the data-generation mechanisms, so predictions outside the observed data range based on GLMM and LME models can be unreliable.

Let $y_i = (y_{i1}, y_{i2}, \cdots, y_{im_i})^T$ denote the longitudinal response $y$ for individual $i$, and let $x_i^* = (x_{i1}^*, x_{i2}^*, \cdots, x_{im_i}^*)^T$ be the error-prone time-varying covariates, with the corresponding (unobserved) true values $x_i$. An NLME model can be written as

$$y_i = g(x_i, a_i, \alpha) + \epsilon_i, \qquad i = 1, 2, \cdots, n,$$

where $g(\cdot)$ is a known nonlinear function, vector $a_i$ contains random effects in the response model, vector $\alpha$ contains fixed effect parameters, and vector $\epsilon_i$ is the error term with $\epsilon_i \sim N(0, R_i)$ and $R_i$ is an $m_i \times m_i$ covariance matrix. Note that, both GLMM and NLME models are nonlinear in the parameters and random effects. However, a main difference between GLMM and NLME models is that, for NLME models, the covariates and random effects need not enter the models in a linear form and function $g(\cdot)$ can be any nonlinear function. Moreover, the error term $\epsilon_i$ in a NLME model is usually assumed to follow a normal distribution.

Methods for parameter estimation and inference are conceptually similar between GLMM and NLME models. So the methods to address measurement errors in time-varying covariates in a NLME model are similar to that for a GLMM described in the previous section. However, different issues may arise in implementation, since the response in a NLME model is assumed to be normal while the response in a GLMM can be discrete and follow non-normal distributions.

### 16.3.2 Survival Models with Measurement Errors in Time-Varying Covariates

In longitudinal studies, survival data or time-to-event data arise frequently. A key characteristic of survival data is that the data may be censored, such as the event of interest not being observed by the end of the study. In a survival model, some covariates may be measured repeatedly over time and may be measured with errors. In this section, we consider survival models with measurement errors in time-varying covariates. The popular joint models for longitudinal and survival data are motivated in these settings.

Let $s_i$ be the survival time for individual $i$, $i = 1, 2, \cdots, n$. Note that some individuals may not experience any events by the end of the study, so their event times may be *right censored.* We assume that the right censoring is random or non-informative. For individual $i$, let $c_i$ be the censoring time, and let $\delta_i = I(s_i \leq c_i)$ be the censoring indicator such that $\delta_i = 0$ if the survival time for individual $i$ is right censored and $\delta_i = 1$ otherwise. The observed survival data are $\{(t_i, \delta_i),\ i = 1, 2, \cdots, n\}$, where $t_i = \min(s_i, c_i)$ is either the event time or the censoring time.

We consider the following Cox model for the survival data, with time-dependent and error-prone covariate $x_i^*(t)$,

$$\lambda_i(t) = \lambda_0(t) \exp(x_i(t)\alpha_1 + \mathbf{w}_i^T \alpha_2), \qquad i = 1, \cdots, n, \tag{16.5}$$

where $\lambda_i(t)$ is the hazard function for individual $i$ at time $t$, $\lambda_0(t)$ is the unspecified baseline hazard function, $x_i(t)$ is the (unobserved) true covariate value for individual $i$ at time $t$ whose observed but mis-measured version is $x_i^*(t)$, $\mathbf{w}_i$ contains (possibly time-dependent) covariates without measurement errors, and $\alpha = (\alpha_1, \alpha_2)$ contains unknown parameters. Model (16.5) assumes that the hazard function $\lambda_i(t)$ depends on the unobserved true covariate values $x_i(t)$ rather than the observed but mis-measured covariate value $x_i^*(t)$. To address measurement errors for covariate $x_i^*(t)$, we may again consider the LME model (16.2).

Parameter estimation can again be based on the two-step method and the joint likelihood method. However, in this case, the longitudinal covariate $x_i(t)$ may be truncated by the events if the events of interest are (say) deaths or dropouts. Then the two-step method may lead to biased results, although it may be possible to reduce such biases with more complex modelling (e.g., Ye et al. 2008). In this case, the joint likelihood method remains valid. The joint likelihood for all the observed data is given by

$$L(\theta) = \prod_{i=1}^{n} \int f(t_i, \delta_i | x_i, \lambda_0, \alpha) f(x_i^* | b_i, \beta, \sigma^2) f(b_i | B)\, db_i, \tag{16.6}$$

where $f(\cdot)$ denotes a generic density function, the covariate model for $x_i^*$ is the same as that in model (16.2), $f(t_i, \delta_i | x_i, \lambda_0, \alpha) = \lambda_i(t_i)^{\delta_i} S(t_i)$, and $S(t_i)$ is the survival function. MLEs of the model parameters can be obtained either by using an EM algorithm or an approximate method. However, the computation becomes more challenging than that discussed in the previous sections, due to the nonparametric hazard functions and censoring.

There has been an extensive literature on joint models for longitudinal and survival data in the past two decades. Rizopoulos (2012) and Elashoff et al. (2015) provided nice reviews. Also see Section 5.6 of Yi (2017). One of the main applications of joint models is survival models with measurement errors in time-dependent covariates. These joint models are also useful in other applications, such as longitudinal models with informative dropouts and joint modelling of a longitudinal process and an event process.

### 16.3.3 Mechanistic Nonlinear Covariate Models for Measurement Errors

In the previous sections, we have used LME models empirically to model the observed error-prone covariate data in order to address measurement errors.

In some cases, the covariate data may be measured infrequently or may even be censored. For example, in HIV/AIDS studies, viral load data may be left censored due to a lower detection limit. In these cases, empirical LME models based on the observed error-prone covariate data may not provide good estimates of the corresponding unobserved true covariate values. In some applications, such as pharmacokinetics and HIV viral dynamics, mechanistic NLME models are available. Since such NLME models are derived based on the underlying data-generation mechanisms, the models should still be valid at times when no data are available or the data are censored. Thus, we can use the mechanistic NLME covariate models to estimate the unobserved true covariate values.

Figure 16.3 shows the individual fitted curves based on an NLME model and an empirical LME (ELM) model for viral load (in $\log_{10}$ scale) data during an anti-HIV treatment respectively (Zhang and Wu, 2018). Some viral loads are left censored (below the detection limit), and they are substituted by half the detection limit in the Figure. We denote the observed viral load data by $x_{ij}^*$, which is subject to measurement error and left censoring, and consider the following mechanistic NLME model derived from biological arguments (Wu and Ding, 1999)

$$
\begin{aligned}
x_{ij}^* &= \log_{10}\{e^{\beta_1+b_{1i}} + e^{(\beta_2+b_{2i})-(\beta_3+b_{3i})t_{ij}}\} + e_{ij}, \\
b_i &= (b_{1i}, b_{2i}, b_{3i})^T \sim N(0, B), \quad e_{ij} \quad \text{i.i.d.} \quad \sim N(0, \sigma^2),
\end{aligned}
$$

where $\beta_j$'s are fixed effects, $b_{ki}$'s are random effects, $B$ is a $3 \times 3$ covariance matrix incorporating the correlations among the random effects $b_{ki}$'s, and $e_{ij}$ represents measurement error. We assume that the $b_i$'s are independent, and $b_i$ is independent of $e_{ij}$ for any $i$ and $j$. For the ELM model, we consider a quadratic polynomial mixed effects model as shown in previous sections.

From Figure 16.3, we see that the individual fitted curves based on an NLME model and an ELM model are different. These fitted curves are used to estimate the (unobserved) true viral load values. The estimated true viral load values based on the NLME model should be better, since the foregoing NLME model is justified biologically so it should hold at times no data are observed. This is confirmed by extensive simulation studies (Zhang and Wu, 2018).

### 16.3.4 Nonparametric Covariate Models for Measurement Errors

Longitudinal data can be highly complex, so parametric models may not provide good fit to the observed data in some cases. In these cases, we may consider nonparametric mixed effects model to fit the observed data (Liu and Wu, 2007). Nonparametric models are flexible and may provide reasonable fit to any observed data.

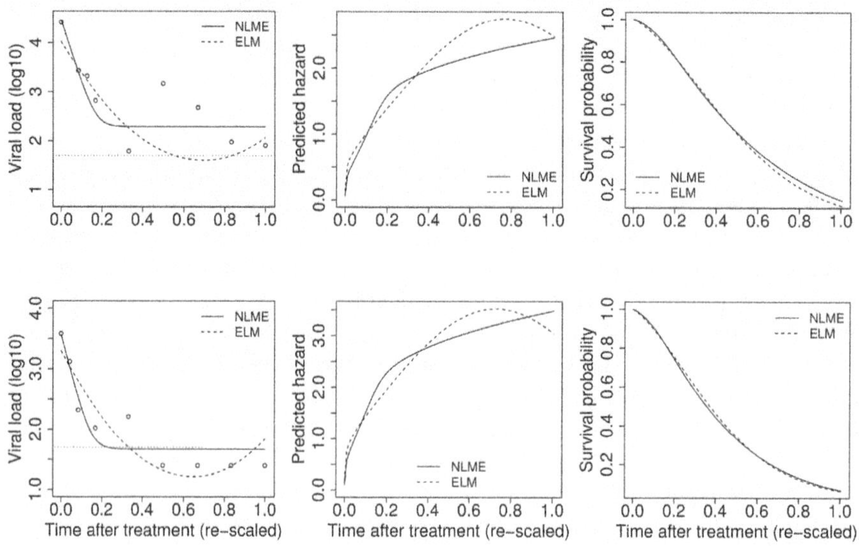


**FIGURE 16.3**
Individual fitted curves based on an NLME model and an ELM model for viral load (in $\log_{10}$ scale) data respectively. The solid fitted curve is based on an NLME model, the dotted fitted curve is based on an ELM model, and the dotted horizontal line is the detection limit.

A general nonparametric mixed effects model can be written as:

$$\begin{aligned} x_{ij}^* &= g(t_{ij}) + u_i(t_{ij}) + e_{ij}, \qquad (16.7)\\ u_i(t) &\sim GP(0,\gamma), \qquad e_i \sim N(0, R_i), \ \ i = 1, \cdots, n; \ j = 1, \cdots, m_i, \end{aligned}$$

where $g(\cdot)$ is an unknown smooth function, $u_i(t)$ is a random smooth process and assumed to follow a Gaussian process with mean 0 and covariance function $Cov(u_i(s), u_i(t)) = \gamma(s,t)$, denoted by $u_i(t) \sim GP(0,\gamma)$, and $e_i = (e_{i1}, \cdots, e_{im_i})^T$. We assume that $u_i(t)$ and $e_i$ are independent for any $t$. Although there are many nonparametric methods, here we consider a regression spline approach. The idea is to approximate model (16.7) by

$$x_i^*(t_{ij}) \approx \sum_{k=0}^{l_1} \beta_k \psi_k(t_{ij}) + \sum_{k=0}^{l_2} b_{ik}\phi_k(t_{ij}) + e_i(t_{ij}), \qquad (16.8)$$

where $\Psi_{l_1}(t) = (\psi_1(t), \cdots, \psi_{l_1}(t))^T$ and $\Phi_{l_2}(t) = (\phi_1(t), \cdots, \phi_{l_2}(t))^T$ are known basis functions, $\beta = (\beta_1, \cdots, \beta_{l_1})^T$ are fixed parameters, and $b_i = (b_{i1}, \cdots, b_{il_2})^T$ are random coefficients. We assume that $b_i \sim N(0, B)$ with $B$ being a $l_2 \times l_2$ covariance matrix. The numbers $l_1$ and $l_2$ of basis functions control the smoothness and goodness of fit of the estimated function.

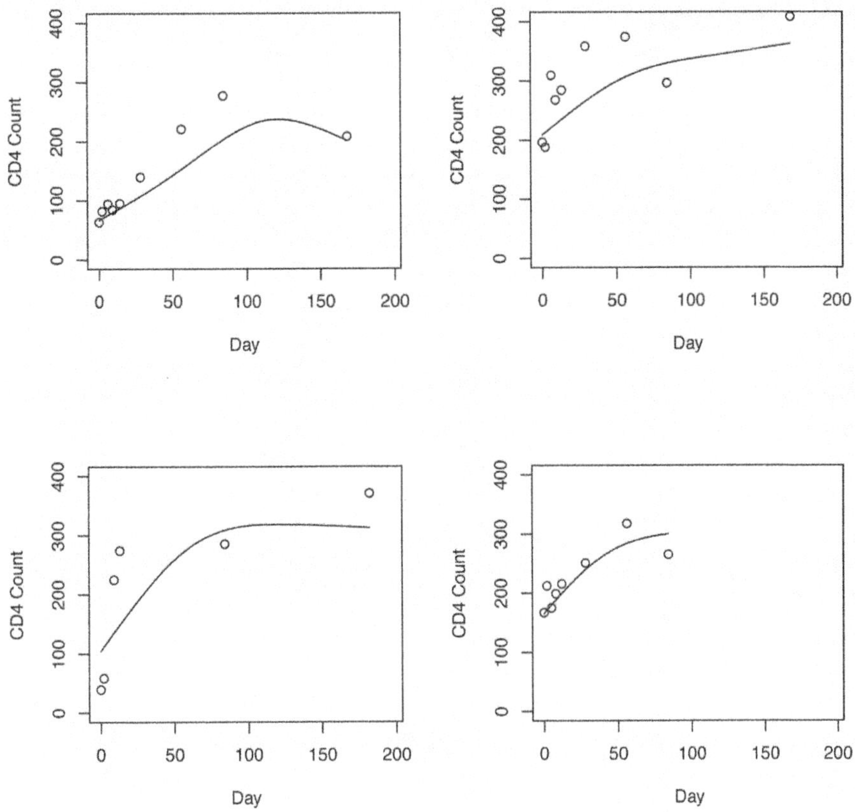


**FIGURE 16.4**
CD4 data fitted by a nonparametric smoothing method for four randomly selected subjects.

Let $\mathbf{w}_{ij} = \Phi_{l_1}(t_{ij})$ and $\mathbf{z}_{ij} = \Psi_{l_2}(t_{ij})$. Model (16.8) can then be written as a standard LME model

$$x_{ij}^* = \mathbf{w}_{ij}^T\beta + \mathbf{z}_{ij}^T b_i + e_{ij}, \tag{16.9}$$

$$b_i \sim N(0, B), \qquad \mathbf{e}_i \sim N(0, R_i). \tag{16.10}$$

So standard estimation methods for LME models can be used for approximate inference of the original nonparametric mixed effects model (16.7). The basis functions can be any commonly used ones, and we often choose $\phi_j(t) = \psi_j(t)$ for simplicity. Choices of $l_1$ and $l_2$ are based on the trade-off between goodness of fit and model complexity. Figure 16.4 shows an example of CD4 data fitted by a nonparametric smoothing method for four randomly selected subjects.

## 16.4 Example

As an illustration, we consider an AIDS dataset which includes 46 HIV infected patients receiving an anti-HIV treatment (Zhang and Wu, 2018). Viral loads and CD4 cell counts were repeatedly measured during the treatment. The number of repeated measurements for each individual varies from 4 to 10. About 11% viral load measurements are left censored or below the detection limit of 100 copies/mL. We call the viral loads below the detection limit as "viral suppression". Our objective is to check if the initial CD4 trajectories are associated with the time to viral suppression.

We consider a survival model for the time to viral suppression, i.e., the time from the start of the treatment to the first scheduled time when the viral load drops below the detection limit. The viral suppression times for patients whose viral loads never dropped below detection limit may be considered as right censored, with the study end time as the censoring time. We consider the following Cox model for the times to viral suppression

$$\lambda_i(t) = \lambda_0(t) \exp(x_i(t)\alpha_1),$$

where $x_i(t)$ is the (true) CD4 value for individual $i$ at time $t$, and other covariates are not included to keep the model simple.

To address the measurement error in the time-dependent covariate CD4 cell count, we use the LME model to model the CD4 trajectories

$$x^*_{ij} = (\beta_0 + b_{i1}) + (\beta_1 + b_{i2})t_{ij} + \epsilon_{ij}, \qquad \epsilon_{ij} \sim N(0, \sigma^2), \tag{16.11}$$

where the notation and assumptions are the same as those described in the previous sections. To avoid very small (large) estimates, which may be unstable, we standardize the CD4 cell counts and rescale the original time $t$ (in days) so that the new time scale is between 0 and 1. We estimate the model parameters using the joint model (likelihood) method and the two-stage method. The analyses were done using the R functions *coxph*(), *lme*(), and *jointModel*().

Table 16.1 presents the resulting estimates of parameters of interest and their standard errors. We see that both the two-stage and the joint model

**TABLE 16.1**
Analysis results of the AIDS data.

| Method | | $\alpha_1$ | $\beta_0$ | $\beta_1$ | $\sigma$ |
|---|---|---|---|---|---|
| Two-stage | Estimate | 0.315 | −0.233 | 1.345 | 0.605 |
| | Standard Error | 0.208 | 0.113 | 0.154 | – |
| | $p$-value | 0.129 | 0.040 | $< 0.001$ | – |
| Joint model | Estimate | 0.648 | −0.201 | 1.342 | 0.603 |
| | Standard Error | 0.234 | 0.135 | 0.162 | – |
| | $p$-value | 0.006 | 0.137 | $< 0.001$ | – |

methods produce similar estimates for the covariate (CD4) longitudinal model. However, the two-stage method may underestimate the standard errors of the parameter estimates. The parameter $\alpha_1$ in the survival model measures the effect of the true time-dependent covariate CD4 values on event times, so its estimate and the associated $p$-value can be used to check if the true CD4 values are predictive for the times to viral suppression. For the joint model method, there is some evidence that covariate CD4 is associated with the time to viral suppression, after measurement error has been addressed. On the other hand, the two-stage method may severely under-estimate the covariate CD4 effect.

## 16.5 Discussion

In this chapter, we have discussed mixed effects models with measurement errors in time-dependent covariates. A main advantage of time-dependent covariates is that the longitudinal measurements of the covariates can be used to estimate the magnitudes of measurement errors since these repeated measurements may be viewed as replicates of the covariates. For *time-independent* covariates with measurement errors, we need replicates or external data to estimate the magnitudes of the measurement errors. In the absence of replicates or external data, we may perform sensitivity analysis by assuming various magnitudes of the measurement errors and check how sensitive the analysis results are to the assumed magnitudes of measurement errors.

For time-dependent covariates, we have assumed models for the longitudinal covariate data. If the assumed models hold, a joint model for the longitudinal covariate data and the response data is desirable, since it simultaneously estimate all model parameters so a joint likelihood method may provide most efficient inference. There are other models for longitudinal data, such as generalized estimating equation models, and other methods for measurement errors (Carroll et al., 2006; Yi, 2017). Due to space limitation, we will not discuss those models and methods.

## Bibliography

Carroll, R., Ruppert, D., Stefanski, L., and Crainiceanu, C. (2006). *Measurement Error in Nonlinear Models: A Modern Perspective.* 2nd ed., Chapman and Hall, London.

Liu, W. and Wu, L. (2007). Simultaneous inference for semiparametric nonlinear mixed-effects models with covariate measurement errors and missing respones. *Biometrics*, 63(4), 342-350.

Elashoff, R., Li, G., and Li, N. (2015). Joint modeling of longitudinal and time-to-event data. Chapman & Hall.

Rizopoulos, D. (2012). *Joint Models for Longitudinal and Time-to-Event Data: with Applications in R.* Chapman & Hall/CRC.

Wu, H. and Ding, A. (1999). Population HIV-1 dynamics in vivo: Applicable models and inferential tools for virological data from AIDS clinical trials. *Biometrics*, 55, 410-418.

Wu, L. (2009). *Mixed Effects Models for Complex Data.* CRC Press.

Ye, W., Lin, X., and Taylor, J. (2008). Semiparametric modeling of longitudinal measurements and time-to-event data – a two-stage regression calibration approach. *Biometrics*, 64, 1238-1246.

Yi, G. Y. (2017). *Statistical Analysis with Measurement Error or Misclassification: Strategy, Method and Application.* Springer.

Zhang, H. and Wu, L. (2018). A non-linear model for censored and mismeasured time varying covariates in survival models, with applications in human immunodeficiency virus and acquired immune deficiency syndrome studies. *Journal of the Royal Statistical Society, Series C*, 67, 1437-1450.

# 17

# *Estimation in Mixed-effects Models with Measurement Error*

**Liqun Wang**

## CONTENTS



## 17.1 Introduction

Measurement error is common in longitudinal data analysis. For example, in epidemiologic studies covariates such as blood pressure, cholesterol level, exposure to air pollutants, dietary intakes, etc. are often measured with error. In HIV trials, the viral load and CD4+ T-cell counts are also subject to measurement error. It is well-known that simply substituting a proxy variable for the unobserved covariate in a model will generally lead to biased and inconsistent estimates of regression coefficients and variance components (e.g., Wang and Davidian, 1996; Tosteson, Buonaccorsi and Demidenko, 1998; Wang et al., 1998; Carroll et al., 2006). To account for the measurement error as

DOI: 10.1201/9781315101279-17

well as the intra-unit correlation in the longitudinal data, Wang et al (1998) proposed the simulation extrapolation (SIMEX) method to correct for the bias of the naive penalized quasi-likelihood estimator in a generalized linear mixed model, while Wang, Lin and Guitierrez (1999), and Bartlett, de Stavola and Frost (2009) used the regression calibration (RC) approach under the availability of validation data. Although both RC and SIMEX approaches may produce satisfactory results when the measurement errors are small, in general they yield approximate but inconsistent estimators.

On the other hand, Buonaccorsi, Demidenko and Tosteson (2000) studied the likelihood based methods, and Zhong, Fung and Wei (2002) used the corrected score approach. However, the likelihood methods typically entail computational difficulties due to intractability of the likelihood function that involves multiple integrals. Consequently, one usually relies on normality assumption for random effects, measurement error and regression random error term. Non- or semi-parametric approaches have also been considered for models with normal measurement error (Tsiatis and Davidian, 2001; Pan, Zeng and Lin, 2009). Moreover, Liu and Wu (2007), Wang et al. (2008), Yi, Liu and Wu (2011), and Yi, Ma and Carroll (2012) studied the joint problem of covariate measurement error and missing response in longitudinal data models. Most of the above mentioned methods assume that the measurement error variance is known or can be estimated by using validation or replicate data. However, note that the repeated longitudinal measurements taken at different time points cannot be used as replicate data in this context unless the mismeasured covariates are time-invariant.

The instrumental variable (IV) method has been used by many researchers to overcome measurement error problems in cross-sectional data analysis (e.g., Fuller, 1987; Buzas and Stefanski, 1996; Carroll et al., 2006; Wang and Hsiao, 2011; Abarin and Wang, 2012; Xu, Ma and Wang, 2015; Guan et al., 2019). It is also used in the longitudinal data models with measurement error by, e.g., Li and Wang (2012a) and Abarin et al (2014). In practice, any variable that is correlated with the error-prone covariates and independent of the measurement error can serve as valid IV, e.g., a second independent measurement, or repeated measurements at different time points in longitudinal studies. Hence the IV assumption is weaker than that of replicate data because IV can be a biased observation for the true covariates (Carroll and Stefanski, 1994; Carroll et al., 2006).

In this chapter, we introduce a semiparametric estimation approach for the generalized linear mixed models with measurement error based on the methods of moments and instrumental variables. This method is easy to implement when the closed forms of the moments exist. We also propose a simulation-based estimator for the case where the marginal moments do not admit closed forms. The proposed estimators are root-n consistent and do not require the parametric assumptions for the distributions of the unobserved covariates or of the measurement errors. Further, these estimators have bounded influence functions so they are robust to data outliers (Li and Wang, 2012b).

The rest of this chapter is organized as follows. In Section 17.2 we introduce the IV estimation method in the linear mixed measurement error model. This method is extended to the generalized linear mixed measurement error model in Section 17.3. In Section 17.4 we introduce the simulation-based estimation for the case where the closed forms of the marginal moments are not available. In Section 17.5 we deal with numerical computation issues and present Monte Carlo simulation examples. The asymptotic theories and mathematical proofs are given in Sections 17.6 and 17.7 respectively. Finally, conclusions and discussion are given in Section 17.8.

## 17.2 Linear Mixed Measurement Error Model

Let $Y_{ij}$ be the response variable of individual $i$ at time $j$, where $i = 1, 2, ..., n$, $j = 1, 2, ..., m$, $X_{ij} \in I\!R^{p_x}$ and $Z_{ij} \in I\!R^{p_z}$ be the covariates measured with and without measurement error respectively. Then the linear mixed model is defined as

$$Y_{ij} = X_{ij}^\top \beta_x + Z_{ij}^\top \beta_z + B_{ij}^\top b_i + \varepsilon_{ij}, \tag{17.1}$$

where $B_{ij}$ is a vector of predictors, $b_i$ is the vector of unobserved random effects and $\varepsilon_{ij}$ is the random error. Throughout this chapter we assume that $Z_{ij}$ and $B_{ij}$ are exogenous and all expectations are taken conditional on them, however, they are suppressed to simplify notation. Further, we assume that the random effects $b_i$ have mean $E(b_i|X_i) = 0$ and variance $E(b_i b_i^\top|X_i) = \Sigma_b$, where $X_i = (X_{i1}, X_{i2}, ..., X_{im})^\top$, and the random errors $\varepsilon_i = (\varepsilon_{i1}, \varepsilon_{i2}, ..., \varepsilon_{im})^\top$ satisfy $E(\varepsilon_i|X_i, b_i) = 0$ and $E(\varepsilon_i\varepsilon_i^\top|X_i, b_i) = \phi I$, where $I$ is the identity matrix.

Thus, under the model assumptions the first two marginal moments of the response variables are given by

$$E(Y_{ij}|X_i) = X_{ij}^\top \beta_x + Z_{ij}^\top \beta_z \tag{17.2}$$

and

$$E(Y_{ij}Y_{ik}|X_i) = (X_{ij}^\top \beta_x + Z_{ij}^\top \beta_z)(X_{ik}^\top \beta_x + Z_{ik}^\top \beta_z) + B_{ij}^\top \Sigma_b B_{ik} + d_{jk}\phi, \tag{17.3}$$

where $d_{jk} = 1$ if $j = k$ and zero otherwise.

For the error-prone covariates $X_{ij}$ we assume an additive classical measurement error model, so that its observed surrogate is

$$X_{ij}^* = X_{ij} + U_{ij}, \tag{17.4}$$

where $U_{ij}$ is the vector of measurement errors satisfying $E(U_{ij}|X_{ij}) = 0$. Further, we assume that instrumental variables $W_{ij} \in I\!R^{p_w}$ are available that are related to $X_{ij}$ through

$$X_{ij} = \Gamma_w W_{ij} + \delta_{ij}, \tag{17.5}$$

where $\Gamma_w \in I\!R^{p_x \times p_w}$ is a matrix of unknown parameters, $\delta_{ij}$ is the random error with $E(\delta_{ij}|W_i) = 0$ and $E(\delta_{ij}\delta_{ik}^\top|W_i) = d_{jk}\Sigma_\delta$, and $W_i = (W_{i1}, W_{i2}, ..., W_{im})^\top$. In order to ensure model identifiability, one needs to have at least as many IVs as the number of unobserved variables $X_{ij}$, so it is assumed that $p_w \geq p_x$ and $\Gamma_w$ has full row rank (Wang 2021). Moreover, the IV $W_{ij}$ may contain extra variables such as constant 1 and components of $Z_{ij}$ that are highly correlated with $X_{ij}$. It is further assumed that the random effects and errors satisfy $E(U_{ij}|X_i, W_i) = 0$, $E(\epsilon_{ij}|X_i, X_i^*, W_i) = 0$ and $E(b_i|X_i, X_i^*, W_i) = 0$ . These assumptions imply that

$$E(Y_{ij}|X_i, W_i) = E(Y_{ij}|X_i) \tag{17.6}$$

and

$$E(Y_{ij}Y_{ik}|X_i, W_i) = E(Y_{ij}Y_{ik}|X_i). \tag{17.7}$$

Note that in model (17.1), (17.4) and (17.5), there is no assumption on the functional forms of the distributions of unobserved variables, random effects and errors. The observed variables are $(Y_{ij}, X_{ij}^{*\top}, W_{ij}, Z_{ij}^\top, B_{ij}^\top)^\top$ and the parameters of main interest are $\psi = (\beta_x^\top, \beta_z^\top, \theta^\top, \alpha^\top, \phi)^\top$, where $\theta$ is the vector of unknown variance parameters in $\Sigma_b$ and $\alpha$ is the vector of unknown variance parameters in $\Sigma_\delta$. Throughout this chapter, we denote the parameter space of $\psi$ by $\Omega_\psi$.

The parameter estimation is based on the first two conditional moments of the responses and observed covariates given the instrumental variables. Specifically, by equation (17.6) and the law of iterated expectation, the conditional expectation of $Y_{ij}$ given $W_i$ is given by

$$\begin{aligned}
\mu_{ij}(\psi) &= E(Y_{ij}|W_i) \\
&= E\left[E(Y_{ij}|X_i, W_i)|W_i\right] \\
&= E\left[E(Y_{ij}|X_i)|W_i\right] \\
&= E(X_{ij}|W_i)^\top\beta_x + Z_{ij}^\top\beta_z \\
&= (\Gamma_w W_{ij})^\top\beta_x + Z_{ij}^\top\beta_z.
\end{aligned} \tag{17.8}$$

Similarly, the second conditional moments are given by

$$\begin{aligned}
\nu_{ijk}(\psi) &= E(Y_{ij}Y_{ik}|W_i) \\
&= E\left[E(Y_{ij}Y_{ik}|X_i)|W_i\right] \\
&= E\left[(X_{ij}^\top\beta_x + Z_{ij}^\top\beta_z)(X_{ik}^\top\beta_x + Z_{ik}^\top\beta_z)|W_i\right] + B_{ij}^\top\Sigma_b B_{ik} + d_{jk}\phi \\
&= (\Gamma_w W_{ij})^\top\beta_x + Z_{ij}^\top\beta_z)((\Gamma_w W_{ik})^\top\beta_x + Z_{ik}^\top\beta_z) + B_{ij}^\top\Sigma_b B_{ik} \\
&\quad + d_{jk}(\beta_x^\top\Sigma_\delta\beta_x + \phi) \\
&= \mu_{ij}(\psi)\mu_{ik}(\psi) + B_{ij}^\top\Sigma_b B_{ik} + d_{jk}(\beta_x^\top\Sigma_\delta\beta_x + \phi),
\end{aligned} \tag{17.9}$$

and

$$\begin{aligned}\kappa_{ijk}(\psi) &= E(Y_{ij}X_{ik}^*|W_i) \\ &= E(Y_{ij}X_{ik}|W_i) \\ &= E\left[E(Y_{ij}|X_i)X_{ik}|W_i\right] \\ &= E\left[(X_{ij}^\top\beta_x + Z_{ij}^\top\beta_z)X_{ik}|W_i\right] \\ &= \left[(\Gamma_w W_{ij})^\top\beta_x + Z_{ij}^\top\beta_z\right](\Gamma_w W_{ik}) + d_{jk}\Sigma_\delta\beta_x \\ &= \mu_{ij}(\psi)(\Gamma_w W_{ik}) + d_{jk}\Sigma_\delta\beta_x. \end{aligned} \tag{17.10}$$

Next we construct semiparametric IV estimator for $\psi$ based on these conditional moments. First, note that substituting (17.5) into (17.4) results in a usual regression equation

$$E(X_{ij}^*|W_{ij}) = \Gamma_w W_{ij}, \tag{17.11}$$

and therefore $\Gamma_w$ can be estimated by the least squares estimator

$$\widehat{\Gamma}_w = \left(\sum_{i=1}^n X_i^{*\top} W_i\right)\left(\sum_{i=1}^n W_i^\top W_i\right)^{-1}, \tag{17.12}$$

where $X_i^* = (X_{i1}^*, X_{i2}^*, ..., X_{im}^*)^\top$ and $W_i = (W_{i1}, W_{i2}, ..., W_{im})^\top$. Then we substitute $\widehat{\Gamma}_w$ for $\Gamma_w$ in (17.8)-(17.10) and denote the conditional moments correspondingly as $\widehat{\mu}_{ij}, \widehat{\nu}_{ijk}$, and $\widehat{\kappa}_{ijk}$. Finally, the IV estimator (IVE) for $\psi$ is defined as

$$\widehat{\psi}_n = \arg\min_{\psi\in\Omega_\psi} Q_n(\psi) := \sum_{i=1}^n \widehat{\rho}_i^\top(\psi) A_i \widehat{\rho}_i(\psi), \tag{17.13}$$

where $\widehat{\rho}_i^\top(\psi) = (Y_{ij} - \widehat{\mu}_{ij}(\psi), Y_{ij}Y_{ik} - \widehat{\nu}_{ijk}(\psi), Y_{ij}X_{ik}^* - \widehat{\kappa}_{ijk}(\psi), j = 1, ..., m; k = j, ..., m)$ and $A_i = A(W_i)$ is a nonnegative definite matrix that may depend on $W_i$. A numerical example of this estimator is given in Section 17.5.

## 17.3 Generalized Linear Mixed Model

Generalized linear mixed models (GLMM) have been widely used to analyze longitudinal data where the response variable can be either discrete or continuous. Various estimation methods for GLMM have been developed in the literature (e.g., Breslow and Clayton, 1993; Durbin and Koopman, 1997; Rabe-Hesketh, Skrondal and Pickles, 2002). However, estimation and inference in a GLMM remain very challenging when some of the covariates are measured with error.

In this section we study the model

$$E(Y_{ij}|X_i, b_i) = g(\eta_{ij}), \tag{17.14}$$
$$V(Y_{ij}|X_i, b_i) = \phi h(\eta_{ij}), \tag{17.15}$$

where $\eta_{ij} = X_{ij}^\top \beta_x + Z_{ij}^\top \beta_z + B_{ij}^\top b_i$ is the linear predictor, $\beta_x \in I\!R^{p_x}$ and $\beta_z \in I\!R^{p_z}$ are vectors of fixed effects, $b_i$ is the random effect having mean zero and distribution $f_b(b;\theta)$ with unknown variance parameters $\theta \in I\!R^{p_b}$. The link function $g(\cdot)$ and variance function $h(\cdot)$ are known functions and $\phi \in I\!R$ is a scale parameter that may be known or unknown. Note that the estimation methods in this chapter do not require the conditional distribution of $Y_{ij}$ given $b_i$ to belong to an exponential family. However, we assume that $Y_{ij}, j = 1, 2, ..., m$ are conditionally independent given $b_i$ and, therefore, we have

$$E(Y_{ij}^2|X_i, b_i) = g^2(\eta_{ij}) + \phi h(\eta_{ij}) \tag{17.16}$$

and for $j \neq k$,

$$E(Y_{ij}Y_{ik}|X_i, b_i) = E(Y_{ij}|X_i, b_i)E(Y_{ik}|X_i, b_i) = g(\eta_{ij})g(\eta_{ik}). \tag{17.17}$$

Model (17.14)–(17.15) has been studied by various authors, e.g., Wang et al (1998), Buonaccorsi, Demidenko and Tosteson (2000), Zhong, Fung and Wei (2002) and Carroll et al. (2006).

Again, suppose that $X_{ij}$ is not observable and we assume the measurement error model (17.4) and instrumental model (17.5). We further assume that $W_i, \delta_i, b_i$ are mutually independent and, similar to (17.6) and (17.7), that

$$E(Y_{ij}|X_i, b_i, W_i) = E(Y_{ij}|X_i, b_i) \tag{17.18}$$

and

$$E(Y_{ij}Y_{ik}|X_i, b_i, W_i) = E(Y_{ij}Y_{ik}|X_i, b_i). \tag{17.19}$$

We extend the estimation method in the previous section to model (17.14)-(17.15). To simplify notation, let $g_{ij}(b, t, \beta, \gamma) = g((\Gamma_w W_{ij} + t)^\top \beta_x + Z_{ij}^\top \beta_z + B_{ij}^\top b)$, where $\gamma = \operatorname{vec}\Gamma_w$ is the vector consisting of the columns of $\Gamma_w$, and $h_{ij}(b, t, \beta, \gamma)$ is defined similarly. First, by model assumptions and the law of iterated expectation, the first conditional moments of $Y_{ij}$ given $W_i$ are given by

$$\begin{aligned} \mu_{ij}(\psi) &= E(Y_{ij}|W_i) \\ &= E\left[E(Y_{ij}|X_i, b_i)|W_i\right] \\ &= \int g_{ij}(b, t, \beta, \gamma) f_b(b;\theta) f_\delta(t;\alpha)\, db\, dt. \end{aligned} \tag{17.20}$$

Similarly, the second moments are given by

$$\begin{aligned} \nu_{ijj}(\psi) &= E(Y_{ij}^2|W_i) \\ &= \int [g_{ij}^2(b, t, \beta, \gamma) + \phi h_{ij}(b, t, \beta, \gamma)] f_b(b;\theta) f_\delta(t;\alpha)\, db\, dt, \end{aligned} \tag{17.21}$$

and for $j \neq k$,

$$\nu_{ijk}(\psi) = E(Y_{ij}Y_{ik}|W_i)$$
$$= \int g_{ij}(b,t,\beta,\gamma)g_{ik}(b,t',\beta,\gamma)f_b(b;\theta)f_\delta(t;\alpha)f_\delta(t';\alpha)\, db\, dt\, dt'. \tag{17.22}$$

Further, we have

$$\begin{aligned}\kappa_{ijj}(\psi) &= E(Y_{ij}X_{ij}^*|W_i)\\ &= E\left[E(Y_{ij}|X_i,b_i)X_{ij}|W_i\right]\\ &= \int g_{ij}(b,t,\beta,\gamma)(\Gamma_w W_{ij}+t)f_b(b;\theta)f_\delta(t;\alpha)\, db\, dt\\ &= \mu_{ij}(\psi)(\Gamma_w W_{ij}) + \int t g_{ij}(b,t,\beta,\gamma)f_b(b;\theta)f_\delta(t;\alpha)\, db\, dt, \end{aligned} \tag{17.23}$$

and for $j \neq k$,

$$\begin{aligned}\kappa_{ijk}(\psi) &= E(Y_{ij}X_{ik}^*|W_i)\\ &= E\left[E(Y_{ij}|X_i,b_i)X_{ik}|W_i\right]\\ &= E\left[E(Y_{ij}|X_i,b_i)(\Gamma_w W_{ik})|W_i\right]\\ &= \mu_{ij}(\psi)(\Gamma_w W_{ik}). \end{aligned} \tag{17.24}$$

Again, we substitute the least squares estimator $\widehat{\Gamma}_w$ for $\Gamma_w$ in (17.20)-(17.24) and denote the resulting moments as $\widehat{\mu}_{ij}, \widehat{\nu}_{ijk}$, and $\widehat{\kappa}_{ijk}$ correspondingly. Then the IV estimator (IVE) for $\psi = (\beta_x^\top, \beta_z^\top, \theta^\top, \alpha^\top, \phi)^\top$ is given by

$$\widehat{\psi}_n = \arg\min_{\psi\in\Omega_\psi} Q_n(\psi) := \sum_{i=1}^{n} \widehat{\rho}_i^{\top}(\psi)A_i\widehat{\rho}_i(\psi), \tag{17.25}$$

where $\widehat{\rho}_i^\top(\psi) = (Y_{ij} - \widehat{\mu}_{ij}(\psi), Y_{ij}Y_{ik} - \widehat{\nu}_{ijk}(\psi), Y_{ij}X_{ik}^* - \widehat{\kappa}_{ijk}(\psi), j = 1,...,m; k = j,...,m)$ and $A_i = A(W_i)$ is the weight matrix. The asymptotic properties of the IVE $\widehat{\psi}_n$ are given in Section 17.6 while a numerical example is given in Section 17.5.

## 17.4 Simulation-based Estimation

The conditional moments in (17.20)–(17.24) involve multiple integrals. In the case where these integrals admit explicit forms, the numerical optimization of the objective function $Q_n(\psi)$ in (17.25) is straightforward. However, sometimes it is difficult or impossible to obtain closed forms of these integrals, e.g., in a logistic model. In this case, the integrals can be estimated using the following importance sampling technique. First, choose some known densities $f_{0b}(b)$ and $f_{0\delta}(t)$ such that their supports cover the supports of $f_b(b,\theta)$ and $f_\delta(t,\alpha)$ respectively. Then generate independent samples $b_s \sim f_{0b}(b)$ and $t_s, r_s \sim f_{0\delta}(t)$, $s = 1, 2, ..., S$, and let

$$\mu_{ij,1}(\psi) = \frac{1}{S}\sum_{s=1}^{S} g_{ij}(b_s, t_s, \beta, \gamma)\frac{f_b(b_s;\theta)f_\delta(t_s;\alpha)}{f_{0b}(b_s)f_{0\delta}(t_s)}, \tag{17.26}$$

$$\nu_{ijk,1}(\psi) = \frac{1}{S}\sum_{s=1}^{S} g_{ij}(b_s, t_s, \beta, \gamma)g_{ik}(b_s, r_s, \beta, \gamma)\frac{f_b(b_s;\theta)f_\delta(t_s;\alpha)f_\delta(r_s;\alpha)}{f_{0b}(b_s)f_{0\delta}(t_s)f_{0\delta}(r_s)}, j \neq k, \tag{17.27}$$

further, generate another set of samples $b_s \sim f_{0b}(b)$ and $t_s, r_s \sim f_{0\delta}(t)$, $s = S+1, S+2, ..., 2S$ to calculate $\mu_{ij,2}(\psi)$ and $\nu_{ijk,2}(\psi)$ respectively. Other moments are estimated similarly. It is easy to see that such simulated moments $\mu_{ij,l}(\psi)$, $\nu_{ijk,l}(\psi)$ and $\kappa_{ijk,l}(\psi)$, $l = 1, 2$ are unbiased estimators for $\mu_{ij}(\psi)$, $\nu_{ijk}(\psi)$ and $\kappa_{ijk}(\psi)$ respectively. Finally, the simulation-based IV estimator (SIVE) for $\psi$ is defined as

$$\widehat{\psi}_{n,S} = \arg\min_{\psi\in\Omega_\psi} Q_{n,S}(\psi) := \sum_{i=1}^{n} \widehat{\rho}_{i,1}^{\top}(\psi)A_i\widehat{\rho}_{i,2}(\psi), \tag{17.28}$$

where $\widehat{\rho}_{i,l}^{\top}(\psi) = (Y_{ij} - \widehat{\mu}_{ij,l}(\psi), Y_{ij}Y_{ik} - \widehat{\nu}_{ijk,l}(\psi), Y_{ij}X_{ik}^* - \widehat{\kappa}_{ijk,l}(\psi), j = 1, ..., m; k = j, ..., m)$, $l = 1, 2$. Note that, since $\widehat{\rho}_{i,1}(\psi)$ and $\widehat{\rho}_{i,2}(\psi)$ are constructed by using two independent importance samples, they are conditionally independent given the observed data $(Y_i, X_i^*, W_i, Z_i, B_i)$. Therefore $Q_{n,S}(\psi)$ is an unbiased simulator for $Q_n(\psi)$ in (17.25) for finite $S$. A numerical example of this estimator is given in Section 17.5.

## 17.5 Numerical Computation and Simulations

In principle, the estimators IVE and SIVE can be computed using Newton-Raphson algorithm as

$$\widehat{\psi}^{(\tau+1)} = \widehat{\psi}^{(\tau)} - \left(\frac{\partial^2 Q_n(\widehat{\psi}^{(\tau)})}{\partial\psi\partial\psi^{\top}}\right)^{-1}\frac{\partial Q_n(\widehat{\psi}^{(\tau)})}{\partial\psi},$$

where $\widehat{\psi}^{(\tau)}$ denotes the estimate of $\psi$ at the $\tau^{th}$ iteration, and the gradient and Hessian matrix are given by

$$\frac{\partial Q_n(\psi)}{\partial\psi} = 2\sum_{i=1}^{n}\frac{\partial\rho_i(\psi)^{\top}}{\partial\psi}A_i\rho_i(\psi), \tag{17.29}$$

and

$$\frac{\partial^2 Q_n(\psi)}{\partial\psi\partial\psi^\top} = 2\sum_{i=1}^{n}\left[\frac{\partial\rho_i(\psi)^\top}{\partial\psi}A_i\frac{\partial\rho_i(\psi)}{\partial\psi^\top} + (\rho_i(\widehat{\psi})^\top A_i \otimes I)\frac{\partial \mathrm{vec}(\partial\rho_i(\psi)^\top/\partial\psi)}{\partial\psi^\top}\right] \tag{17.30}$$

$$\approx 2\sum_{i=1}^{n}\left[\frac{\partial\rho_i(\psi)^\top}{\partial\psi}A_i\frac{\partial\rho_i(\psi)}{\partial\psi^\top}\right].$$

respectively. The last approximation holds because the second term in (17.30) has expectation zero at the true value of the parameters and therefore can be omitted for computational simplicity.

Another issue is the choice of the weight matrix $A_i = A(W_i)$ in the objective functions $Q_n(\psi)$ and $Q_{n,S}(\psi)$. Although any nonnegative definite matrix satisfying the regularity conditions in Section 17.6 will result in consistent estimators, the optimal choice that yields most efficient estimator is $A_i^{opt} = E[\rho_i(\psi_0)\rho_i^\top(\psi_0)|W_i]^{-1}$ (Abarin and Wang 2006, Wang 2007). Since the optimal weight depends on the unknown parameters to be estimated, it needs to be pre-estimated by plugging in a first-stage estimator such as the naive estimator that ignores measurement error or by the IVE (SIVE) calculated using the identity weight $A_i = I$. All numerical examples in this section used the following estimate

$$\widehat{A}^{opt} = \left(\frac{1}{n}\sum_{i=1}^{n}\rho_i(\widehat{\psi}_n^{(1)})\rho_i^\top(\widehat{\psi}_n^{(1)})\right)^{-1}, \tag{17.31}$$

where $\widehat{\psi}_n^{(1)}$ is the first-stage estimator. A more detailed discussion on the choice of $A_i^{opt}$ can be found in Li and Wang (2012b, 2013).

In the rest of this section, we calculate some numerical examples to demonstrate the proposed estimation procedures and carry out Monte Carlo simulation studies to evaluate their finite sample performance. For comparison we also calculate the naive maximum likelihood estimate (nMLE) that ignores measurement error. In each example, we carry out 1000 Monte Carlo runs and report the biases (BIAS) and the mean absolute errors (MAE) of the estimators. All computations are done using statistical programming language `R` (R Development Core Team 2009). The numerical optimization was done using function `nlm()` and the nMLE are calculated using package `lme4`.

### 17.5.1 Linear Mixed Model

First we consider the linear mixed model

$$Y_{ij} = \beta_x X_{ij} + \beta_z Z_{ij} + b_i + \varepsilon_{ij}, \tag{17.32}$$

where $X_{ij}, Z_{ij}$ are scalars, $B_{ij} \equiv 1$, $b_i \sim (0,\theta)$ (any distribution with mean 0 and variance $\theta$), and $\varepsilon \sim (0,\phi)$. Further, suppose $X_{ij} = \gamma_1 + \gamma_w W_{ij} + \delta_{ij}$

**TABLE 17.1**
BIAS (MAE) of the naive MLE and IVE for the linear model in Example 17.5.1.

| | $n = 100$ | | $n = 300$ | |
|---|---|---|---|---|
| Parameter | nMLE | IVE | nMLE | IVE |
| $\beta_0 = 1.5$ | -0.001 (0.084) | -0.020 (0.095) | 0.003 (0.048) | -0.006 (0.055) |
| $\beta_x = 1$ | -0.144 (0.144) | -0.072 (0.080) | -0.144 (0.144) | -0.028 (0.037) |
| $\beta_z = -0.2$ | 0.000 (0.028) | 0.003 (0.030) | -0.001 (0.016) | 0.000 (0.018) |
| $\theta = 0.2$ | 0.002 (0.040) | -0.013 (0.049) | -0.000 (0.022) | -0.005 (0.028) |
| $\phi = 0.5$ | 0.085 (0.086) | -0.015 (0.045) | 0.085 (0.086) | -0.006 (0.027) |

with $\delta_{ij} \sim (0, \alpha)$, and $X^*_{ij} = X_{ij} + U_{ij}$ with $U_{ij} \sim (0, \sigma^2_u)$. For this model the conditional moments (17.8)–(17.10) become

$$\mu_{ij}(\psi) = \beta_x(\gamma_1 + \gamma_w W_{ij}) + \beta_z Z_{ij},$$

$$\nu_{ijk}(\psi) = \mu_{ij}(\psi)\mu_{ik}(\psi) + \theta + d_{jk}(\alpha\beta_x^2 + \phi),$$

and

$$\kappa_{ijk}(\psi) = \mu_{ij}(\psi)(\gamma_1 + \gamma_w W_{ij}) + d_{jk}\alpha\beta_x.$$

In the simulation study, the data are generated as follows. First generate independent variates $W_{ij} \sim N(0,1)$ and $X_{ij} = 0.7W_{ij} + \delta_{ij}$ with $\delta_{ij} \sim N(0, \alpha = 0.1)$. Then, generate $X^*_{ij} = X_{ij} + U_{ij}$ with $U_{ij} \sim N(0, 0.1)$. The covariate $Z_{ij} = j, j = 1, 2, ..., m$. Finally, generate $b_i \sim N(0, \theta = 0.2)$ and the responses $Y_{ij}$ according to (17.32) with $\varepsilon_{ij} \sim N(0, \phi = 0.5)$ and parameter values $(\beta_0, \beta_x, \beta_z) = (1.5, 1, -0.2)$. The sample sizes are $n = 100, 300$ respectively with repetition $m = 4$ in each case.

The simulation results are reported in Table 17.1. These results show clearly that the naive MLE for $\beta_x$ is biased and the bias persists when the sample size increases. In contrast, the proposed IVE corrects the bias effectively. In addition, when the sample size increases, both the bias and mean absolute error of the IVE decrease rapidly. For the dispersion parameter $\phi$, The IVE has significantly smaller bias and mean absolute error than the naive MLE. In some cases, the IVE has slightly larger MAE than the naive MLE, which is due to the numerical variability of the optimization algorithm used.

### 17.5.2 Mixed Poisson Model

Next we consider a mixed Poisson model where $g(\eta_{ij}) = h(\eta_{ij})$, $\phi = 1$ and

$$E(Y_{ij}|X_i, b_i) = \exp(\beta_0 + \beta_x X_{ij} + \beta_z Z_{ij} + b_i). \tag{17.33}$$

Further, suppose that $b_i \sim N(0, \theta)$ and $X_{ij} = \gamma_1 + \gamma_w W_{ij} + \delta_{ij}$ with $\delta_i \sim N(0, \alpha I)$. Then the moments (17.20)–(17.24) have the following closed forms.

First, using the formula of the normal moment generating function, we obtain

$$\begin{aligned}\mu_{ij}(\psi) &= E(Y_{ij}|W_i) \\ &= \exp(\beta_0+\beta_x(\gamma_1+\gamma_w W_{ij})+\beta_z Z_{ij})E\exp(\beta_x\delta_{ij})E\exp(b_i) \\ &= \exp(\beta_0+\beta_x(\gamma_1+\gamma_w W_{ij})+\beta_z Z_{ij}+\beta_x^2\alpha/2+\theta/2). \quad (17.34)\end{aligned}$$

Similarly, we have

$$\begin{aligned}\nu_{ijj}(\psi) &= E(Y_{ij}^2|W_i) \\ &= \mu_{ij}(\psi)+\exp[2(\beta_0+\beta_x(\gamma_1+\gamma_w W_{ij})+\beta_z Z_{ij})]E\exp(2\beta_x\delta_{ij})E \\ &\quad \times\exp(2b_i) \\ &= \mu_{ij}(\psi)+\mu_{ij}^2(\psi)\exp(\alpha\beta_x^2+\theta) \quad (17.35)\end{aligned}$$

and, for $j \neq k$,

$$\begin{aligned}\nu_{ijk}(\psi) &= E(Y_{ij}Y_{ik}|W_i) \\ &= \exp(\beta_0+\beta_x(\gamma_1+\gamma_w W_{ij}) \\ &\quad +\beta_z Z_{ij})\exp(\beta_0+\beta_x(\gamma_1+\gamma_w W_{ik})+\beta_z Z_{ik}) \\ &\quad \times E\exp(\beta_x\delta_{ij})E\exp(\beta_x\delta_{ik})E\exp(2b_i) \\ &= \mu_{ij}(\psi)\mu_{ik}(\psi)\exp(\theta). \quad (17.36)\end{aligned}$$

Finally,

$$\begin{aligned}\kappa_{ijk}(\psi) &= E(Y_{ij}X_{ik}^*|W_i) \\ &= E(Y_{ij}|W_i)(\gamma_1+\gamma_w W_{ik}) \\ &\quad +\exp(\beta_0+\beta_x(\gamma_1+\gamma_w W_{ik})+\beta_z Z_{ik})E[\delta_{ik}\exp(\beta_x\delta_{ij})]E\exp(b_i) \\ &= \mu_{ij}(\psi)(\gamma_1+\gamma_w W_{ik}+d_{jk}\alpha\beta_x). \quad (17.37)\end{aligned}$$

In the simulations the covariates are generated similarly as in Example 17.5.1, except now $X_{ij} = 1.5+0.5W_{ij}+\delta_{ij}$ and the responses $Y_{ij}$ are generated from Poisson distribution with conditional mean (17.33) and true parameter values $(\beta_0, \beta_x, \beta_z) = (1.2, 0.9, -0.2)$. The sample sizes are $n = 100, 300$ and $m = 4$.

The simulation results are given in Table 17.2. Again, these results show clearly that the naive MLE for $\beta_0$ and $\beta_x$ are severely biased and the biases persist for the large sample. In contrast, the proposed IVE corrects the bias effectively, and its bias and mean absolute error decrease significantly when sample size increases. Again, in some cases the IVE has slightly larger MAE than the naive MLE due to the numerical instability in the optimization algorithm.

### 17.5.3 Mixed Logistic Model

In the third example we consider a mixed logistic model for a binary response $Y_{ij}$ taking values 0 or 1 with probability

$$P(Y_{ij} = 1|X_{ij}, b_i) = g(\beta_0+\beta_x X_{ij}+\beta_z Z_{ij}+b_i), \quad (17.38)$$

**TABLE 17.2**
BIAS (MAE) of the naive MLE and IVE for the Poisson model in Example 17.5.2.

| | $n = 100$ | | $n = 300$ | |
|---|---|---|---|---|
| Parameter | nMLE | IVE | nMLE | IVE |
| $\beta_0 = 1.2$ | 0.324 (0.324) | 0.120 (0.142) | 0.318 (0.318) | 0.083 (0.098) |
| $\beta_x = 0.9$ | -0.200 (0.200) | -0.112 (0.117) | -0.200 (0.200) | -0.074 (0.076) |
| $\beta_z = -0.2$ | -0.001 (0.017) | 0.002 (0.020) | 0.001 (0.009) | 0.003 (0.014) |
| $\theta = 0.2$ | 0.017 (0.031) | -0.054 (0.063) | 0.018 (0.023) | -0.056 (0.058) |

**TABLE 17.3**
BIAS (MAE) of the naive MLE and SIVE for the logistic model in Example 17.5.3.

| | $n = 200$ | | $n = 400$ | |
|---|---|---|---|---|
| Parameter | nMLE | SIVE | nMLE | SIVE |
| $\beta_0 = 0.4$ | -0.002 (0.144) | 0.017 (0.182) | -0.007 (0.100) | 0.015 (0.133) |
| $\beta_x = 0.6$ | -0.141 (0.153) | 0.018 (0.139) | -0.139 (0.142) | 0.012 (0.106) |
| $\beta_z = -0.2$ | 0.002 (0.051) | -0.007 (0.064) | 0.002 (0.037) | -0.003 (0.046) |
| $\theta = 0.2$ | -0.029 (0.100) | 0.049 (0.224) | -0.042 (0.079) | 0.000 (0.185) |

where $g(\eta_{ij}) = 1/(1 + \exp(-\eta_{ij}))$. In this model the variance function $h(\eta_{ij}) = g(\eta_{ij})(1 - g(\eta_{ij}))$ and $\phi = 1$. For this model the conditional moments in (17.20)–(17.24) do not have closed forms and therefore we apply the simulation-based procedure in Section 17.4. In addition, since $Y_{ij}$ is binary, $E(Y_{ij}^2|X_i, b_i) = E(Y_{ij}|X_i, b_i)$ and, therefore, the moments $\nu_{ijj}$ in (17.21) are not included in the objective function $Q_{n,S}(\psi)$.

In the simulation study, the covariates are generated similarly as in Example 17.5.1, except now $X_{ij} = 0.5W_{ij} + \delta_{ij}$ and the response $Y_{ij}$ are generated from Bernoulli distribution with conditional probability (17.38) and true parameter values $(\beta_0, \beta_x, \beta_z) = (0.4, 0.6, -0.2)$. The sample sizes are $n = 200, 400$ and $m = 4$. To compute the SIVE, we chose the normal density of $N(0, 2)$ for both $f_{0b}(b)$ and $f_{0\delta}(t)$, and generate independent samples $b_s, t_s, r_s$, $s = 1, ..., 2S$ with $S = 5000$.

The simulation results are shown in Table 17.3. Similar to the previous examples, these results show that the naive MLE for $\beta_x$ is biased and the bias persists for the large sample. In contrast, the proposed IVE corrects the bias effectively, and the its bias and mean absolute error decrease significantly when sample size increases. Again, in some cases the IVE has larger MAE than the naive MLE due to the numerical instability in the optimization algorithm.

## 17.6 Asymptotic Theory

In this section we outline the asymptotic theories for the proposed estimators and the associated regularity conditions. For the sake of generality, we present the conditions and results in terms of the generalized linear mixed models, however, some of these conditions can be simplified for the linear mixed models. As in Section 17.2 and 17.3, let $\psi$ and $\Omega_\psi$ be the parameter vector and its parameter space respectively. Similarly, let $\gamma = \operatorname{vec}\Gamma_w$, $\Omega_\gamma$ be the corresponding parameter space, and $\Omega = \Omega_\psi \times \Omega_\gamma$ be the joint parameter space. Finally, let $\psi_0$ and $\gamma_0$ denote the true values with which the observed data are generated.

To obtain the consistency and asymptotic normality for the IVE and SIVE, we make the following assumptions.

**Assumption 17.1** $g(\cdot)$ and $h(\cdot)$ are continuously differentiable functions.

**Assumption 17.2** $(Y_i, X_i^*, W_i, Z_i, B_i)$, $i = 1, ..., n$ are independent and identically distributed and satisfy $E\left[\|A_i\|\left(Y_{ij}^4 + \|Y_{ij}W_{ij}\|^2 + 1\right)\right] < \infty$. Further,

$$E\left[\|A_i\| \int \sup_\Omega g_{ij}^2(b, t, \beta, \gamma) f_b(b; \theta) f_\delta(t; \alpha)\, db\, dt\right] < \infty \tag{17.39}$$

and

$$E\left[\|A_i\| \int \sup_\Omega h_{ij}(b, t, \beta, \gamma) f_b(b; \theta) f_\delta(t; \alpha)\, db\, dt\right] < \infty. \tag{17.40}$$

**Assumption 17.3** The parameter space $\Omega_\psi$ is compact.

**Assumption 17.4** $E[(\rho_i(\psi) - \rho_i(\psi_0))^\top A_i(\rho_i(\psi) - \rho_i(\psi_0))] = 0$ if and only if $\psi = \psi_0$.

**Assumption 17.5** $g(\cdot)$ and $h(\cdot)$ are twice continuously differentiable; $f_b(b;\theta)$ and $f_\delta(t;\alpha)$ are twice continuously differentiable with respect to $\theta$ and $\alpha$ respectively around their true values; all first and second order partial derivatives of $g_{ij}(b, t, \beta, \gamma) f_b(b;\theta) f_\delta(t;\alpha)$ and $h_{ij}(b, t, \beta, \gamma) f_b(b;\theta) f_\delta(t;\alpha)$ with respect to $(\psi^\top, \gamma^\top)^\top$ satisfy similar conditions as in (17.39) and (17.40).

**Assumption 17.6** The matrix

$$D = E\left[\frac{\partial \rho_i^\top(\psi_0)}{\partial \psi} A_i \frac{\partial \rho_i(\psi_0)}{\partial \psi'}\right] \tag{17.41}$$

is nonsingular.

Then we have the following results.

**Theorem 17.1** Let $\widehat{\psi}_n$ be the IVE defined in (17.25). Then, as $n \to \infty$,

1. under Assumption 17.1-17.4, $\widehat{\psi}_n \xrightarrow{a.s.} \psi_0$; and
2. under Assumption 17.1-17.6, $\sqrt{n}(\widehat{\psi}_n - \psi_0) \xrightarrow{d} N(0, D^{-1}CD^{-1})$, where

$$C = \operatorname*{plim}_{n\to\infty} \frac{1}{4n} \frac{\partial Q_n(\psi_0)}{\partial \psi} \frac{\partial Q_n(\psi_0)}{\partial \psi^\top}. \tag{17.42}$$

Further, for the simulation-based IVE of Section 17.4, we have the following results.

**Theorem 17.2** Suppose that the supports of $f_b(b,\theta)$ and $f_\delta(t,\alpha)$ are contained in the supports of $f_{0b}(b)$ and $f_{0\delta}(t)$ respectively for all $\theta$ and $\alpha$ in the neighborhood of their true values. Let $\widehat{\psi}_{n,S}$ be the SIVE defined in (17.28). Then for any fixed $S > 0$, as $n \to \infty$,

1. under Assumptions 17.1-17.4, $\widehat{\psi}_{n,S} \xrightarrow{a.s.} \psi_0$;
2. under Assumptions 17.1-17.6, $\sqrt{n}(\widehat{\psi}_{n,S} - \psi_0) \xrightarrow{d} N(0, D^{-1}C_S D)$, where

$$C_S = \operatorname*{plim}_{n\to\infty} \frac{1}{4n} \frac{\partial Q_{n,S}(\psi_0)}{\partial \psi} \frac{\partial Q_{n,S}(\psi_0)}{\partial \psi^\top}. \tag{17.43}$$

Note that the above asymptotic results do not require the simulation size $S$ to tend to infinity because the objective function $Q_{n,S}(\psi)$ is constructed using the simulation-by-parts technique. This is fundamentally different from other simulation-based methods in the literature which typically require $S$ tend to infinity to obtain consistent estimators. However, due to the Monte Carlo approximation of the marginal moments, $\widehat{\psi}_{n,S}$ is generally less efficient than $\widehat{\psi}_n$. In general, it can be shown that the efficiency loss caused by simulation decreases at the rate $O(1/S)$ (Wang, 2004, 2007).

## 17.7 Mathematical Proofs

In this section we give a sketch of the proof of Theorem 17.1. Theorem 17.2 can be similarly proved. For more details, see Wang (2004, 2007) and Wang and Hsiao (2011).

### 17.7.1 Proof of Theorem 17.1.1

By Assumption 17.1 and the Dominated Convergence Theorem (DCT), we have the first-order Taylor expansion about $\gamma_0$

$$Q_n(\psi) = \sum_{i=1}^n \rho_i^\top(\psi) A_i \rho_i(\psi) + 2\sum_{i=1}^n \rho_i^\top(\psi,\widetilde{\gamma}) A_i \frac{\partial \rho_i(\psi,\widetilde{\gamma})}{\partial \gamma^\top}(\widehat{\gamma}_n - \gamma_0), \tag{17.44}$$

where $\|\widetilde{\gamma} - \gamma_0\| \leq \|\widehat{\gamma}_n - \gamma_0\|$ and $\widehat{\gamma}_n = \mathrm{vec}\,\widehat{\Gamma}_w$. Further, for any $1 \leq i \leq n$, by Assumption 17.1–17.3 and the uniform law of large numbers (ULLN), we have

$$\sup_{\psi \in \Omega_\psi} \left| \frac{1}{n} \sum_{i=1}^{n} \rho_i^\top(\psi) A_i \rho_i(\psi) - Q(\psi) \right| \xrightarrow{a.s.} 0, \tag{17.45}$$

where $Q(\psi) = E[\rho_i^\top(\psi) A_i \rho_i(\psi)]$. Similarly, by Assumption 17.1-17.3 we have

$$\begin{aligned} &\sup_{\Omega_\psi} \left\| \frac{1}{n} \sum_{i=1}^{n} \rho_i^\top(\psi, \widetilde{\gamma}) A_i \frac{\partial \rho_i(\psi, \widetilde{\gamma})}{\partial \gamma^\top} (\widehat{\gamma}_n - \gamma_0) \right\| \\ &\leq \sup_{\Omega} \left\| \frac{1}{n} \sum_{i=1}^{n} \rho_i^\top(\psi, \gamma) A_i \frac{\partial \rho_i(\psi, \gamma)}{\partial \gamma^\top} \right\| \|\widehat{\gamma}_n - \gamma_0\| \xrightarrow{a.s.} 0. \end{aligned} \tag{17.46}$$

Therefore it follows from (17.44)–(17.46) that

$$\sup_{\Omega_\psi} \left| \frac{1}{n} Q_n(\psi) - Q(\psi) \right| \xrightarrow{a.s.} 0. \tag{17.47}$$

Furthermore, since $Q(\psi) = Q(\psi_0) + E[\rho_i(\psi) - \rho_i(\psi_0))^\top A_i(\rho_i(\psi) - \rho_i(\psi_0)]$, by Assumption 17.4, $Q(\psi) \geq Q(\psi_0)$ and the equality holds if and only if $\psi = \psi_0$. Thus, by Amemiya (1973, Lemma 3) we have $\widehat{\psi}_n \xrightarrow{a.s.} \psi_0$, as $n \to \infty$.

### 17.7.2 Proof of Theorem 17.1.2

By Assumption 17.5 and the DCT, the first derivative $\partial Q_n(\psi)/\partial\psi$ exists and has the first-order Taylor expansion in the neighborhood of $\psi_0$. Since $\widehat{\psi}_n \xrightarrow{a.s.} \psi_0$, for sufficiently large $n$ we have

$$\frac{\partial Q_n(\widehat{\psi}_n)}{\partial \psi} = \frac{\partial Q_n(\psi_0)}{\partial \psi} + \frac{\partial^2 Q_n(\widetilde{\psi}_n)}{\partial \psi \partial \psi^\top} (\widehat{\psi}_n - \psi_0) = 0, \tag{17.48}$$

where $\left\|\widetilde{\psi}_n - \psi_0\right\| \leq \left\|\widehat{\psi}_n - \psi_0\right\|$, and the first and second derivatives of $Q_n(\psi)$ are given in (17.29) and (17.30) respectively.

Analogous to the proof of Theorem 17.1.1, by Assumption 17.1–17.5, the ULLN and Amemiya (1973, Lemma 4) we can show that

$$\frac{1}{2n} \frac{\partial^2 Q_n(\widetilde{\psi}_n)}{\partial \psi \partial \psi^\top} \xrightarrow{a.s.} E\left[ \frac{\partial \rho_i^\top(\psi_0)}{\partial \psi} A_i \frac{\partial \rho_i(\psi_0)}{\partial \psi^\top} \right] = D, \tag{17.49}$$

where $D$ is given in (17.41). Since $D$ is nonsingular by Assumption 17.6, for sufficiently large $n$, we can rewrite (17.48) as

$$\sqrt{n}(\widehat{\psi}_n - \psi_0) = -\left( \frac{1}{2n} \frac{\partial^2 Q_n(\widetilde{\psi}_n)}{\partial \psi \partial \psi^\top} \right)^{-1} \left( \frac{1}{2\sqrt{n}} \frac{\partial Q_n(\psi_0)}{\partial \psi} \right). \tag{17.50}$$

Further, similar to Wang (2007) and Wang and Hsiao (2011), it can be shown that

$$\frac{1}{2\sqrt{n}} \frac{\partial Q_n(\psi_0)}{\partial \psi} \xrightarrow{d} N(0, C), \tag{17.51}$$

where $C$ is given in (17.42). Finally, the theorem follows from (17.48)–(17.51) and Slutsky's Theorem.

## 17.8 Conclusions and Discussion

In this chapter we proposed an instrumental variable approach to estimation of the generalized linear mixed models with measurement error. This approach is based on the first two conditional moments of the responses given the instrumental variables, and it does not require distributional assumption for the unobserved covariates and measurement error. The random effects can have any parametric distribution that is not necessarily normal. A simulation-based estimator is developed to overcome the computational difficulty when the marginal moments do not have closed forms. The proposed estimators are consistent and asymptotically normally distributed under general conditions. Numerical examples demonstrate that the proposed estimators effectively correct the attenuation bias in the naive maximum likelihood estimator caused by the measurement error. The computation of the estimators is done through numerical optimization. Therefore developing more efficient numerical optimization procedure will be very helpful.

## Acknowledgements

I am grateful to co-editor Paul Gustafson for his kind invitation to write this chapter and for his helpful comments and suggestions on the previous drafts. I am also thankful to Zhiyong Jin and Lin Xue for their assistance in R programming for the computation of the numerical examples. This research is supported by the Natural Sciences and Engineering Research Council of Canada (NSERC).

## References

Abarin, T. and Wang, L. (2006). Comparison of GMM with second-order least squares estimator in nonlinear models. *Far East Journal of Theoretical Statistics*, 20, 179-196.

Abarin, T. and Wang, L. (2012). Instrumental variable approach to covariate measurement error in generalized linear models. *Annals of the Institute of Statistical Mathematics*, 64, 475-493.

Abarin, T., Li, H., Wang, L., and Briollais, L. (2014). On method of moments estimation in linear mixed effects models with measurement error on covariates and response with application to a longitudinal study of gene-environment interaction. *Statistics in Biosciences*, 6, 1-18.

Amemiya, T. (1973). Regression analysis when the dependent variable is truncated normal. *Econometrica*, 41, 997-1016.

Bartlett, J.W., de Stavola, B.L., and Frost, C. (2009). Linear mixed models for replication data to efficiently allow for covariate measurement error. *Statistics in Medicine*, 28, 3158-3178.

Breslow, N.E. and Clayton, D.G. (1993). Approximate inference in generalized linear mixed models. *Journal of American Statistician Association*, 88, 9-25.

Buonaccorsi, J., Demidenko, E., and Tosteson T. (2000). Estimation in longitudinal random effects models with measurement error. *Statistica Sinica*, 10, 885-903.

Buzas, J.S. and Stefanski L.A. (1996). Instrumental variable estimation in generalized measurement error models. *Journal of American Statistical Association*, 91, 999-1006.

Carroll, R.J. and Stefanski, L.A. (1994). Measurement error, instrumental variables and corrections for attenuation with applications to meta-analyses. *Statistics in Medicine*, 13, 1265-1282.

Carroll, R.J., Ruppert, D., Stefanski, L.A., and Crainiceanu, C. (2006). *Measurement Error in Nonlinear Models: A Modern Perspective.* 2nd Edition, Chapman & Hall, London.

Durbin, J. and Koopman, S.J. (1997). Monte Carlo maximum likelihood estimation for non-Gaussian state space models. *Biometrika*, 84, 669-684.

Fuller, W. (1987). *Measurement Error Models*, New York: John Wiley & Sons.

Guan, J., Cheng, H., Bollen, K.A., Thomas, D.R., and Wang, L. (2019). Instrumental variable estimation in ordinal Probit models with mismeasured predictors. *Canadian Journal of Statistics*, 47, 653-666.

Li, D. and Wang, L. (2013). A semiparametric estimation approach for linear mixed models. *Communications in Statistics – Theory and Methods*, 42, 1982-1997.

Li, H. and Wang, L (2012a). Consistent estimation in generalized linear mixed models with measurement error. *Journal of Biometrics and Biostatistics*, S7:007, doi:10.4172/2155-6180.S7-007.

Li, H. and Wang, L. (2012b). A consistent simulation-based estimator in generalized linear mixed models. *Journal of Statistical Computation and Simulation*, 82, 1085-1103.

Liu, W. and Wu, L. (2007). Simultaneous inference for semiparametric nonlinear mixed?effects models with covariate measurement errors and missing responses. *Biometrics*, 63, 342-350.

Pan, W., Zeng, D., and Lin, X. (2009). Semiparametric transition measurement error models for longitudinal data. *Biometrics*, 65, 728-736.

R Development Core Team (2009). R: A language and environment for statistical computing. R Foundation for Statistical Computing, Vienna, Austria. ISBN 3-900051-07-0, http://www.R-project.org.

Rabe-Hesketh, S., Skrondal, A., and Pickles, A. (2002). Reliable estimation of generalized linear mixed models using adaptive quadrature. *The Stata Journal*, 2, 1-21.

Tsiatis, T. and Davidian, M. (2001) A semiparametric estimator for the proportional hazards model with longitudinal covariates measured with error. *Biometrika*, 88, 447 - 458.

Tosteson, T., Buonaccorsi, J., and Demidenko, E. (1998). Covariate measurement error and the estimation of random effect parameters in a mixed model for longitudinal data. *Statistics in Medicine*, 17, 1959-1971.

Wang, C.Y., Huang, Y, Chao, E.C., and Jeffcoat, M.K. (2008). Expected estimating equations for missing data, measurement error, and misclassification, with application to longitudinal nonignorable missing data. *Biometrics*, 64, 85-95.

Wang, L. (2004). Estimation of nonlinear models with Berkson measurement errors. *Annals of Statistics*, 32, 2559-2579.

Wang, L. (2007). A unified approach to estimation of nonlinear mixed effects and Berkson measurement error models. *The Canadian Journal of Statistics*, 35, 233-248.

Wang, L. (2021). Identifiability in measurement error models. In G. Y. Yi, A. Delaigle, and P. Gustafson (Eds.), *Handbook of Measurement Error Models*, Chapter 3. Chapman & Hall/CRC.

Wang, L. and Hsiao, C. (2011). Method of moments estimation and identifiability of semiparametric nonlinear errors-in-variables models. *Journal of Econometrics*, 165, 30-44.

Wang, N. and Davidian, M. (1996). A note on covariate measurement error in nonlinear mixed effects models. *Biometrics*, 83, 801-812.

Wang, N., Lin, X., and Guttierrez, R. G. (1999). A bias correction regression calibration approach in generalized linear mixed measurement error models. *Communication in Statistics – Theory and Methods*, 28, 217-233.

Wang, N., Lin, X., Gutierrez, R. G., and Carroll, R. J. (1998). Bias analysis and SIMEX approach in generalized linear mixed measurement error models. *Journal of the American Statistical Association*, 93, 249-261.

Xu, K., Ma, Y. and Wang, L. (2015). Instrument assisted regression for errors in variables models with binary response. *Scandinavian Journal of Statistics* 42, 104-117.

Yi, G. Y., Liu, W., and Wu, L. (2011). Simultaneous inference and bias analysis for longitudinal data with covariate measurement error and missing responses. *Biometrics*, 67, 67-75.

Yi, G. Y., Ma, Y., and Carroll, R. J. (2012). A functional generalized method of moments approach for longitudinal studies with missing responses and covariate measurement error. *Biometrika*, 99, 151-165.

Zhong, X.P., Fung, W.K., and Wei, B.C. (2002). Estimation in linear models with random effects and errors-invariables. *Annals of the Institute of Statistical Mathematics*, 54, 595-606.

# 18

## *Measurement Error in Dynamic Models*

**John P. Buonaccorsi**

CONTENTS



## 18.1 Introduction

As with many other types of data, time series data are prone to measurement error since the main variable of interest frequently needs to be estimated at each point in time. Examples include the mismeasurement of population abundances or densities, air pollution or temperatures levels, disease rates, medical indices (e.g., Scott et al., 1977), the labor force in Israel (e.g., Pfeffermann et al., 1998) and retail sales figures (e.g., Bell and Wilcox, 1993).

The two main ingredients involved here are a dynamic model for the true (but unobserved) values and a measurement error model. The random true value at time $t$ will be denoted $X_t$, and it's realized value by $x_t$. Measurement

DOI: 10.1201/9781315101279-18

error arises where instead of $x_t$ we observe the outcome of $X_t^*$, which is an estimator or, sometimes, a general index of $x_t$. Measurement error models are introduced in detail in Section 18.2. While a large proportion of the previous literature on this topic proceeds under the assumption of constant measurement error variance this is rarely realistic with time series since the measurement error often changes over time for various reasons, as discussed further there.

The focus in this chapter will be on estimation of the parameters in a specified dynamic model, with an emphasis on autoregressive models. This is a logical first step since these parameters provide the building blocks for other objectives including forecasting or estimating probabilities about the process in the future and in many problems (especially in ecological applications) the parameters have specific meaning and are the main object of interest. It is easiest to first present a treatment of the important, but simpler, linear autoregressive models in Section 18.3, along with some comments about more general linear stationary models. Section 18.4 then provides an overview for handling general models with an emphasis on non-linear autoregressive models. This last section also includes a look at some other techniques, borrowed from regression problems, that serve as alternatives to the likelihood methods that have tended to dominate the time series literature and provides a brief overview of bootstrapping, something that has received limited attention in this context.

The goal of this chapter is to provide an introduction to the behavior of "naive" approaches which ignore the measurement error and how to correct for it in time series settings. It is assumed that the reader has had some prior exposure to time series. Good introductions can be found in Brockwell and Davis (2002) or Box et al. (1994), among others. There is a large literature that connects to the problems discussed here, including in the traditional statistics and econometrics literature as well as in a burgeoning ecological literature focused on population dynamics (where measurement error is called observation error). With both the introductory nature of the chapter and space limitations both the number of references as well as the topics covered are limited, including no discussion of model selection. A large number of other important references, in addition to discussion of some other problems can be found in Buonaccorsi (2013) and Chapter 12 of Buonaccorsi (2010).

The reader will notice that despite a long history and large literature addressing certain aspects of this problem, there are still a number of areas ripe for future work. We will identify a number of these as we move through the chapter, although the coverage is certainly not meant to be exhaustive.

## 18.2 Measurement Error Models

To describe the measurement error (ME) model broadly, we collect the realized values of the true series in $\mathbf{x} = (x_1, \ldots, x_T)'$ and the random error prone values in $\mathbf{X}^* = (X_1^*, \ldots, X_T^*)'$. The measurement error model is then a model for the conditional behavior of the observable $\mathbf{X}^*$ given $\mathbf{x}$. This can take many forms depending on the context and sampling scheme(s) employed. A convenient representation is

$$\mathbf{X}^* = \mathbf{x} + \mathbf{U}, \quad E(\mathbf{U}|\mathbf{x}) = \mathbf{B}_c, \quad \text{and} \quad Cov(\mathbf{U}|\mathbf{x}) = Cov(\mathbf{X}^*|\mathbf{x}) = \mathbf{\Sigma}_{uc}. \tag{1}$$

The $\mathbf{B}_c' = (B_{1c}, \ldots, B_{Tc})$ contains any conditional biases, while $\mathbf{\Sigma}_{uc}$ is the conditional covariance matrix. The $c$ is a reminder that these are conditional on $\mathbf{x}$. The commonly used/assumed *additive model*, assumes

$$E(\mathbf{X}^*|\mathbf{x}) = \mathbf{x} \text{ or } E(\mathbf{U}|\mathbf{x}) = \mathbf{0}, \tag{2}$$

so each $X_t^*$ is an unbiased estimator of the corresponding $x_t$. This is frequently a realistic (although approximate) assumption. Models with bias have been considered including ones with constant bias, $E(X_t^*|x_t) = x_t + \theta$, or proportional bias, $E(X_t^*|x_t) = \theta x_t$; see Buonaccorsi et al. (2006) and Stenseth et al. (2003) for motivation. Even richer bias models can be considered as in Lillegard et al. (2008).

The bulk of the literature proceeds under the assumption that the measurement errors are *conditionally uncorrelated*; i.e.,

$$Cov(\mathbf{X}^*|\mathbf{x}) = \mathbf{\Sigma}_{uc} = diag(\sigma^2_{u1c}, \ldots, \sigma^2_{uTc}), \tag{3}$$

a diagonal matrix with $(t,t)$ element $V(X_t^*|x_t) = \sigma^2_{utc}$. The assumption of conditionally uncorrelated measurement errors is reasonable when there is independent sampling at each time point. There are many settings, however, where some common sampling units occur over time, leading to correlated measurement errors. This occurs, for example, in many biological and climatological monitoring schemes and is also a key feature in large national repeated sample surveys use block resampling (where fairly general dynamic models have been used for the measurement error itself; see for example Pfefferman et al. (1998), Feder(2001) and references therein). Most of our attention here is on the case of conditionally uncorrelated measurement errors.

The model in (3) allows for heteroscedastic measurement errors where $\sigma^2_{utc}$ is conditional measurement error variance for the tth observation. This may depend on $x_t$ in some manner, although the nature of that dependence need not be specified. The unconditional variance (over random $X_t$) is denoted by $\sigma^2_{ut}$. Suppose, for example, that $\sigma^2_{utc} = h(x_t, \boldsymbol{\theta})$ and there is additive error or constant bias. Then, unconditionally, $\sigma^2_{ut} = V(U_t) = E[V(U_t|X_t)] + V[E(U_t|X_t)] = E[h(X_t, \boldsymbol{\theta})]$. Note that if the conditional variance only changes over $t$ as a function of $x_t$ and the process for $X_t$ is stationary then $h(X_t, \boldsymbol{\theta})$ is stationary and unconditionally $\sigma^2_{ut} = \sigma^2_u$. Hence, we can have conditional heteroscedasticity but unconditional homescedasticity.

To make the above more concrete (and show that some of the definitions can be a bit subtle) suppose at time $t$ the population of interest consists of $N_t$ units with a true value $x_{tj}$ associated with unit $j$. The true value at time $t$ is $x_t$, the mean of the $N_t$ values. If a random sample of size $n_t$ is taken at time $t$ then $X^*_t$ will be the sample mean and (ignoring a finite population correction factor for simplicity) the variance of $X^*_t$ at that time is $\tau^2_t/n_t$ where $\tau^2_t$ is the population variance at time $t$. Formally, since the preceding writes the model conditional on $x_t$, the $\sigma^2_{utc}$ is $E(\tau^2_t|x_t)/n_t$. Fortunately, this doesn't need to be modeled explicitly for our discussion here.

## 18.3 Linear Autoregressive Models

In this section we we treat linear autoregressive models under additive measurement error in some detail, while also commenting on some aspects of handling more general stationary linear models (e.g., autoregressive-moving average (ARMA) and auto-regressive integrated (ARIMA) models). The linear autoregressive model of order $p$, denoted AR(p), assumes

$$X_t = \phi_0 + \phi_1 x_{t-1} + \ldots + \phi_p x_{t-p} + \epsilon_t,$$

where $\epsilon_t$ is random (so-called process error) with mean 0. The linear AR(p) models have long been a workhorse in time series analysis. We assume the model is stationary (e.g. Box et al., 1994 Chapter 3). In an AR(1) model this means $|\phi_1| < 1$. In the population ecology literature the AR models are referred to as the Gompertz model, with the AR(1) or AR(2) models often being employed. There, based on multiplicative models, $X_t = log(N_t)$ where $N_t$ is population abundance or density at time $t$, and the primary objective is estimation of $\phi_1$ and/or $\phi_2$, interpreted as measures of density dependence and delayed density dependence, respectively; see Stenseth et al. (2003), Solow (2001) and references therein. The AR(p) models can also be extended to multivariate autoregressive (MAR) models (e.g., Ives et al., 2003) or to models involving other predictors; see, for example, Williams et al. (2003), Viljugrein et al. (2005), and Schmid et al. (1996).

One advantage of the AR(p) model is that the parameters of interest can be related to the moments of the underlying process. Under stationary $E(X_t) = \mu_X$ and $V(X_t) = \sigma^2_X$ (these are unconditional expected value and variance, both constant over $t$), while the lag $k$ covariance, $Cov(X_t, X_{t+k}) = \gamma_k$, is a function only of the lag $k$. Note that $\gamma_0 = V(X_t)$. The autoregressive

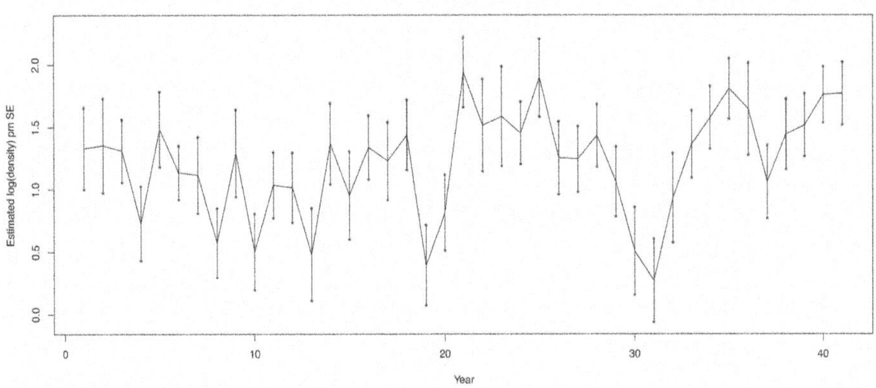


**FIGURE 18.1**
Mallard data for stand 3. Estimated log(densities) as a function of year, plus and minus two standard errors.

coefficients can be expressed as

$$\boldsymbol{\phi} = \begin{pmatrix} \phi_1 \\ \cdot \\ \cdot \\ \phi_p \end{pmatrix} = \boldsymbol{\Gamma}^{-1}\boldsymbol{\gamma}, \text{ with } \boldsymbol{\Gamma} = \begin{pmatrix} \gamma_0 & \cdots & \gamma_{p-1} \\ \vdots & \ddots & \vdots \\ \gamma_{p-1} & \cdots & \gamma_0 \end{pmatrix} \text{ and } \boldsymbol{\gamma} = \begin{pmatrix} \gamma_1 \\ \cdot \\ \cdot \\ \gamma_p \end{pmatrix}. \tag{4}$$

For the rest of this section we assume the additive measurement error model with uncorrelated measurement errors; see (2) and (3). Unconditionally

$$V(X_t^*) = \gamma_0 + \sigma_{ut}^2 \text{ and } cov(X_t^*, X_{t+k}^*) = \gamma_k, k > 1. \tag{5}$$

Note that with uncorrelated measurement errors for a lag greater than 1 the covariance for the observed series is the same as the original series.

For a motivating example, Figure 18.1 presents data from the North American duck survey (see Viljugrein et al. (2005) for some background). This shows the estimated log(density) of mallard ducks on one stand $\pm$ an estimated standard error. The original data has an estimated density $\widehat{D}_t$ and associated standard error $SE_t$. Following the ecological literature we will fit an autoregressive model to the log density so $X_t^* = log(\widehat{D}_t)$ with estimated measurement error variance (based on the delta method) of $\widehat{\sigma}_{ut}^2 = SE_t^2/\widehat{D}_t^2$. The biases from the use of logs here are considered negligible so the measurement error is treated as additive. We analyze these data in Section 18.3.4.

### 18.3.1 Properties of Naive Estimators

The "naive" approach just analyzes the observed $X^*$ values as if they were the true values. There are a variety of estimation methods employed without measurement error, and hence a variety of naive estimators to consider. The primary ones are maximum likelihood (ML), restricted maximum likelihood (REML) and Yule-Walker (YW). The latter, which is closely related to simple least squares, is often used to get preliminary estimates. The ML method assume normality and maximizes the likelihood of $\mathbf{X}$ assumed to be $N(\mu\mathbf{1}, \mathbf{\Sigma}_X)$ where $\mathbf{\Sigma}_X$ has the structure imposed by the AR(p) model, while REML, which has shown to reduce small sample bias (e.g., Cheang and Reinsel, 2000) maximizes a modified likelihood. Section 18.4 has a broader discussion of likelihood methods.

The ML, REML and YW estimators are equivalent asymptotically, but it is easiest to assess the asymptotic behavior via the naive YW estimators since they have closed form. The estimated lag $k$ correlation using the observed values $\widehat{\gamma}_{k,naive} = \sum_{t=1}^{T-k}(X_t^* - \bar{X}^*)(X_{t+k}^* - \bar{X}^*)/T$ for $k = 0, \ldots p$ and, consistent with notation in (4), define $\widehat{\boldsymbol{\gamma}}_{naive}$ and $\widehat{\mathbf{\Gamma}}_{naive}$ computing using the $\widehat{\gamma}_{k,naive}$'s. (One could use $T - k - 1$ to estimate $\gamma_k$ but following Brockwell and Davis (1996) we use $T$ throughout to ensure the overall estimated covariance matrix is non-negative. This doesn't alter the general arguments here.) The YW estimator is given by $\widehat{\boldsymbol{\phi}}_{naive} = \widehat{\mathbf{\Gamma}}_{naive}^{-1}\widehat{\boldsymbol{\gamma}}_{naive}$, with $\widehat{\phi}_{1,naive} = \widehat{\gamma}_{1,naive}/\widehat{\gamma}_{0,naive}$ for the case of $p = 1$. These are closely related to ordinary least squares estimates.

For assessing the large sample properties under heteroscedastic measurement error we assume that $Lim_{T\to\infty}\sum_{t=1}^{T}\sigma_{ut}^2/T = \sigma_u^2$, which corrals the average measurement error variance. The limit is in probability if the conditional ME variances depend on the true values. Under some regularity conditions the estimated lag $k$ covariance using the observed values, $\widehat{\gamma}_{k,naive}$, converges to $\gamma_k$ for $k \geq 1$. However, $\widehat{\gamma}_{0,naive}$ converges to $\gamma_0 + \sigma_u^2$. Hence the naive estimator $\widehat{\boldsymbol{\phi}}_{naive}$ converges in probability to $\boldsymbol{\phi}^* = (\mathbf{\Gamma} + \sigma_u^2\mathbf{I}_p)^{-1}\mathbf{\Gamma}\boldsymbol{\phi}$

When $p = 1$, the naive estimator is consistent for $\phi_1^* = \kappa\phi_1 = \kappa\phi_1$, where $\kappa = \gamma_0/(\gamma_0 + \sigma_u^2)$. Surprisingly the attenuation in the naive estimator here is the same as in simple linear regression (under certain conditions). Surprisingly since from a regression perspective the model here has error in both the predictor and response with what is the error in the response at time $t$ becoming the error in the predictor at time $t+1$. Similar to multiple linear regression, for $p > 1$ the asymptotic/approximate biases are more complicated. For instance, with $p = 2$ the naive estimators of $\phi_1$ and $\phi_2$ are consistent for

$$\frac{1}{1 - \kappa^2\rho_1^2}\begin{pmatrix} \kappa\rho_1 - \kappa^2\rho_1\rho_2 \\ \kappa\rho_2 - \kappa^2\rho_1^2 \end{pmatrix},$$

where $\rho_k = \gamma_k/\gamma_0$ is the lag $k$ correlation in the true series, $\rho_1 = \phi_1/(1 - \phi_2)$ and $\rho_2 = (\phi_1^2 + \phi_2 - \phi_2^2)/(1 - \phi_2)$. The asymptotic bias in either element can be either attenuating (smaller in absolute value) or accentuating (larger in absolute value), and the bias depends on both the amount of measurement error and the true values for $\phi_1$ and $\phi_2$. See Staudenmayer and Buonaccorsi( 2005) (hereafter referred to as SB(2005)) for further illustration and for a proof the naive estimator of $\sigma^2$ has an asymptotic bias of $\boldsymbol{\gamma}'\left\{\mathbf{\Gamma}^{-1} - (\mathbf{\Gamma} + \sigma_u^2\mathbf{I})^{-1}\right\}\boldsymbol{\gamma} > 0$.

How useful are the above bias expressions for "small" samples? Even without measurement error, the issue of bias in small samples is an important one. To illustrate data was generated from the AR(1) model with $X_t = \phi_1 X_{t-1} + \epsilon_t$ and $X_t^* = x_t + U_t$, where the $\epsilon_t$ are iid $N(0, \sigma^2)$, the $U_t$ are iid $N(0, \sigma_u^2)$ and $X_1 \sim N(0, \sigma_X^2)$ where $\sigma_X^2 = \sigma^2/(1 - \phi_1^2)$ (as holds for an AR(1) model). The process variance was held to $\sigma^2 = .8$, while $\phi_1 = 2., .5$ or $.8$ and $\sigma_u^2 = .15, .4$ and $.8$. The case with $\phi_1 = .5$ and $\sigma_u^2 = .15$ is based roughly on an analysis of mouse dynamics given in Buonaccorsi (2010, Ch. 12). For each combination 1000 simulations were run and YW, ML and REML estimators obtained, using the true $X$'s and the error prone $X^*$'s. Partial results appear in Table 18.1. The analysis with true values is given for two reasons. First it shows the clear superiority of REML to ML estimation, especially at smallish sample sizes, with the ML only being modestly better than the YW estimator. Notice that even using true values all of the estimators are attenuated towards zero, sometimes dramatically with $n = 10$. Secondly it gives a baseline to compare the performance of the naive estimators to. The measurement error leads to further attenuation, increasing in $\sigma_u^2$, as expected.The REML estimator obviously provides some extra protection against measurement error compared to ML and YW, especially at small sample sizes. The variable $\phi_1^*$ is the limiting value of the naive estimator (whether YW, ML or REML). The asymptotic bias associated with this can be substantially different than the simulated bias, sometimes even with samples of size 50. The upshot of this is that one cannot always rely on the approximate bias expressions, a problem that can possibly be addressed in data analysis through the use of bootstrap methods to estimate bias.

**TABLE 18.1**

Performance of estimators of $\phi_1$ based on true and mismeasured values in the AR(1) model. $\phi_1^* = \kappa\phi_1$ = limiting value of naive estimator.

| | | | True (using $X$) | | | | Naive (using $X^*$) | | |
|---|---|---|---|---|---|---|---|---|---|
| $\phi_1$ | $\sigma_u^2$ | $n$ | YW | ML | REML | $\phi_1^*$ | YW | ML | REML |
| 0.2 | 0.15 | 10 | 0.023 | 0.029 | 0.176 | 0.169 | 0.006 | 0.009 | 0.152 |
| 0.2 | 0.15 | 50 | 0.161 | 0.164 | 0.188 | 0.169 | 0.136 | 0.139 | 0.163 |
| 0.2 | 0.15 | 100 | 0.179 | 0.180 | 0.192 | 0.169 | 0.149 | 0.150 | 0.162 |
| 0.2 | 0.6 | 10 | 0.031 | 0.040 | 0.185 | 0.116 | -0.022 | -0.020 | 0.120 |
| 0.2 | 0.6 | 50 | 0.171 | 0.174 | 0.198 | 0.116 | 0.090 | 0.092 | 0.115 |
| 0.2 | 0.6 | 100 | 0.185 | 0.187 | 0.199 | 0.116 | 0.101 | 0.102 | 0.113 |
| 0.8 | 0.15 | 10 | 0.356 | 0.435 | 0.623 | 0.749 | 0.290 | 0.354 | 0.536 |
| 0.8 | 0.15 | 50 | 0.710 | 0.731 | 0.768 | 0.749 | 0.650 | 0.669 | 0.705 |
| 0.8 | 0.15 | 100 | 0.756 | 0.765 | 0.783 | 0.749 | 0.701 | 0.709 | 0.727 |
| 0.8 | 0.6 | 10 | 0.357 | 0.444 | 0.641 | 0.630 | 0.195 | 0.235 | 0.410 |
| 0.8 | 0.6 | 50 | 0.709 | 0.729 | 0.766 | 0.630 | 0.526 | 0.540 | 0.572 |
| 0.8 | 0.6 | 100 | 0.756 | 0.766 | 0.785 | 0.630 | 0.574 | 0.582 | 0.598 |

### 18.3.2 Correcting Using Just Observed Values

Unlike many regression problems, the parameters in many dynamic models, including the AR(p) models, can be estimated using just the observed $X_t^*$ values, typically under the assumption of constant ME variance. Not surprisingly, estimating all of the parameters, including the ME variance, with no additional data may be difficult to do efficiently, especially with short series.

**ARMA method:** This is based on the fact (see, for example, Box *et al.* (1994) and Ives et al. (2010)) that if the true values follow an ARMA(p,p) and the measurement error model is an $MA(q)$ process ($q = 0$ corresponding to the $U_t$'s being i.i.d. $N(0, \sigma_u^2)$) then the model for the $X^*$ is an ARMA(p,p + q) and the autoregressive parameters are unchanged. This suggests we could estimate the autoregressive coefficients in $\boldsymbol{\phi}$ by simply fitting an ARMA$(p,q)$ model. This is the hybrid approach of Wong and Miller (1990). For an AR(p) model where the $U_t$ are i.i.d. with mean 0 and constant variance $\sigma_u^2$, this means using the inferences for the autoregressive parameters from fitting an $ARMA(p,p)$ process to $X^*$. For $p = 1$ this actually yields the ML estimate of $\phi_1$. For higher order models this is not an efficient way to proceed as restrictions on the moving average parameters in the induced model are not accounted for, something which is accounted for in the likelihood approach below. See Buonaccorsi (2010, Ch.12) or Buonaccorsi (2013) for further discussion and references for the ARMA method and also of a modified Yule-Walker approach which was found to not perform very well in practice.

**Likelihood methods under normality:** Under a normal model for $\mathbf{X}$ and $\mathbf{U}$ and constant $\boldsymbol{\Sigma}_u$, then $\mathbf{X}^*$ is $N(\boldsymbol{\mu}_X, \boldsymbol{\Sigma}_X + \boldsymbol{\Sigma}_u)$, with structure on $\boldsymbol{\Sigma}_X$ following from the assumed model for the true values. With a finite number of parameters in $\boldsymbol{\Sigma}_u$ (in many cases $\boldsymbol{\Sigma}_u = \sigma_u^2\mathbf{I}$ although some authors allow $\boldsymbol{\Sigma}_u$ to itself come from an ARMA or ARIMA model) this is a classic state-space formulation of a time series model for which a large literature exists. For the normal linear stationary models here, computational methods typically use the Kalman Filter or some variation on it; see, for example, Harvey (1990) Brockwell and Davis (1996), Ives et al. (2003), Ives et al. (2010), and, for the AR(1) models, SB(2005), Dennis et al. (2006), and Knape (2008). These last two papers touch on the important problem that even in the simple AR(1) model there may be issues with local maxima and/or the maximum occurring on the boundary. These models can also be cast as mixed models, which often compute using the EM algorithm and modifications of it, although only the AR(1) model is typically available through this route in most software.

### 18.3.3 Correcting Using Estimated ME Variances

Recall that $\widehat{\sigma}_{ut}^2$ is the estimated measurement error variance at time $t$ and define $\widehat{\sigma}_u^2 = \sum_{t=1}^{T} \widehat{\sigma}_{ut}^2/T$, the average estimated measurement error variance. Here we look at methods that utilize the estimated variance(s). We limit the discussion here to a moment correction approach and pseudo-maximum likelihood under normality with additional approaches touched on in Section 18.4.3.

**Moment approach.** The problem with the naive estimators stems from the fact that $\widehat{\gamma}_{0,naive}$ estimates $\gamma_0 + \sigma_u^2$ rather than $\gamma_0$. This suggests using $\widehat{\gamma}_0 = \widehat{\gamma}_{0,naive} - \widehat{\sigma}_u^2$ leading to

$$\widehat{\boldsymbol{\phi}}_{CEE} = (\widehat{\boldsymbol{\Gamma}} - \widehat{\sigma}_u^2 \mathbf{I}_p)^{-1}\widehat{\boldsymbol{\gamma}}. \tag{6}$$

When $p = 1$, $\widehat{\phi}_1 = \widehat{\kappa}^{-1}\widehat{\phi}_{1,naive}$ where $\widehat{\kappa} = \widehat{\gamma}_{0,naive}/\widehat{\gamma}_0$, the same type of correction used in simple linear regression. This is a moment estimator which can also be viewed as correcting the naive YW estimating equations (hence the CEE). One could also try to modify the naive estimating equations associated with other methods (ML, REML, etc). One advantage of the $\widehat{\boldsymbol{\phi}}_{CEE}$ is that is trivial to compute. Like moment estimators in linear regression $\widehat{\phi}_{CEE}$ can have problems for small samples since the estimate of $\gamma_0$ may be negative, in which case a modification is needed.

Detailed expressions for the asymptotic covariance of $\widehat{\boldsymbol{\phi}}_{CEE}$ are complicated, both in final expression and in derivation, especially when trying to fully account for the uncertainty in the measurement error variances. SB(2005) show that under certain conditions $\widehat{\boldsymbol{\phi}}_{CEE}$ is consistent for $\boldsymbol{\phi}$ and asymptotically normal and provide expressions for the asymptotic covariance matrix and discuss ways to estimate it. These results do not require the measurement error or the unobserved time series to have a normal distribution, but the asymptotic variances do have slightly simpler forms when that is the case. Consider the AR(1) model. Assuming the estimated measurement error variances are independent of the $X_t^*$'s, the approximate variance of $\widehat{\phi}_1$ is

$$\frac{1}{T}\left[\frac{(1-\phi_1^2)(2-\kappa)}{\kappa} + \frac{(1-\phi_1^2)\overline{\sigma_u^4} + \phi_1^2\overline{E(u^4)}}{\gamma_0^2}\right] + \frac{\phi_1^2 V(\widehat{\sigma}_u^2)}{T\gamma_0^2}, \tag{7}$$

where $\overline{\mathrm{E}(u^4)} = \sum_t E(U_t^4)/T$ and $\overline{\sigma_u^4} = \sum_t \sigma_{ut}^4/T$. Recall that $\widehat{\sigma}_u^2 = \sum_{t-1}^{T}\widehat{\sigma}_{ut}^2/T$. If the $\widehat{\sigma}_u^2$ and $X_t^*$ are not independent, additional terms involving the covariance of $\widehat{\sigma}_u^2$ with $\widehat{\gamma}_0$ and $\widehat{\gamma}_1$ are needed. Under normality $E(U_t^4) = 3\sigma_{ut}^4$, which can be estimated using $3\widehat{\sigma}_{ut}^4$. Otherwise $E(U_t^4)$ must be estimated in some manner from the data at time $t$.

If we treat $\widehat{\sigma}_u^2$ as fixed then the last term in (7) can be ignored. This last term will be roughly of order $1/T^2$ and hopefully negligible relative to the first term. Otherwise we need some way to robustly estimate $V(\widehat{\sigma}_u^2)$. This is touched on further in discussing the example in Section 18.3.4, where we find that this second term is in fact negligible.

**Pseudo-likelihood methods.** If $\mathbf{X}$ and $\mathbf{U}$ are both normal and independent of each other, and $Cov(\mathbf{U}) = \boldsymbol{\Sigma}_u$ is constant, then $\mathbf{X}^* = \mathbf{X} + \mathbf{U}$ is normal with covariance $\boldsymbol{\Sigma}_X + \boldsymbol{\Sigma}_u$. As noted earlier ML estimation (not using the estimated ME variances) estimates the parameters under the assumption that $\boldsymbol{\Sigma}_u = \sigma_u^2\mathbf{I}$. Here we replace $\boldsymbol{\Sigma}_u$ with an estimate $\widehat{\boldsymbol{\Sigma}}_u$ and then maximize the likelihood over the rest of the parameters. In our examples and explicit discussion we treat the case where $\mathbf{\Sigma}_u$ is diagonal (3) but it is easy to see that the method here can accommodate correlated measurement errors as long as we can estimate $\mathbf{\Sigma}_u$. These lead to what we'll call a pseudo-ML estimator, $\widehat{\phi}_{PML}$. Bell and Wilcox (1993), for example, took this approach when both $X_t$ and $U_t$ are assumed to follow ARIMA models, while Wong et al.(2001) used this approach for ARMA models allowing different variances at each point in time. These papers illustrate how to obtain the covariance of $\widehat{\boldsymbol{\phi}}$ when $\widehat{\mathbf{\Sigma}}_u$ is treated as known and fixed. Obtaining the covariance of $\widehat{\boldsymbol{\phi}}_{PML}$ when accounting for the uncertainty of the estimated measurement error variances is more difficult. With constant ME variance and the use of $\widehat{\sigma}_u^2$, SB(2005) provide a general expression for the approximate variance of $\widehat{\phi}_{pml}$. See also equation (11) from Section 18.4.2 from which the approximate covariance matrix of the pseudo-ML is $Acov(\widehat{\boldsymbol{\phi}}_{PML}) \approx Acov(\widehat{\boldsymbol{\phi}}_{PML,K}) + V(\widehat{\sigma}_u^2)\mathbf{\Omega}$ where $Acov(\widehat{\boldsymbol{\phi}}_{PML,K})$ is the asymptotic covariance of the PML if $\sigma_u^2$ were known and $\mathbf{\Omega}$ is a function of the parameters. As with the CEE estimator, the second term involves the variance of $\widehat{\sigma}_u^2$ and will frequently be small compared to the first term.

We note that with heteroscedasticity and without modeling the measurement error variances parametrically the number of parameters increase with the sample size and the asymptotic properties of pseudo ML estimators have not been fully explored. In addition, with heteroscedasticity the distribution of of $\mathbf{X}^*$ is not normal even if $\mathbf{X}$ and $\mathbf{U}$ are normal, so the normal based likelihoods are only approximations.

### 18.3.4 Example

We return to the mallard duck data introduced earlier (see Figure 18.1), where we fit an AR(1) model in various ways to the log(density). These data are over T = 41 years, where at time t the estimated log(density) is $X_t^*$ and the estimated measurement error variance is $\widehat{\sigma}_{ut}^2$. There is substantial measurement error here with an average estimated measurement error variance of $\widehat{\sigma}_u^2 = .0911$. Table 18.2 displays results for a variety of estimators.

Under naive methods that ignore the measurement error we have simple least squares regression, the Yule-Walker estimate, then conditional least squares(CLS), maximum likelihood (ML) and restricted maximum likelihood (REML). The CLS and ML are fit using standard time series method (in this case proc ARIMA in SAS) for fitting an AR(1) model. These are labeled AR. The ML and REML can also be fit with a suitable implementation of a mixed model procedure (in this case proc MIXED in SAS). Note that the standard errors for the ML estimate differ due to different ways of estimating the standard error in the two procedures. The time series program also estimates $\sigma^2$ directly while the mixed model approach gives an estimate of $\sigma_X^2 = \gamma_0$ from which we can find $\widehat{\sigma}^2 = (1 - \widehat{\phi}_1^2)\widehat{\sigma}_X^2$.

**TABLE 18.2**
AR(1) fits to Mallard data, stand 3.

| Method | $\widehat{\phi}_1$ | SE | $\widehat{\sigma}^2$ | $\widehat{\sigma}_u^2$ |
|---|---|---|---|---|
| | Naive fits | | | |
| LS | .3387 | .1563 | .1677 | |
| YW | .3243 | | | |
| CLS(AR) | .3394 | .1545 | .1637 | |
| ML(AR) | .3314 | .1542 | .1637 | |
| ML(Mixed) | .3315 | .1485 | | |
| REML(Mixed) | .3654 | .1543 | | |
| | Assuming constant ME variance | | | |
| ARMA-CLS | .5054 | .4230 | .167 | |
| ARMA-ML | .4936 | .4351 | .167 | |
| ML | .4936 | .3458 | .0902 | .0561 |
| REML | .5896 | .3301 | .0793 | .0663 |
| | Correcting with estimate ME variances | | | |
| CEE | .6771 | .3199 | .0454 | |
| PREML | .7089 | 2188 | .0473 | |
| PML | .6333 | .2155 | .0485 | |

Shown next are estimates based on methods assuming additive measurement error with constant variance, but not utilizing any estimate of the measurement error variance. These include the ARMA and likelihood approaches (see Section 18.3.2) where the likelihood approaches also automatically produce an estimate of the common $\sigma_u^2$. Lastly, pseudo-estimates based on the use of the estimated measurement error variances are given. The CEE, which corrects the naive Yule-Walker estimate uses just the average ME variance of .0911 while the likelihood approaches use the individual measurement error variances. Although we omit details, the pseudo-REML (PREML) and pseudo-ML (PML) were readily computed with the appropriate implementation of mixed model software.

The CEE and PREML estimates of $\phi_1$ are quite similar, and both substantially larger than the others that use just the estimated log(densities), with the correction in the expected direction. The associated estimates of the process variance $\sigma^2$ also agree and are less than the naive estimates, also as expected. The standard errors associated with these estimates of $\phi_1$ are rather different however. This may be due to PREML being more efficient or the methods used in estimating the standard error. It remains to be seen. The standard errors here initially did not account for the variability in $\widehat{\sigma}_u^2$ (which, recall is a mean of estimated ME variances). We did, however try to account for this in the CEE estimator by estimating the second term in (7). This was done by estimating $V(\widehat{\sigma}_u^2)$ using $S_v^2/T$ where $S_v^2$ is simply the sample variance of the $\widehat{\sigma}_{ut}^2$s (see Buonaccorsi(2005) for why this is valid). The change was tiny with the estimated standard error still .3199 to four decimal places. We expect the additional contribution to the SE for the PREML estimate may also be negligible. Lastly we note that we have focused on the PREML estimate here since without measurement error the REML approach outperforms simple maximum likelihood

Similar comparisons occurred using data from another stand. However, the analyses are not so clean with very short series; see the example in Buonaccorsi (2010, Ch. 12).

### 18.3.5 Comments

Even in this simplest of settings, the problem is complicated and the methodology still emerging. It is difficult to provide definitive statements about the properties of various estimators, especially with the ME variances changing. SB(2005) provide some analytical comparisons of the asymptotic efficiency of the CEE, PML,ARMA/ML and modified Yule-Walker estimators for the AR(1) model with constant ME variance. They conclude that the PML or CEE estimator are better than the estimators not using the estimated ME variance. But further comparisons and simulations are still needed, including ones that examine REML estimators, with and without estimated ME variances.

The other thing that needs to be investigated further is using just average estimated ME variance, $\widehat{\sigma}_u^2$ in place of each $\sigma_{ui}^2$ in the pseudo methods even if the model is heteroscedastic. While this seems contradictory there is evidence from some regression settings that doing so might lead to a better behaved estimator, even in the presence of some heteroscedasticity. This same suggestion applies to the more general discussion of pseudo methods in Section 18.4.2

## 18.4 General Models

This section provide a broad survey of some strategies for handling general dynamic models with a focus on nonlinear autoregressive models which are frequently employed in practice. There are more challenges here than in the preceding section where the linearity simplified things somewhat. The general autoregressive model is $X_t|\mathbf{x}_{t-1} = m(\mathbf{x}_{t-1}, \boldsymbol{\phi}) + \epsilon_t$, where, $E(\epsilon_t) = 0$ and $V(\epsilon_t) = v(\mathbf{x}_{t-1}, \boldsymbol{\phi}, \boldsymbol{\sigma})$. with $\mathbf{x}_{t-1} = (...., x_{t-2}, x_{t-1})$ containing past values and $\boldsymbol{\sigma}$ contains any variance parameters. The process error $\epsilon_t$ is frequently assumed to be normal with constant variance $\sigma^2$.

There are many non-linear models (either in the $x$'s or the parameters) that are of interest. For example two non-linear (in $x$) models that have been used, especially in ecology where $X_t$ is often $log(N_t)$, with $N_t$ being abundance or density, are the Ricker model with $X_t = \phi_0 + x_{t-1} + \phi_1 e^{x_{t-1}} + \epsilon_t$ and the Beaverton-Holt model with $X_t = x_{t-1} + log(\phi_0) - log(1 + \phi_1 n_{t-1}) + \epsilon_t$, among many others. Notice that in these problems once could also work directly with other non-linear models where $X_t$ is the abundance directly, typically multiplicative versions of the ones just given. For example, consider the Ricker model. With $X_t$ being abundance itself we could work directly with a model where $E(X_t|x_{t-1}) = \phi_0 x_{t-1}e^{\phi_1 x_{t-1}}$ with some suitable structure on the error variance. For example if $X_t$ was distributed Poisson the variance would equal $E(X_t|x_{t-1}))$ (or proportional to it allowing over-dispersion). These types of models are accommodated by the general discussion that follows.

Even without measurement error a full discussion on fitting non-linear time series is certainly beyond the scope of this chapter and, in addition, non-stationary models raise additional concerns. So, we only sketch some general ideas. For likelihood based approaches, assumptions are made about the distribution for both the true values and the measurement error. The joint density of $\mathbf{X}$ (the true values) is denoted $f_X(\mathbf{x}; \boldsymbol{\phi}, \boldsymbol{\sigma})$. The term density is used here for either the continuous or discrete case with summations replacing integration below for the discrete case. The ML estimate maximizes $L(\boldsymbol{\phi}, \boldsymbol{\sigma}|\mathbf{x})$ arising from $f_X(\mathbf{x}; \boldsymbol{\phi}, \boldsymbol{\sigma})$. For conditional likelihood approaches, assuming an autoregressive model suppose the distribution of $X_t|\mathbf{x}_{t-1}$ depends on just the past $p$ values. Partitioning $\mathbf{x}$ into $\mathbf{x}' = (\widetilde{\mathbf{x}}_1', \widetilde{\mathbf{x}}_2')$, where $\widetilde{\mathbf{x}}_1' = (x_1, \ldots, x_p)$ and $\widetilde{\mathbf{x}}_2' = (x_{p+1}, \ldots, x_T)$, then the conditional density, of $\widetilde{\mathbf{X}}_2$ given $\widetilde{\mathbf{x}}_1$ is $f_c(\widetilde{\mathbf{x}}_2|\boldsymbol{\phi}, \boldsymbol{\sigma}, \widetilde{\mathbf{x}}_1) = \prod_{t=p+1}^{T} f(x_t|\mathbf{x}_{t-1}, \boldsymbol{\phi}, \boldsymbol{\sigma})$, where $f(x_t|\mathbf{x}_{t-1}, \boldsymbol{\phi}, \boldsymbol{\sigma})$ is the density of $X_t$ given $\mathbf{x}_{t-1}$. Here, the $\widetilde{\mathbf{x}}_1$ (including the first $p$ values of the series), is treated as fixed. If we also assumed an unconditional density, $f(\widetilde{\mathbf{x}}_1)$, for $\widetilde{\mathbf{X}}_1$ (which can depend on some parameters) then the unconditional likelihood for $\mathbf{X}$ can be built via $f(\mathbf{x}; \boldsymbol{\phi}, \boldsymbol{\sigma}) = \int_{\widetilde{x}_1} f_c(\widetilde{\mathbf{x}}_2|\boldsymbol{\phi}, \boldsymbol{\sigma}, \widetilde{\mathbf{x}}_1) f(\widetilde{\mathbf{x}}_1) d\widetilde{\mathbf{x}}_1$.

Using the true values conditional maximum likelihood (CML) estimates maximize $L(\boldsymbol{\phi}, \boldsymbol{\sigma}|\widetilde{x})$ arising from $f_c(\widetilde{\mathbf{x}}_2|\boldsymbol{\phi}, \boldsymbol{\sigma}, \widetilde{\mathbf{x}}_1)$ This avoids making any assumption about the marginal distribution of $\mathbf{X}_1$ and usually leads to easier computing. For a normal autoregressive model with the $\epsilon_t$ assumed iid $N(0, \sigma^2)$ this leads to *conditional least squares (CLS)*, where $\widehat{\boldsymbol{\phi}}_{LS}$ minimizes $\sum_{t=p+1}^{T}(x_t - m(\mathbf{x}_{t-1}, \boldsymbol{\phi}))^2$. This is an easy approach to treating nonlinear time series which enjoys some popularity and for our purposes here, leads to the easiest way to try and assess bias and correct for measurement error. As described here this is ordinary least squares. The term conditional least squares, however, will sometimes have a slightly different meaning leading to slightly different estimates; see Brockwell and Davis (1996) and Box et al. (1994). Obviously if $m(\mathbf{x}_{t-1}, \boldsymbol{\phi})$ is linear in the $\phi$'s, as it is for the Ricker model, this leads to simple linear least squares More generally this leads to non-linear least squares with estimating equations of the form

$$\sum_{t=p+1}^{t} (x_t - m(\mathbf{x}_{t-1}, \boldsymbol{\phi}))\Delta(\mathbf{x}_{t-1}, \boldsymbol{\phi}) = \mathbf{0}, \tag{8}$$

where the *jth* element of the $\Delta(\mathbf{x}_{t-1}, \boldsymbol{\phi})$ is $\partial m(\mathbf{x}_{t-1}, \boldsymbol{\phi})/\partial \phi_j$. Similar estimating equations arise using the conditional approach for other models, including some involving discrete distributions, similar to what happens with generalized linear models in standard regression settings.

For the measurement error model, $\mathbf{X}^*|\mathbf{x}$ is assumed to have density $f(\mathbf{x}^*|\mathbf{x},\boldsymbol{\theta})$, where $\boldsymbol{\theta}$ includes any measurement error parameters. There are two densities for the observable $\mathbf{X}^*$ that will be used later, the unconditional

$$f_X^*(\mathbf{x}^*;\phi,\sigma,\boldsymbol{\theta}) = \int_{\mathbf{x}} f(\mathbf{x}^*|\mathbf{x},\boldsymbol{\theta}) f_{\mathbf{X}}(\mathbf{x};\boldsymbol{\phi},\boldsymbol{\sigma})d\mathbf{x} \tag{9}$$

or the conditional density for the autoregressive models

$$f_c^*(\mathbf{x}^*|\phi,\sigma,\boldsymbol{\theta},\widetilde{\mathbf{x}}_1) = \int_{\widetilde{\mathbf{x}}_2} f(\mathbf{x}^*|\mathbf{x},\boldsymbol{\theta}) f_c(\widetilde{\mathbf{x}}_2|\boldsymbol{\phi},\boldsymbol{\sigma},\widetilde{\mathbf{x}}_1)d\widetilde{\mathbf{x}}_2. \tag{10}$$

### 18.4.1 Performance of Naive Estimators

Based on the earlier discussion it is not surprising that measurement error will lead to biases in naive estimators. Obtaining analytical expressions, however, for the asymptotic or approximate bias of the naive estimators is challenging. The strategy of using an explicit expression for the estimators helped for the AR(p) models and will for models (e.g., the Ricker model) that are linear in the parameters, but is not helpful for models nonlinear in the parameters. The preceding section also showed that the strategy of using an "induced model for $X_t^*|\mathbf{x}_{t-1}^*$ (which was ARMA(p,p) if the true series was AR(p)) leads to a question of performance of the naive estimator under model misidentification. So, using an induced model is not really helpful here. This really leaves us with two approaches, simulation or utilizing estimating equations.

While it can be challenging to fully characterize the nature of the biases from simulations this can be a very useful approach and has been widely used. It also helps to characterize small sample biases where any analytical approximations may not hold. (Buonaccorsi (2013) summarizes a number of papers where simulations have been utilized.) Table 18.3 shows some simulation results from Resendes (2011) for the naive estimators using the Ricker model where $K = -\phi_0/\phi_1$ is the carrying capacity and $\phi_0$ is an intrinsic growth rate. The settings are based on parameter values similar to those used by DeValpine and Hastings (2002) but with some larger measurement error variances. The magnitude and direction of the biases depend heavily on $\phi_0$ with naive estimators of $\phi_0$ tending to be overestimates at small $\phi_0$ and underestimates as $\phi_0$ increases. The same thing happens for the naive estimator of $K$ but with less sensitivity to the measurement error variance. These results also show overestimation of the process standard deviation $\sigma$, although the bias is somewhat modest at the smaller measurement error variances.

For illustrating the estimating equation approach, suppose the naive estimators solve $S(\mathbf{X}^*,\boldsymbol{\phi},\boldsymbol{\sigma}) = \mathbf{0}$, as in using (8) for example with $\mathbf{x}^*$ in place of $\mathbf{x}$. Under some conditions the naive estimators will converge to $\boldsymbol{\phi}^*$ and $\boldsymbol{\sigma}^*$ which

**TABLE 18.3**
Simulation means for naive estimator from the Ricker model with $\epsilon_t \sim N(0, \sigma^2)$ with $K = 100$ and $\sigma = 0.2$.

| | True $\phi_0$ | | | | | |
|---|---|---|---|---|---|---|
| | 0.2 | 0.75 | 1.5 | 2.4 | 2.6 | $\sigma_u^2$ |
| $\widehat{\phi}_0$ | 0.413 | 0.822 | 1.444 | 2.381 | 2.575 | 0.05 |
| | 0.593 | 0.939 | 1.266 | 2.206 | 2.427 | 0.2 |
| | 0.813 | 0.983 | 1.053 | 1.628 | 1.855 | 0.5 |
| $\widehat{K}$ | 97.54 | 100.09 | 100.00 | 100.20 | 100.04 | 0.05 |
| | 94.77 | 102.04 | 102.32 | 101.52 | 101.67 | 0.2 |
| | 100.69 | 113.06 | 113.29 | 111.58 | 112.37 | 0.5 |
| $\widehat{\sigma}$ | 0.202 | 0.206 | 0.205 | 0.226 | 0.231 | 0.05 |
| | 0.301 | 0.291 | 0.294 | 0.456 | 0.536 | 0.2 |
| | 0.586 | 0.566 | 0.573 | 0.906 | 1.069 | 0.5 |

satisfy $E_{\boldsymbol{\phi},\boldsymbol{\sigma}}[S(\mathbf{X}^*, \boldsymbol{\phi}^*, \boldsymbol{\sigma}^*)]/T \to \mathbf{0}$. This approach first used for regression by Stefanski (1985), is often the only realistic analytical strategy in time series when the estimators do not have a closed form. Expanding the estimating equations leads to

$$\boldsymbol{\phi}^* \approx \boldsymbol{\phi} - (Lim_{T\to\infty} \sum_t E[\dot{S}(X_t^*, \boldsymbol{\phi})]/T)^{-1} Lim_{t\to T} \sum_t E(S(X_t^*, \boldsymbol{\phi}))/T,$$

assuming the limits exist and where $\dot{S}$ denotes partial derivatives with respect to the parameters. The second term will give an asymptotic bias but the problem here is in finding the expected values and limits. We can outline some of the issues with the Ricker model, which was extensively examined by Resendes (2011). Although non-linear in $x$, the Ricker model is linear in the parameters, leading to simple linear least squares. Defining, $D_t = X_{t+1}^* - X_t^*$ and $C_t = e^{X_t^*}$, $S_{DC} = \sum_{t=1}^{T-1}(D_t - \bar{D})(C_t - \bar{C})/T$ and $S_{CC} = \sum_{t=1}^{T-1}(C_t - \bar{C})^2/T$, then the naive estimator of $\phi_1$ is $\widehat{\phi}_{1,naive} = S_{DC}/S_{CC}$ and asymptotically $\widehat{\phi}_{1,naive} \Rightarrow LimE(S_{DC})/LimE(S_{CC})$, if the limits exists. We faced two problems here; finding the expected values involving non-linear functions and determining whether the sums converge and to what. Whether the series is stationary or not will enter into these considerations. The Ricker model, in particular, is not necessarily stationary and in general the dynamic behavior may be complex.

### 18.4.2 Correcting for Measurement Error

As earlier, we use two strategies, using just the observed $X^*$ values (under suitable assumptions) and pseudo-methods utilizing estimated measurement error parameters.

**Using the observed $X^*$ values.** As earlier, this approach assumes a model for the original time series along with a measurement error model involving a fixed number of parameters, for which all parameters are identifiable. A large amount of the work on correcting for measurement error in dynamic settings has attacked the problem from this perspective. As noted Section 18.3, these are state-space models and the methods can be applied to either linear or non-linear models. The approach is standard in principle but there can be computational challenges. The shortcomings of this approach are the potential restrictive nature of the measurement error model and the fact that identifiability does not guarantee good estimators. Of course, with no estimates of the ME parameters, this is the only option.

There are two likelihoods of interest here, $L(\boldsymbol{\phi}, \boldsymbol{\sigma}, \boldsymbol{\theta}|\mathbf{x}^*) = f(\mathbf{x}^*|\boldsymbol{\phi}, \boldsymbol{\sigma}, \boldsymbol{\theta})$ and $L^*(\boldsymbol{\phi}, \boldsymbol{\sigma}, \boldsymbol{\theta}, \widetilde{\mathbf{x}}_1|\mathbf{x}^*) = f_c(\mathbf{x}^*|\boldsymbol{\phi}, \boldsymbol{\sigma}, \boldsymbol{\theta}, \widetilde{\mathbf{x}}_1)$, from (9) and (10), respectively. The ML estimator maximizes the former and the CML the latter. The computational challenges are more severe for non-linear models both in the integration required to obtain the likelihood, and in getting the information matrix or other quantities for use in inference. Note that the full likelihood specifies a marginal distribution for $X_1$, while in working with the conditional likelihood $\widetilde{\mathbf{x}}_1$ is treated as another parameter. This would seem to argue more for the use of the conditional approach. For overviews and references see DeValpine and Hastings (2002), DeValpine (2002), DeValpine and Hilborn (2005), and Wang (2007). More recent methods that have been developed to try an overcome some of the computational challenges include the Monte Carlo Kernel Likelihood (MCKL) (DeValpine, 2004), a method called data cloning, which borrows from Bayesian computing (Lele et al., 2007; Poincano et al., 2009) and composite maximum likelihood estimation (ComML) (Lele, 2006).

Bayesian approaches here use the likelihoods above along with priors for the parameters ($\boldsymbol{\phi}, \boldsymbol{\sigma}$ and $\boldsymbol{\theta}$) and base inferences on the posterior distribution of the parameters with the main focus being on estimating $\boldsymbol{\phi}$. One has to be cautious about simply using a Bayesian approach with a prior on $\boldsymbol{\theta}$ to avoid identifiability problems. The computational challenges here are similar to those in the likelihood setting but there are some formulations that can be easily fit using Winbugs; see, for example, Bolker (2008, Section 11.6.2) and Viljugrein et al. (2005). General discussion of the Bayesian approach can be found in Calder et al. (2003), Clark and Bjornstad (2004), Wang (2007), and Jungbacker and Koopman (2007). Viljugrein et al. (2005) is really a pseudo-Bayesian approach in using estimated measurement error variances from each point in time. Clark and Bjornstad (2004) is notable for its treatment of unequal measurement error variances by incorporating different priors on each of the $\sigma^2_{utc}$ to reflect the amount of information about them. Additional applications of the Bayesian method can be found in Stenseth et al. (2003), Saether et al. (2008), and Lillegard et al. (2008), among others.

**Pseudo methods:** Here we assume we have $\widehat{\boldsymbol{\theta}}$ which estimates the measurement error parameters. This may include estimated variances as well as biases and/or correlations if they are part of the model. With additive uncorrelated measurement errors, allowing changing variance over time then $\widehat{\boldsymbol{\theta}}$ contains an estimate, $\widehat{\sigma}^2_{ut}$, at each time point $t$, typically arising from the same data that produces $X^*_t$. The pseudo-methods set $\boldsymbol{\theta} = \widehat{\boldsymbol{\theta}}$ and then estimate the parameters in the dynamic model. While it seems natural to exploit estimates about the measurement error parameters, this strategy has been seriously underutilized. We subsume under pseudo methods methods approaches that simply assume that the measurement error parameters are given.

The pseudo ML estimates maximize either $L(\boldsymbol{\phi}, \boldsymbol{\sigma}, \widehat{\boldsymbol{\theta}}|\mathbf{w})$ or $L_2(\boldsymbol{\phi}, \boldsymbol{\sigma}, \widehat{\boldsymbol{\theta}}, \mathbf{x}^*_1|\mathbf{w})$ where $\widehat{\boldsymbol{\theta}}$ contains estimated, or assumed known, measurement error parameters. These methods also have a long history of use in modeling with repeated samples surveys where the true values are ARIMA (and special cases thereof) or follow a basic structural model (BSM) and the sampling error also may follow a dynamic model(AR, MA, etc.), which is first estimated and then held fixed. See Bell and Wilcox (1993), Koons and Foutz (1990), Wong and Miller (1990), Miazaki and Dorea (1993), Lee and Shin (1997) and Feder (2001) and references therein. Many pseudo-approaches treat stationary normal models assuming $\mathbf{X}^* \sim N(\mu\mathbf{1}, \boldsymbol{\Sigma}_X + \widehat{\boldsymbol{\Sigma}}_u)$, but recall the earlier caution about non-normality of $\mathbf{X}^*$ if the measurement error covariance change with $X_t$.

For the most part, the pseudo likelihood approaches face the same computational demands as the non-pseudo likelihood methods. An added challenge lies in finding the covariance matrix for the estimated dynamic parameters which accounts for uncertainty in $\widehat{\boldsymbol{\theta}}$. To illustrate, let $\omega' = (\boldsymbol{\phi}', \boldsymbol{\sigma}')$ for the collection of dynamic parameters and $I(\boldsymbol{\omega})$ the corresponding information matrix, with submatrices $I_\phi$, etc. If $\widehat{\boldsymbol{\theta}}$ is treated as fixed, the asymptotic covariance matrix of $\widehat{\boldsymbol{\omega}}_{ML}$ is $I(\boldsymbol{\omega})^{-1}$, leading to an asymptotic covariance matrix of $\widehat{\boldsymbol{\phi}}_{ML}$ of $Acov(\widehat{\boldsymbol{\phi}}_{ML,K}) = (I_\phi - I_{\phi,\sigma}I_\sigma^{-1}I'_{\phi,\sigma})^{-1}$, $K$ for known. This covariance can be estimated in standard fashion, computational issues aside.

What about accounting for the uncertainty in $\widehat{\boldsymbol{\theta}}$, say with covariance $\boldsymbol{\Sigma}_{\widehat{\theta}}$? This part has been essentially ignored, an exception being SB(2005). If $\boldsymbol{\theta}$ is of fixed dimension and $\widehat{\boldsymbol{\theta}}$ is consistent and asymptotically normal with covariance matrix $\boldsymbol{\Sigma}_{\widehat{\theta}}$, then as shown by Parke (1986), often

$$Acov(\widehat{\boldsymbol{\omega}}_{ML}) = I(\boldsymbol{\omega})^{-1} + I(\boldsymbol{\omega})^{-1}I_{\omega,\theta}\boldsymbol{\Sigma}_{\widehat{\theta}}I'_{\omega,\theta}I(\boldsymbol{\omega})^{-1}. \tag{11}$$

Hence, $Acov(\widehat{\boldsymbol{\phi}}_{ML}) = Acov(\widehat{\boldsymbol{\phi}}_{ML,K}) + \mathbf{Q}$, where $\mathbf{Q}$ is the upper left $p \times p$ block of the second matrix in (11) and $p$ is the size of $\boldsymbol{\phi}$. The $\mathbf{Q}$ will involve $V(\widehat{\sigma}^2_u)$ in the case where the measurement errors are uncorrelated and $\widehat{\boldsymbol{\Sigma}}_u = \widehat{\sigma}^2_u\mathbf{I}$ is used. The hope is that this second term above in negligible as it was in our AR(1) example in Section 18.3.4. However this remains to be fully explored.

The expression in (11) depends on $\widehat{\boldsymbol{\theta}}$ being asymptotically uncorrelated with $\widehat{\boldsymbol{\omega}}$. This certainly holds if $\widehat{\boldsymbol{\theta}}$ is independent of $\mathbf{X}^*$, but see Buonaccorsi (2013) for a generalization of the above result in a general estimating equation context. We also note that asymptotic arguments will be delicate if the number of measurement error parameters increases with $T$.

### 18.4.3 SIMEX, MEE and RC

Here we briefly present three other correction methods, SIMEX, modifying/correcting estimating equations and regression calibration, all of which have been successful in regression settings. All three use information about the measurement error parameters and are designed to both ease the computational burden and, more importantly, relax some of the distributional assumptions underlying likelihood and Bayesian techniques.

**SIMEX.** Originally due to Stefanski and Cook (1995), it has been used mainly with additive measurement error but can also accommodate multiplicative errors (e.g, Solow, 1998; Resendes, 2011). Briefly it proceeds here as follows. At each of a number of values of $c$ and for $k = 1$ to some large number $K$, the estimated variances are used to generate values $X_{tkc}$ such that they have approximate variance $(1 + c)\sigma^2_{ut}$ . The naive fit is obtained for each $k$ and then the estimated coefficients are averaged over $k$ for each $c$. One then fits a curve for how the average naive estimator behaves as a function of $c$ and projects back to no measurement error ($c = -1$). It has seen some, but rather, limited use in dynamic settings; see Solow (1998) Ellner et al. (2002) and Bolker (2011, Ch. 11). While certainly not bullet proof, SIMEX has proven itself to perform quite well across a variety of regression models. Its great advantage is the need to only have to be able to fit the naive estimator. Getting analytical standard errors is more challenging, and has not been examined thoroughly in dynamic contexts. This is another place where the bootstrap will come in handy. Resendes (2011) evaluated the performance of SIMEX in fitting the Ricker model via simulation and obtained bootstrap standard errors and confidence intervals. He found that except for large (and unreasonable) levels of measurement error, SIMEX was quite successful in removing bias and bootstrap based inferences performed fairly well. One problem with SIMEX in combination with the bootstrap was the huge number of fits that need to be done. This was easy for the version of the Ricker model that leads to linear least squares but was more problematic when needing to use root finding methods for solving non-linear equations for the multiplicative version.

SIMEX does hold promise but may need fine tuning. For example in the mallard density example in Section 18.3.4 the use of SIMEX based on the naive Yule-Walker estimates produced an estimate of .4945, considerably smaller than the CEE and PML estimates. It is anticipated however that the SIMEX would be improved here with the use of REML, rather than Yule-Walker to get naive estimates.

**Modified estimating equations.** This is closely related to finding corrected scores and is also motivated by minimizing distributional assumptions. The idea is to use the estimated measurement error parameters and try to modify the naive estimating equations so the corrected equations have asymptotic mean **0**. While attractive in principle, for time series it is often difficult to implement for the same reasons associated with using the estimating equations to assess bias. Approximate corrections are most easily found for the least squares type estimators. One convenience of getting explicit corrected equations is the ability to build from them to get analytical expressions for the approximate covariance matrix of the estimators. While a promising approach in general, an extensive investigation into its use for the Ricker model (the easiest of the "nonlinear" models) by Resendes (2011) found that the resulting estimators can be erratic, were outperformed by SIMEX and it was difficult to get good standard errors. Perhaps further fine tuning might alleviate some of these issues.

**Regression calibration.** Finally we briefly mention regression calibration, which is extremely popular method in regression contexts. For an autoregressive model, consider $E(X_t^*|\mathbf{X}_{t-1}^*) = E[E(X_t^*|\mathbf{X}_{t-1}^*, \mathbf{X}_{t-1}] = E[E(X_t^*|\mathbf{X}_{t-1}|\mathbf{X}_{t-1}^*)] = E[m(\boldsymbol{\phi}, \mathbf{X}_{t-1})|\mathbf{X}_{t-1}^*] \approx m(\boldsymbol{\phi}, E(\mathbf{X}_{t-1}|\mathbf{X}_{t-1}^*))$, where the approximation is exact if the model is linear in the $X$'s. (The last step of running the expectation through the $m$ function is what motivates RC methods in regression.) This suggests finding an estimate $\widehat{\mathbf{X}}_{t-1}$ of $E(\mathbf{X}_{t-1}|\mathbf{X}_{t-1}^*)$ and then estimating $\boldsymbol{\phi}$ by regressing $X_t^*$ on $\widehat{\mathbf{X}}_{t-1}$. Notice that this is *not* the same as running the usual time series analysis on the $\widehat{X}_t$s since we are leaving $X_t^*$ as is when it is the "outcome" but modifying "predictors" by using $\widehat{\mathbf{X}}_{t-1}$ in place of $\mathbf{X}_{t-1}^*$. For the linear autoregressive model and using estimated best linear predictors, this leads essentially to the CEE estimator in Section 18.3. This approach, quite successful in regression problems, has not been investigated in the time series setting yet.

### 18.4.4 Bootstrapping

The preceding sections provide a number of reasons why the bootstrap could be useful in these models, both for getting standard errors and assessing remaining bias in corrected estimators. The parametric bootstrap, based on an assumed distribution for both the measurement errors and the true values is relatively easy to implement. For an autoregressive model depending on the past $p$ values, for each bootstrap sample $b$ $(= 1$ to $B)$, we can set $x_{b1} = (x_{b1}, \ldots, x_{bp})'$, where $x_{bj} = X_j^*$ for $j = 1$ to $p$. We would then generate (sequentially) $X_{bt} = m(\widehat{\boldsymbol{\phi}}, \mathbf{x}_{b,t-1}) + e_{bt}$, where $e_{bt}$ is based on the distribution of $\epsilon_t$ with estimated parameters. Measurement error is then added to generate $\mathbf{X}_b^*$ from $\mathbf{x}_b$ according to the estimated model for $\mathbf{X}^*|\mathbf{x}$. If a pseudo-method is being used and we want to account for uncertainty from estimating the measurement error parameters, then we also would generate $\widehat{\boldsymbol{\theta}}_b$, based on a distributional assumption. For each bootstrap sample, the corrected estimators are obtained and standard bootstrap inferences obtained using the $B$ bootstrap values. This approach resamples from the dynamic model explicitly. (There are some methods for bootstrap time series via block resampling, e.g., but these are of limited value with short series and their use needs to be carefully considered if there are measurement errors present with changing properties over time). While in general non-parametric bootstrapping is preferred, it is difficult to get an estimate of the process error distribution; i.e., the distribution of the $\epsilon_t$. To see the problem suppose we knew the dynamic parameters exactly and examine residuals $r_t = X_t^* - m(\boldsymbol{\phi}, X_{t-1}^*) = X_t + u_t - m(\boldsymbol{\phi}, \mathbf{X}_{t-1}) + (m(\boldsymbol{\phi}, \mathbf{X}_{t-1}) - m(\boldsymbol{\phi}, X_{t-1}^*) = \epsilon_t + u_t + (m(\boldsymbol{\phi}, \mathbf{X}_{t-1}) - m(\boldsymbol{\phi}, X_{t-1}^*)$. This is contaminated by the measurement errors and some type of "unmixing" (related to deconvolution) is needed to get a nonparametric estimate of the distribution of $\epsilon_t$. The problem is exacerbated further with non-linear models and use of the estimated coefficients.

### 18.4.5 Non-linear Example

For illustration, we take a brief look at analyzing data shown in Figure 18.2 which shows the estimated log(abundance) from annual censuses of moose in the Bialowsieza Primeval Forest (Jedrzejewska et al., 1997). This was analyzed by Clark and Bjornstad (2004) as a measurement error in time series problem from a Bayesian perspective. A handful of missing values have been imputed (since treating missing values is another topic beyond the scope of this chapter). The series is obviously non-stationary. The Ricker model is used with $x$ =log(abundance), where recall $\phi_0$ is a growth rate and $K = -\phi_0/\phi_1$ a carrying capacity. For this model $x_t - x_{t-1}$ is linear in $e^{x_{t-1}}$. This is no longer exactly the case with $x_t^*$ in place of $x_t$ but the second part of the figure is still useful for a rough diagnostic for whether the Ricker model is reasonable. Resendes (2011) carried out an extensive analysis of these data. No estimates of the measurement error variances were available so he explored fitting over different values of $\sigma_u$ assuming the ME variance was constant. Table 18.4 shows just a few of his results with $\sigma_u = .05$ or .2 using SIMEX and modifiying the naive estimating equations (MEE) based on least squares. The bootstrapping was as described in the previous section assuming normal process error and measurement error. The main points to make here are 1) there is little change with modest measurement error ($\sigma_u = .05$) and SIMEX and MEE are in pretty close agreement and 2) with larger measurement error the estimates differ substantially from the naive analysis and SIMEX and MEE have noticable differences. SIMEX is the preferred method here based on the simulation results of Resendes. We also note the large amount of uncertainty in the estimate of $K$.

## 18.5 Acknowledgments

I am very grateful to David Resendes for allowing use of some results from his dissertation, to Hildegunn Viljugrein for providing the Mallard data, and to to Springer and Chapman & Hall for permission to use some material from Buonaccorsi (2013) and Buonaccorsi(2010), respectively.

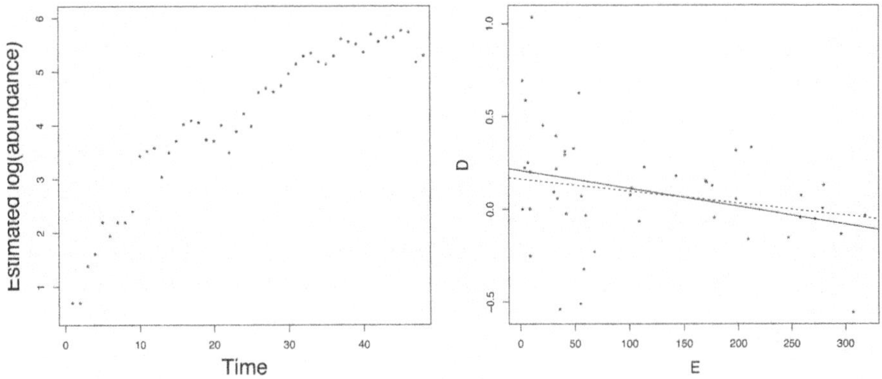


**FIGURE 18.2**
Plot of $x_t$ = estimated log(abudance) of moose over the period 1946-1993 (Time = 1 to 48) and $D_t = x_t^* - x_{t-1}^*$ versus $E_t = e^{x_{t-1}}$. on right with naive (solid) and SIMEX using the larger measurement error variance (dashed) fits.

**TABLE 18.4**
Estimates of parameters fitting Ricker model to the moose data. Bootstrap standard errors in parentheses.

| | | SIMEX | | MEE | |
|---|---|---|---|---|---|
| | Naive | $\sigma_u = 0.05$ | $\sigma_u = .2$ | $\sigma_u = 0.05$ | $\sigma_u = .2$ |
| $\phi_0$ | .208 (.079) | .205 (.069) | .162 (.047) | .208 (.070) | .164 (.020) |
| $K$ | 216.15 (72.9) | 218.94 (76.8) | 249.72 (83.2) | 216.39 (76.8) | 278.68 (83.1) |
| $\sigma$ | .289 (.03) | .282 (.031) | .161 (.060) | .281 (.031) | .081 (.078) |

## References

Bell, W. R., and Wilcox, D. W. (1993). The effect of sampling error on the time series behavior of consumption data. *Journal of Econometrics*, 55, 235-265.

Bolker (2008). *Ecological Models and Data in R*. Princeton University.

Box, G., Jenkins, G., and Reinsel, G. (1994). *Time Series Analysis, Forecasting and Control*, 3rd ed., Prentice Hall.

Brockwell, P. and Davis, R. (2002). *Introduction to Time Series and Forecasting*. Springer-Verlag Inc.

Buonaccorsi (2006). Estimation in two-stage models with heteroscedasticity. *International Statistical Review*, 74(3), 403-415.

Buonaccorsi, J. P. (2010). *Measurement Error, Models, Methods, and Applications*. Chapman & Hall.

Buonaccorsi, J.P. (2013) Measurement error in dynamic models. In *ISS-2012 Proceedings Volume On Longitudinal Data Analysis Subject to Measurement Errors, Missing Values, and/or Outliers.* Lecture Notes in Statistics. Sutradhar, B. (eds), vol 211. Springer, New York, NY.

Buonaccorsi, J.P., Staudenmayer, J., and Carreras, M. (2006). Modeling observation error and its effects in a random walk/extinction model. *Theoretical Population Biology*, 70, 322-335.

Calder, C., Lavine, M., Muller, P., and Clark, J. (2003). Incorporating multiple sources of stochasticity into dynamic population models, *Ecology*, 84, 1395-1402.

Cheang, W. and Reinsel, G. C. (2000). Bias reduction of autoregressive estimates in time series regression model through restricted maximum likelihood. *Journal of the American Statistical Association*, 95, 1173-1184.

Clark, J. S. and Bjornstad, O. N. (2004). Population time series, process variability, observation errors, missing values, lags, and hidden states. *Ecology*, 85, 3140-3150.

Dennis, B., Ponciano, J., Lele, S., Taper, M., and Staples, D. (2006). Estimating density dependence, process noise, and observation error. *Ecological Monographs*, 76, 323-341.

De Valpine, P. (2002). Review of methods for fitting time-series models with process and observation error and likelihood calculations for nonlinear non-gaussian state-space models. *Bulletin of Marine Science*, 70, 455-471.

De Valpine, P. (2004). Monte-Carlo state-space likelihoods by weighted posterior kernel density estimation. *Journal of the American Statistical Association*, 99, 523-536.

De Valpine, P. and Hastings, A. (2002). Fitting population models incorporating process noise and observation error. *Ecological Monographs*, 72, 57-76.

De Valpine, P. and Hilborn, R. (2005). State-space likelihoods for nonlinear fisheries time series. *Canadian Journal of Fisheries and Aquatic Science*, 62, 1937-1952.

Ellner, S., Yodit, S., and Smith, R. (2002). Fitting population dynamic models to time-series by gradient matching. *Ecology*, 83, 2256- 2270.

Feder, M. (2001). Time series analysis of repeated surveys, The state-space approach, *Statistica Neerlandica*, 55 (2), 182-199.

Harvey, A. C. (1990), *Forecasting, Structural Time Series Models, and the Kalman Filter.* Cambridge University Press.

Ives, A.R., Dennis, B., Cottingham, K. L., and Carpenter, S.R. (2003). Estimating community stability and ecological interactions from time-series data. *Ecological Monographs*, 73, 301-330.

Ives, A.R, Abbott, K., and Ziebarth, N. (2010). Analysis of ecological time series with ARMA(p,q) models. *Ecololgy*, 91, 858-871.

Jungbacker, B. and Koopman, S. J. (2007). Monte Carlo estimation for nonlinear non-Gaussian state space models. *Biometrika*, 94, 827-839.

Knape J. (2008). Estimability of density dependence in models of time series data. *Ecology*, 89, 2994-3000.

Koons, B. K. and Foutz, R. V. (1990). Estimating moving average parameters in the presence of measurement error. *Communications in Statistics*, 19, 3179-3187.

Lele, S. R. (2006). Sampling variability and estimates of density dependence, a composite-likelihood approach. *Ecology*, 87, 189-202.

Lele, S. R., Dennis, B., and Lutscher, F. (2007). Data cloning, easy maximum likelihood estimation for complex ecological models using Bayesian Markov chain Monte Carlo methods. *Ecology Letters*, 10, 551-563.

Lillegard, M., Engen, S., Saether, B. E., Grotan, V., and Drever, M. (2008). Estimation of population parameters from aerial counts of North American mallards: A cautionary tale. *Ecological Applications*, 18, 197-207.

Miazaki, E. S., and Dorea, C. C. Y. (1993). Estimation of the parameters of a time series subject to the error of rotation sampling, *Communications in Statistics, Part A – Theory and Methods*, 22, 805-825.

Parke, W. (1986). Pseudo-maximum likelihood estimation: The asymptotic distribution. *Annals of Statistics*, 14, 355-357.

Pfeffermann, D., Feder, M., and Signorelli, D. (1998). Estimation of autocorrelations of survey errors with application to trend estimation in small areas. *Journal of Business and Economic Statistics*, 16, 339-348.

Resendes, D. (2011). Statistical methods for nonlinear dynamic models with measurement error using the Ricker model. Ph.D. thesis, University of Massachusetts, Amherst.

Saether B., Lilligard M., Grotan V., Drever M., Engen S., Nudds T., and Podruzny K. (2008). Geographical gradients in the population dynamics of North American prairie ducks. *Journal of Animal Ecology*, 77, 869-882.

Schmid, C. H., Segal, M. R., and Rosner, B. (1994). Incorporating measurement error in the estimation of autoregressive models for longitudinal data. *Journal of Statistical Planning and Inference*, 42, 1-18.

Scott, A. J., Smith, T. M. F., and Jones, R. G. (1977). The application of time series methods to the analysis of repeated surveys. *International Statistical Review*, 45, 13-28.

Solow A.R. (1998). On fitting a population model in the presence of observation error. *Ecology*, 79, 1463-1466.

Solow A.R. (2001). Observation error and the detection of delayed density dependence. *Ecology*, 82, 3263-3264.

Staudenmayer, J. and Buonaccorsi, J. P. (2005). Measurement error in linear autoregressive models. *Journal of the American Statistical Association*, 100, 841-852.

Stefanski, L. (1985). The effects of measurement error on parameter estimation. *Biometrika*, 72, 583-592.

Stefanski, L. and Cook, J. (1995). Simulation-extrapolation: The measurement error jackknife. *Journal of the American Statistical Association*, 90, 1247-1256.

Stenseth N. C., Viljugrein, H., Saitoh, T., Hansen, T. F., Kittilsen, M. O., Bolviken, E. and Glockner, F. (2003). Seasonality, density dependence, and population cycles in Hokkaido voles. *PNAS*, 100, 11478-11483.

Viljugrein, H., Stenseth, N. C., Smith, G. W., and Steinbakk, G. H. (2005). Density Dependence in North American Ducks. *Ecology*, 86, 245-254.

Wang G. (2007). On the latent state estimation of nonlinear population dynamics using Bayesian and non-Bayesian state-space models. *Ecological Modeling*, 20, 521-528.

Williams, C. K., Ives, A. R., and Applegate, R. D. (2003). Population dynamics across geographical ranges, time-series analyses of three small game species. *Ecology*, 84, 2654-2667.

Wong, Wing-keung, and Miller, R. B. (1990). Repeated time series analysis of ARIMA-noise models. *Journal of Business and Economic Statistics*, 8, 243-250.

Wong, Wing-keung, Miller, R. B., and Shrestha, K. (2001), Maximum likelihood estimation of ARMA models with error processes for replicated observations, *Journal of Applied Statistical Science*, 10, 287-297.

# 19

# *Spatial Exposure Measurement Error in Environmental Epidemiology*

**Howard H. Chang and Joshua P. Keller**

## CONTENTS



## 19.1 Introduction

The field of environmental epidemiology aims to determine and quantify adverse health effects related to exposures that humans encounter via the air, water and land. Environmental exposures include toxic contaminants from

DOI: 10.1201/9781315101279-19

anthropogenic sources (e.g. agricultural, industrial and transportation operations), as well as risk factors such as high temperatures, the built environment and ecological changes. Advancing our understanding of how environmental exposures affect human health continues to be an important area of research for several reasons. Pollutants, especially those released into the atmosphere and the water system, can affect large populations. Health impact assessments are made often in response to emerging concerns (e.g., hydraulic fracturing) or disasters (e.g. oil spills). Under a changing climate, hurricanes, heat waves, wildfires and other extreme events are projected to increase in frequency and intensity in the future. Most importantly, because environmental exposures are often involuntary, particularly among vulnerable subpopulations, regulatory standards and policies that are informed by epidemiologic studies can play an important role in protecting public health.

Environmental epidemiologic studies are predominantly observational because study participants generally cannot be easily or ethically assigned to receive a specific exposure. These studies can be broadly classified into two types based on exposure duration, which impacts how exposures are linked to health outcomes. First, studies of *chronic* exposures can be conducted by cohort or case-control designs where exposure during a hypothesized long-term period (e.g. year, decade) is of interest (Berhane et al., 2004). Examples include studies on long-term exposure to air pollution and the risk of developing neurological disorders, and life-time cumulative exposure to occupational contaminants and cancer incidence. In contrast, studies of *acute* exposures are interested in exposures during a short-term window (typically a few days) prior to an adverse health event. Examples include studies on daily pollen counts and asthma exacerbation, and heat waves and mortality. The two most commonly used approaches for acute exposure studies are: (1) the time-series design where cases are aggregated and analyzed as counts over time (Gasparrini et al., 2013) and (2) the case-crossover design where control time periods are identified for each event case (Carracedo-Martinez et al., 2010). Short-term effects of environmental exposures are typically smaller in magnitude compared to long-term effects. Hence studies of acute exposures often leverage large administrative databases using a case-only design to achieve sufficient sample size.

The ability to accurately assign exposures to health data is a crucial component in any environmental health study. However, it is generally not possible to measure exposures continuously for all study participants during the long follow-up period in chronic exposure studies, nor is measuring exposures for the large number of adverse events in acute exposure studies. Moreover, population-based studies are often retrospective, where exposures are not collected concurrently with health outcomes. In practice, exposure measurements are only available at a limited number of spatial locations and time points, and their values need to be interpolated to perform exposure assessment. For example, air pollution measurements at a few monitors may be spatially interpolated to assign exposures to participants based upon their residential addresses in chronic exposure studies, or averaged to represent exposures for all cases in acute exposure studies within a geographical area.

Uncertainty arising from the *spatial-temporal misalignment* of environmental exposure measurements and health data is the focus of this chapter. Challenges in accounting for environmental exposure error center around the use of spatial-temporal models to estimate exposures without complete spatio-temporal coverage. Moreover, a person's exposure can be affected by activity patterns. For example, personal exposure to air pollution is determined by the amount of time spent at different locations and how much air pollution is present at each microenvironment (e.g., residence, workplace, mode of commute). Most of the time, a validation sub-study with gold-standard measurements is also unavailable. Environmental exposures can exhibit complex spatial and temporal trends because they may be released from common sources; and the fate and transport of pollutants are governed by atmospheric and hydrological processes. Environmental measurements are also usually conducted sparsely in space and time, with potential selection bias. For example, monitors for meteorology are often located at airports and monitors for regulating pollution are often preferentially located in areas where the at-risk population is large and the pollution level is high.

This chapter aims to provide an overview of methods to account for exposure uncertainty in the context of environmental epidemiology. Statistical approaches presented here are drawn largely from air pollution research because of the rich literature on exposure modeling and health effect estimation. We will first introduce common modeling approaches to estimate environmental exposures. This sets the stage for a discussion on the different types of exposure measurement errors that arise when estimates from these models are assigned to individual-level and aggregated health outcomes. Then a review of methods to account for exposure measurement error will be presented. Finally, we will describe several important issues and research directions in this field, including multipollutant exposures, model selection for estimating exposure, and linking environmental measurements to personal exposures.

## 19.2 Modeling Environmental Exposures

An environmental exposure model uses available point-level measurements at sparse locations to estimate the unobserved spatio-temporal exposure surface. Population-based environmental health studies have mostly adopted a *two-stage* approach where an exposure model is constructed first and its predictions are then used to fit health models. Joint modeling between exposure and health data (commonly done in other error-in-covariate applications) is challenging because of the spatial-temporal misalignment between observed exposure and health data. Specifically, the modeled exposure surface often needs to be averaged in space and/or time to match the exposure window of interest for each health outcome. Additionally, the same estimated exposure surface is often used in analyses of multiple distinct health outcomes. The need to conduct extensive sensitivity analyses in most environmental health studies further increases the computational demand of a joint modeling approach of exposure and health outcomes

The general model form and parameters of a two-stage analysis can be written as:

$$\text{Exposure Model:} \quad \mathbf{W}_o \,|\, \boldsymbol{\Omega}; \tag{19.1}$$

$$\text{Prediction Model:} \quad \mathbf{X} \,|\, \mathbf{W}_o, \boldsymbol{\Omega}; \tag{19.2}$$

$$\text{Heath Model:} \quad \mathbf{Y} \,|\, \mathbf{X}^*, \beta_X \,. \tag{19.3}$$

Observed data in an analysis include exposure measurements $\mathbf{W}_o$ and health outcomes $\mathbf{Y}$. Expression (19.1) represents the exposure model with unknown parameters $\boldsymbol{\Omega}$. Expression (19.2) describes the distribution of the unknown exposure $\mathbf{X}$ at a set of locations required for alignment with health outcomes (e.g., at unique point locations of $\mathbf{Y}$ or a set of grid points). Expression (19.3) is the health model where $\mathbf{X}^*$ is the estimated exposure assigned to health outcomes. For example, $\mathbf{X}^*$ can be the conditional mean of $[\mathbf{X}|\mathbf{W}_o, \boldsymbol{\Omega}]$ or some pre-defined spatial-temporal averages of $\mathbf{X}$. Our main parameter of interest is the health association $\beta_X$. Additional covariates can enter the health model as confounders, but are left out here for notational ease.

### 19.2.1 Defining Exposures from Spatial Interpolation

Let $W_o(\mathbf{s}_i)$ denote the pollutant concentration measurement at the $i^{\text{th}}$ *observed* point-location $\mathbf{s}_i$ with coordinates $(s_{1i}, s_{2i})$ (e.g., projected x-y coordinate). We assume $W_o(\mathbf{s}_i)$ is an error-prone version of an unobserved true exposure $X_o(\mathbf{s}_i)$. A typical spatial exposure model $\mathbf{W}_o \,|\, \boldsymbol{\Omega}$ is given by:

$$W_o(\mathbf{s}_i) = X_o(\mathbf{s}_i) + \epsilon(\mathbf{s}_i); \tag{19.4}$$

$$X_o(\mathbf{s}_i) = \mathbf{Z}_o^{\mathrm{T}}(\mathbf{s}_i)\boldsymbol{\alpha} + v(\mathbf{s}_i), \tag{19.5}$$

where $\mathbf{Z}_o(\mathbf{s}_i)$ is a vector of covariates that are predictive of the exposure with corresponding regression coefficient $\boldsymbol{\alpha}$, component $v(\mathbf{s}_i)$ represents a smooth residual spatial trend, and component $\epsilon(\mathbf{s}_i)$ represents independent residual variation due to instrumental error or fine-scale spatial variation not captured by $v(\mathbf{s}_i)$. Both $\epsilon(\mathbf{s}_i)$ and $v(\mathbf{s}_i)$ are assumed to have mean zero.

The latent variable $v(\mathbf{s}_i)$ is typically modeled as a Gaussian process (GP). A mean-zero GP assumes that the joint distribution of $v(\mathbf{s}_i)$ at a finite set of $n$ locations is multivariate Normal:

$$\mathbf{v} = [v(\mathbf{s}_1), v(\mathbf{s}_2), \ldots, v(\mathbf{s}_n)]^{\mathrm{T}} \sim N\left[\mathbf{Zero},\ \boldsymbol{\Sigma}(\boldsymbol{\theta})\right],$$

where $\boldsymbol{\Sigma}(\boldsymbol{\theta})$ is the covariance matrix parameterized by $\boldsymbol{\theta}$. The entries of $\boldsymbol{\Sigma}(\boldsymbol{\theta})$ are given by a covariance function $C(\cdot|\boldsymbol{\theta})$. Let $d_{ij} = ||\mathbf{s}_i - \mathbf{s}_j||$ denote the Euclidean distance between locations $\mathbf{s}_i$ and $\mathbf{s}_j$. One popular covariance function is the Matérn:

$$C(d_{ij}|\boldsymbol{\theta}) = \theta_1 \frac{1}{\Gamma(\theta_3)2^{\theta_3 - 1}} \left(\frac{d_{ij}}{\theta_2}\right)^{\theta_3} K_{\theta_3}\left(\frac{d_{ij}}{\theta_2}\right),$$

where $\boldsymbol{\theta} = (\theta_1, \theta_2, \theta_3)^{\mathrm{T}}$ with $\theta_1, \theta_2, \theta_3 > 0$, and $K_{\theta_3}(\cdot)$ is the modified Bessel function of the second kind (Abrahamsen, 1997). The Matérn covariance function contains two important special cases. When $\theta_3 = 0.5$, it corresponds to the exponential covariance function: $C(d_{ij}|\boldsymbol{\theta}) = \theta_1 e^{-d_{ij}/\theta_2}$; as $\theta_3 \to \infty$, it gives the double-exponential covariance function $C(d_{ij}|\boldsymbol{\theta}) = \theta_1 e^{-d_{ij}^2/\theta_2^2}$. In the above covariance functions $\theta_1$ corresponds to the value when when $d_{ij} = 0$. Hence, $\theta_1$ is known as the *marginal variance* which describes the variability at any location across independent realizations of the GP. Parameter $\theta_2$ is known as the *range* parameter and describes the correlation as a function of distance. Finally, $\theta_3$ determines the *smoothness* of the covariance function. The Matérn family is an example of *isotropic* covariance function because its value only depends on the distance between locations, regardless of direction and regions of the modeling domain.

Modeling the spatial dependence in $v(\mathbf{s}_i)$ allows us to perform spatial interpolation using values at observed locations to locations without measurements. Let $\mathbf{X} = [X(\mathbf{s}'_1), \ldots, X(\mathbf{s}'_m)]^{\mathrm{T}}$ denote a vector of $m$ exposures to be interpolated at locations $\mathbf{s}'_1, \ldots, \mathbf{s}'_m$ with covariate matrix $\mathbf{Z} = [\,\mathbf{Z}(\mathbf{s}'_1)\ \ldots\ \mathbf{Z}(\mathbf{s}'_m)\,]^{\mathrm{T}}$. Similarly define $\mathbf{X}_0$ and $\mathbf{Z}_0$ as the vector of exposure measurements and covariate matrix at observed locations. Consider the joint distribution

$$\begin{bmatrix} \mathbf{X}_o \\ \mathbf{X} \end{bmatrix} \sim N\left( \begin{bmatrix} \mathbf{Z}_0\boldsymbol{\alpha} \\ \mathbf{Z}\boldsymbol{\alpha} \end{bmatrix}, \begin{bmatrix} \boldsymbol{\Sigma}_{11}(\boldsymbol{\theta}) & \boldsymbol{\Sigma}_{12}(\boldsymbol{\theta}) \\ \boldsymbol{\Sigma}_{21}(\boldsymbol{\theta}) & \boldsymbol{\Sigma}_{22}(\boldsymbol{\theta}) \end{bmatrix} \right),$$

where the block covariance matrix is governed by the same covariance function. Assuming the residual error $\epsilon(\mathbf{s}_i) \sim N(0, \sigma_\epsilon^2)$ and letting $\boldsymbol{\Omega} = (\boldsymbol{\alpha}^{\mathrm{T}}, \boldsymbol{\theta}^{\mathrm{T}}, \sigma_\epsilon^2)^{\mathrm{T}}$, the conditional distribution of $\mathbf{X}$ can be derived with respect to observations $\mathbf{W}_o = [W_o(\mathbf{s}_1), \ldots, W_o(\mathbf{s}_n)]^{\mathrm{T}}$:

$$\begin{aligned} \mathbf{X}|\mathbf{W}_o, \boldsymbol{\Omega} \sim N\big[\, & \mathbf{Z}\boldsymbol{\alpha} + \boldsymbol{\Sigma}_{21}(\boldsymbol{\Sigma}_{11} + \sigma_\epsilon^2\mathbf{I}_n)^{-1}(\mathbf{W}_o - \mathbf{Z}_o\boldsymbol{\alpha}), \\ & \boldsymbol{\Sigma}_{22} - \boldsymbol{\Sigma}_{21}(\boldsymbol{\Sigma}_{11} + \sigma_\epsilon^2\mathbf{I}_n)^{-1}\boldsymbol{\Sigma}_{12}\big], \end{aligned} \tag{19.6}$$

where the $\boldsymbol{\theta}$ index in $\boldsymbol{\Sigma}(\boldsymbol{\theta})$ is suppressed for notational ease and $\mathbf{I}_n$ is an $n \times n$ identity matrix. The mean of the Gaussian distribution in (19.6) is also known as the kriging predictor.

In chronic exposure studies, the conditional mean $E[\mathbf{X}|\mathbf{W}_o, \boldsymbol{\Omega}]$ is used as the *plug-in* exposure estimate in a two-stage analysis. For acute exposures where short-term variation is of interest, the desired exposure metric may be $W(\mathbf{s}_i) = X(\mathbf{s}_i) + \epsilon(\mathbf{s}_i)$. Let $\mathbf{W} = [W(\mathbf{s}'_1), \ldots, W(\mathbf{s}'_m)]^{\mathrm{T}}$. The conditional distribution $[\mathbf{W}|\mathbf{W}_o, \boldsymbol{\Omega}]$ can be derived by considering the joint Normal distribution of $\mathbf{W}$ and $\mathbf{W}_0$. Though the plug-in estimator is the same: $E[\mathbf{W}|\mathbf{W}_o, \boldsymbol{\Omega}] = E[\mathbf{X}|\mathbf{W}_o, \boldsymbol{\Omega}]$ since $\epsilon(\mathbf{s}_i) \perp v(\mathbf{s}_i)$ for all $i = 1, \ldots, m$. In the special case of no spatial dependence, i.e., $v(\mathbf{s}_i) = 0$ for all $\mathbf{s}$, we will use the fitted values (mean trend) $\mathbf{Z}\boldsymbol{\alpha}$ from the exposure regression model as the plug-in estimate of exposure. In another special case where we have no covariates,

$$E[\mathbf{X}|\mathbf{W}_o, \boldsymbol{\Omega}] = \boldsymbol{\Sigma}_{21}(\boldsymbol{\Sigma}_{11} + \sigma^2 \mathbf{I}_n)^{-1}\mathbf{W}_o \,,$$

which can be viewed as an average of observed measurements $\mathbf{W}_o$ with optimal simple kriging weights.

### 19.2.2 Common Regression Models for Environmental Exposures

We now review several commonly used regression approaches for modeling environmental exposures using different forms of model (19.5), other than kriging described in the previous sub-section. First, if we assume $v(\mathbf{s}_i) = 0$ for all $i = 1, \ldots, m$, then the model becomes a standard multiple regression model and $E[\mathbf{X}|\mathbf{W}] = \mathbf{Z}\boldsymbol{\alpha}$. This is also known as a *land use regression* model where the exposure surface is driven only by spatially-varying predictors, such as elevation, roadway density, and distance to pollution sources (Ryan and LeMasters, 2007). One challenge with land use regression models is that predictions can only capture spatial variation represented by the selected land use variables. Often additional measurement campaigns are conducted to enrich the observation dataset and the distribution of predictor variables (Clougherty et al., 2013).

One way to extend the exposure model in (19.5) is to consider spatially-varying coefficients. Here regression coefficients are allowed to vary spatially:

$$X_0(\mathbf{s}_i) = \mathbf{Z}_0(\mathbf{s}_i)^{\mathrm{T}}\boldsymbol{\alpha}(\mathbf{s}_i) + v(\mathbf{s}_i) \,,$$

capturing different associations between pollutant level and predictors across the modeling domain. These coefficients $\boldsymbol{\alpha}(\mathbf{s}_i)$ can be modeled as random effects using a GP under a hierarchical framework (Gelfand et al., 2004), or local regression via geographically weighted regression (Brunsdon et al., 1998). Typically $\alpha(\mathbf{s}_i)$ and $v(\mathbf{s}_i)$ are also allowed to be correlated. One particular application of recent interest is the use of gridded predictors that are informative of exposure but exhibit complex spatial biases. Examples include numerical model simulations (Berrocal et al., 2010) or satellite retrievals (Chang et al., 2013). These models with spatially-varying coefficients are often referred to as *statistical downscalers* because by linking point-level measurements and gridded inputs using continuous surfaces of regression coefficients, predictions can be made at the point-level.

Instead of specifying the residual spatial trend using a GP, $v(\mathbf{s}_i)$ can also be modeled parametrically using functions of coordinates directly, for example by including terms $s_{1i}, s_{2i}, s_{1i}^2$, and $s_{2i}^2$. More generally, one can use spatial basis functions:

$$v(\mathbf{s}_i) = \mathbf{S}(\mathbf{s}_i)^{\mathrm{T}}\boldsymbol{\theta}\,,$$

where $\mathbf{S}(\mathbf{s}_i) \equiv [S_1(\mathbf{s}_i), \ldots, S_r(\mathbf{s}_i)]^{\mathrm{T}}$ is a vector of $r$ basis functions evaluated at location $\mathbf{s}_i$. If the coefficient vector $\boldsymbol{\theta}$ is assumed to be mean-zero Gaussian random effects with covariance matrix $\mathbf{K}$, then $v(\mathbf{s}_i)$ is Gaussian with the covariance between $\mathbf{s}_i$ and $\mathbf{s}_j$ given by $\mathbf{S}(\mathbf{s}_i)^{\mathrm{T}}\mathbf{K}\mathbf{S}(\mathbf{s}_j)$. The above formulation has two main advantages. First, the choice of basis functions and covariance matrix $\mathbf{K}$ can allow for flexible non-stationary structures. Second, when the number of basis functions $r$ is smaller than the number of spatial locations, one can avoid large matrix inversions in the kriging solution, which can be computational burdensome for large datasets. This approach is also known as *fixed rank* kriging (Cressie and Johannesson et al., 2008). Different basis functions have been proposed using pre-specified covariance function (Kammann and Wand, 2003), thin-plate splines (Wood, 2003), and compact kernels (Nychka et al., 2015). In place of a model with random effects, the spline coefficients can also be directly penalized (Bergen and Szpiro, 2015; Keller and Peng, 2019). This results in a penalized regression model of the form

$$\widehat{\boldsymbol{\Omega}}_\lambda = \underset{\boldsymbol{\theta}}{\arg\min}\, \frac{1}{n}\sum_{i=1}^{n}\left[\, W_o(\mathbf{s}_i) - \mathbf{S}(\mathbf{s}_i)^{\mathrm{T}}\boldsymbol{\theta}\,\right]^2 + \lambda\boldsymbol{\theta}^{\mathrm{T}}\mathbf{D}\boldsymbol{\theta}, \tag{19.7}$$

where $\lambda$ controls the global amount of penalization and matrix $\mathbf{D}$ governs the relative penalization of the coefficients. This approach not only allows for flexible choice of spatial basis functions, but it is also reduces computationally burden associated with analyzing large spatial datasets.

### 19.2.3 Spatial-Temporal Models

Spatial-temporal models are used for exposures that are measured across both space and discrete time points. Let $t_i$ index the time point for the $i^{\mathrm{th}}$ observation, spatial-temporal covariates $\mathbf{Z}(\mathbf{s}_i, t_i)$ often include short-term meteorological variables such as temperature and precipitation. For exposures with smooth temporal trends, including them in the mean via temporal splines or cyclic functions may be sufficient; otherwise, additional temporal autocorrelation can built into the random effect $v(\mathbf{s}_i, t_i)$. There is a rich literature on how to model spatial-temporal data with different covariance functions (Gneiting et al., 2006). The simplest covariance function assumes that correlation due to spatial and temporal proximity are *separable*, i.e., Corr $[v(\mathbf{s}_i, t_i), v(\mathbf{s}_j, t_j)] = h_1(||\mathbf{s}_i - \mathbf{s}_j||) \times h_2(|t_i - t_j|)$, where $h_1(\cdot)$ and $h_2(\cdot)$ are correlation functions in space and time, respectively, for $i \neq j$. A dynamic model is another popular formulation where the spatial process evolves through time. For example, let $\rho \in [0, 1]$, we can assume that $v(\mathbf{s}_i, t_i) = \rho \times v(\mathbf{s}_i, t_i - 1) + \eta(\mathbf{s}_i, t_i)$, where $\eta(\mathbf{s}_i, t_i)$ is a second GP that is independent across time points. Alternatively, one might consider modeling spatial-temporal data as time-series data with spatial dependence; for example, see Szpiro et al. (2010) and Lindström et al. (2014).

## 19.3 Sources of Exposure Measurement Error

The previous section describes regression models for estimating unobserved exposures, exploiting spatial and temporal dependence in the exposure field. Let $\mathbf{X}^*$ denote the estimated exposures that are assigned to health outcomes, in place of the unobserved true exposures $\mathbf{X}$. Here we define $\mathbf{X}^*$ as the conditional mean $E[\mathbf{X}|\mathbf{W}_o, \widehat{\boldsymbol{\Omega}}]$ given observed measurements $\mathbf{W}_o$ and point estimate $\widehat{\boldsymbol{\Omega}}$, which can correspond to the maximum likelihood estimate or the posterior mean under Bayesian inference. In a two-stage analysis, $\mathbf{X}^*$ is used as a covariate in the health model. This section describes the various potential sources of error in using $\mathbf{X}^*$ and their impacts on estimating health effect associations.

### 19.3.1 Errors from Exposure Modeling

Error arising from the exposure modeling is captured in the difference between $\mathbf{X}^*$ and the true exposure $\mathbf{X}$. Following the framework of Szpiro et al. (2011a) and Szpiro and Paciorek (2013), the exposure error can be decomposed as

$$\begin{aligned} \mathbf{X} - \mathbf{X}^* &= (\,\mathbf{X} - E[\mathbf{X}|\mathbf{W}_o, \boldsymbol{\Omega}]\,) + (\,E[\mathbf{X}|\mathbf{W}_o, \boldsymbol{\Omega}] - E[\mathbf{X}|\mathbf{W}_o, \widehat{\boldsymbol{\Omega}}]\,) \\ &= \mathbf{U}_b + \mathbf{U}_c\,. \end{aligned} \tag{19.8}$$

The first component $\mathbf{U}_b$ represents error due to *smoothing* induced by the exposure regression model, assuming the exposure model is correct with known $\boldsymbol{\Omega}$. Smoothing error occurs because $E[\mathbf{X}|\mathbf{W}_o, \boldsymbol{\Omega}]$ does not account for the variability associated with the full distribution $[\mathbf{X}|\mathbf{W}_o, \boldsymbol{\Omega}]$. Conditional on known exposure model parameters $\boldsymbol{\Omega}$, $\mathbf{U}_b$ is unbiased. Hence, $\mathbf{U}_b$ is often interpreted as *Berkson-like*. The second error component $\mathbf{U}_c$ in Equation (19.8) describes error due to estimation uncertainty in the exposure model (i.e., $\widehat{\boldsymbol{\Omega}}$ versus $\Omega$). Sampling variability in $\mathbf{W}_o$ results in variability in $E[\mathbf{X}|\mathbf{W}_o, \widehat{\boldsymbol{\Omega}}]$; hence this error component can be viewed as *Classical-like*.

To examine impacts of these exposure error components on health effect estimation, consider the following simple true health model:

$$\mathbf{Y} = \beta_0 \mathbf{1} + \beta_X \mathbf{X} + \mathbf{e},$$

where $\mathbf{Y}$ is the vector of health outcomes with corresponding vector of estimated exposures $\mathbf{X}$, $\mathbf{1}$ is a vector of ones representing the intercept, $\beta_X$ is the parameter of interest, and $\mathbf{e} \sim N(\mathbf{0}, \sigma_e^2 \mathbf{I})$. If we assume $\mathbf{U}_c = \mathbf{0}$, using the plug-in estimator gives

$$\begin{aligned} \mathbf{Y} &= \beta_0 \mathbf{1} + \beta_X \mathbf{X} + \mathbf{e} \\ &= \beta_0 \mathbf{1} + \beta_X (\mathbf{X}^* + \mathbf{U}_b) + \mathbf{e} \\ &= \beta_0 \mathbf{1} + \beta_X \mathbf{X}^* + \mathbf{e}^* \end{aligned}$$

where $\mathbf{e}^* \sim N\left(\mathbf{0}, \beta_X^2 \mathbf{V} + \sigma_e^2 \mathbf{I}\right)$ and $\mathbf{V} = \mathbf{\Sigma}_{22} - \mathbf{\Sigma}_{21}(\mathbf{\Sigma}_{11} + \sigma_\epsilon^2 \mathbf{I}_n)^{-1}\mathbf{\Sigma}_{12}$. While the error induced by spatial smoothing alone does not result in bias, the residual error becomes larger, spatially correlated, and nonhomoscedastic, resulting in a reduction in precision and incorrect inference. Simulation studies by Lopiano et al. (2013) show that when $\mathbf{V}$ is assumed known, the least-square estimate $\widehat{\beta}_X$ is unbiased. However, the standard error of $\widehat{\beta}_X$ is under-estimated, especially when there is a small number of locations with measurements, or the sample size of $\mathbf{Y}$ is large.

Alexeef et al. (2016) examined the bias in the least-square estimate $\widehat{\beta}_X$ due to the classical measurement error component $\mathbf{U}_c$ using a second-order Taylor's expansion. With the error-prone interpolated exposure $\mathbf{X}^*$, $\widehat{\beta}_X$ is asymptotically unbiased if $E[\widehat{\mathbf{\Omega}} - \mathbf{\Omega}] \to \mathbf{0}$ as the number of monitors $n \to \infty$. Because $\widehat{\beta}_X$ is not a linear function of the spatial parameters, even if $\widehat{\mathbf{\Omega}}$ is unbiased, some attenuation will be present. Simulation studies by Alexeef et al. (2016), Gryparis et al. (2009), and Szpiro et al. (2011a) have shown that attenuation is stronger when the number of monitors is smaller and the true exposure surface $\mathbf{X}$ is more heterogeneous, corresponding to situations where estimating $\mathbf{\Omega}$ is more difficult.

In the penalized regression model framework using the minimizer in Equation (19.7), Bergen and Szpiro (2015) presented a related decomposition of the exposure measurement error:

$$\begin{aligned} \mathbf{X} - \mathbf{X}^* &= (\mathbf{X} - E[\mathbf{X}|\mathbf{W}_o, \mathbf{\Omega}_\lambda]) + (E[\mathbf{X}|\mathbf{W}_o, \mathbf{\Omega}_\lambda] - E[\mathbf{X}|\mathbf{W}_o, \widehat{\mathbf{\Omega}}_\lambda]) \quad (19.9) \\ &\equiv \mathbf{U}_{\lambda b} + \mathbf{U}_{\lambda c}. \end{aligned}$$

Here, $\mathbf{\Omega}_\lambda$ are the optimal model parameters from calculating Equation (19.7) with infinite number of monitoring locations ($\widehat{\mathbf{\Omega}} - \mathbf{\Omega}$ as $n \to \infty$). However, unlike $\mathbf{U}_b$, the expected value of $\mathbf{U}_{\lambda b}$ is non-zero due to the difference between $\mathbf{\Omega}_\lambda$ and $\mathbf{\Omega}$ arising from the penalization. Bergen and Szpiro (2015) and Bergen et al. (2016) showed that $\mathbf{U}_{\lambda b}$ can yield bias in the health effect estimates in this setting and presented analytic approaches that are based on asymptotic results to correct for it.

### 19.3.2 Errors from Areal Exposure Averages

Ideally, for each observed health outcome $Y(\mathbf{s}_i)$, we can assign a corresponding exposure estimate $X^*(\mathbf{s}_i)$ using the exposure model. However, sometimes the spatial information of the participant may only be available at coarser spatial resolutions. For example, during the process of geocoding a participant's residential address, we may only be able to identify the geographical administrative unit (e.g., postal/ZIP code or census units), instead of the longitude-latitude coordinate. Reasons for this type of spatial uncertainty can arise because of incomplete addresses, errors in reporting, or confidentiality issues.

Let $B_i$ denote the spatial unit or block to which the health data is georeferenced. Because the exposure model provides predictions at point-level, one common exposure assessment approach is to define exposure as the block-average:

$$X(B_i) = |B_i|^{-1} \int_{\mathbf{s} \in B_i} X(\mathbf{s})\, d\mathbf{s}, \tag{19.10}$$

where $|B_i|$ is the area of $B_i$. This average can be weighted by a spatial density to obtain, for example, a population-weighted average. The need to "upscale" the exposure estimate to the areal-level in order to match the health outcome is an example of the *change-of-support* problem (Gelfand et al., 2001).

The integral in (19.10) is typically evaluated by overlaying a fine grid of prediction locations in $B_i$. Let $\{\mathbf{s}_1, \ldots \mathbf{s}_K\}$ be a set of $K$ grid points in $B_i$. The plug-in estimator of $X(B_i)$ is

$$X^*(B_i) = K^{-1} \sum_{k=1}^{K} X^*(\mathbf{s}_k)\ .$$

From the conditional distribution of $\mathbf{X}|\mathbf{W}_0$ given in (19.6), we have

$$E[X^*(B_i)] = K^{-1} \sum_{k=1}^{K} \mu^*(\mathbf{s}_k) \quad \text{and} \quad \text{Var}\,[X^*(B_i)] = K^{-2} \sum_{k=1}^{K} \sum_{k'=1}^{K} \mathbf{V}^*_{[k,k']}, \tag{19.11}$$

where $\mu^*(\mathbf{s}_k)$ is the conditional mean $E[\mathbf{X}(\mathbf{s}_k)|\mathbf{W}_0, \widehat{\boldsymbol{\Omega}}]$ at grid point $\mathbf{s}_k$ and $\mathbf{V}^*_{[k,k']}$ is the covariance of $\mathbf{X}|\mathbf{W}_0, \widehat{\boldsymbol{\Omega}}$ between grid points $\mathbf{s}_k$ and $\mathbf{s}'_k$. Note that the exposure estimate variance uses the covariance matrix $\mathbf{V}^*$, which is not diagonal and has unequal diagonal elements. This reflects the locations of monitoring measurements in relation to the area being estimated. Spatial correlation between blocks can also be derived similarly using $\mathbf{V}^*$. The effect of upscaling point-level estimates to areal averages to health effect estimation is only recently receiving attention in a measurement error context (Keller and Peng, 2019). Heuristically, point-level exposure should be more variable than the areal average, resulting in Berkson-type measurement error in the areal average.

The use of areal exposures also arises in the setting of acute environmental exposures where health outcomes are aggregated counts. Let $Y_t$ denote the total count of an adverse health outcome (e.g., death) on day $t$ over a geographical area. A basic time-series model without confounders is given by

$$\log E[\,Y_t\,] = \beta_0 + \beta_X X_t\,. \tag{19.12}$$

The main source of potential exposure measurement error here is the need to assign an exposure $X_t$ for the area. Most studies have used measurements from monitors located in the area by defining $X_t$ as the measurement at the most central location or the average of measurements when multiple monitors are present. However, when the exposure field is heterogeneous, exposure measurement error may be present when there is insufficient monitoring locations. Simulation studies by Shaddick et al. (2013) and Sheppard et al. (2005) have shown that this measurement error can lead to bias (not necessarily attenuation) and increased variability.

To better elucidate challenges associated with modeling aggregated health outcomes, we follow the framework of ecologic bias (Wakefield and Salway, 2001). First, consider the following risk model of a binary disease outcome for any individual $i$ among a total of $N$ at-risk individuals on day $t$:

$$Y_{it} \sim \text{Binomial}\ (p_{it}) \quad \text{and} \quad p_{it} = \lambda_0 \exp\{\beta_X X_{it}(\mathbf{s}_i)\}\,,$$

where $p_{it}$ is the probability of the event and $\lambda_0$ is a common baseline risk shared among all individuals. Assuming outcomes are independent (e.g., after controlling for other covariates in the model), the log-linear model for counts $Y_t = \sum_{i=1}^N Y_{it}$ entails a mean structure given by

$$\log E[Y_t] = \log\left(\sum_{i=1}^{N} \lambda_0 \exp\{\beta_X X_{it}(\mathbf{s}_i)\}\right)\,.$$

Hence, the coefficient $\beta_X$ estimated in model (19.12) will not be the same as $\beta_X$ on the individual-level. This bias due to aggregation and the logarithmic link function is known as *pure specification bias.* However, if $\beta_X$ is small (typical of acute environmental health exposures), we can approximate the exponential term linearly:

$$\begin{aligned}\log E[Y_t] &\approx \log\left(\sum_{i=1}^{N}\lambda_0[1+\beta_X X_{it}(\mathbf{s}_i)]\right)\\ &= \log\lambda_0 N + \log\left(1+\beta_X\sum_{i=1}^{N}X_{it}(\mathbf{s}_i)/N\right)\\ &\approx \log\lambda_0 N + \beta_X\sum_{i=1}^{N}X_{it}(\mathbf{s}_i)/N\,.\end{aligned}$$

The above implies that to estimate the individual-level risk association $\beta_X$, the target exposure $X_t$ is the average of all individuals' exposures (population-averaged). Second-order approximation will further highlight how the variance of $X_{it}(\mathbf{s}_i)$ impacts aggregation bias (Richardson et al., 1987).

## 19.4 Methods to Account for Exposure Measurement Error

The main goals of applying methods to account for exposure measurement error are to provide more valid uncertainty measures and reduce bias in the health association estimate. We again focus on methods developed for two-stage analysis, where exposures are often derived from a spatial-temporal model to address misalignment between health outcomes and available exposure measurements. In applications where data from validation studies are available, approaches (e.g., regression calibration) discussed in other chapters can be utilized. We refer readers to a few references here in air pollution epidemiology: Dominici et al. (2000), Van Roosbroeck et al. (2008), and Liao et al. (2018). While the previous section details various components of exposure measurement error (i.e., Berkson versus classical) and is useful to conceptually evaluate impacts of measurement error, methods reviewed below generally aim to address them jointly.

### 19.4.1 Parametric Bootstrap

Szpiro et al. (2011a) proposed a parametric bootstrap approach with the following algorithm. First, carry out the entire two-stage analysis and obtain estimates $\widehat{\mathbf{\Omega}}$ and $\widehat{\beta}_X$. The $l$-th bootstrap sample is obtained by the following steps.

1. Simulate $\mathbf{W}_o^{(l)}$ and $\mathbf{X}^{(l)}$ from the joint distribution $[\mathbf{W}_o^{(l)}, \mathbf{X}^{(l)} \mid \widehat{\mathbf{\Omega}}]$.

2. Simulate $\mathbf{Y}^{(l)}$ from $[\mathbf{Y}|\mathbf{X}^{(l)}, \widehat{\beta}_X]$.
3. Conduct the two-stage analysis with $\mathbf{Y}^{(l)}$ and $\mathbf{W}_o^{(l)}$ to obtain $\beta_X^{(l)}$.

The empirical distribution of $\beta_X^{(l)}$ can then be used to bias-corrected the estimate $\widehat{\beta}_X$ and estimate its standard error. In essence, the bootstrap approach uses variability in realizations of both $\mathbf{W}_o$ and $\mathbf{Y}$ to assess variability associated with model parameter estimation and spatial interpolation. If the number of measurements is large, computation can become burdensome because the spatial exposure model needs to be fitted for every bootstrap iteration. Szpiro et al. (2011a) also described a *parameter bootstrap* approach where in Step 3, instead of fitting the exposure model again, $\mathbf{\Omega}^{(l)}$ is drawn from the asymptotic distribution of $\widehat{\mathbf{\Omega}}$.

### 19.4.2 Non-Parametric Bootstrap

An alternative modeling framework for long-term exposure concentrations is to consider the monitor and subject locations as the source of variability in repeated samples of the experiment (Szpiro and Paciorek, 2013). This contrasts with the typical kriging formulation that considers monitor and subject locations fixed, with variation arising from different realizations of a GP. The practical impact of this framework is that the bootstrap correction involves re-sampling monitor and subject locations, instead of simulating new values of $\mathbf{W}_o$ and $\mathbf{Y}$ (Keller et al., 2017a; Keller and Peng, 2019; Szpiro and Paciorek, 2013). Let $n$ and $N$ denote the number of monitor and subject locations, respectively. The non-parametric bootstrap procedure is:

1. Sample, with replacement, a set of $n$ monitor locations, including the measurement $\mathbf{W}_o$ and predictor variables $\mathbf{Z}_o$.
2. Sample, with replacement, a set of $N$ subjects, including their location, health outcome, and any associated confounder measurements.
3. Conduct the two-stage analysis with the resampled subjects and monitors to obtain $\beta_X^{(l)}$.

Inference then proceeds using the empirical distribution of $\beta_X^{(l)}$ in the same manner as the parametric bootstrap.

In the penalized regression framework, Bergen and Szpiro (2015) and Bergen et al. (2016) presented analytic bias corrections that can be combined with this non-parametric bootstrap in a complete paradigm for exposure measurement error correction. However, the analytic corrections they presented are limited to linear health models and do not apply to generalized linear model settings.

### 19.4.3 Simulation Extrapolation

Alexeef et al. (2016) proposed a simulation extrapolation (SIMEX) approach for the spatial exposure setting. Let $[\lambda_1, \ldots, \lambda_P]^{\mathrm{T}}$ be an increasing sequence of non-negative numbers starting with $\lambda_1 = 0$. In the *simulation* step, pseudo-exposure datasets are generated by adding spatially correlated errors to the estimated exposures. Specifically, for each $l$-th sample ($l = 1, \ldots, L$) given a $\lambda$ value, simulate

$$\widehat{\mathbf{X}}^{(l)}(\lambda_p) \sim N(\widehat{\mathbf{X}}, (1 + \lambda_p)\boldsymbol{\Sigma}_{\mathrm{U}}\,),$$

where $\boldsymbol{\Sigma}_{\mathrm{U}}$ is a known covariance matrix approximated by out-of-sample cross-validation experiments and $\widehat{\mathbf{X}}$ corresponds to the exposure model estimated for health analysis. To estimate $\boldsymbol{\Sigma}_{\mathrm{U}}$, residuals are first calculated between held-out observations and predictions from the exposure model fitted using training observations. Then a spatial model is used to estimate the spatial covariance structure of the error. The simulated pseudo-exposures $\widehat{\mathbf{X}}^{(l)}(\lambda_p)$ are then used to fit the health model and obtain $\beta_X^{(l)}(\lambda_p)$.

In the *extrapolation step*, a linear or quadratic function is estimated between $\widehat{\beta}_X(\lambda_p)$ and $\lambda_p$, where $\widehat{\beta}_X(\lambda_p)$ is the average of $\beta_X^{(l)}(\lambda_p)$ across $L$ simulations. The point estimate of the measurement error-corrected health effect is obtained by setting $\lambda = -1$. Finally, standard error is calculated using bootstrap where measurements $\mathbf{W}_o$ is sampled with replacement and the entire SIMEX procedure is conducted for each bootstrap iteration. One important advantage of SIMEX is that $\boldsymbol{\Sigma}_{\mathrm{U}}$ includes error that may be due to exposure model mis-specification, in additional to smoothing and parameter estimation.

### 19.4.4 Bayesian Approaches

For Bayesian approaches, inference is made on the marginal posterior distribution $[\beta_X|\mathbf{Y}, \mathbf{W}_o]$ that accounts for (i.e., integrates out) uncertainties associated with $\boldsymbol{\Omega}$ and $\mathbf{X}$. In a two-stage analysis, given prior distribution $[\boldsymbol{\Omega}]$, the posterior predictive distribution of the exposures is given by

$$\begin{aligned}[\mathbf{X}^* \mid \mathbf{W}_o\,] &= \int [\mathbf{X}^*, \mathbf{X}, \boldsymbol{\Omega}|\, \mathbf{W}_o]\, d\boldsymbol{\Omega}\, d\mathbf{X} \\ &= \int [\mathbf{X}^* \mid \mathbf{X}, \mathbf{W}_o]\ \times [\mathbf{X}, \boldsymbol{\Omega} \mid \mathbf{W}_o\,]\, d\boldsymbol{\Omega}\, d\mathbf{X},\end{aligned}$$

where

$$[\mathbf{X}, \boldsymbol{\Omega} \mid \mathbf{W}_o\,] \propto [\,\mathbf{X} \mid \boldsymbol{\Omega}, \mathbf{W}_o\,] \times [\,\mathbf{W}_o \mid \boldsymbol{\Omega}\,] \times [\boldsymbol{\Omega}].$$

The above also assumes that $[\mathbf{X}^* \mid \mathbf{X}, \mathbf{W}_o, \boldsymbol{\Omega}] = [\mathbf{X}^* \mid \mathbf{X}, \mathbf{W}_o]$, i.e., parameters in the exposure model have no influence on $\mathbf{X}^*$ conditioned on the observed ($\mathbf{W}_0$) and interpolated ($\mathbf{X}$) exposure data. Note that $[\mathbf{X}^* \mid \mathbf{X}]$ is often a deterministic function, for example the conditional mean of $[\mathbf{X} \mid \boldsymbol{\Omega}, \mathbf{W}_o]$ or the population-weighted average exposure for aggregated health outcomes.

In the second-stage, the posterior predictive distribution of the exposure is treated as a prior distribution in fitting the health model:

$$[\beta_X, \mathbf{X}^* \mid \mathbf{Y}, \mathbf{W}_o] \propto [\,\mathbf{Y} \mid \mathbf{X}^*, \beta_X\,] \times [\,\mathbf{X}^* \mid \mathbf{W}_o\,],$$

and finally,

$$[\,\beta_X | \mathbf{Y}, \mathbf{W}_o] = \int [\beta_X, \mathbf{X}^* \mid \mathbf{Y}, \mathbf{W}_o]\, d\mathbf{X}\,.$$

First note that in this setup the health outcome $\mathbf{Y}$ is also used to inform exposure $\mathbf{X}$. This draws similarity to an imputation-like approach where multiple imputations of $\mathbf{X}$ needs to be conditioned on $\mathbf{Y}$. However, this differs from a fully-Bayesian joint analysis because estimation of $\boldsymbol{\Omega}$ does not depend on $\mathbf{Y}$. In practice, Markov chain Monte Carlo techniques are used to simulate samples from the joint posterior distribution and perform marginal inference. The use of posterior samples from the exposure model facilitates straightforward calculations of $[\mathbf{X}^* \mid \mathbf{X}]$. Hence, this approach is typically adopted when summary exposure metrics are needed, as in the case when health outcomes are aggregated in time-series analysis. For examples, see Peng et al. (2010), Chang et al. (2011), and Lee et al. (2017).

## 19.5 Additional Issues

The goal of this section is to highlight several additional challenges relevant to environmental epidemiologic research. These topics also represent active areas of research in estimating environmental exposures and linking them to health outcomes.

### 19.5.1 Estimating Personal Exposures

Environmental measurements, especially those from monitoring networks, often do not reflect an individual's *personal* exposure. For example, air pollution studies routinely use measurements from outdoor stationary monitors, while humans are mobile and spend the majority of their times indoor. Even though quantifying health associations with outdoor levels can provide important information for regulatory purposes, focusing on personal exposures may help further identify vulnerable sub-populations and methods to reduce exposure on the individual-level. Previous studies in air pollution have generally found larger health effect estimates when using personal exposures on a per unit increase scale; however, it is important to note that often the exposure variability is different between the two different exposure definitions.

Because continual monitoring of personal exposure is infeasible in most population-based environmental health studies, additional data sources are needed to account for discrepancies between personal exposures and measurements taken by the study. Data may come from panel studies where personal exposures are characterized among a small number of participants. Then by treating personal exposures as the gold standard, measurement error methods can be applied (Huang et al., 2018; Kioumourtzoglou et al., 2014b). Another approach of increasing interest in the area of exposure science is to use stochastic simulations to better characterize the *distribution* of personal exposures in a population. Here we briefly describe the Stochastic Human Exposure and Dose Simulation (SHEDS) model developed by the US Environmental Protection Agency to estimate human exposure to air pollution and other chemicals (Burke et al., 2001).

Let $X_i(\mathbf{s}, t)$ denote the personal exposure to air pollution for individual $i$ on day $t$ at location $\mathbf{s}$. Also let $C_{ik}(\mathbf{s}, t)$ and $T_{ikh}(\mathbf{s}, t)$ denote the outdoor concentration and time spent in environment $k$ during hour $h$. Example environments include outdoor, home, office, school, store, restaurant, bar, and in-vehicle. Daily personal exposure is then calculated by averaging time-weighted exposure to outdoor concentration in $K$ environments across a 24-hour period:

$$X_i(\mathbf{s}, t) = \sum_{k=1}^{K} \sum_{h=1}^{24} b_k(\mathbf{s}) C_{ik}(\mathbf{s}, t) T_{ikh}(\mathbf{s}, t),$$

where $b_k(\mathbf{s})$ determines how much outdoor concentration the individual is exposed to in different microenvironments. For example, $b_k(\mathbf{s}) = 1$ for the outdoor microenvironment and $b_k(\mathbf{s}) < 1$ for the home microenvironment. Note that $b_k(\mathbf{s})$ is spatially-varying because indoor exposure from outdoor sources depends on building type that have different pollutant penetration and deposition rates. SHEDS simulates a distribution of $X_i(\mathbf{s}, t)$ by (1) assigning probabilistic distribution to each $b_k(\mathbf{s})$ based on state-of-the-art exposure science knowledge and (2) sampling daily time-activity patterns, i.e., $T_{ikh}(\mathbf{s}, t)$, from a database that match some characteristics of individual $i$, e.g., age, sex, and occupation. The distribution of simulated $X_i(\mathbf{s}, t)$ can then be used to estimate health effects; for example, see Shaddick et al. (2008), Calder et al. (2008), Berrocal et al. (2011), and Chang et al. (2012).

### 19.5.2 Model Selection for Exposure Estimation

As described in Section 19.2, statistical models for estimating environmental exposures are complex because of spatial-temporal dependence and the large number of candidate predictors. Model selection is typically based on predictive performance evaluated in cross-validation experiments using metrics such as $R^2$, mean squared error, and prediction interval coverage probability. However, this approach does not take into consideration that predictions from the exposure model will ultimately be used in health effect estimation. Szpiro et al. (2011b) described a simulation study where using the true exposure model actually results in poorer health effect estimate when compared to a mis-specified exposure model with fewer predictors and a smaller $R^2$ value. This result can be explained under an exposure measurement error framework. Specifically, the inclusion of a larger set of predictors can lead to larger uncertainty in parameter estimation, which translates to larger amount of classical-type measurement error in subsequent predictions. This issue motivates the work of Bergen and Szpiro (2015) that selects the exposure model by minimizing the mean squared error of the health effect estimate. Szpiro and Paciorek (2013) further discussed the impact of the *spatial compatibility* between the distribution of monitor and subject locations. Large deviations between these spatial distributions can lead to additional measurement error in the estimated health effect coefficients. This problem is closely related to *preferential sampling* of monitor locations near areas of high concentration, which can further impact inference (Antonelli et al., 2016; Lee et al., 2015). These challenges motivate the use of spatial restriction, in which health analyses are limited to areas near a monitor, even when exposure predictions are available for a larger domain (Keller and Peng, 2019). Additionally, unmeasured confounders with spatial or spatiotemporal structures can bias health effect estimates (Keller and Szpiro, 2020)

A related problem in selecting covariates for the exposure model is whether confounders for the health model should be considered as predictors. For example, often meteorological variables are excellent predictors of environmental exposures; but they are also causally related to the health outcome. While meteorological variables improve prediction by explaining additional variations in the exposure, this variation is then removed in estimating health associations when the same meteorological variables are included in the health model. Hence, the use of meteorological variables in the exposure model not only does not contribute to estimating exposure effects, but they also potentially incur uncertainty due to estimation. In practice, sets of potential covariates for predicting exposures and controlling for residual confounding in the health model are likely to overlap. Cefalu and Dominici (2014) provided an analysis that focuses on impacts of different model mis-specifications on health effect estimation when the exposure and health models share similar covariates.

### 19.5.3 Multipollutant Exposures

Humans are exposed to a diverse mixture of environmental pollutants simultaneously. There is increasing interest in understanding health effects of the mixture as a whole, identifying constituents that may be driving etiologic associations, and assessing complex nonlinear interactions between constituents. Multipollutant exposure models need to account for correlated pollutants due to their common sources, fate, and transport. Other analytic challenges include that pollutants can be measured with different spatial-temporal availability and are subject to different levels of instrumental error and limits of detection. Developing separate exposure models for each pollutant can be feasible when the number of pollutants is relatively small, while multivariate kriging and regression models can directly account for the correlation between pollutants.

One particular concern is *effect transfer* (Zeger et al., 2000; Zidek et al., 1996). This occurs when the causal pollutant is measured with greater error compared to a non-causal pollutant. However, if the non-causal pollutant is correlated with the causal pollutant, it may serve as a proxy and exhibit positive health association. Hence, the causal pollutant will be incorrectly identified, resulting in negative implications for intervention or regulatory strategies. The degree of effect attenuation and/or effect transfer is complex because they depend on both the correlation between pollutants and their errors. In air pollution epidemiology, simulation studies have showed that impacts can very across pollutant pairs (Dionisio et al., 2016).

Previous investigations have focused predominantly on methods with two exposures, which are subject to heterogeneous and *correlated* measurement errors. Examples include Bergen et al. (2016) and Huang et al. (2018) for long-term air pollution exposures and Chang et al. (2011) for short-term air pollution exposures in a time-series analysis. When health effect estimates are available from multiple studies and the measurement error variances are identical across studies, Schwartz and Coull (2003) described a meta-analysis approach to correct for biases.

Another approach to examine mixture is via dimension reduction techniques such as principle component analysis (Jandarov et al., 2017), clustering (Austin et al., 2012; Keller et al., 2017b), factor analysis, or source apportionment. However, most applications of these approaches have ignored the role of measurement error. Source apportionment is a specific type of dimension reduction to infer exposures emitted from different sources by incorporating external source-specific information and constraints. Impacts of measurement errors in source apportionment results are limited (Gass et al., 2015; Kioumourtzoglou et al., 2014a), mainly because uncertainties in source-specific exposure estimates are difficult to quantify.

## 19.6 Concluding Remarks

This chapter has reviewed several analytic issues related to exposure measurement error commonly encountered in environmental health studies. Exposure measurement errors arise mainly from the use of spatially and temporally sparse measurements for estimating exposures and linking them to health outcomes. Various statistical methods have been developed that are motivated by different types of exposures (e.g., long-term versus short-term), study designs, and health endpoints. While the issue of exposure measurement error is well-recognized, methods to account for this source of uncertainty in health effect estimates are not routinely applied in practice. This may be because these methods require advanced computational techniques and there is a lack of user friendly implementations. Moreover, as exposure assessment becomes more advanced with the use of computer model simulations and satellite imagery, exposure modeling and health effect estimation are often conducted by different research groups. Specifically, epidemiologists may utilize publicly available data products where uncertainty metrics are not provided and cannot be ascertained. Finally, the development of new measurement techniques (e.g., low-cost sensors) and more refined hypotheses in health research (e.g., identification of susceptible exposure windows) will continue to require new statistical techniques to ensure results from health studies to be accurate, reliable and reproducible.

## References


Abrahamsen, P. A review of Gaussian random fields and correlation functions. Technical Report 917, Norwegian Computing Center.

Alexeef, S. E., Carroll, R. J., and Coull, B. (2016). Spatial measurement error and correction by spatial SIMEX in linear regression models when using predicted air pollution exposures. *Biostatistics*, 17, 377-389.

Antonelli, J., Cefalu, M., and Bornn, L. (2016). The positive effects of population-based preferential sampling in environmental epidemiology. *Biostatistics*, 17, 764-778.

Austin, E., Coull, B., Thomas, D., and Koutrakis, P. (2012). A framework for identifying distinct multipollutant profiles in air pollution data. *Environment International*, 45, 112-121.

Bergen, S. and Szpiro, A. (2015). Mitigating the impact of measurement error when using penalized regression to model exposure in two-stage air pollution epidemiology studies. *Environmental and Ecological Statistics*, 22, 601-631.

Bergen, S., Sheppard, L., Kaufman, J.D., and Szpiro, A. (2016). Multipollutant measurement error in air pollution epidemiology studies arising from predicting exposures with penalized regression splines. *Journal of the Royal Statistical Socieity, Series C*, 65, 731-753.

Berhane, K., Gauderman, W.J., Stram, D.O., and Thomas, D.C. (2004). Statistical issues in studies of long-term effects of air pollution: the Southern California Children's Health Study. *Statistical Science*, 19, 414-449.

Berrocal, V.J., Gelfand, A.E., and Holland, D.M. (2010). A spatio-temporal downscaler for output from numerical models. *Journal of Agricultural, Biological, and Environmental Statistics*, 15, 176-197.

Berrocal, V.J., Gelfand, A.E., Holland, D.M., Burke, J., and Miranda, M.L. (2011). On the use of a $PM_{2.5}$ exposure simulator to explain birthweight. *Environmetrics*, 22, 553-571.

Burke, J.M., Zufall, M.J., and Ozkaynak, H. (2001). A population exposure model for particulate matter: case study results for $PM_{2.5}$ in Philadelphia, PA. *Journal of Exposure Analysis and Environmental Epidemiology*, 11, 470-489.

Bhaskaran, K., Gasparrini, A., Hajat, S., Smeeth, L., and Armstrong, B. (2013). Time series regression studies in environmental epidemiology. *International Journal of Epidemiology*, 42, 1187-1195.

Brunsdon, C., Fotheringham, S., and Charlton, M. (1998). Geographically weighted regression - modelling spatial non-stationarity. *Journal of the Royal Statistical Socieity, Series D*, 47, 431-443.

Calder, C.A., Holloman, C.H., Bortnick, S., Strauss, W., and Morara, M. (2008). Relating ambient particulate matter concentration levels to mortality using an exposure simulator. *Journal of the American Statistical Association*, 103, 137-148.

Carracedo-Martnez, E., Taracido, M., Tobias, A., Saez, M., and Figueiras, A. (2010). Case-crossover analysis of air pollution health effects: A systematic review of methodology and application. *Environmental Health Perspectives*, 118, 1173-1182.

Cefalu, M. and Dominici, F. (2014). Does exposure prediction bias health effect estimation? The relationship between confounding adjustment and exposure prediction. *Epidemiology*, 25, 583-590.

Chang, H.H., Peng, P.D., and Dominici, F. (2011). Estimating the acute health effects of coarse particulate matter accounting for exposure measurement error. *Biostatistics*, 12, 637-653.

Chang, H.H., Fuentes, M., and Frey, H.C. (2012). Time series analysis of personal exposure to ambient air pollution and mortality using an exposure simulator. *Journal of Exposure Science and Environmental Epidemiology*, 22, 483-488.

Chang, H.H., Xu, X., and Liu, Y. (2013). Calibrating MODIS aerosol optical depth for predicting daily $PM_{2.5}$ concentrations via statistical downscaling. *Journal of Exposure Science and Environmental Epidemiology*, 24, 398-404.

Clougherty, J.E., Kheirbek, I., Eisl, H.M., Ross, Z., Pezeshki, G., Gorczynski, J.E., Johnson, S., Markowitz, S., Kass, D., and Matte, T. (2013). Intra-urban spatial variability in wintertime street-level concentrations of multiple combustion-related air pollutants: the New York City Community Air Survey (NYCCAS). *Journal of Exposure Science and Environmental Epidemiology*, 23, 232-240.

Cressie, N. and Johannesson, G. (2008). Fixed rank kriging for very large spatial data sets. *Journal of the Royal Statistical Society, Series B*, 70, 209-226.

Dionisio, K.L., Chang, H.H., and Baxter, L.K. (2016). A simulation study to quantify the impacts of exposure measurement error on air pollution health risk estimates in copollutant time-series models. *Environmental Health*, 15, 114.

Dominici, F., Zeger, S.L., and Samet, J.M. (2000). A measurement error model for time-series studies of air pollution and mortality. *Biostatistics*, 1, 157-175.

Gass, K., Balachandran, S., Chang, H.H., Russell, A.G., and Strickland, M.J. (2015). Ensemble-based source apportionment of fine particulate matter and emergency department visits for pediatric asthma. *American Journal of Epidemiology*, 181, 504-512.

Gelfand, A., Zhu, Li., and Carlin, B.P. (2001). On the change of support problem for spatio-temporal data. *Biostatistics*, 13, 31-45.

Gelfand, A.E., Schmidt, A.M., Banerjee, S., and Sirmans, C.F. (2004). Nonstationary multivariate process modeling through spatially varying coregionalization. *Test*, 13, 263-312.

Gneiting, T., Genten, M.G., and Guttorp (2004). Geostatistical space-time models, stationarity, separability, and full symmetry. *In Statistical Methods for Spatio-Temporal Systems*, Finkenstadt, B., Held, L., and Isham, V., (Eds). 151-172.

Gryparis, A., Paciorek, C., Zeka, A., Schwartz, J., and Coull, B.A. (2009). Measurement error caused by spatial misalignment in environmental epidemiology. *Biostatistics*, 10, 258-274.

Huang, G., Lee, D., and Scott, E.M. (2018). Multivariate space-time modelling of multiple air pollutants and their health effects accounting for exposure uncertainty. *Statistics in Medicine*, 7, 1134-1148.

Jandarov, R.A., Sheppard, L.A., Sampson, P.D., and Szpiro, A.A. (2017). A novel principal component analysis for spatially misaligned multivariate air pollution data. *Journal of the Royal Statistical Society, Series C*, 66, 3-28.

Kammann, E.E. and Wand, M. (2003). Geoadditive models. *Journal of the Royal Statistical Society, Series C*, 51, 1-18.

Kioumourtzoglou, M.A., Coull, B.A., Dominici, F., Koutrakis, P., Schwartz, J.D., and Suh, H. (2014a). The impact of source contribution uncertainty on the effects of source specific $PM_{2.5}$ on hospital admissions: a case study in Boston, MA. *Journal of Exposure Science and Environmental Epidemiology*, 24, 365-371.

Kioumourtzoglou, M.A., Spiegelman, D., Szpiro, A.A., Sheppard, L., Kaufman, J.D., Yanosky, J.D., Williams, R., Laden, F., Hong, B., and Suh, H.H. (2014b). Exposure measurement error in $PM_{2.5}$ health effects studies: A pooled analysis of eight personal exposure validation studies. *Environmental Health*, 12, 2.

Keller, J.P., Chang, H.H., Strickland, M.J., and Szpiro, A.A. (2017a). Measurement error correction for predicted spatiotemporal air pollution exposure. *Epidemiology*, 28, 338-345.

Keller, J.P., Drton, M., Larson, T., Kaufman, J.D., Sandler, D.P., and Szpiro, A.A. (2017b). Covariate-adaptive clustering of exposures for air pollution epidemiology cohorts. *Annals of Applied Statistics*, 11, 93-113.

Keller, J.P. and Peng, R.D. (2019). Error in estimating area-level air pollution exposures for epidemiology. *Environmetrics*, 30, e273.

Keller, J.P. and Szpiro, A.A. (2020). Selecting a scale for spatial confounding adjustment. *Journal of the Royal Statistical Society, Series A*, 183, 1121-1143.

Lee, A., Szpiro, A., Kim, S.Y., and Sheppard, L. (2015). Impact of preferential sampling on exposure prediction and health effect inference in the context of air pollution epidemiology. *Environmetrics*, 26, 255-267.

Lee, D., Mukhopadhyay, S., Rushworth, A., and Sahu, S.K. (2017). A rigorous statistical framework for spatio-temporal pollution prediction and estimation of its long-term impact on health. *Biostatistics*, 2017, 370-385.

Liao, X., Zhou, X., Wang, M., Hart, J.E., Laden, F., and Spiegelman, D. (2018). Survival analysis with functions of mismeasured covariate histories: The case of chronic air pollution exposure in relation to mortality in the nurses health study. *Journal of the Royal Statistical Socieity, Series C*, 67, 307-337.

Lindström, J., Szpiro, A.A., Sampson, P.D., Oron, A., Richards, M., Larson, T., and Sheppard, L. (2014). A flexible spatio-temporal model for air pollution with spatial and spatio-temporal covariates. *Environmental and Ecological Statistics*, 21, 411-433.

Lopiano, K.K., Young, L.J., and Gotway, C.A. (2013). Estimated generalized least squares in spatially misaligned regression models with Berkson error. *Biostatistics*, 14, 737-751.

Nychka, D., Bandyopadhyay, S., Hammerling, D., Lindgren, F., and Sain, S. (2015). A multiresolution Gaussian process model for the analysis of large spatial datasets. *Journal of Computational and Graphical Statistics*, 24, 579-599.

Peng, R.D. and Bell, M.L. (2010). Spatial misalignment in time series studies of air pollution and health data. *Biostatistics*, 11, 720-740.

Richardson, S., Stucker, I., and Hemon, D. (1987). Comparison of relative risks obtained in ecological and individual studies: some methodological considerations. *International Journal of Epidemiology*, 16, 111-120.

Ryan, P.H. and LeMasters, G.K. (2007). A review of land-use regression models for characterizing intraurban air pollution exposure. *Inhalation Toxicology*, 19, Suppl 1:127-133.

Schwartz, J. and Coull, B.A. (2003). Control for confounding in the presence of measurement error in hierarchical models. *Biostatistics*, 4, 539-553.

Shaddick, G., Lee, D., Zidek, J.V., and Salway, R. (2008). Estimating exposure response functions using ambient pollution concentrations. *Annals of Applied Statistics*, 2, 1249-1270.

Shaddick, G., Lee, D., and Wakefield, J. (2013). Ecological bias in studies of the short-term effects of air pollution and health. *International Journal of Applied Earth Observation and Geoinformation*, 22, 65-74.

Sheppard, L., Slaughter, J.C., Schildcrout, J., Liu, L.J.S., and Lumley, T. (2005). Exposure and measurement contributions to estimates of acute air pollution effects. *Journal of Exposure Analysis and Environmental Epidemiology*, 15, 366-376.

Szpiro, A.A., Sampson, P.D., Sheppard, L., Lumley, T., Adar, S.D., and Kaufman, J.D. (2010). Predicting intra-urban variation in air pollution concentrations with complex spatio-temporal dependencies. *Environmetrics*, 21, 606-631.

Szpiro, A.A., Sheppard, L., and Lumley, T. (2011a). Efficient measurement error correction with spatially misaligned data. *Biostatistics*, 12, 610-623.

Szpiro, A.A., Paciorek, C.J., and Sheppard, L. (2011b). Does more accurate exposure prediction improve health effect estimates? *Epidemiology*, 22, 680-685.

Szpiro, A.A. and Paciorek, C.J. (2013). Measurement error in two-stage analyses, with application to air pollution epidemiology. *Environmetrics*, 24, 501-517.

Van Roosbroeck, S., Li, R., Hoek, G., Lebret, E., Brunekeef, B., and Spiegelman, D. (2008). Traffic-related outdoor air pollution and respiratory symptoms in children: The impact of adjustment for exposure measurement error. *Epidemiology*, 19, 409-416.

Wakefield, J. and Salway, R. (2001). A statistical framework for ecological and aggregate studies. *Journal of the Royal Statistical Society, Series A*, 164, 119-137.

Wood, S. (2003). Thin plate regression splines. *Journal of the Royal Statistical Socieity, Series B*, 65, 95-114.

Zeger, S.L., Thomas, D., Dominici, F., Samet, J.M., Schwartz, J., Dockery, D., and Cohen, A. (2000). Exposure measurement error in time-series studies of air pollution: concepts and consequences. *Environmental Health Perspectives*, 108, 419-426.

Zidek, J.V., Wong, H., Le, N.D., and Burnett, R. (1996). Causality, measurement error and multicollinearity in epidemiology. *Environmetrics*, 7, 441-451.

# Part VI

# Other Features

# 20

# *Measurement Error as a Missing Data Problem*

**Ruth H. Keogh and Jonathan W. Bartlett**

## CONTENTS



## 20.1 Introduction

Studies with variables measured with error can be considered as studies in which the true variable is missing, for either some or all study participants. This chapter focuses on measurement error in covariates in regression analyses in which the aim is to estimate the association between one or more covariates

DOI: 10.1201/9781315101279-20

and an outcome, adjusting for confounding. Error in covariate measurements, if ignored, results in biased estimates of parameters representing the associations of interest. We make the link between measurement error and missing data and describe methods for correcting this bias. By considering covariate measurement error as a missing data problem, we can take advantage of statistical methods developed for handling missing data. Interest is assumed to be in the regression of an outcome $Y$ on two correlated covariates, $X$ and $Z$, using the generalized linear model

$$g\{E(Y|X,Z)\} = \alpha + \beta_X X + \beta_Z Z. \tag{20.1}$$

We refer to this as the outcome model or substantive model. We shall also consider models for censored failure time outcomes. We consider a cohort of $n$ individuals and the outcome $Y$ is observed without error on the complete cohort. Covariate $X$ is measured with error, and the error prone variable is denoted $X^*$. Covariate $Z$ is measured without error for all individuals. A naive analysis uses $X^*$ in place of $X$, with $X^*$ observed for all individuals:

$$g\{E(Y|X^*,Z)\} = \alpha^* + \beta_X^* X^* + \beta_Z^* Z. \tag{20.2}$$

Estimates of $\beta_X^*$ and $\beta_Z^*$ are not consistent estimates of the parameters of interest, $\beta_X$ and $\beta_Z$. The direction of the bias in these parameter estimates depends on the form of the error in $X^*$, and the relation between $X$ and $Z$. Different forms of error in $X^*$ and their impact on parameter estimates are discussed in the next section.

To make any correction for the impact of measurement error in $X^*$ information is needed about the relationship between $X$ and $X^*$. We consider three types of sub-study within the cohort from which this information can be obtained:

*Validation study:* In a validation study the true value of $X$ is observed for a subset of individuals in the cohort. A validation study permits a wider range of possible error models to be used.

*Replication study:* In a replication study two or more error-prone measures of $X$ are observed for at least a subset of the cohort, and we denote the repeated measures $X_j^*$ $j = 1, \ldots, J$, with all individuals having one measure $X_1^*$. The true value of $X$ is not observed for any individuals in the cohort. A replication study is appropriate if the $X_j^*$ are subject only to independent error such that $E(X_j^*|X) = X$.

*Calibration study:* A calibration study is appropriate if $X^*$, assumed to be observed for all individuals in the cohort, is subject to systematic error, that is $E(X^*|X) \neq X$. As in a replication study, the true value of $X$ is not observed for any individuals in the cohort. In a calibration study, a second error prone measure of $X$, denoted $X^{**}$, which is subject only to mean zero independent error is observed in at least a subset of individuals. In some situations, two

**TABLE 20.1**
Summary of what is observed in different study types.

| Study type | $R_i = 1$ | $R_i = 0$ |
|---|---|---|
| Validation study | $\{Y_i, Z_i, X_i, X_i^*\}$ | $\{Y_i, Z_i, X_i^*\}$ |
| Replication study | $\{Y_i, Z_i, X_{1i}^*, X_{2i}^*\}$ | $\{Y_i, Z_i, X_{1i}^*\}$ |
| Calibration study (i) | $\{Y_i, Z_i, X_i^*, X_i^{**}\}$ | $\{Y_i, Z_i, X_i^*\}$ |
| Calibration study (ii) | $\{Y_i, Z_i, X_i^*, X_{1i}^{**}, X_{2i}^{**}\}$ | $\{Y_i, Z_i, X_i^*\}$ |

or more repeated measures, $X_j^{**}$ $j = 1, \ldots, J$, may be obtained for some individuals.

In a validation, replication and calibration study a subset of the study cohort has more information on the true value $X$, with the form of this information differing in the three study types. We let $R_i = 1$ for individuals with all possible measurements observed and $R_i = 0$ for individuals with a minimal set of measurements. Table 20.1 summarises what is observed for individuals with $R_i = 1$ and $R_i = 0$ in the three study types assuming $J = 2$.

In Section 20.2 we discuss missing data mechanisms and how they relate to the measurement error setting, considering different forms of error. Sections 20.3-20.5 outline methods for measurement error correction using regression calibration, maximum likelihood estimation, and Bayesian analysis. In Section 20.6 we discuss the extension of multiple imputation to the measurement error setting. Section 20.7 compares the properties of the methods, and Section 20.8 presents a comparison of the methods through an application to data from the Third National Health and Nutrition Examination Survey (NHANES), and we conclude with a discussion in Section 20.9

## 20.2 Missing Data and Measurement Error Mechanisms

### 20.2.1 Sources of Missingness

There are two sources of missingness, or coarsening, in our setting. The first is due to the error in the observed covariates, and the second is the selection of only a subset of individuals to the validation, replication or calibration substudy ($R_i = 1$ in Table 20.1). The form and degree of measurement error in the measures $X^*$ (and $X^{**}$ in a calibration study) determines the extent to which the true covariate values are 'missing' or coarsened and hence the degree of potential bias in naive analyses ignoring measurement error. We can view the coarsening due to measurement error as a continuum: if the measurement error is small, the error prone values $X^*$ contain substantial information about $X$, and as the degree of error increases this information is reduced. Missingness due to selection to the sub-study can be considered as regular missing data.

The individuals selected to the sub-study are used to learn about the extent of error in $X^*$ and hence make corrections for it.

When there is a validation study in which $X$ is observed for a subset of individuals, we can consider ourselves to be in a standard missing data setting: the true $X$ is observed for some individuals and missing for others. Though a difference from the standard missing data setting is that we have an observed error-prone exposure measure $X^*$ for all individuals. Such variables are sometimes referred to as *auxiliary variables* in the standard missing data setting.

### 20.2.2 Missing Data and Selection Mechanisms

In the missing data context, the missingness mechanism can be classified as one of three types, as proposed by Rubin (Rubin, 1987). Data are described as missing completely at random (MCAR) when the probability of the true value being observed for a given individual is unrelated to the observed and unobserved data for that individual. In the context of a validation study this can be expressed as $\Pr(R_i = 1|Y_i, X_i, Z_i, X_i^*) = \Pr(R_i = 1)$. Data are missing at random (MAR) when the probability of the true value being observed depends on the fully observed variables and conditional on these, not on the partially observed variable $X$, which can be expressed as $\Pr(R_i = 1|Y_i, X_i, Z_i, X_i^*) = \Pr(R_i = 1|Y_i, Z_i, X_i^*)$. The third possibility is that data are missing not at random (MNAR), meaning that the probability of the true value being observed depends on $X$, even after conditioning on the fully observed variables, so that $\Pr(R_i = 1|Y_i, X_i, Z_i, X_i^*) \neq \Pr(R_i = 1|Y_i, Z_i, X_i^*)$. We refer to Rubin (1987), Carpenter and Kenward (2013) and Seaman et al. (2013) for discussion and definition of missing data mechanisms. In a replication study the missingness mechanism corresponds to the mechanism that determines which subset of subjects has a replicate measure taken, and in a calibration study to the mechanism that determines which subset of subjects has the superior measurement. The MAR assumption therefore corresponds to $\Pr(R_i = 1|Y_i, X_{1i}^*, Z_i, X_{2i}^*) = \Pr(R_i = 1|Y_i, X_{1i}^*, Z_i)$ in a replication study and to $\Pr(R_i = 1|Y_i, X_i^*, Z_i, X_i^{**}) = \Pr(R_i = 1|Y_i, X_i^*, Z_i)$ in a calibration study.

Within the context of regular missing data, the naive analysis approach is a 'complete case' analysis, in which the regression is based on the subset of individuals with no missing data. A major concern is that the probability that a variable is missing is conditionally or unconditionally related to the underlying value of that variable (MAR or MNAR). If this is the case, a complete case analysis may lead to biased inferences. Even if the data are missing completely at random (MCAR) it is usually inefficient to restrict the analysis to the complete case subset, because for individuals with incomplete data, there is often some information about the parameters of interest contained in the incomplete cases' data.

In the case of measurement error, the selection mechanism is typically known because the subset with $R_i = 1$ is chosen by design. The subset is almost always chosen completely at random, although alternative designs have been proposed, for example where those with an extreme first measurement are selected to have a second measurement (Berglund et al., 2007). When, as is usually the case, the selection is completely at random, the missingness process can be ignored for the purposes of inference. This feature renders this aspect of the problem much easier than in the usual case of missing data. If the subset $R_i = 1$ arises in a non-random fashion, attention should be paid to the missing data mechanism. We primarily focus on the MCAR setting.

### 20.2.3 Measurement Error Models

In the case where a validation study is available, unbiased estimates of the parameters in model (20.1) could be obtained by fitting the model within the subset of individuals with $X$ observed ($R = 1$). However, this would be highly inefficient because the size of the validation sample is usually small and methods that make use of all the data should be used. This is not even an option in a replication or calibration study were $X$ is not observed for anyone, and hence other approaches are needed to obtain unbiased estimates of the parameters of interest. For most measurement error correction methods we need to understand the form and degree of the measurement error. In subsequent sections we will discuss several methods with reference to common forms of error.

The simplest form of error is classical random error, such that the observed value is the true value plus independent random error:

$$X_i^* = X_i + U_i. \tag{20.3}$$

where $E(U_i|X_i) = 0$ and the $U_i$ have constant variance $\sigma_U^2$, and are independent of $X$, $Y$ and $Z$. An extension includes systematic error components as well as the random component:

$$X_i^* = \delta_0 + \delta_1 X_i + U_i. \tag{20.4}$$

An assumption often made is that measurement errors are *non-differential*, meaning that the errors and outcome $Y$ are conditionally independent given $X$ and $Z$. A consequence of this assumption is that $E(Y|X, Z, X^*) = E(Y|X, Z)$.

There are many other types of measurement error. These include multiplicative error, in which $X^*$ is equal to $X$ multiplied by a random component, such that the classical error model may hold on the log scale. Some error-prone measures are subject to a threshold effect or to an excess number of zero measures. Under Berkson error the error-prone measures $X^*$ are less variable than the true values $X$, with $X = X^* + U$, $E(U|X^*) = 0$, which raises specific issues for analysis.

In a validation study, the form of the measurement error can be investigated directly because the true values are known for some individuals alongside the error prone values. In contrast, in a replication or calibration study, it is necessary to make assumptions about the form of the error in order to make progress in correcting for it.

## 20.3 Regression Calibration and Conditional Mean Imputation

Regression calibration is the most commonly applied method for measurement error correction (Armstrong, 1985; Shaw et al., 2018). It involves replacing $X$ in the regression model of interest (20.1) with its expectation conditional on the error-prone measure and the fully observed covariates $E(X|X^*, Z)$:

$$g\{E(Y|X^*, Z)\} = \alpha + \beta_X E(X|X^*, Z) + \beta_Z Z. \tag{20.5}$$

In the case of a linear regression model this is justified by the result that

$$\begin{aligned} E(Y|X^*, Z) &= E\{E(Y|X, Z, X^*)|X^*, Z\} \\ &= E\{E(Y|X, Z)|X^*, Z\} \\ &= \alpha + \beta_X E(X|X^*, Z) + \beta_Z Z \end{aligned}$$

which makes the assumption that the measurement error is non-differential $(E(Y|X, Z, X^*) = E(Y|X, Z))$. Regression calibration therefore relies on the assumption of non-differential error. The justification of this method for non-linear outcome models, for example logistic regression, uses approximations (Rosner et al., 1989, 1992). Regression calibration also extends approximately to survival studies (Hughes, 1993).

To apply regression calibration requires estimation of the expectation $E(X|X^*, Z)$. In a validation study the expectation $E(X|X^*, Z)$ can be estimated directly, using a regression of $X$ on $X^*$ and $Z$ using the subset of individuals with $R = 1$. For example, assuming this conditional mean is linear in $X^*$ and $Z$,

$$X = \gamma_0 + \gamma_X^* X^* + \gamma_Z Z + \epsilon, \tag{20.6}$$

giving $\widehat{E}(X|X^*, Z) = \widehat{\gamma}_0 + \widehat{\gamma}_X^* X^* + \widehat{\gamma}_Z Z$. It is inefficient to use $E(X|X^*, Z)$ when $X$ is actually observed, and so in this case $X$ is used when it is observed $(R = 1)$.

In a replication study, and when $X_1^*$ and $X_2^*$ are assumed to be have classical error as defined in (20.3), the unobserved $X$ is replaced by $E(X|X_1^*, Z)$ (or rather an estimate of this). This can be estimated from a linear regression of $X_2^*$ on $X_1^*$ and $Z$ in the $R = 1$ group. A more efficient approach is to replace $X$ in the outcome model by $E(X|X_1^*, Z)$ for those with $R = 0$ and $E(X|X_1^*, X_2^*, Z)$ for those with $R = 1$. These expectations can be in turn be estimated efficiently by fitting a random intercepts model to the data (Bartlett et al., 2009).

In a calibration study, the expectation $E(X|X^*, Z)$ can be estimated from a linear regression of $X^{**}$ on $X^*$ and $Z$ in the $R = 1$ group, under the assumption that $X^{**}$ follows the classical error model and $X^*$ has systematic error of the form in (20.4). As in a replication study, more efficient use of the data could be made by making additional distributional assumptions. Only one measure $X^{**}$ is needed in a subset of individuals to perform regression calibration in a calibration study; other methods, as we will discuss below, require more than one measure $X^{**}$ in a subset of individuals.

Regression calibration can be viewed as a 'conditional mean imputation' approach. For individuals with the true value of $X$ missing, which is *all* individuals in a replication or calibration study, a value is imputed as the estimated conditional mean given $Z$ and the error-prone measurements. In Section 20.6 we contrast this single imputation approach with a multiple imputation approach.

After using $\widehat{E}(X|X^*, Z)$ in place of $X$ in the outcome model, standard errors can be obtained using standard methods. However, these do not take into account the uncertainty in the estimation of $\widehat{E}(X|X^*, Z)$, that is the uncertainty in the estimates of the parameters in the model used to estimate $E(X|X^*, Z)$. In the above example given for a validation study (20.6), this is the parameters $\gamma_0, \gamma_X^*, \gamma_Z$. If this uncertainty is ignored, the confidence intervals for estimate of the parameters in (20.5) will be too narrow and therefore have too-low coverage. This can be resolved in one of two ways. In simple settings with a small number of covariates, such as that focused on in this chapter, a 'delta method' approximation can be made to obtain correct estimated standard error (Rosner et al., 1989). More generally, bootstrapping can be used, in which the regression calibration model (e.g., (20.6)) and the outcome model (20.5) are both fitted within each bootstrap sample.

In more recent work, some authors have extended the use of regression calibration to include additional variables, $V$ say, in the set of predictors so that the focus is on estimating $E(X|X^*, Z, V)$ (Freedman et al., 2011; Prentice et al., 2009). The $V$ should be predictors of $X$ but not independently associated with the outcome. This approach has been applied in nutritional epidemiology, where $X$ represents a true long term average intake of a given nutrient, $X^*$ is a self-reported measure and $V$ denotes a biomarker measure. Thinking of the measurement error in the missing data context, the additional variables $V$ take the role of auxiliary variables.

## 20.4 Maximum Likelihood

In this section we briefly review the likelihood approach to measurement error correction. We refer to Carroll et al. (2006) and Chapter 6 of this Handbook for detailed overviews. In the likelihood approach a joint model for the full data vector must first be specified, with parameter $\omega$. The model is almost always specified conditional on the error-free covariates $Z_i$, to avoid having to model their distribution. In a validation study contributions to the likelihood function are thus of the form $p(Y_i, X_i, X_i^*, R_i = 1|Z_i; \omega)$ and $p(Y_i, X_i^*, R_i = 0|Z_i; \omega)$, with corresponding expressions in the cases of replication or calibration studies. When the selection into the sub-study is MCAR or MAR, there is no need to model the missingness indicator $R_i$.

The observed data likelihood involves integrating over the unobserved $X$ in those portions of the study sample in which $X$ is unobserved. The likelihood in the setting of a validation study is

$$L_V = \prod_{i:R_i=1} p(Y_i, X_i, X_i^*|Z_i; \omega) \prod_{i:R_i=0} \int p(Y_i, X_i^*, X|Z_i; \omega) dX. \tag{20.7}$$

If the measurement error is assumed to be non-differential, so that $p(Y_i|X_i, Z_i, X_i^*) = p(Y_i|X_i, Z_i)$, then the likelihood can be factorised as

$$\begin{aligned} L_V = &\prod_{i:R_i=1} p(Y_i|X_i, Z_i; \beta)p(X_i^*|X_i, Z_i; \delta)p(X_i|Z_i; \gamma) \\ &\times \prod_{i:R_i=0} \int p(Y_i|X, Z_i; \beta)p(X_i^*|X, Z_i; \delta)p(X|Z_i; \gamma)dX. \end{aligned} \tag{20.8}$$

In the above, we have used $\beta$ to denote the parameters of the outcome model, $\delta$ the parameters of the measurement error model ($\delta = \sigma_U^2$ in the case of classical error), and $\gamma$ the parameters describing the distribution of $X$ given $Z$.

Assuming again that error is non-differential, and suppressing dependence on parameters in the notation, in a replication study the observed data likelihood is

$$\begin{aligned} L_R = &\prod_{R_i=1} \int p(Y_i|X, Z_i)p(X_{i1}^*|X, Z_i)p(X_{i2}^*|X, Z_i)p(X|Z_i)dX \\ &\times \prod_{R_i=0} \int p(Y_i|X, Z_i)p(X_{i1}^*|X, Z_i)p(X|Z_i)dX. \end{aligned} \tag{20.9}$$

The likelihood in the case of a calibration study is the same as that of a replication study, except the model and corresponding likelihood component for the first measurement must account for the assumed systematic measurement error.

The integrals in the observed data likelihoods over the unobserved $X$ are generally intractable except for certain special cases. One such special case is where the outcome is continuous and the full data vector is assumed to be multivariate normal, for which in the case of a replication study maximum likelihood estimates can be obtained by fitting an appropriate linear mixed model (Bartlett et al., 2009). More generally, the integrals must be approximated using quadrature or Monte-Carlo methods. The observed data likelihood (or an estimate of it) can then be maximised using gradient type methods. In Stata the gllamm command implements Newton-Raphson with adaptive quadature (Rabe-Hesketh et al. (2004)), and the same can be readily implemented in SAS using PROC NLMIXED. In R and Stata the merlin package provides a flexible approach to this problem (Crowther, 2018)

A natural concern with using fully parametric maximum likelihood is the robustness of inferences to misspecification of various parts of the joint model. To try and mitigate such concerns, a number of authors (Hu et al., 1998; Rabe-Hesketh et al., 2004; Schafer, 2001) have proposed and investigated a semiparametric likelihood approach which avoids specification of a parametric model for $X$ (or the residuals in the $X|Z$ model).

## 20.5 Bayesian Approach

In the Bayesian approach a joint model is chosen as described in the preceding section. To this, prior distributions are added for the model parameters, and inference is based on the implied posterior distributions. Assuming *a priori* independence between the parameters of the sub-models, we can do this by specifying separate priors for each sub-model parameter, i.e. $\beta$, $\delta$, $\gamma$. Bayesian inference is then based on the posterior distribution of the model parameters, which is proportional to the product of the prior and the observed data likelihood. Usually primary interest is in the parameters $\beta$ indexing the outcome model, in which case we would focus on the marginal posterior of $\beta$.

Analogous to the situation with maximum likelihood, the posterior distribution(s) are typically not available in closed form, and so we must resort to numerical methods to obtain estimates of them. In recent decades the most popular approach to this has been Markov Chain Monte Carlo (MCMC) which use Gibbs and/or Metropolis-Hastings sampling. This can be performed readily in software such as BUGS or JAGS.

Several authors have discussed Bayesian analysis for measurement error correction, including Gustafson (2003) and Richardson and Gilks (1993a,b). Chapters 23 and 24 of this handbook provides an overview.

In the last decade there have been a number of developments in terms of improved computational methods for obtaining Bayesian inferences when the posterior is analytically intractable, with direct relevance to measurement error correction. One is the development of Hamiltonian Monte-Carlo (HMC) methods, and its implementation in the software Stan (Carpenter et al., 2017). HMC samplers usually converge to their stationary distribution faster and require less iterations for inference because the autocorrelations within chains tend to be much lower.

A second is inference based on the integrated Laplace approximation (INLA) approach (Muff et al., 2015). The INLA approach numerically approximates the required posteriors by using numerical integration together with Laplace approximations used to approximate the integrands. INLA has been shown to provide accurate and computationally fast estimates of the posteriors for so called latent Gaussian models. The latter includes GLMs with covariates subject to normal measurement errors.

Aside from any philosophical considerations, a practical strength of the Bayesian approach in general, and in the context of measurement error correction in particular, is the ability to bring external knowledge or information in to the analysis, via the specification of the priors.

## 20.6 Multiple Imputation for Measurement Error Correction

Multiple imputation (MI) has become arguably the most popular principled approach for the handling of missing data in practice. It involves generation of multiple imputations for each missing value, resulting in multiple completed datasets. As originally formulated, imputations are generated as independent draws from the posterior distribution of the missing data from an appropriate Bayesian model. The outcome/substantive model of interest (20.1) is then fitted to each completed dataset. Estimates and standard errors from each analysis are then combined as we describe below.

MI can be transferred directly from the traditional missing data setting to the measurement error setting when there is a validation study in which the true exposure $X$ is observed for a subset of individuals. There are, however, two ways in which this measurement error setting differs from the usual missing data setting. First, the proportion of individuals with $X$ unobserved will typically be smaller than the proportion of individuals with fully observed data in the missing data context. Second, all individuals have the error prone value $X^*$ observed. This takes the role of an auxiliary variable in the missing data context. MI can also be used for measurement error correction in the context of a replicates study or a calibration study, though the steps required to obtain the imputations are different from in the missing data context, and software for MI for missing data mostly cannot handle this situation.

The use of MI as a method for measurement error correction was probably first described by Brownstone and Valletta (1996) in an economics context. They wished to correct for the impact of non-random error in measures of individual earnings, when used as a dependent variable in a regression, and had access to validation data. Cole et al. (2006), Freedman et al. (2008) and Keogh and White (2014) focused on MI of covariates in the epidemiological context, and their work is discussed further below. More recently, MI for measurement error correction has been discussed in the sociological literature by Blackwell et al. (2017a,b), who viewed measurement error as partially missing data, and in turn viewed missing data as an extreme form of measurement error. Their approach accommodates both measurement error and missing values, but is restricted by requiring a multivariate normal distribution for the variables with missing values and measurement error.

In this section, we provide an overview of the use of MI for measurement error correction, considering validation, replicate and calibration studies.

### 20.6.1 General Procedure

The general procedure is the same across settings. The aim is to draw values of the true exposure $X$ from its distribution conditional on the error prone measure $X^*$, the outcome $Y$, and any covariates $Z$. Let $p(X|X^*, Z, Y; \theta)$ denote a model for this distribution, parameterized by $\theta$. MI consists of the following steps:

1. Fit the model $p(X|X^*, Z, Y; \theta)$ by maximum likelihood to obtain estimates $\widehat{\theta}$ and a corresponding variance-covariance matrix $\Sigma_\theta$. Then for $m = 1, \ldots, M$:
2. Obtain draws $\theta^{(m)}$ of the parameters from their approximate joint posterior distribution.
3. For each individual $i$ with $X$ unobserved, obtain a draw of $X_i^{(m)}$ from $p(X_i|X_i^*, Z_i, Y_i; \theta^{(m)})$. This gives an imputed data set in which the true exposure is available for all individuals.
4. Fit the substantive model using the imputed $X$ values to obtain estimates $\widehat{\beta}^{(m)} = (\widehat{\alpha}^{(m)}, \widehat{\beta}_X^{(m)}, \widehat{\beta}_Z^{(m)})^T$ and their estimated variance-covariance matrix $\Sigma^{(m)}$.

The estimates $\widehat{\beta}^{(m)}$ and $\Sigma^{(m)}$ $(m = 1, \ldots, M)$ are then combined using Rubin's Rules (Rubin, 1987) to give an overall estimate of $\beta$ and corresponding variance-covariance matrix.

According to Rubin's Rules the pooled estimate is

$$\widehat{\beta} = M^{-1} \sum_{m=1}^{M} \widehat{\beta}^{(m)},$$

and its estimated variance-covariance matrix is

$$\text{var}\,\widehat{\beta} = \mathbf{W} + (1 + M^{-1})\mathbf{B},$$

where $\mathbf{W}$ is the within-imputation variance and $\mathbf{B}$ the between-imputation variance. Rubin's rules should be applied on a scale for which the full data estimator is as close as possible to normal.

Although in principle any model $p(X|X^*, Z, Y; \theta)$ could be used to perform the imputation, potentially serious bias could arise in the estimates of $\beta$ and their variance-covariance matrix if the imputation model is mis-specified. In particular, the imputation model should be compatible with the substantive model that is used for the analysis, i.e. model (20.1), which is assumed to be correctly specified (Meng, 1994). When the substantive model is a normal linear regression with linear effects of $X$, a conditional normal model for $p(X|X^*, Z, Y; \theta)$ meets the compatibility requirement. This also holds when the substantive model is a logistic regression. However, if the substantive model is a more complex model, such as a Cox regression, then standard parametric imputation models are not strictly compatible (Bartlett et al., 2015). Issues of compatibility also arise in general if the substantive model includes non-linear terms in $X$, including interaction terms.

### 20.6.2 Validation Study

As noted above, MI can be transferred directly from the traditional missing data setting to the measurement error setting when there is a validation study, with the error-prone variable $X^*$ treated as an auxiliary variable. MI for measurement error correction in covariates was described by Cole et al. (2006), who focused on a validation study, though this was only made explicit in a commentary by White (2006). Cole et al. (2006) describe their method in the context of a single misclassified binary variable and where the substantive model is Cox regression. They suggested an imputation model which is a logistic regression of $X$ on $X^*$, $D$ (the binary event indicator) and $\log T$ (where $T$ denotes the smaller of the event and censoring time). This model can be fitted within the validation study. The remainder of their MI procedure is as described above. Subsequent work in the missing data context showed that an approximately compatible imputation model would be a logistic regression of $X$ on $X^*$, $D$ and $\widehat{H}(T)$, the Nelson-Aalen estimate of the cumulative hazard (White and Royston, 2009). For continuous $X$, the logistic regression is replaced by a linear regression. The substantive model compatible method of Bartlett et al. (2015) can also be used directly.

MI using standard software in the validation setting can be used to impute $X$ using a model for $p(X|X^*, Z, Y; \theta)$, which allows for the measurement error to be differential. To utilise the non-differential error assumption the substantive model compatible approach can be adopted, whereby $X^*$ is used as an auxiliary variable to impute $X$ but is not included in the outcome/substantive model.

### 20.6.3 Replicates and Calibration Studies

MI for measurement error correction in the context of a replicates study was described by Keogh and White (2014). In a replicates study we do not observe the true exposure $X$ for any individuals, and so the imputation model $p(X|X^*, Z, Y; \theta)$ must be fitted indirectly. This requires repeated measures (e.g. $X_1^*, X_2^*$) and some additional distributional assumptions. We assume a multivariate normal distribution for $(X, X_1^*, X_2^*)$ conditional on $Z$ and $Y$. This enables us to derive the implied model $p(X|X_1^*, X_2^*, Y, Z; \theta)$, required for step 1 of the general imputation procedure. Repeated measures are needed on a subset of individuals to identify the variance of the errors $U_i$ in the classical error model $X_{ij}^* = X + U_{ij}$ $(j = 1, 2)$. In step 3, for individuals in the sub-study with the replicate measure $X_2^*$ observed $(R_i = 1)$, a draw $X_i^{(m)}$ is taken from $p(X|X_1^*, X_2^*, Y, Z; \theta^{(m)})$, while for individuals with only $X_1^*$ observed $(R_i = 0)$, a draw is taken from $p(X|X_1^*, Y, Z; \theta^{(m)})$.

Under the classical error model for $X_1^*$ and $X_2^*$ and the multivariate distribution for $(X, X_1^*, X_2^*)$ conditional on $Z$ and $Y$ it can be shown that $X|X_1^*, X_2^*, Z, Y$ is normally distributed with mean and variance:

$$E(X|X_1^*, X_2^*, Z, Y) = E(X|Y, Z) + (X_1^* + X_2^* - 2E(X|Y, Z)) \frac{2\text{var}(X|Y, Z)}{\text{var}(X|Y, Z) + \sigma_U^2} \tag{20.10}$$

$$\text{var}(X|X_1^*, X_2^*, Z, Y) = \frac{\text{var}(X|Y, Z)}{2\text{var}(X|Y, Z) + \sigma_U^2}. \tag{20.11}$$

Similarly it can be shown that $X|X_1^*, Z, Y$ is normally distributed with mean and variance:

$$E(X|X_1^*, Z, Y) = E(X|Y, Z) + (X_1^* - E(X|Y, Z)) \frac{\text{var}(X|Y, Z)}{\text{var}(X|Y, Z) + \sigma_U^2} \tag{20.12}$$

$$\text{var}(X|X_1^*, Z, Y) = \frac{\text{var}(X|Y, Z)}{\text{var}(X|Y, Z) + \sigma_U^2}. \tag{20.13}$$

After the paper of Cole et al. (2006), the idea of using MI for measurement error correction was taken up again in 2008 by Freedman et al. (2008), though they referred to their method as *stochastic imputation*. Their focus was on the calibration study setting in which the error prone measure $X^*$ is subject to systematic error, but a second measure, $X^{**}$, which is subject only to classical error $(X_i^{**} = X_i + U_i)$ is available for a subset of individuals. In fact, two measures of the second type, $X_1^{**}, X_2^{**}$, are needed for at least some individuals. Unlike Cole et al. (2006), who focused on a binary mismeasured covariate, Freedman et al. (2008) considered a continuous mismeasured covariate, alongside a continuous or binary outcome. The model $p(X|X^*, X_1^{**}, X_2^{**}, Y, Z; \theta)$ can be derived by assuming that $(X, X^*, X_1^{**}, X_2^{**})$ have a multivariate normal distribution conditional on $Z$ and $Y$, as in the replicates study setting.

The above results for the replicates study rely on the assumption of a multivariate normal distribution for $(X, X_1^*, X_2^*)$ conditional on $Z$ and $Y$. When the substantive model is a linear regression of $Y$ on $X$ and $Z$, this is straightforward to justify. However, for other types of outcome model, for example logistic or time-to-event models, the distribution of $(X, X_1^*, X_2^*)$ conditional on $Z$ and $Y$ no longer takes on a standard form. The substantive model compatible method of Bartlett et al. (2015), which was designed to address this problem in the missing data context, was extended to the setting of measurement error correction with a replicates study by Gray (2018), and is implemented in the R package SMCFCS (Bartlett and Keogh, 2019). We give a brief overview of the steps used in this procedure:

1. Draw a candidate value for each individual for whom the true exposure $X$ is missing from a 'proposal distribution' $p(X|X^*, Z)$. While this step is straightforward for a validation study, in a replicates study, it requires indirect estimation of the parameters of a model for the proposal distribution $p(X|X^*, Z; \gamma, \delta)$, derived from the measurement error model and a model for $X$ given $Z$. Parameter values $\gamma^*, \delta^*$ are first drawn from their approximate joint posterior and proposed values $X^c$ are then drawn from the distribution $p(X|X^*, Z; \gamma^*, \delta^*)$.
2. A rejection rule is used to determine whether the proposed value $X^c$ for a given individual is accepted as a value from the target posterior distribution $p(X|X_1^*, X_2^*, Y, Z; \beta, \gamma, \delta)$. The rejection rule is derived based on the form of the substantive model and uses draws of the substantive model parameters, $\beta$. Steps 1 and 2 are repeated until a candidate value of $X$ is accepted for every individual. The algorithm is then repeated iteratively until the imputed $X$ values have converged to a stationary distribution. The last cycle of imputed values is retained to create an imputed data set.
3. Steps 1 and 2 are repeated to create several imputed data sets. The outcome model of interest is then fitted to each imputed data set and Rubin's rules are applied as described above.

The proposal distribution used in step 1 is a posterior distribution and as such is based on both a prior distribution and the likelihood. Following Gustafson (2003) proper inverse-Gamma priors are recommended for the variances in formulating the proposal distribution and the priors for regression coefficients are independent normal distributions with zero means and infinite variance. The substantive model compatible approach could also be extended to the setting of a calibration study, but this has not been considered to date.

## 20.7 Comparison of Methods

We have described several approaches to measurement error correction. In this section we compare some of their properties and summarise results from authors who have compared the methods.

Regression calibration, a mean-imputation approach, is attractive in its simplicity, and this has led to it becoming the most commonly applied measurement error correction approach (Shaw et al., 2018). However, it is restricted to non-differential error. It also has a number of additional drawbacks. These include that it requires an approximation when the substantive model is not a linear regression. Extra steps, such as bootstrapping, are required to obtain correct standard errors for estimated parameters in the substantive model, which are not obtained directly in regression calibration. Further, the error prone variable must be entered in the substantive model as a linear term. Extensions to including transformations $f(X)$ in the substantive model are not in general straightforward as they would require derivation of $E(f(X)|X^*, Z)$.

The maximum likelihood approach is attractive in that the resulting estimators are consistent, asymptotically normal and efficient. However, in the measurement error context, a maximum likelihood analysis typically requires numerical integration, and, while some software is available for doing this, it is not straightforward for all outcome models, e.g., time-to-event models. A number of authors have compared regression calibration to maximum likelihood (Bartlett et al., 2009; Messer and Natarajan, 2008; Schafer and Purdy, 1996). They show that in certain settings, e.g., large measurement error and/or strong association between $X$ and $Y$, maximum likelihood estimators can have superior efficiency to regression calibration. Moreover, since measurement error corrected estimators typically have skewed distributions, inferences based on likelihood ratio tests and intervals typically perform better than Wald type tests and intervals. Bartlett et al. (2009) also showed that the maximum likelihood estimator when the outcome model is normal linear regression and $X$ is assumed normal is consistent regardless of whether the latter assumption is true.

Relative to a maximum likelihood based analysis, a Bayesian analysis requires specification of priors for the model parameters. This can be very useful when only external information is available regarding the measurement error model parameters, which can be encoded into the priors. Even when information about these is available within the study, as demonstrated by Bartlett and Keogh (2018), mildly informative priors can be used to stabilise inferences in settings where non-Bayesian methods such as regression calibration or maximum likelihood estimation may be highly variable. They showed that in the internal replication study setting, Bayes estimators can have lower bias and less variability than regression calibration, and Bayes 95% credible intervals performed well with regards frequentist coverage.

MI can be viewed as an approximation to a full Bayesian analysis (Carpenter and Kenward, 2013). From the Bayesian perspective, application of MI and Rubin's rules can be viewed as a particular route to performing a Bayesian analysis, in which one effectively assumes that the posterior distributions for the parameters are normally distributed. Like a maximum likelihood or fully Bayesian approach, MI can accommodate differential measurement error. MI is an attractive option for measurement error correction in the context of a validation studies, as the analyst can then take advantage of the many packages that have been developed in different software for the standard missing data setting. MI is less attractive in the context of a replicates or calibration study because of the lack of software. The simpler multivariate normal approach described above for implementation could be applied without specialized software. However, for a more general situation, such as the inclusions of non-linear terms for $X$ in the substantive model, the researcher would need to derive the appropriate form for the imputation model, e.g. $p(X|X_1^*, X_2^*, Z, Y; \theta)$ in a replicates study, raising complex issues of compatibility. The substantive model compatible approach outlined for a replicates study resolves this problem, but it has been found to be computationally intensive and may be inefficient relative to a direct Bayesian analysis (Gray, 2018). Lastly, the use of Rubin's rules to obtain pooled estimates assumes normality of the estimators. In the measurement error context the estimators are not in general normally distributed, which calls into question the validity of Rubin's rules. For these reasons, Bartlett and Keogh (2018) argued that a direct Bayesian approach may in many cases be preferable to use of MI.

Freedman et al. (2008) compared the MI approach with regression calibration and another imputation-based approach called 'moment-adjusted imputation'. They found that regression calibration can be more efficient than MI when the measurement error is non-differential, but importantly their implementation of MI did not exploit the non-differential error assumption. They reported that in further simulations an implementation of MI that did utilise the non-differential error assumption had similar efficiency to regression calibration. Under differential error, regression calibration gave biased estimates while their differential MI implementation delivered approximately unbiased estimates.

## 20.8 Example: Risk Factors for Cardiovascular Disease

### 20.8.1 Data Description

To illustrate the methods outlined in this chapter, we consider how they can be applied to a research question using data from the Third National Health and Nutrition Examination Survey (NHANES III). These data were used by Bartlett and Keogh (2018) in an empirical comparison of a Bayesian analysis with regression calibration. The data are freely available at `https://wwwn.cdc.gov/nchs/nhanes/Default.aspx` and example code is made available alongside the data set used at `https://github.com/ruthkeogh/meas_error_handbook`.

NHANES III was a survey conducted in the United States between 1988 and 1994 in 33,994 individuals aged two months and older. We consider a model relating known risk factors for cardiovascular disease (CVD) measured at the original survey to subsequent hazard of CVD. Mortality status at the end of 2011 is available through linkage to the US National Death Index, with cause of death classified using the ICD-10 system. We restricted to individuals aged 60 years and above at the time of the original survey.

The error-prone variable in this example is systolic blood pressure (SBP) and the covariates $Z$ to be adjusted for are age, sex, diabetes status, and smoking status. The true SBP measure of interest, $X$, is assumed to be the underlying average SBP, which is unobserved. The first error-prone measurement, $X_1^*$, is the SBP measurement taken at the original survey and this is assumed to be subject to classical measurement error. An approximate 5% subset of individuals was (non-randomly) selected to participate in a second examination, during which SBP was again measured. This second exam took place on average 17.5 days after the first exam. We assume this second measurement of SBP, $X_2^*$, to be an independent error-prone measurement of each individuals underlying SBP. We are therefore in the setting of a replicates study.

After deleting seven individuals who were missing diabetes status, data were available on 6519 individuals. Age and sex were observed for all individuals. The SBP measurement from the first examination, $X_1^*$, was available for 5033 (77.2%) individuals, and the second SBP measurement $X_2^*$ was available in 401 (6.2%) of individuals. Unfortunately, smoking status was only recorded in 3433 (52.3%) of individuals. The analysis thus required handling of both the measurement error in the SBP measurements and the substantial missingness in the smoking and SBP variables.

By the end of 2011 1469 (22.5%) had died due to CVD, 3641 had died from other causes, and 1409 were still alive. The analysis is based on a Weibull model for hazard for CVD: $h(t) = rt^{r-1}\exp\{\beta_0 + \beta_1\text{SBP} + \beta_2\text{sex} + \beta_3\text{age} + \beta_4\text{smoker} + \beta_5\text{diabetes}\}$. Deaths from causes other than CVD were treated as censorings.

### 20.8.2 Analysis Methods

The combination of both measurement error and missing data is a challenge for the analysis. The time-to-event outcome also presents a challenge for some methods.

If using regression calibration to address the measurement error, missing data could in principle be handled using MI by first obtaining multiply imputed datasets in which smoking status and SBP at the original survey are imputed, and secondly applying regression calibration within each imputed dataset. However, to implement Rubin's rules requires estimates of the variance of estimates of substantive model parameters obtained through regression calibration, which can only be obtained through bootstrapping or by deriving analytical expressions. This approach has not been investigated and is impractical without readily available software. We therefore did not pursue the combination of regression calibration and MI further.

With a Weibull model for the CVD hazard, a maximum likelihood analysis is challenging to implement because numerical integration is required to perform the integration over $X$ in equation (20.9). While there exist general software solutions to this problem, as noted in Section 20.4, they do not extend easily to the measurement error setting according to our investigations. There are practical software difficulties in incorporating any one of a time-to-event outcome, a replicate measure being available in only a subset of participants, and missing data in addition to measurement error. We therefore did not pursue a maximum likelihood analysis for these data.

Using a fully Bayesian analysis it is straightforward, given the flexible JAGS software, to incorporate both measurement error and missing data simultaneously, as well as the Weibull hazard model. We assumed that each individual's true underlying SBP around the time at which the first measurement was obtained, $X_1^*$, was normally distributed conditional on smoking, sex, age, and diabetes, with $N(0, 10^4)$ priors on the regression coefficients and a $Ga(0.5, 0.5)$ prior on the precision parameter. We assumed the classical error model for the two SBP measurements, $X_{ij}^* = X_i + U_{ij}$ $(j = 1, 2)$. The measurement errors $U_{i1}$ and $U_{i2}$ were considered normally distributed with means 0, a common variance $\sigma_U^2$ and zero correlation. The prior for $\sigma_U^{-2}$ was $Ga(0.5, 0.5)$. To accommodate missingness in the smoking and SBP variables under a missing at random assumption, we assumed a model for the distribution of smoking, conditional on the fully observed error-free covariates sex, age, and diabetes. In our analysis, we assumed a logistic model for this conditional distribution and used independent mean zero normal priors for the regression coefficients, each with variance $10^4$. For the shape parameter of the Weibull hazard model, $r$, we assumed an exponential prior with parameter 0.001. We used independent $N(0, 10^6)$ priors for the scaled regression coefficients $-\beta_k/r$ $(k = 0, \ldots, 5)$. We refer to Bartlett and Keogh (2018) and Gustafson (2004) for further discussion of suitable priors in the measurement error setting.

MI naturally accommodates both measurement error and missing data, though we are not aware of any prior applications to this setting. The first MI approach outlined in Section 20.6 for measurement error correction in a replicates study relies on the assumption of a multivariate normal distribution for $(X, X_1^*, X_2^*)$ conditional on $Z$ and $Y$. In our setting of a time-to-event, the outcome $Y$ for each individual is comprised of the earlier of their event or censoring time, $T$, and the event indicator $D$. The multivariate normality assumption is not compatible with a Weibull model for the hazard. We therefore considered the substantive model compatible approach outlined in steps 1-3 in section 20.6.3. Missing data in smoking status is assumed to depend on the other covariates through a logistic model. The SMCFCS package in R was used to perform MI, assuming a Cox proportional hazards outcome model (Bartlett and Keogh, 2019). A Cox regression model for the hazard was considered for the direct Bayesian analysis (Bartlett and Keogh, 2018), however the computation was found to be prohibitively slow.

### 20.8.3 Results

We first implemented a naive analysis ignoring both measurement error and missing values. This uses $X_1^*$ as the SBP measurement and is restricted to the subset of 2667 individuals (the 'complete cases') with both $X_1^*$ and smoking status observed. On the same subset of individuals, i.e. ignoring missing data, measurement error correction was then performed, using regression calibration, a direct Bayesian analysis, and MI. Lastly, the direct Bayesian analysis and MI were applied to additionally incorporate the missing data. These analyses are based on the full set of 6519 individuals. The results are shown in Table 20.2.

The results from regression calibration, the direct Bayesian analysis, and MI in which the missing data in SBP and smoking status is ignored are very similar. Compared to the naive analysis, all three correction methods results in a larger estimated coefficient for SBP. The estimates for sex, age, smoking status and diabetes are also very similar across these three analyses, and similar to those from the naive analysis. The direct Bayesian and MI analyses that additionally incorporate the missing data give very similar results to each other for the covariates measured without error, though the coefficients for SBP are somewhat different. This may be because the substantive model compatible MI approach assumed a Cox rather than Weibull outcome model. Changes in the estimated coefficients may be indicative of bias in the complete cases analyses. The widths of confidence/credible intervals are substantially reduced in the direct Bayesian and MI analyses that make use of all available data.

**TABLE 20.2**
Application of measurement error correction methods to NHANES III data. Log hazard ratio estimates and 95% confidence intervals (naive, regression calibration (RC) and MI) or credible intervals (Bayes). The Bayesian estimates are posterior means.

| Covariate | Naive | Bayes[c] | Bayes[d] |
|---|---|---|---|
| SBP[a] | 0.085 (0.014, 0.157) | 0.114 (0.015, 0.211) | 0.121 (0.055, 0.186) |
| Male | 0.49 (0.30, 0.67) | 0.49 (0.30, 0.68) | 0.47 (0.36, 0.57) |
| Age[b] | 0.88 (0.77, 0.99) | 0.87 (0.75, 0.98) | 1.02 (0.94, 1.09) |
| Smoker | 0.26 (0.07, 0.46) | 0.26 (0.07, 0.45) | 0.25 (0.08, 0.42) |
| Diabetes | 0.50 (0.29, 0.72) | 0.50 (0.27, 0.72) | 0.68 (0.55, 0.82) |
| | RC[c] | MI[c] | MI[d] |
| SBP | 0.114 (0.011, 0.222) | 0.120 (0.020, 0.219) | 0.104 (0.035, 0.173) |
| Male | 0.49 (0.32, 0.68) | 0.49 (0.30, 0.67) | 0.46 (0.35, 0.56) |
| Age | 0.87 (0.76, 0.99) | 0.88 (0.77, 0.99) | 1.04 (0.97, 1.11) |
| Smoker | 0.26 (0.07, 0.45) | 0.26 (0.07, 0.46) | 0.26 (0.09, 0.43) |
| Diabetes | 0.50 (0.28, 0.72) | 0.50 (0.29, 0.72) | 0.69 (0.56, 0.83) |

[a]per 20mmHg.
[b]per 10 years.
[c]Without handling of missing data in SBP and smoking status.
[d]With handling of missing data in SBP and smoking status.

## 20.9 Discussion

In this chapter we have outlined how measurement error in covariates can be viewed as a type of missing or 'coarsened' data. This has the advantage of enabling the analyst to exploit existing methods and potentially software developed for handling missing data. We considered three different settings: validation studies, replicates studies and calibration studies (Table 20.1) in which different sources of information about error-prone variables are available. The common approach of regression calibration for measurement error correction can be viewed as a mean imputation approach. This was contrasted with likelihood based methods of maximum likelihood estimation, a direct Bayesian approach and MI, all of which are well-developed for their use in the traditional missing data setting. These methods offer greater flexibility in terms of modelling assumptions and in some settings more accurate inferences. They can also naturally incorporate missing data in addition to measurement error. As discussed in Section 20.2, the assumptions required for use of these approaches in the measurement error setting may be more plausible than they are in the traditional missing data setting, because the set of individuals on whom gold standard or replicate measures are available is often a random subset or has been selected by some other design known to the analyst.

Likelihood based methods are particularly appropriate for measurement error correction in the setting of a validation study in which the 'true' value of an error-pone variable is measured on some individuals. This is very close to a traditional missing data problem, with the special feature that an auxiliary variable $X^*$ is available on everyone, meaning that methods and software for traditional missing data can be applied directly.

In Section 20.8 we discussed the application of measurement error correction methods to investigate the association between cardiovascular disease risk factors and the hazard of CVD death using data from NHANES III. Repeated measures of the error-prone variable of systolic blood pressure were available from a replicates study. The setting is representative of many studies in epidemiology, involving a time-to-event outcome and missing values in covariates as well as measurement error. This highlighted some of the challenges faced in applying measurement error correction methods in practice, notably that other features of the analysis need to be accommodated alongside the measurement error correction. While regression calibration is an attractively simple approach to measurement error correction, it does not extend easily to enable the analyst to simultaneously address missing values. A maximum likelihood approach is conceptually straightforward and accommodates both measurement error and missing values, but there is a lack of software for flexible implementation that allows the analyst to handle both of these issues at the same time, especially alongside a time-to-event outcome. A direct Bayesian analysis was the most flexible approach and by far the most straightforward to apply to accommodate both measurement error and missing data. MI, while attractive due to its now common use in handling missing data, was not straightforward to implement for measurement error correction in a replicates study, or to combine with missing values.

We have focused on measurement error in a single covariate. In some settings we face error in multiple covariates, which may include both continuous and categorical variables. Regression calibration extends to the setting of multiple covariates measured with error, though its other limitations discussed above remain. Similarly maximum likelihood estimation extends directly to this setting in theory, but the practical implementation becomes further complicated by the need for multivariate numerical integration. A Bayesian approach remains straightforward both conceptually and from a practical standpoint when there are multiple covariates measured with error. MI using SMCFCS in R can accommodate multiple covariates measured with error, each of which has two or more error-prone replicates, assuming normally distributed independent errors.

In conclusion, we recommend a Bayesian analysis for measurement error correction due to its flexibility to handle several issues simultaneously and due to the readily available software for straightforward practical implementation. While initially seeming attractive, MI is currently impractical as a measurement error correction method in many realistic problems. There is a need for development of software to enable implementation of maximum likelihood estimation, particularly for those who may object on philosophical grounds to a Bayesian analysis.

## Bibliography


Armstrong, B. (1985). Measurement error in generalized linear models. *Communications in Statistics, Series B*, 16, 529-544.

Bartlett, J., De Stavola, B., and Frost, C. (2009). Linear mixed models for replication data to efficiently allow for covariate measurement error. *Statistics in Medicine*, 28, 3158-3178.

Bartlett, J. and Keogh, R. (2018). Bayesian correction for covariate measurement error: A frequentist evaluation and comparison with regression calibration. *Statistical Methods in Medical Research*, 27, 1695-1708.

Bartlett, J. and Keogh, R. (2019). smcfcs: Multiple imputation of covariates by substantive model compatible fully conditional specification.

Bartlett, J., Seaman, S., White, I., and Carpenter, J. (2015). Multiple imputation of covariates by fully conditional specification: accommodating the substantive model. *Statistical Methods in Medical Research*, 24, 462-487.

Berglund, L., Garmo, H., Lindbäck, J., and Zethelius, B. (2007). Correction for regression dilution bias using replicates from subjects with extreme first measurements. *Statistics in Medicine*, 26, 2246-2257.

Blackwell, M., Honaker, J., and King, G. (2017a). A unified approach to measurement error and missing data: Details and extensions. *Sociological Methods and Research*, 46, 342-369.

Blackwell, M., Honaker, J., and King, G. (2017b). A unified approach to measurement error and missing data: Overview and applications. *Sociological Methods and Research*, 46, 303-341.

Brownstone, D. and Valletta, R. (1996). Modeling earnings measurement error: a multiple imputation approach. *The Review of Economics and Statistics*, 78, 705-717.

Carpenter, B., Gelman, A., Hoffman, M., Lee, D., Goodrich, B., Betancourt, M., Brubaker, M., Guo, J., Li, P., and Riddell, A. (2017). Stan: A probabilistic programming language. *Journal of Statistical Software*, 76.

Carpenter, J. and Kenward, M. (2013). *Multiple Imputation and Its Application.* Wiley, New York.

Carroll, R., Ruppert, D., Stefanski, L., and Crainiceanu, C. (2006). *Measurement Error in Non-linear Models* (2nd ed.). Chapman and Hall/CRC.

Cole, S., Chu, H., and Greenland, S. (2006). Multiple-imputation for measurement-error correction. *International Journal of Epidemiology*, 35, 1074-1081.

Crowther, M. (2018). Extended multivariate generalised linear and non-linear mixed effects models. *arXiv:1710.02223.*

Freedman, L., Midthune, D., Carroll, R., and Kipnis, V. (2008). A comparison of regression calibration, moment reconstruction and imputation for adjusting for covariate measurement error in regression. *Statistics in Medicine*, 27, 5195-5216.

Freedman, L., Midthune, D., Carroll, R., Tasevska, N., Schatzkin, A., Mares, J., Tinker, L., Potischman, N., and Kipnis, V. (2011). Using regression calibration equations that combine self-reported intake and biomarker measures to obtain unbiased estimates and more powerful tests of dietary associations. *American Journal of Epidemiology*, 174, 1238-1245.

Gray, C. (2018). Use of the Bayesian family of methods to correct for effects of exposure measurement error in polynomial regression models. *PhD thesis, London School of Hygiene & Tropical Medicine. DOI: https://doi.org/10.17037/PUBS.04649757.*

Gustafson, P. (2004). *Measurement Error and Misclassification in Statistics and Epidemiology: Impacts and Bayesian Adjustments.* Chapman and Hall/CRC, Boca Raton.

Hu, P., Tsiatis, A. and Davidian, M. (1998). Estimating the parameters in the Cox model when covariate variables are measured with error. *Biometrics*, 54, 1407-1419.

Hughes, M. (1993). Ignorability and coarse data. *Biometrics*, 49, 1056-1066.

Keogh, R. and White, I. (2014). A toolkit for measurement error correction, with a focus on nutritional epidemiology. *Statistics in Medicine*, 33, 2137-2155.

Meng, X. (1994). Multiple-imputation inferences with uncongenial sources of input. *Statistical Science*, 9, 538-558.

Messer, K. and Natarajan, L. (2008). Maximum likelihood, multiple imputation and regression calibration for measurement error adjustment. *Statistics in Medicine*, 27, 6332-6350.

Muff, S., Riebler, A., Held, L., Rue, H., and Saner, P. (2015). Bayesian analysis of measurement error models using integrated nested laplace approximations. *Journal of the Royal Statistical Society, Series C*, 64, 231-252.

Prentice, R., Shaw, P., Bingham, S., Beresford, S., Caan, B., Neuhouser, M., Patterson, R., Stefanick, M., Satterfield, S., Thomson, C., Snetselaar, L., Thomas, A., and Tinker, L. (2009). Biomarker-calibrated energy and protein consumption and increased cancer risk among postmenopausal women. *American Journal of Epidemiology*, 169, 977-989.

Rabe-Hesketh, S., Skrondal, A., and Pickles, A. (2004). Maximum likelihood estimation of generalized linear models with covariate measurement error. *The Stata Journal*, 3, 386-411.

Richardson, S. and Gilks, W. (1993a). A Bayesian approach to measurement error problems in epidemiology using conditional independence models. *American Journal of Epidemiology*, 138, 430-442.

Richardson, S. and Gilks, W. (1993b). Conditional independence models for epidemiological studies with covariate measurement error. *Statistics in Medicine*, 12, 1703-1722.

Rosner, B., Spiegelman, D., and Willett, W. (1992). Correction of logistic regression relative risk estimates and confidence intervals for random within person measurement error. *American Journal of Epidemiology*, 136, 1400-1413.

Rosner, B., Willett, W., and Spiegelman, D. (1989). Correction of logistic regression relative risk estimates and confidence intervals for systematic within-person measurement error. *Statistics in Medicine*, 8, 1051-1069.

Rubin, D. (1987). *Multiple Imputation for Nonresponse in Surveys.* Wiley, New York.

Schafer, D. (2001). Semiparametric maximum likelihood for measurement error model regression. *Biometrics*, 57, 53-61.

Schafer, D. and Purdy, K. (1996). Likelihood analysis for errors-in-variables regression with replicate measurements. *Biometrika*, 83, 813-824.

Seaman, S., Galati, J., Jackson, D., and Carlin, J. (2013). What is meant by "missing at random"? *Statistical Science*, 28, 257-268.

Shaw, P., Deffner, V., Keogh, R., Tooze, J., Kuchenhoff, H., Kipnis, V., and Freedman, L. (2018). Epidemiologic analyses with error-prone exposures: review of current practice and recommendations. *Annals of Epidemiology*, 28, 821-828.

White, I. (2006). Commentary: Dealing with measurement error: multiple imputation or regression calibration? *International Journal of Epidemiology*, 35, 1081-1082.

White, I. and Royston, P. (2009). Imputing missing covariate values for the Cox model. *Statistics in Medicine*, 28, 1982-1998.

# 21

## *Measurement Error in Causal Inference*

**Linda Valeri**

### CONTENTS



## 21.1 Introduction

Valid causal inference, the pursuit of explanation of phenomena and evaluation of treatment effects (Lewis, 1973), relies on several testable and untestable assumptions (Pearl, 2009). Among those, one that is often disregarded is that all the variables involved in the analyses are correctly measured. Conversely,

DOI: 10.1201/9781315101279-21

it is often ignored that employing a causal inference framework in the study of measurement error can allow us to better characterize the source, the impact, and the remedies to this ever present issue in data science.

The literature at the intersection of measurement error and causal inference is very rich, albeit relatively recent. The purpose of this chapter is to provide a series of points of reflection, by no means exhaustive, to bridge these two vast fields of research. It describes uses of the causal inference framework to communicate assumptions about the measurement error mechanism and the impact of measurement error in the estimation of some of the most popular causal contrasts. The chapter also describes causal inference principles that should guide measurement error correction to improve upon causal inferences.

This chapter is organized as follows. The second section introduces the potential outcomes framework for causal inference, causal estimands, conditions of identifiability of causal effects and directed acyclic graphs. The third section connects measurement error to common biases in causal inference and describes how directed acyclic graphs can be used to encode assumptions about the measurement error mechanism. The fourth section describes the impact of measurement error and misclassification on the average causal effect, direct and indirect effects estimation. The fifth section discusses approaches to correcting for measurement error in light of the goal of improving validity of causal interpretations.

## 21.2 Overview of Causal Inference

The goal of this section is to review the potential outcomes framework for causal inference, including relevant causal contrast of interest, and directed acyclic graphs.

### 21.2.1 Causal Estimands

Questions about cause-effect relationship constitute us as human beings (Hume, 1748). A milestone advancement in our pursuit of causal understanding involved the introduction of a mathematical framework to formalize concepts of causality by Neyman (Rubin, 1990). The potential outcomes framework (Rubin, 1974) provides a rigorous, model-free, definition of causal questions that can be translated in target parameters for statistical inference, under certain identifiability assumptions (Pearl, 2009; Robins, 1986).

The *potential outcome* is the fundamental element of causal inference: the value that the outcome would take under a certain level of the exposure or treatment under study, when such level of exposure is potentially different to what was observed in data (arising from an experimental or observational study). Therefore, the potential outcome is also referred to as counterfactual (Lewis, 1973).

Let $Y$ denote the observed outcome, $A$ the observed exposure, $M$ an intermediate variable (or mediator), in that is temporally after $A$ and temporally before $Y$, and $C$ additional covariates of interest in the study. For this introduction the response variable $Y$ is correctly measured and the vector of covariates $X = (C^T, A, M)^T$ is assumed to be error-free as well. The potential outcomes $Y_a$ denote the value of outcome that would have been observed had the exposure $A$ been set to level $a$. The counterfactual $Y_{am}$ for a joint intervention on $A$ and $M$ denote the value of the outcome that would have been observed had the exposure, $A$, and mediator, $M$, been set to levels $a$ and $m$, respectively. Often, the exposure has effects on the mediator and we denote $M_a$ as the value of the mediator that would have been observed had the exposure $A$ been set to level $a$.

Given this notation, we define four causal estimands popular in the causal inference literature. Valid estimation of these causal contrasts in the presence of error-prone response and covariates will be the focus of this chapter.

The average treatment effect (ATE) comparing exposure level $a$ to $a^*$ is defined by (Rubin, 1974)

$$ATE_{a,a^*} = E[Y_a - Y_{a^*}]. \tag{21.1}$$

**Example:** Consider the setting in which $A$ and $Y$ are binary variables. Investigators are interested in studying the causal effect of maternal smoking during pregnancy on child mortality. The average causal effect of maternal smoking on child mortality is the change in the mean of potential mortality status had all mothers in our study were smokers relative to the scenario in which all mothers had not been smokers. Table 21.1 provides a toy example where, say, we have a population of 8 mothers (assumed to be independent). Given the information in this table $ATE = E[Y_1] - E[Y_0] = 5/8 - 4/8 = 1/8$.

**TABLE 21.1**
A population of 8 individuals in the hypothetical setting when both potential outcomes $Y_a$ for $a = 0, 1$ are observed.

| Individual | $Y_1$ | $Y_0$ |
|---|---|---|
| 1 | 1 | 0 |
| 2 | 0 | 1 |
| 3 | 1 | 1 |
| 4 | 0 | 0 |
| 5 | 1 | 1 |
| 6 | 0 | 0 |
| 7 | 1 | 1 |
| 8 | 1 | 0 |
| Total | 5 | 4 |

**TABLE 21.2**
A population of 8 individuals in the realistic setting when only one of the potential outcomes $Y_a$ for $a = 0, 1$ are observed and the exposure $A$ is assigned to be either zero or one for each individual.

| Individual | $Y_1$ | $Y_0$ | A |
|---|---|---|---|
| 1 | 1 | ? | A=1 |
| 2 | 0 | ? | A=1 |
| 3 | ? | 1 | A=0 |
| 4 | 0 | ? | A=1 |
| 5 | ? | 1 | A=0 |
| 6 | ? | 0 | A=0 |
| 7 | ? | 1 | A=0 |
| 8 | 1 | ? | A=1 |
| Total | ? | ? | |
| Observed | 2 | 3 | |

However, in general we do not have information on the potential outcome under both smoking status levels. Mothers are going to be either smokers or non-smokers and we will instead observe Table 21.2. Comparing the mean of the observed mortality outcomes between the exposed and unexposed groups will not in general deliver the correct $ATE$, rather a measure of association. We here can compute $E[Y|A = 1] - E[Y|A = 0] = 2/4 - 3/4 = -1/4$, which is different from the true causal effect. This is the fundamental problem of causal inference (Rubin, 1974), that not all the potential outcomes are observed. Additional assumptions are required to validly estimate the causal effect of interest from the observed data.

We might be interested in evaluating the effect of interventions that involve more than one factor. Consider intervening on two causally related factors $A$ and $M$. The average controlled direct effect (CDE) comparing exposure level $a$ to $a^*$ and fixing the mediator to level $m$ is defined by (Robins and Greenland, 1992):

$$CDE_{a,a^*}(m) = E[Y_{am} - Y_{a^*m}]. \tag{21.2}$$

**Example:** Consider the setting in which $A$ , $M$, and $Y$ are binary variables. Investigators are interested in studying the causal effect of maternal smoking during pregnancy on child mortality if we further intervened on pre-term birth status. The average causal effect of maternal smoking on child mortality if all babies were born on term $m = 0$ (i.e., $E[Y_{10} - Y_{00}]$), is the change in the mean of potential mortality status had all mothers in our study were smokers relative to the scenario in which all mothers had not been smokers, while further intervening fixing the intermediate factor, preterm-birth, to zero so that all babies were born on term. This is a type of direct effect because the intermediate variable, preterm birth, is held fixed so that smoking cannot change it. Therefore, $CDE(m)$ captures an effect of smoking on mortality directly, not through pre-term birth.

Mediation contrasts express the scientific question of how and why a treatment effect arises (VanderWeele, 2015). For example we might be interested in quantifying the role of pre-term birth as potential mediator of the relationship between smoking and mortality. Controlled direct effects, albeit involving an intervention on $A$ while keeping the mediator $M$ fixed, cannot in general be used for this purpose. This is because we can define as many controlled direct effects as many are the levels that the mediator can take (e.g., if $M$ is binary, then two controlled direct effects $CDE(m = 1)$ and $CDE(m = 0)$ can be defined). Natural effects have been proposed to decompose the total effect of the treatment in two parts: the indirect effects through a mediator and direct effects not through the mediator (Robins and Greenland, 1992; Pearl, 2001). For example, we can quantify how much of the smoking effect on mortality operates directly, i.e., independently of preterm birth, and how much smoking affects mortality indirectly, i.e., through preterm birth. Robins and Greenland (1992) provide the formal definitions of natural direct and indirect effects. The average natural direct effect (NDE) compares the average potential responses for a change in the exposure $a$ to $a^*$ on the outcome when the mediator is set to its potential value $M_a^*$ when $A$ is set to $a^*$:

$$NDE_{a,a^*}(a^*) = E[Y_{aM_{a^*}} - Y_{a^*M_{a^*}}]. \tag{21.3}$$

The average natural indirect effect (NIE) compares the effect of the mediator at levels $M_a$ and $M_{a^*}$ on the outcome when exposure $A$ is set to $a$:

$$NIE_{a,a^*}(a) = E[Y_{aM_a} - Y_{aM_{a^*}}]. \tag{21.4}$$

For a dichotomous outcome the effects can be defined on the odds ratio scale or risk ratio scale and for failure time outcomes the effects can be defined on the hazard difference or ratio or survival probability difference scales, for instance.

The causal contrasts are functions of potential outcomes which are not in general observed from the real data. Identifiability assumptions are required to recover potential outcomes using data arising from randomized or observational studies.

### 21.2.2 Identifiability

This section reviews conditions under which we can hope to recover the causal estimands defined in the previous section from observational data. We refer to these as identifiability conditions. Hernán and Robins (2020) provide the following definition for identifiability of causal effects: "An average causal effect is (non-parametrically) identifiable under a particular set of assumptions if these assumptions imply that the distribution of the observed data is compatible with a single value of the effect measure. Conversely, we say that an average causal effect is non-identifiable under the assumptions when the distribution of the observed data is compatible with several values of the effect measure." (Hernán and Robins, 2020, p.27).

Identifiability conditions for causal estimands require that counterfactuals are well defined (*consistency*), the exposure levels considered in the causal contrast are realistic (*positivity*), individuals in the study are exchangeable (*exchangeability*) and non-interfering (*no interference*). In what follows conditions for identifiability of $ATE$, $CDE(m)$, natural direct ($NDE$) and indirect ($NIE$) effects are considered (Hernán and Robins, 2020; Pearl, 2009; VanderWeele, 2015).

**Consistency (CA)** is the fundamental assumption in causal inference that links the observed data to the latent counterfactuals. Formally, if consistency holds, the observed outcome is a function of the potential outcomes:

$$Y = AY_1 + (1 - A)Y_0$$

so that if in the data sample, you happen to be a person with $A = 1$, we observe $Y_1$, and vice versa for a person with $A = 0$. The observed outcome is the counterfactual corresponding to the treatment you did indeed take.

The consistency assumption is implied by:

1. The intervention is well defined and therefore there is only one version of the potential outcome.
2. A person's outcome is not influenced by another person's exposure or treatment (i.e., units are *non-interfereing*). That is,

$$Y_i(A_1, A_2, ..., A_n) = Y_i(A_i).$$

These two conditions are typically known as the Stable Unit Treatment Value Assumption (SUTVA) (Imbens and Rubin, 2015).

**Exchangeability (RA)** assumption, also referred to randomization or no unmeasured confounding, requires that the assignment to $A$ does not depend on the potential outcomes. If we let $X \perp Y|Z$ denote that $X$ is independent of $Y$ conditional on $Z$, the randomization assumption can be formalized as:

$$\{Y_0, Y_1\} \perp A.$$

An unconfounded assignment of the exposure satisfies the exchangeability assumption. A randomized controlled study is the gold standard design to achieve exchangeability, whereby the random assignment in a sufficiently large sample should achieve balance in the potential outcome response types across exposed and unexposed groups.

In observational studies full randomization is unlikely to hold and is replaced by a conditional randomization assumption, also called conditional exchangeability:

$$\{Y_0, Y_1\} \perp A|C.$$

**Positivity** assumption holds when across all levels of the confounding factors there is a positive probability to observe each exposure or treatment level under study. Formally, $Pr(A = a|C = c)$ is positive for all $c$ such that $Pr(C = c)$ is nonzero. This condition is guaranteed to hold in conditionally randomized experiments. Positivity is only required for the variables $C$ that are required for exchangeability.

Under these conditions the $ATE$ is identified by the following function of the observed data:

$$ATE = E[Y_1 - Y_0]$$
$$= \sum_c \{E[Y_1|A = 1, C = c] - E[Y_0|A = 0, C = c]\}p(c)$$
$$= \sum_c \{E[Y|A = 1, C = c] - E[Y|A = 0, C = c]\}p(c),$$

where the second equality is due to the conditional exchangeability assumption and the last step follows from the consistency assumption.

**Example:** Consider the example in Table 21.2 and let us reason on why comparing the mean of the response between exposed and unexposed group does not produce a valid estimate of the causal effects. Both exchangeability and positivity assumptions are violated in this example. Exchangeability is violated because response types $(Y_1, Y_0) = (0, 1)$, $(Y_1, Y_0) = (1, 0)$, and $(Y_1, Y_0) = (1, 1)$ are not balanced between the group of individuals assigned to $A = 1$ and those assigned to $A = 0$. The positivity assumption is violated because response type (1,1) has zero probability to be assigned to $A = 1$ and response types (0,1) and (1,0) have zero probability of being assigned to $A = 0$.

Identification assumptions for the causal effects involving intermediate variables are slightly more complex and for an extensive discussion the reader can refer to VanderWeele (2015).

To identify controlled direct effects we require exchangeability of assignment to both exposure and mediator (Robins and Greenland, 1992). Formally,

(i) $Y_{am} \perp A|C$;

(ii) $Y_{am} \perp M|\{A, C\}$.

In addition, natural direct and indirect effects require the assumption of no exposure-mediator confounding and that no confounders of the mediator-outcome relationship are affected by the exposure (Pearl, 2001; Avin et al., 2005):

(iii) $M_a \perp A|C$;

(iv) $Y_{am} \perp M_{a^*}|C$.

The intuitive interpretation of these assumptions follows from the theory of causal diagrams (Pearl, 2001), which we review in the next section. Alternative identification assumptions for mediation estimands have also been proposed (Imai et al., 2010).

Study design and analyses should take into careful consideration these assumptions. The more the investigator can be in control of the exposure assignment the more these assumptions are likely to be met. There are however several circumstances when exposure assignment cannot be under the control of the investigator, such as in observational studies, and these are also the situations when measurement error is more likely to arise. One of the purposes of this chapter is to illustrate how the validity of each of these conditions is potentially threatened by measurement error.

### 21.2.3 Directed Acyclic Graphs

A causal graph is a directed acyclic graph (DAG) in which the vertices (nodes) of the graph represent variables; the directed edges (arrows) represent direct causal relations between variables; and there are no directed cycles, because no variable can cause itself. For a DAG to be causal, the variables represented on the graph must include the measured variables and additional unmeasured variables, such that if any two variables on the graph have a cause in common, that common cause is itself included as a variable on the graph (Pearl, 1995).

DAGs are useful to classify sources of bias and to identify potential problems in study design and analysis. DAGs and the counterfactual approach are intimately linked (Spirtes, 2001).

Modern theory of causal diagrams mainly arose within the disciplines of computer science and artificial intelligence. Comprehensive books include Pearl (2009) and Spirtes, Glymour, Scheines and Heckerman (2000).

DAGs encode conditional and marginal independence assumptions and are the graphical representation of non parametric structural equation models (NPSEM) with independent errors (Pearl, 1995 and 1998). For a node $V$, the NPSEM specifies a non-parametric function $f_v(pa_v, \epsilon_v)$ which encodes dependencies with parent nodes ($pa_v$) and conditional independence assumptions. Figure 21.1 represents a causal diagram for the study of the causal effect of $A$ on $Y$ and Figure 21.2 represents a causal diagram where further intervention on $M$ is sought either to recover a CDE or direct and indirect pathways.

Consider Figure 21.1. The NPSEM represented in the DAG is: $Y = f_y(A, C, \epsilon_y); A = f_a(C, \epsilon_a); C = f_c(\epsilon_c)$. $Y$ is a *descendant* of $A$ and $C$, $A$ is a *mediator* of the $C - Y$ relationship and $C$ is a confounder of the $A - Y$ relationship.

The NPSEM represented in the DAG in Figure 21.2 is instead $Y = f_y(M, A, C_1, C_2, \epsilon_y); M = f_m(A, C_2, C_1, \epsilon_m); A = f_a(C_1, \epsilon_a); C_2 = f_{c_2}(\epsilon_{c_2}); C_1 = f_{c_1}(\epsilon_{c_1})$.

From this representation we realize that DAGs completely describe marginal and conditional independence for all the variables. In particular,

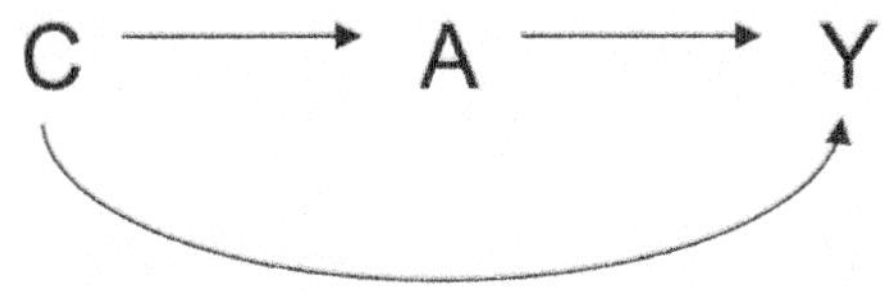


**FIGURE 21.1**
Directed acyclic graph for $ATE$

the absence of an arrow in the DAG linking two nodes encodes a conditional independence.

The most important use of DAGs is to understand whether the causal contrast of interest can be identified by satisfying the conditional exchangeability assumption. The theorem of *d-separation* (Pearl, 2009; Geiger, Verma and Pearl, 1990) is the key tool that can be used, provided we believe what represented in the causal diagram, to reason about confounding adjustment and unmeasured confounding.

**D-separation:** A path is said to be blocked if and only if it contains a non-collider that has been conditioned on (i.e., a confounder), or it contains a collider (a node to which two arrows point to) that has not been conditioned on and has no descendants that have been conditioned on. Two variables are said to be d-separated if all paths between them are blocked (otherwise, they are said to be d-connected). Two sets of variables are said to be d-separated if each variable in the first set is d-separated from every variable in the second set.

In order to identify the causal effect under study a careful strategy can be laid out to block all spurious paths using the rule of d-separation.

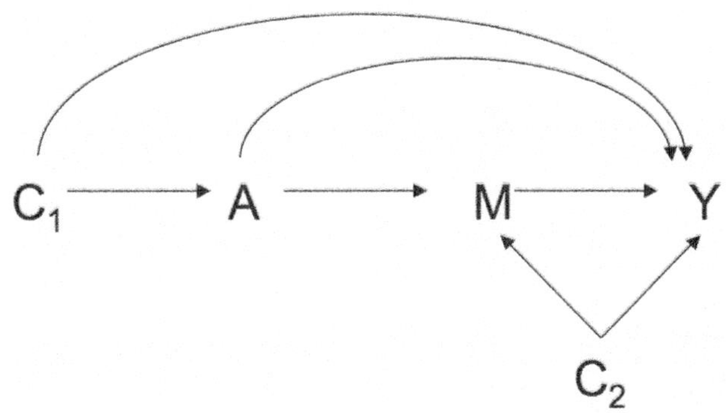


**FIGURE 21.2**
Mediation directed acyclic graph

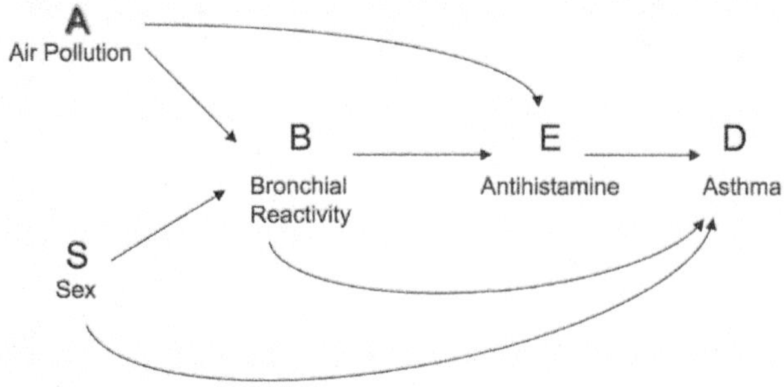


**FIGURE 21.3**
Example of directed acyclic graph for the study of the effect of anthistamine on asthma from Greenland et al. (1999)

**Example:** Consider the DAG in Figure 21.3 and say interest lies in quantifying the effect of anthistamine on asthma (Greenland, Pearl and Robins, 1999). We can use the theorem of d-separation to reason about possible sets of confounding adjustment that would suffice to meet the exchangeability assumption.

Provided that we believe that this is the causal graph including all the parents of the nodes, and correctly specifiying the conditional independences among the nodes, to control for confounding it suffices to condition on air pollution ($A$), bronchial reactivity ($B$) and sex ($S$). Alternatively, it suffices to condition on only air pollution ($A$) and bronchial reactivity ($B$) or it suffices to condition on only sex ($S$) and bronchial reactivity ($B$). However, it does not suffice to condition on sex alone (as this adjustment would leave a confounding path opened) nor bronchial reactivity alone (as this adjustment would leave a collider path opened). It does not suffice to condition on $S$ only because $B$ is a confounder. It does not suffice to condition on $B$ only because $B$ is a collider on the path $E - A - B - S - D$.

Concluding remark. DAGs do not encode any assumption about the qualitative nor quantitative relationship between variables represented in the graph.

## 21.3 The Structure of Measurement Error and Implications on Identifiability

The counterfactual framework and DAGs are very useful in characterizing and communicating assumptions about the sources of measurement error. Furthermore, a clear representation of the measurement error mechanism can better inform its potential impact on the identifiability of the causal effects under study.

This section focuses on the structural characterization of measurement error in exposure and outcome, when interest lies in the quantification of the average treatment effect and the setting in which the mediator is measured with error when interest lies in estimating direct and indirect effects.

As seen in previous chapters, measurement error can be non-differential or related to some of the variables under study. Moreover, if more than one variable under study is measured with error, measurement errors can be independent or dependent. Each of these scenarios has different implications on causal effects identifiability.

### 21.3.1 Structural Representation of Measurement Error in the Exposure and Outcome

Consider the setting in which we are interested in the causal effect of an exposure $A$ on an outcome $Y$. This situation is depicted in Figure 21.4. Hernán and Cole (2009) and Edwards et al. (2015a) propose a DAG representation of various types of measurement error mechanisms in the exposure and outcome. Figure 21.4A-F encode assumptions on measurement error, ignoring confounding for simplicity. In the figures, $A^*$ and $Y^*$ are the observed exposure and outcome measured with error and $U_A$ and $U_Y$ denote all factors other than the latent true $A$ and $Y$ that influence the observed measures. The graphs represent different combinations of conditional independence assumptions that characterize non-parametrically the measurement error mechanism.

In Figure 21.4A,C,D the measurement errors $U_A$ and $U_Y$ are independent, while in the other cases measurement error in the exposure and outcome are dependent. Study design will influence the nature of these dependences. For example, in retrospectives studies it is likely that the measurement errors are dependent, say because memory ability is one of the factors influencing measurement of both outcome and exposure and therefore present in both $U_A$ and $U_Y$. Differential measurement error is represented by an arrow originating from a variable pointing to the measurement error of another variable. DAGs in Figures 21.4C-F encode assumptions of differential measurement error. Figures 21.4A-B assume instead independence between the true variables and the error term. Note that when the outcome is assumed to influence exposure measurement error $U_A$, the study must be of retrospective nature, as causal diagrams are always acyclic. Causal diagrams do not provide quantitative information, and therefore they can be used to describe the structure of the bias but not its magnitude or direction. We can use these graphical representations and the rule of d-separation to understand whether estimated associations between the exposure and the outcome could potentially be attributed to measurement error (i.e., we are under the null hypothesis and measurement error leads us to incorrectly rejecting it.)

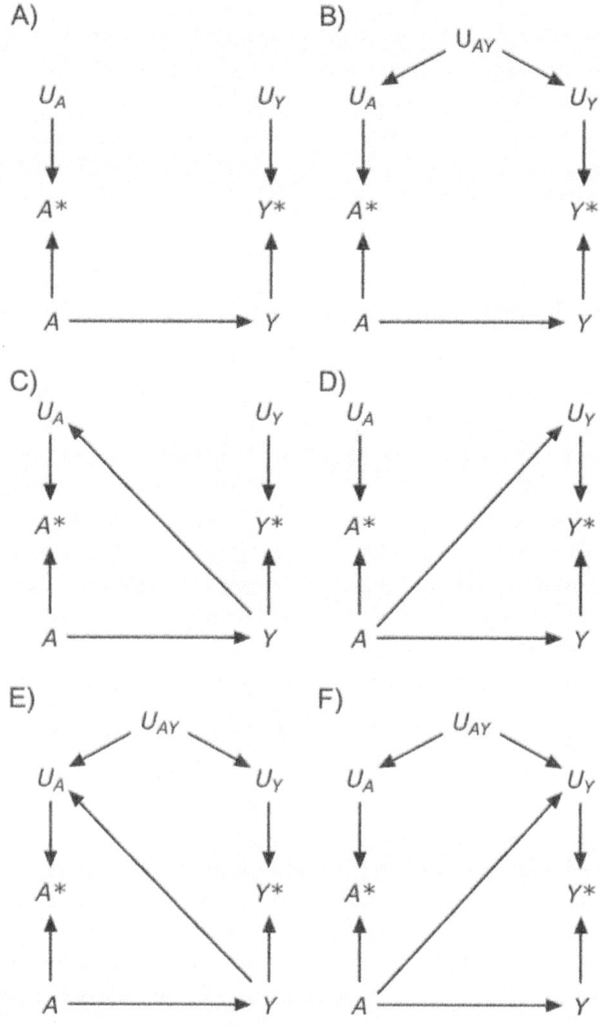


**FIGURE 21.4**
DAGs for measurement error impact on the identifiability of $ATE$ from Hernán and Cole (2009)

Figure 21.4A represents the case of non-differential and independent measurement error. In this scenario, there are no unblocked backdoor paths from the outcome to the exposure. Therefore, if an exposure outcome association is detected, it shall not be attributable solely to measurement error. In all other scenarios, if we do not correct for measurement error, observed associations could instead be partly attributable to measurement error since unblocked backdoor paths involving the measurement error are present.

When measurement error is represented in graphical form we can easily recognize its connection with other well studied biases in the causal inference literature such as confounding bias, collider bias and reverse causation. Design and analytic strategies to address these biases could be adopted to tame measurement error bias and viceversa.

**Example:** Investigators conduct a retrospective case-control study to quantify the effect of smoking on lung cancer. The measured exposure is self-reported average number of cigarettes smoked per day. Measurement error can impact the identifiability of the average causal effect in this study in several ways (Figure 21.5). Recall bias might be differential with respect to lung cancer status, introducing reverse causation. Consistency might also be violated because average number of cigarettes smoked per day might not correctly represent the smoking causal factor. Differential misclassification opens a back door path through $U_A$ because of adjustment for the collider $A^*$.

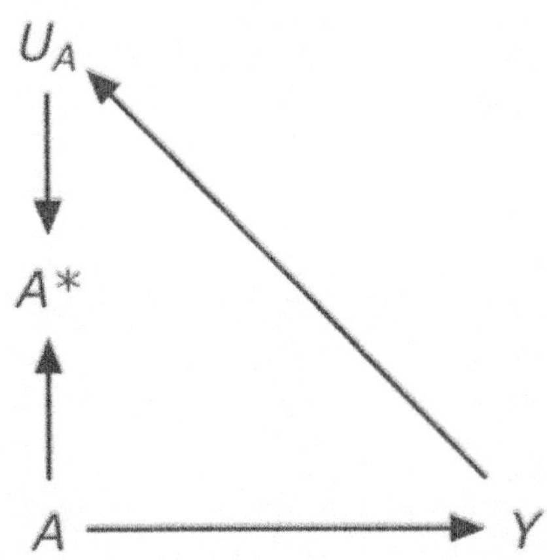


**FIGURE 21.5**
DAGs for differential exposure measurement error in a retrospective case-control study of lung cancer.

### 21.3.2 Structural Representation of Measurement Error in the Mediator

Measurement error in the mediator can severely impact the identifiability of direct and indirect effects. le Cessie et al. (2012) proposed a structural representation of measurement error in this context. Again, since DAGs do not encode information about the magnitude of the associations we are interested in reasoning on whether we would be detecting a spurious association under the null hypothesis due to measurement error. Even under non-differential and independent measurement error in the mediator the direct effect might not be identifiable. This is because conditioning on $M^*$ instead of $M$ will not completely block the path between $A$ and $Y$, that is, $A$ and $Y$ will still be indirectly connected via the true $M$. This part of the indirect effect would be incorrectly attributed to the direct effect (Figure 21.6A). In the instance of differential measurement error, adjusting for $M^*$ opens spurious collider paths between $A - M$ and $M - Y$ (Figure 21.6B). In general, this impacts the identifiability of both direct and indirect effects.

**Example:** Investigators conduct a retrospective case-control study to quantify how much of the effect of genetic variants on chromosome 15q25.1 on lung cancer operate through smoking and how much directly, independently of smoking behavior (VanderWeele et al., 2012). The measured mediator variable is self-reported average number of cigarettes smoked per day. Measurement error can impact the identifiability of the average causal direct and indirect effect in complex ways. Again consistency is questionable. The mediator-outcome association could be partly attributable to differential measurement error. This would lead to the indirect effect to be partly attributable to differential measurement error. Finally, even if the measurement error were non-differential, identifiability of the direct effect is questionable because adjusting for the mismeasured mediator will not completely block the indirect pathway through $M$, which could therefore be erroneously partly attributed to the direct effect.

In conclusion, a structural representation of measurement error using DAGs can help us understanding the impact of different measurement error mechanisms on the identifiability of total, direct and indirect causal effects. Measurement error can at times be due to inaccurate conceptualization of the variables under study, mining the validity of the consistency assumptions. Measurement error can also frequently arise in retrospective study design. In particular, dependent and differential measurement error have the potential of opening spurious channels of association, similar to what unmeasured confounding and collider bias induce. Measurement error in confounding variables can also be characterized as residual unmeasured confounding (Hernán et al., 2002; Pearl, 2012). In some instances, unless information on measurement error can be gathered, one cannot rule out that the estimates of the causal effects could be at least in part attributable to exposure, outcome or mediator measurement error.

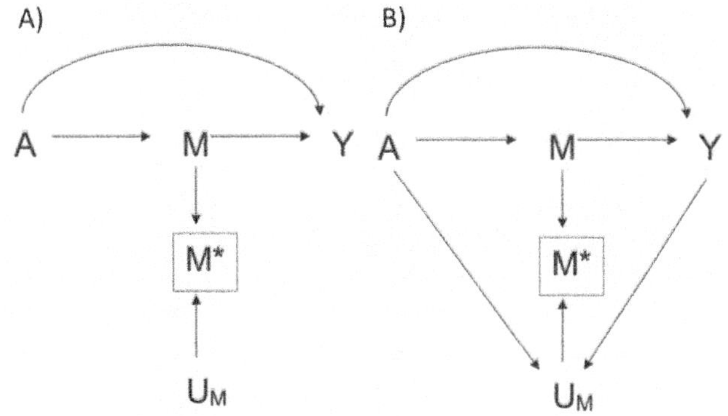


**FIGURE 21.6**
DAGs for measurement error impact on the identifiability of direct and indirect effects from le Cessie et al. (2012)

## 21.4 Estimation of Causal Effects in the Presence of Non-Differential Measurement Error in Non-Linear Models

The previous section focused on the impact of measurement error on the identifiability of causal effects in a non-parametric setting. This section reviews recent studies on the impact of measurement error on validity of the estimates obtained ignoring measurement error when non-linear parametric regression models are employed to estimate average causal effect, direct and indirect effects.

The majority of the section will be devoted to present recent studies of the impact of classical and additive non-differential measurement error of a continuous variable and of non-differential misclassification of a binary variable.

### 21.4.1 Estimation of *ATE* when the Exposure Is Measured with Error

It is often thought that non-differential measurement error is benign, biasing the effects conservatively. This popular claim is not generally true when the relationship among the variables under study are non-linear, or only partially linear and when the variables under study are strongly correlated (Carroll et al., 2006; Buonaccorsi, 2010).

Suppose that a continuous exposure $A$ is subject to non-differential measurement error (i.e., the error does not depend on the outcome conditional on the true exposure and covariates). The outcome $Y$ and covariates $C$ are error-free. Therefore, $X = (A, C^T)^T$ denotes the true latent design matrix and

$X^* = (A^*, C^T)^T$ denotes the observed design matrix, where $A^* = A+U$, with $E(U) = 0$ and $Var(U) = \sigma_u^2$.

For a continuous outcome $Y$, consider the linear model:

$$E[Y|A^*, C] = \phi_0^* + \phi_1^* A^* + \phi_2^{*T} C. \tag{21.5}$$

Parameter estimators obtained by ignoring the error in $X^*$ as measurement of $X$ and fitting the regression model to the observed data, are referred to as naive estimators. These are generally biased and inconsistent estimators of the true parameters in the regression of $Y$ given $X$ (Carroll et al., 2006; Buonaccorsi, 2010). In linear regression naive estimators of the regression coefficient of variables measured with error are biased toward zero. This type of bias is called attenuation and the amount of attenuation is called the reliability ratio (Fuller, 1987), denoted by $\lambda = \frac{\sigma^2_{a|c}}{(\sigma^2_{a|c}+\sigma^2_u)}$, where $\sigma_a^2$ is the variance of the true $A$ and $\sigma_u^2$ is the measurement error variance. Non-differential misclassification of binary variables can be characterized by sensitivity ($SN$) and specificity ($SP$) (Aigner, 1973).

The naive estimate of the average treatment effect, $\widehat{ATE^*} = \widehat{\phi_1^*}$, will provide a conservative estimate of the true treatment effect $\phi_1$.

The bias of the naive estimator for $ATE$ due to non-differential measurement error of a continuous exposure is given by:

$$ATE^* - ATE = \phi_1^* - \phi_1 = \lambda\phi_1$$

Consider now the setting in which a partially linear model is more appropriate, so that the exposure interacts with one of the confounders, $C_k$.

For a continuous outcome $Y$ we would fit the linear model:

$$E[Y|A^*, C] = \phi_0^* + \phi_1^* A^* + \phi_2^{*T} C + \phi_3^* A^* C_k \tag{21.6}$$

Under this model specification the conditional causal effect of the exposure on the outcome is estimated as $\widehat{ATE^*} = \widehat{\phi^*}_1 + \widehat{\phi^*}_3 c_k$. Evaluating the bias due to exposure measurement error is more challenging in this setting. The error in the interaction term includes a product of two covariate errors, which will not be normally distributed even when the covariate errors are normal. Furthermore, when the covariate errors are correlated, the interaction error will not have mean zero (Murad and Freedman, 2007; Buonaccorsi, 2010), even when the covariate errors have mean zero. Thus, errors in interaction terms have unusually complex structure, affecting the bias of $\widehat{ATE^*}$ in this setting. Wang et al. (1998) show that $\phi_1^*$ and $\phi_3^*$ are complex functions of the reliability ratio $\lambda$, the true latent parameters and the covariance among the variables in the design matrix, which can lead to attenuation or inflation of the $ATE$ estimates.

In the setting of non-differential exposure misclassification, Aigner (1973) and Kristensen (1992) have similarly shown that in the presence of correlated errors and/or exposure-covariates interactions $ATE$ might be either over-estimated or under-estimated.

In conclusion, in non-linear models the bias of the naive estimate of $ATE$ that ignores non-differential measurement error could lead to either inflation or attenuation of the causal effect. A measurement correction analysis is warranted to assess whether the causal effect estimated could be attributed solely to measurement error bias.

### 21.4.2 Estimation of Direct and Indirect Effects when the Mediator is Measured with Error

In mediation analysis it is often believed that non-differential measurement error or misclassification of the mediator bias naive estimators of mediated effects towards the null and of direct effects away from the null. It is important to know when this well-known heuristic is valid.

le Cessie (2012), Blakely et al. (2013), Valeri et al. (2014) and Valeri and VanderWeele (2014) have shown that this intuition will hold in generalized linear models provided that the mediator has a linear effect on the outcome.

Suppose that a continuous mediator $M$ is subject to non-differential measurement error (i.e., the error does not depend on the outcome, exposure and covariates). The outcome $Y$, the exposure $A$ and covariates $C$ are error-free. Therefore, $X = (A, M, C^T)^T$ denotes the true latent design matrix and $X^* = (A, M^*, C^T)^T$ denotes the observed design matrix, where $M^* = M + U$, with $E(U) = 0$ and $Var(U) = \sigma_u^2$. For a continuous outcome $Y$ and continuous mediator $M^*$ consider the linear models:

$$E[Y|A, M^*, C] = \theta_0^* + \theta_1^* A + \theta_2^* M^* + \theta_3^{*T} C; \tag{21.7}$$

$$E[M^*|A, C] = \beta_0 + \beta_1 A + \beta_2^T C. \tag{21.8}$$

The naive estimates of direct and indirect effects are given by $\widehat{NDE^*} = \widehat{\theta_1^*}$ and $\widehat{NIE^*} = \widehat{\beta_1}\widehat{\theta_2^*}$. The bias due to non-differential measurement error for direct and indirect effects is given by le Cessie (2012) and Valeri et al. (2014):

$$NDE^* - NDE = \theta_1^* - \theta_1 = \theta_2\beta_1(1 - \lambda);$$

$$NIE^* - NIE = \beta_1\theta_2^* - \beta_1\theta_2 = \theta_2\beta_1(\lambda - 1).$$

Since $0 \leq \lambda = \frac{\sigma_{a|c}^2}{(\sigma_{a|c}^2 + \sigma_u^2)} \leq 1$ the naive estimator for $NDE$ overestimates the true effect while the naive estimator for $NIE$ understimates the true effect. This result is similarly shown by Valeri and VanderWeele (2014) in the setting in which a binary mediator is misclassified and logistic regression is employed to model the mediator. In this context the bias is more complex because the parameter estimators in the mediator regression are biased as well.

Conversely, non-differential misclassification of a polytomous mediator does not always result in biases that follow these patterns (Ogburn and VanderWeele, 2013).

As discussed for the estimation of $ATE$, when the effect of the mediator is non-linear or only partially linear, such as in the setting of exposure-mediator interaction, Valeri et al. (2014) and Valeri and VanderWeele (2014) show that non-differential measurement error in a continuous or binary mediator will not always result in biases that follow the commonly believe pattern of underestimation of the indirect effect and over-estimation of the direct effects. Zhao and Prentice (2014) show similar results in the context of survival analysis.

### 21.4.3 Estimation of Direct and Indirect Effects when the Exposure Is Measured with Error

Consider now a binary exposure measured with non-differential error. Bias of direct and indirect effects again is impacted by model specification and the true underlying parameters. Valeri et al. (2017) show the impact of non-differential exposure misclassification in a parametric setting.

When the mean outcome conditional on exposure, mediator and covariate is modeled using linear regression, in the absence of exposure-mediator interaction the naive estimator of the natural direct effect is biased toward the null. Let $X^y = (1, A, M, C^T)^T$ and $X^{y*} = (1, A^*, M, C^T)^T$ denote the matrix of the true and observed centered covariates of the outcome regression, where $A^* = A + U$. When the latent variable is binary the measurement error, $U$, can take values $(1, 0, 1)$ under certain probabilities and restrictions. Moreover, in the case of misclassification of a binary variable, $Cov(U, A) \neq 0$ and $Cov(U, A^*) \neq 0$, that is the error must be correlated with both the true and the observed level of the exposure (Carroll et al., 2006). The moments of the error can be completely characterized by the knowledge of the prevalence of the true exposure, the sensitivity and specificity parameters. Let $X^m = (1, A, C^T)^T$ and $X^{m*} = (1, A^*, C^T)^T$ denote the matrix of the true and observed centered covariates of the mediator regression. Let $\Delta^* = E[X^{y*T} X^{y*}]$ and $\Delta^* = E[X^{m*T} X^{m*}]$ denote the variance-covariance matrix of the observed centered covariates; $\delta^y(i, j)$ and $\delta^m(i, j)$ denote an element of the inverse of the variance-covariance matrix for the outcome and mediator regression respectively. For a continuous outcome $Y$ and continuous mediator $M$ consider the following models:

$$E[Y|A^*, M, C] = \theta_0^* + \theta_1^* A^* + \theta_2^* M + \theta_3^{*T} C; \tag{21.9}$$

$$E[M = 1|A^*, C] = \beta_0^* + \beta_1^* A^* + \beta_2^{*T} C. \tag{21.10}$$

The naive estimates of direct and indirect effects are given by $\widehat{NDE^*} = \widehat{\theta}_1^*$ and $\widehat{NIE^*} = \widehat{\beta}_1^* \widehat{\theta}_2^*$.

The asymptotic bias of $NDE$ for misclassified exposure is given by:

$$NDE^* - NDE = -\theta_1 \delta^y_{A^*,A^*} Cov(A^*, U).$$

From the result above we notice that under the special case of no direct effect, the naive estimator of the direct effect is unbiased.

Exposure misclassification biases the estimator of the exposure coefficient in the mediator model ($\beta_1$) downward but also biases the estimator of the coefficient for the mediator in the outcome model ($\theta_2$) upward. Therefore, in theory, the bias of the naive indirect effect estimator can be in either direction. However, when the mediator is very strongly correlated with the exposure (i.e., $\beta_1 \neq 0$), the bias of the total effect estimator is larger than the bias of the natural direct effect estimator, leading to overestimation of the indirect effect.

The asymptotic bias of the indirect effect for misclassified exposure is given by:

$$NIE^* - NIE = Cov(A^*, U)\beta_1\{-\theta_2 \delta^m_{A^*,A^*} + \theta_1 \delta^y_{A^*,M}(\delta^m_{A^*,A^*} Cov(A^*, U) - 1)\}.$$

Exposure measurement error will lead to an overestimation of the indirect effect if $\theta_2 \delta^m_{A^*,A^*} < \theta_1 \delta^y_{A^*,M}(\delta^m_{A^*,A^*} Cov(A^*, U) - 1)$.

The case of no indirect effect should be taken in careful consideration. Note that the $NIE$ is zero if either (a) there is no effect of exposure on the mediator and no effect of the mediator on the outcome ($\theta_2 = 0$ and $\beta_1 = 0$); or if (b) there is no effect of exposure on the mediator, but there is an effect of the mediator on the outcome (i.e., $\beta_1 = 0, \theta_2 \neq 0$); or if (c) there is an effect of exposure on the mediator, but there is no effect of the mediator on the outcome (i.e., $\beta_1 \neq 0, \theta_2 = 0$). Inspecting the bias of the $NIE$ above, we see that under the null hypothesis of $NIE = 0$ when $\beta_1 \neq 0$ and $\theta_2 = 0$ the bias is not equal to zero. In particular, the indirect effect is potentially overestimated due to the overestimation of the parameter $\theta_2$. In this setting, measurement error undermines the validity of the Sobel test (Sobel, 1982) for mediation, which has inflated type I error.

Therefore, even when the relationship among variables is linear, non-differential exposure measurement error could lead to over-estimation of the indirect effect, against the common belief that measurement error will dilute estimates of effects.

In the presence of exposure-mediator interaction the direct effect will be either bias towards or against the null as well. Taken together these results indicate that measurement error correction is warranted to obtain correct conclusions in mediation analyses.

**Example:** Consider a study investigating whether the effect of maternal smoking effect on birth weight is mediated by DNA methylation. DNA methylation is one of several epigenetic mechanisms that cells use to control gene expression (Robertson, 2005). Self-reported smoking status during pregnancy is potentially misclassified and in particular we would suspect that smoking mothers are more likely than non smoking mothers to mis-report smoking status (i.e. specificity likely to be 1 but sensitivity likely to be $< 1$). Moreover, DNA methylation is precisely measured a known strong biomarker for smoking behavior (Shenker et al., 2013). In this setting, investigators should be concerned about potential over-estimation of the effect of DNA methylation on birthweight. The causal role of the mediator might be confused with its role as a proxy for the imprecisely measured exposure (Valeri et al., 2017).

## 21.5 Measurement Error Correction in Causal Inference

A wealth of approaches for measurement error correction from a statistical perspective have been reviewed in this book and elsewhere (Carroll et al., 2006; Buonaccorsi, 2010; Fuller, 1987; Yi, 2017). Causal inference methodologists have also relatively recently started contributing to development of methods for measurement error correction. Simulation Extrapolation (SIMEX; Stefanski and Cook, 1995) and regression calibration (Spiegelman et al., 1997) approaches have been employed for measurement error correction in the estimation of time-varying causal effects (Kyle et al., 2016) and mediation analysis (Valeri et al., 2014; Valeri and VanderWeele, 2014; Valeri et al., 2017). A prolific line of research focuses on translating measurement error as a missing data problem and uses inverse probability weighting (McCaffrey et al., 2013; Gravel and Platt, 2018; Shu and Yi, 2019), multiple imputation (Webb-Vargas et al., 2017; Edwards et al., 2015b) or the EM algorithm (Wulfsohn and Tsiatis, 1997; Valeri and VanderWeele, 2014) for measurement error correction. Another interesting perspective is to consider measurement error as a causal inference problem akin to unmeasured confounding and using either sensitivity analyses for unmeasured confounding (Rudolph and Stuart, 2018) or instrumental variables approaches to correct for measurement error (Miles et al., 2018).

The purpose of this section is to highlight that validity of remedies for measurement error can be evaluated from either a statistical or causal viewpoint.

From a statistical perspective, once the causal estimand is defined, if the NPSEM encodes valid assumptions on the measurement error mechanism, and effect is identified in terms of the latent variables, the problem is no longer one of causal inference, but rather of regression analysis.

Pearl (2012) considers the problem of estimating the causal effect of $A$ on $Y$ when a set $C$ of confounders can only be measured with error via a proxy set $C^*$. $C$ suffices to adjust for confounding, $Y_a \perp A|C$. When only $C^*$ is observed, the conditional exchangeability assumption is violated. Assuming non-differential measurement error, if the conditional probability $P(c^*|c)$ that governs the error mechanism is known and a sufficiently large dataset is available, one can perform a modified-adjustment for $C^*$ that would render the causal effect identifiable.

The key point is how one can recover $P(c^*|c)$, or any other, potentially more complex, probability characterizing the measurement error phenomenon under study. Recovering this probability might be extremely difficult, depending on the context. Statistical assumptions are often times not sufficient to support the validity of the estimation of such density and the downstream causal interpretation of the measurement error corrected analyses.

The best case scenarios are when a gold standard measurement for $C$ is collected as an internal validation study for only part of the sample (Carroll et al., 2006) or when multiple internal replicates of mismeasured variables can be obtained. However, in several instances such internal sample measurements are not feasible to obtain.

When $P(c^*|c)$ is not given or cannot be directly estimated in the sample, several approaches can be pursued. One can adopt a Bayesian analysis and assume a prior distribution on the parameters of $P(c^*|c)$, which would yield a distribution over the causal effect of interest (Steenland and Greenland, 2004). Alternatively, sensitivity analysis approaches under a frequentist framework have been widely adopted in causal inference in the presence of measurement error (Lash et al., 2011), which specify bounds for the parameters regulating the measurement error magnitude to obtain bounds for the causal effects.

Finally, combining information from external data sources is often pursued for measurement error correction (Lyles et al., 2007; Siddique et al., 2019). In instances of data integration from external sources, it is necessary to carefully assess the appropriateness of transferring the measurement error mechanism learnt from external data to the original data. *Transportability* is a generalization of the concept of identifiability, critical condition that enables the statistical machinery to deliver valid causal inferences (Pearl and Bareinboim, 2014; Correa and Bareinboim, 2019). This assumption requires that selection into the original or external-validation study does not depend on unobserved covariates after conditioning on observed outcome and covariates.

Depending on the nature of the validation data and specification of the measurement error mechanism the assumption of transportability can be more or less plausible. For example, if internal validation data and internal replicates are available, statistical analyses are more likely to yield transportable inferences of the measurement error probability density than using external data. When external data is used to correct for measurement error effects it is advised to collect information on factors that drive inclusion in both the original study and the external data source. However, even internal validation studies should be carefully planned and controlled. If individuals who contributed to the internal validation/replication sample differ from the overall sample in some unknown features that predict the outcome, validity of the measurement error correction would be questionable. DAGs representation of transportability assumptions can be extremely useful (Pearl and Bareinboim, 2014) to communicate how data integration can help tame measurement error bias or whether validity is questionable depending on the source of information used to estimate the measurement error mechanism.

In conclusion, validity of untestable assumptions will inevitably affect our ability to interpret causally measurement error corrected analyses. A causal inference perspective is valuable to better reason upon such assumptions.

## 21.6 Conclusion

Measurement error can undermine the validity of causal inferences. Correct measurement of all variables in the analysis is a critical assumption often disregarded by causal inference practitioners. This chapter aimed to bridge the fields of causal inference and measurement error. Measurement error induces bias in the estimation of total, direct and indirect effects and, even in the setting of non-differential classical measurement error, the bias can take unintuitive directions. The potential outcomes and causal graphical models frameworks for causal inference can contribute in formalizing assumptions on measurement error mechanism. Moreover, a structural representation of measurement error helps reasoning about the potential impact of measurement error and guiding the choice of measurement error correction approaches. The possibility of correcting for measurement bias may suggest that as long as we know the measurement error magnitude post-hoc analyses can deliver valid causal inferences. If the postulated assumptions for the measurement error mechanism are incorrect estimates will remain biased. For instance, when the conditional probability that characterizes the error mechanism is obtained from an external data source that is not representative of the study population, causal interpretation of the measurement error corrected analyses remains questionable. Therefore, resorting to sensitivity analyses for measurement error correction considering different assumptions underlining the measurement error mechanism may often be advised. Finally, it is important to note that no statistical method for measurement error correction will be able to correct for a poorly designed study where the measured factors do not appropriately represent the scientific question under study, violating the consistency and SUTVA properties for causal effects identifiability.

## References

Aigner, D. J. (1973). Regression with a binary independent variable subject to errors of observation. *Journal of Econometrics*, 1(1), 49-59.

Avin, C., Shpitser, I., and Pearl, J. (2005). Identifiability of path-specific effects. In *Proceedings of the 19th International Joint Conference on Articial*

*Intelligence* Kaelbling, L. P. and Saffiotti, A. (Eds.), 357-363. Morgan Kaufmann, San Francisco, CA.

Blakely, T., McKenzie, S., and Carter, K. (2013). Misclassification of the mediator matters when estimating indirect effects. *J Epidemiol Community Health*, 67(5), 458-466.

Buonaccorsi, J. P. (2010). *Measurement Error: Models, Methods, and Applications.* CRC Press.

Carroll, R. J., Ruppert, D., Stefanski, L. A., and Crainiceanu, C. M. (2006). *Measurement Error in Nonlinear Models: A Modern Perspective.* CRC Press.

Correa, J. D. and Bareinboim, E. (2019). From statistical transportability to estimating the effect of stochastic interventions. In *International Joint Conferences on Artificial Intelligence*, 1661-1667.

Edwards, J. K., Cole, S. R., and Westreich, D. (2015a). All your data are always missing: incorporating bias due to measurement error into the potential outcomes framework. *International Journal of Epidemiology*, 44(4), 1452-1459.

Edwards, J. K., Cole, S. R., Westreich, D., Crane, H., Eron, J. J., Mathews, W. C., Moore, R., Boswell, S. L., Lesko, C. R., and Mugavero, M. J. (2015b). Multiple imputation to account for measurement error in marginal structural models. *Epidemiology (Cambridge, Mass.)*, 26(5), 645.

Fuller, W. A. (1987). *Measurement Error Models.* John Wiley & Sons.

Geiger, D., Verma, T., and Pearl, J. (1990). D-separation: from theorems to algorithms. In *Machine Intelligence and Pattern Recognition*, Vol. 10, 139-148. North-Holland.

Gravel, C. A. and Platt, R. W. (2018). Weighted estimation for confounded binary outcomes subject to misclassification. *Statistics in Medicine*, 37(3), 425-436.

Greenland, S., Pearl, J., and Robins, J. M. (1999). Causal diagrams for epidemiologic research. *Epidemiology*, 10(1), 37-48.

Hernán, M. A. and Cole, S. R. (2009). Invited commentary: causal diagrams and measurement bias. *American Journal of Epidemiology*, 170(8), 959-962.

Hernán, M. A., Hernández-Díaz, S., Werler, M. M., and Mitchell, A. A. (2002). Causal knowledge as a prerequisite for confounding evaluation: an application to birth defects epidemiology. *American Journal of Epidemiology*, 155(2), 176-184.

Hernán, M.A. and Robins, J.M. (2020). *Causal Inference: What If.* Chapman & Hall/CRC, Boca Raton.

Hume, D. (1748). An enquiry concerning human understanding. Reprinted and edited 1993, Indianapolis/Cambridge: Hacket.

Imai, K., Keele, L., and Tingley, D. (2010). A general approach to causal mediation analysis. *Psychological Methods*, 15(4), 309.

Imbens, G. W. and Rubin, D. B. (2015). *Causal Inference in Statistics, Social, and Biomedical Sciences.* Cambridge University Press.

Kristensen, P. (1992). Bias from nondifferential but dependent misclassification of exposure and outcome. *Epidemiology*, 3(3), 210-215.

Kyle, R. P., Moodie, E. E., Klein, M. B., and Abrahamowicz, M. (2016). Correcting for measurement error in time-varying covariates in marginal structural models. *American Journal of Epidemiology*, 184(3), 249-258.

Lash, T. L., Fox, M. P., and Fink, A. K. (2011). *Applying Quantitative Bias Analysis to Epidemiologic Data.* Springer Science & Business Media.

le Cessie, S., Debeij, J., Rosendaal, F. R., Cannegieter, S. C., and Vandenbrouckea, J. P. (2012). Quantification of bias in direct effects estimates due to different types of measurement error in the mediator. *Epidemiology*, 23(4), 551-560.

Lewis, D. (1973). *Counterfactuals and Comparative Possibility.* Springer, Dordrecht.

Lyles, R., Zhang, F., and Drews-Botsch, C. (2007). Combining Internal and external validation data to correct for exposure misclassification: A case study. *Epidemiology*, 18(3), 321-328.

McCaffrey, D. F., Lockwood, J. R., and Setodji, C. M. (2013). Inverse probability weighting with error-prone covariates. *Biometrika*, 100(3), 671-680.

Miles, C. H., Schwartz, J., and Tchetgen, E. J. (2018). A class of semiparametric tests of treatment effect robust to confounder measurement error. *Statistics in Medicine*, 37(24), 3403-3416.

Murad, H. and Freedman, L. S. (2007). Estimating and testing interactions in linear regression models when explanatory variables are subject to classical measurement error. *Statistics in Medicine*, 26(23), 4293-4310.

Ogburn, E. L. and Vanderweele, T. J. (2013). Bias attenuation results for nondifferentially mismeasured ordinal and coarsened confounders. *Biometrika*, 100(1), 241-248.

Pearl, J. (1995). Causal diagrams for empirical research. *Biometrika*, 82(4), 669-688.

Pearl, J. (1998). Graphs, causality, and structural equation models. *Sociological Methods & Research*, 27(2), 226-284.

Pearl, J. (2001). Direct and indirect effects. In Proceedings of UAI-01, 411-420.

Pearl, J. (2009). *Causality.* Cambridge University Press.

Pearl, J. (2012). On measurement bias in causal inference. arXiv preprint arXiv:1203.3504.

Pearl, J. and Bareinboim, E. (2014). External validity: From do-calculus to transportability across populations. *Statistical Science*, 29(4), 579-595.

Robertson, K. (2005). DNA methylation and human disease. *Nature Reviews Genetics*, 6, 597-610.

Robins, J. (1986). A new approach to causal inference in mortality studies with a sustained exposure periodapplication to control of the healthy worker survivor effect. *Mathematical Modelling*, 7(9), 1393-1512.

Robins, J. M. and Greenland, S. (1992). Identifiability and exchangeability for direct and indirect effects. *Epidemiology*, 3(2), 143-155.

Rubin, D. B. (1974). Estimating causal effects of treatments in randomized and nonrandomized studies. *Journal of Educational Psychology*, 66(5), 688-701.

Rubin, D. (1990). [On the Application of Probability Theory to Agricultural Experiments. Essay on Principles. Section 9.] Comment: Neyman (1923) and Causal Inference in Experiments and Observational Studies. *Statistical Science*, 5(4), 472-480.

Rudolph, K. E. and Stuart, E. A. (2018). Using sensitivity analyses for unobserved confounding to address covariate measurement error in propensity score methods. *American Journal of Epidemiology*, 187(3), 604-613.

Shenker, N. S., Ueland, P. M., Polidoro, S., van Veldhoven, K., Ricceri, F., Brown, R., Flanagan, J.M., and Vineis, P. (2013). DNA methylation as a long-term biomarker of exposure to tobacco smoke. *Epidemiology*, 24(5), 712-716.

Shu, D. and Yi, G. Y. (2019). Weighted causal inference methods with mismeasured covariates and misclassified outcomes. *Statistics in Medicine*, 38(10), 1835-1854.

Siddique, J., Daniels, M. J., Carroll, R. J., Raghunathan, T. E., Stuart, E. A., and Freedman, L. S. (2019). Measurement error correction and sensitivity analysis in longitudinal dietary intervention studies using an external validation study. *Biometrics*, 75(3), 927-937.

Sobel, M. E. (1982). Asymptotic intervals for indirect effects in structural equations models. In *Sociological Methodology*, Leinhart, S. (Ed.), 290-312. San Francisco: Jossey-Bass.

Spiegelman, D., McDermott, A., and Rosner, B. (1997). Regression calibration method for correcting measurement-error bias in nutritional epidemiology. *The American Journal of Clinical Nutrition*, 65(4), 1179-1186.

Spirtes, P. (2001). An anytime algorithm for causal inference. In *The Society for AI and Statistics.*

Spirtes, P., Glymour, C. N., Scheines, R., and Heckerman, D. (2000). *Causation, Prediction, and Search.* MIT press.

Steenland, K. and Greenland, S. (2004). Monte Carlo sensitivity analysis and Bayesian analysis of smoking as an unmeasured confounder in a study of silica and lung cancer. *American Journal of Epidemiology*, 160(4), 384-392.

Stefanski, L. A. and Cook, J. R. (1995). Simulation-extrapolation: the measurement error jackknife. *Journal of the American Statistical Association*, 90(432), 1247-1256.

Valeri, L., Lin, X., and VanderWeele, T. J. (2014). Mediation analysis when a continuous mediator is measured with error and the outcome follows a generalized linear model. *Statistics in Medicine*, 33(28), 4875-4890.

Valeri, L., Reese, S. L., Zhao, S., Page, C. M., Nystad, W., Coull, B. A., and London, S. J. (2017). Misclassified exposure in epigenetic mediation analyses. Does DNA methylation mediate effects of smoking on birthweight? *Epigenomics*, 9(3), 253-265.

Valeri, L. and Vanderweele, T. J. (2014). The estimation of direct and indirect causal effects in the presence of misclassified binary mediator. *Biostatistics*, 15(3), 498-512.

VanderWeele, T. (2015). *Explanation in Causal Inference: Methods for Mediation and Interaction.* Oxford University Press.

VanderWeele, T. J., Asomaning, K., Tchetgen Tchetgen, E. J., Han, Y., Spitz, M. R., Shete, S., Wu, X., Gaborieau, V., Wang, Y., McLaughlin, J., Hung, R. J., Brennan, P., Amos C. I., Christiani, D. C., and Lin, X. (2012). Genetic variants on 15q25. 1, smoking, and lung cancer: an assessment of mediation and interaction. *American Journal of Epidemiology*, 175(10), 1013-1020.

Wang, N., Lin, X., Gutierrez, R. G., and Carroll, R. J. (1998). Bias analysis and SIMEX approach in generalized linear mixed measurement error models. *Journal of the American Statistical Association*, 93(441), 249-261.

Webb-Vargas, Y., Rudolph, K. E., Lenis, D., Murakami, P., and Stuart, E. A. (2017). An imputation-based solution to using mismeasured covariates in propensity score analysis. *Statistical Methods in Medical Research*, 26(4), 1824-1837.

Wulfsohn, M. S. and Tsiatis, A. A. (1997). A joint model for survival and longitudinal data measured with error. *Biometrics*, 53(1), 330-339.

Yi, G. Y. (2017). *Statistical Analysis with Measurement Error or Misclassification.* Springer, New York.

Zhao, S. and Prentice, R. L. (2014). Covariate measurement error correction methods in mediation analysis with failure time data. *Biometrics*, 70(4), 835-844.

# 22

## *Measurement Error and Misclassification in Meta-Analysis*

**Annamaria Guolo**

### CONTENTS



## 22.1 Introduction

Meta-analysis is a long-established and diffuse approach to combine and analyze the results from separate studies about the same issue of interest. Meta-analysis studies typically occur in medical and epidemiological investigations, although in recent decades applications in different areas of research, such as sociological and behavioral sciences, economics and ecology, have increased (Roberts, 2005; Sutton and Higgins, 2008; Zeng and Lin, 2015; Koricheva et al., 2013; Gurevitch et al., 2018).

The traditional model for meta-analysis is a linear random-effects model (DerSimonian and Laird, 1986), where the random effect, usually associated to

DOI: 10.1201/9781315101279-22

the intercept, takes into account the heterogeneity among the studies due to subjects' characteristics, study designs, or clinical/treatments interventions (van Houwelingen et al., 2002). Suppose that the meta-analysis involves $n$ studies about the common issue of interest. A typical example is the effect of a new therapy for a certain disease in clinical trials comparing a treated group and a control group. The main information provided by each study is a measure $Y_i$, $i = 1, \ldots, n$, of the treatment effect, typically a log-odds or a difference in mean between treated and control groups, and the variance $\sigma_i^2$ associated to the measure $Y_i$. The simplest random-effects meta-analysis model suggested in DerSimonian and Laird (1986) is

$$Y_i = \beta_i + \varepsilon_i, \quad \varepsilon_i \sim Normal(0, \sigma_i^2), \tag{22.1}$$

with random effect $\beta_i \sim Normal(\beta, \tau^2)$ independent of the within-study error $\varepsilon_i$. Marginally, $Y_i \sim Normal(\beta, \sigma_i^2 + \tau^2)$. The inferential interest is typically on $\beta$, while $\tau^2$ is the between-study variance accounting for the heterogeneity among studies. The within-study variance $\sigma_i^2$ is commonly assumed to be known and equal to the estimate provided by each study included in the meta-analysis, when the sample size of each study is large enough to justify such an approach. A huge literature has discussed effective identification of the heterogeneity among studies and estimation of $\tau^2$ (e.g., Viechtbauer, 2007a, 2007b), as well as appropriate modifications of model (22.1) in order to take into account the nature of the original data $(y_i, \sigma_i^2)$ when the Normal distribution represents just an approximation of the real sampling distribution (e.g., Hamza et al., 2008a; Hoaglin, 2015).

When a covariate is present, it is in form of a summary measure for the information of interest obtained from finite samples in each study included in the meta-analysis. As the meta-analysis data, in terms of either response or covariate, are estimated rather than true values, they are prone to some kind of errors. While the variability due to errors affecting the summary response measure can be accounted for by the variance components of the models, the presence of summary covariates makes the analysis more troublesome. Accordingly, appropriate correction techniques are necessary in order to derive reliable inferential conclusions.

This chapter will focus on two common types of meta-analysis, namely, control risk regression and meta-analysis of diagnostic accuracy studies, where the substantial impact of measurement errors has been faced through different solutions in the literature.

## 22.2 Control Risk Regression

The investigation of between-study heterogeneity is one of the main issues in meta-analysis. In particular, the attention in the literature has been addressed to between-study heterogeneity of treatment effects in meta-analysis of clinical trials, as a consequence of patients' characteristics, study designs, or clinical interventions. Modelling the relationship between a measure of the risk in the treatment group and a measure of the severity of illness in the control group, or underlying risk or baseline risk, has been long recognized as an effective way to account for between-study heterogeneity, e.g., Brand and Kragt (1992), Sharp et al. (1996), van Houwelingen et al. (2002). In this way, emerging differences among studies are a consequence of treatment effects only. A common measure of the baseline risk is provided by the control rate, i.e., the proportion of patients with the event of interest in the control condition. Meta-analysis including such an information is typically referred to as *control risk regression.*

Consider a meta-analysis of $n$ independent studies about the effectiveness of a treatment. Let $Y_i$ indicate the measure of the risk in the treatment group in study $i$ and let $X_i$ denote the risk measure in the control population for the same study. The relationship between $Y_i$ and $X_i$ is commonly assumed linear (e.g., McIntosh, 1996; Schmid et al., 1998; Arends et al., 2000)

$$Y_i = \beta_0 + \beta_x X_i + \varepsilon_i, \ \varepsilon_i \sim \text{Normal}(0, \tau^2), \ i = 1, \ldots, n, \tag{22.2}$$

where parameter $\tau^2$ is the residual variance that describes the variation unexplained by the baseline risk. The linear model is a reasonable option since treatment risks are often monotonically related to the baseline risk, as well as being a computationally convenient choice. Alternative nonlinear relationships are discussed in Wang et al. (2009). The inferential interest is in $\beta_x$, with $\beta_x = 0$ used to represent the constancy of the treatment risk and its independence with respect to $X_i$. Sometimes, it can be of interest to evaluate the relationship between the difference $Y_i - X_i$ and the baseline level $X_i$ (e.g., Ghidey et al., 2013). In this case, $(\beta_0, \beta_x)^{\mathrm{T}} = (0, 1)^{\mathrm{T}}$ represents a claim of no treatment difference, on average.

Inference based on model (22.2) (Brand and Kragt, 1992) is performed through a weighted least squares regression, with weights given by the inverse of the variance of the estimated treatment effect. Such an approach, however, has been long criticized as it does not account for the uncertainty associated to both the available measures of $Y_i$ and $X_i$ provided by each study included in the meta-analysis. In fact, the summary information from each study represents a surrogate for the true unobserved risk measure and consequently is prone to measurement error. Inference relying on the method in Brand and Kragt (1992) can be misleading (e.g., Senn, 1994; McIntosh, 1996; Schmid et al., 1998), the most common consequence being the attenuation phenomenon, which implies the estimation of $\beta_x$ is biased towards zero. More generally, the effects of ignoring measurement errors are unpredictable, since they are related to the model structure as well as the measurement errors characteristics.

**Example:** To illustrate the effect of measurement error on the estimation of $(\beta_0, \beta_x)^{\mathrm{T}}$ in control risk regression consider the following simulation example.

The simulation considers 10 studies, with sample size ranging from 10 to 166. Values of the sample sizes are inspired by the meta-analysis study of randomized controlled trials about a pharmacological therapy in patients with acute renal failure performed in Ho and Sheridan (2006) and later examined in Guolo (2014). Information from each study included in the meta-analysis is reported in terms of log-odds of disease in the treatment group and in the control group. The mortality rate for controls is simulated from a uniform variable on the interval [0.305, 0.964], with values of the interval equal to the range of the mortality rate in the acute renal failure meta-analysis. Let $(\beta_0, \beta_x)^{\mathrm{T}} = (0.003, 0.818)^{\mathrm{T}}$, that is, the value of the Brand and Kragt (1992) regression model on the log-odds for treated and controls. Errors $\varepsilon_i$, $i = 1, \ldots, 10$, are assumed to be generated from a Normal variable with mean zero and variance $\tau^2 = 0.98$. The number of events for the treatment group and the control group are simulated from a Binomial distribution and used to compute the log-odds for treated and controls in each study. Figure 22.1 reports the scatter plot of the simulated data, together with the weighted least squares regression line (solid line). The effects of the measurement error implied by using the summary sample information from each study is highlighted by the weighted least squares regression line with the estimate of $\beta_x$ biased towards zero (dashed line).

### 22.2.1 Measurement Error Models

The literature distinguishes between exact and approximate measurement error models to describe the uncertainty of the summary information of the studies included in the control risk regression. In the following, the summary information about $Y_i$ and $X_i$ provided by study $i$ will be denoted by $Y_i^*$ and $X_i^*$, respectively.

The specification of an *exact measurement error model* is related to the risk measure obtained from study $i$, see, for example, Arends et al. (2000).

*Log-odds as risk measure*

Let log-odds be the risk measure of interest in the treatment group and in the control group. Suppose that each study included in the meta-analysis provides information about the observed number of events $v_{iT}$ and $v_{iC}$ in the treatment group and in the control group, respectively, and the number of treated and controls, $n_{iT}$ and $n_{iC}$, respectively. Thus, the observed values of $Y_i^*$ and $X_i^*$ are $y_i^* = \log\{v_{iT}/(n_{iT} - v_{iT})\}$ and $x_i^* = \log\{v_{iC}/(n_{iC} - v_{iC})\}$, respectively. The exact measurement error model considers the Binomial distribution of the variables $V_{iT}$ and $V_{iC}$ (Arends et al., 2000; Schmid et al., 2004), namely,

$$V_{iT} \sim \text{Binomial}\left(n_{iT}, \frac{e^{y_i}}{1 + e^{y_i}}\right)$$

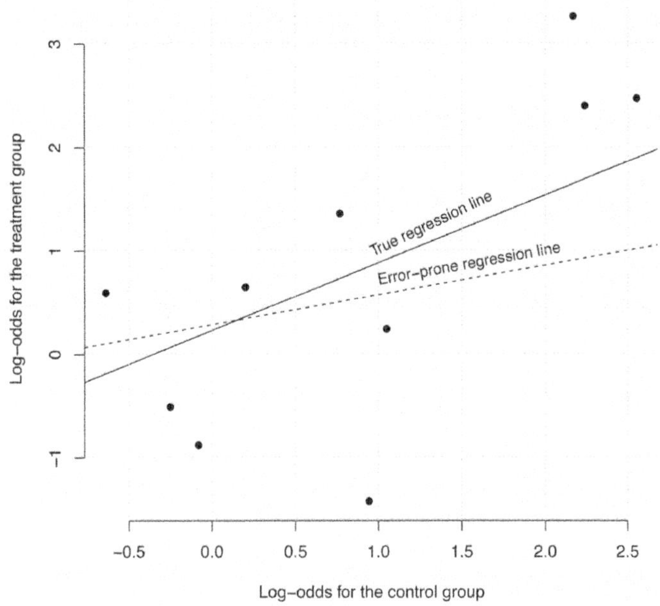


**FIGURE 22.1**
Simulated example. Scatter plot of 10 pairs of simulated log-odds for the treatment group and the control group. Weighted least squares regression lines based on true data (solid line) and summary information (dashed line).

and

$$V_{iC} \sim \text{Binomial}\left(n_{iC}, \frac{e^{x_i}}{1+e^{x_i}}\right).$$

*Log event rate as risk measure*

Let log event rate be the risk measure of interest in the treatment group and in the control group, with study information expressed in terms of observed number of events $v_{iT}$ and $v_{iC}$ and number of person-years $n_{iT}$ and $n_{iC}$, for the treated and the controls, respectively. Thus, $y_i^* = \log(v_{iT}/n_{iT})$ and $x_i^* = \log(v_{iC}/n_{iC})$. The exact measurement error model is obtained by considering the Poisson distribution for the variables $V_{iT}$ and $V_{iC}$ (Arends et al., 2000), namely,

$$V_{iT} \sim \text{Poisson}\left(n_{iT}e^{y_i}\right)$$

and

$$V_{iC} \sim \text{Poisson}\left(n_{iC}e^{x_i}\right).$$

Despite the possibility of specifying the exact measurement error structure, in practice control risk regression is typically based on the approximate solution, mainly for computational convenience. The *approximate error model* follows a bivariate Normal distribution

$$\begin{pmatrix} Y_i^* \\ X_i^* \end{pmatrix} \sim \text{Normal}_2\left(\begin{pmatrix} y_i \\ x_i \end{pmatrix}, \Sigma_i\right), \text{ where } \Sigma_\text{i} = \begin{pmatrix} \sigma^2_{y_i^*} & \sigma_{y_i^* x_i^*} \\ \sigma_{y_i^* x_i^*} & \sigma^2_{x_i^*} \end{pmatrix}, \tag{22.3}$$

with variance/covariance matrix $\Sigma_i$ specified differently on the basis of the outcome measures. As an example, for log-odds measures of risks

$$\Sigma_i = \begin{pmatrix} v_{iT}^{-1} + (n_{iT} - v_{iT})^{-1} & 0 \\ 0 & v_{iC}{}^{-1} + (n_{iC} - v_{iC})^{-1} \end{pmatrix},$$

while for log event rates

$$\Sigma_i = \begin{pmatrix} v_{iT}^{-1} & 0 \\ 0 & v_{iC}^{-1} \end{pmatrix}.$$

### 22.2.2 Correction Techniques

Structural and functional approaches to measurement error correction in control risk regression have been investigated in the literature. In the following, the density function for model (22.2) will be denoted by $f_{Y_i|X_i}(y_i|x_i;\beta_0,\beta_x,\tau^2)$, while the density function for the measurement error model will be denoted by $f_{Y_i^*X_i^*|Y_iX_i}(y_i^*,x_i^*|y_i,x_i;\Sigma_i)$, remembering that $\Sigma_i$ is typically known under the approximate measurement error model.

#### 22.2.2.1 Structural Approaches

The structural approach for measurement error correction requires the specification of a distribution for the risk measure in the control condition $X_i$. Let $f_{X_i}(x_i;\delta)$ denote the density function for $X_i$, depending on a parameter vector $\delta$. The likelihood function $L(\theta)$ for the whole parameter vector $\theta = \left(\beta_0,\beta_x,\tau^2,\delta^\text{T}\right)^\text{T}$ based on the observations $(x_i^*, y_i^*)$ is

$$\begin{aligned} L(\theta) &= \prod_{i=1}^n \int_\mathbb{R}\int_\mathbb{R} f\left(y_i,x_i,y_i^*,x_i^*;\theta\right) dy_i dx_i \\ &= \prod_{i=1}^n \int_\mathbb{R}\int_\mathbb{R} f_{Y_i^*X_i^*|Y_iX_i}\left(y_i^*,x_i^*|y_i,x_i;\Sigma_i\right) f_{Y_i|X_i}\left(y_i|x_i;\beta_0,\beta_x,\tau^2\right) \\ &\qquad f_{X_i}\left(x_i;\delta\right) dy_i dx_i, \end{aligned} \tag{22.4}$$

where the integration is with respect to the unknown $(x_i, y_i)$. A common strategy specifies the model for $X_i$ through a Normal distribution, $X_i \sim$

$Normal(\mu, \nu^2)$, so that $\delta = (\mu, \nu^2)^{\mathrm{T}}$ (e.g., McIntosh, 1996; van Houwelingen et al., 2002). When the approximate measurement error model is used, the Normal specification for the distribution of $X_i$ allows to write the likelihood function in (22.4) in closed-form, as

$$\begin{pmatrix} Y_i^* \\ X_i^* \end{pmatrix} \sim \text{Normal}_2 \left( \begin{pmatrix} \beta_0 + \beta_x \mu \\ \mu \end{pmatrix}, \Sigma_i + \begin{pmatrix} \tau^2 + \beta_x^2 \nu^2 & \beta_x \nu^2 \\ \beta_x \nu^2 & \nu^2 \end{pmatrix} \right). \quad (22.5)$$

The main advantage of such a specification is computational. Limitations are related to the risk of misspecification of the model components. In particular, there is no way to check the normality assumption for the unobserved risk measure in the control condition and common forms of non-normality can often occur in the source population (Lee and Thompson, 2008; Ghidey et al., 2007, 2013). Examples include skewness due to the presence of outliers or bimodality due to patients' characteristics. Again, deviations from normality at the population level can arise as a consequence of a case-control sampling scheme (Guolo, 2008). Although misspecification of the distribution of the unknown measure in the control condition cannot sensibly affect the estimation of the regression coefficient, inference on the variance components can be biased with consequences on the results of all the parameters of the model. See Ghidey et al. (2007, 2013) and Guolo (2013) for discussion in control risk regression and Verbeke and Lesaffre (1997), Zhang and Davidian (2001), Lee and Thompson (2008) for a general discussion about misspecification of latent variables in random-effects models.

The literature in control risk regression has investigated flexible alternatives to the Normal specification for $X_i$ in order to face the risk of misspecification. Arends et al. (2000) and Ghidey et al. (2007) suggest to model the distribution of $X_i$ through a mixture of Normal variables. Inference proceeds within a Bayesian framework in Arends et al. (2000) and according to a semi-parametric approach based on a penalized mixture in Ghidey et al. (2007). The proposals increase the flexibility of the model and can be straightforwardly implemented with existing software. Nevertheless, the applicability is restricted to situations with no outliers and the choice of the number of mixture components is known to be a difficult task, e.g., Lee and Thompson (2008). An alternative strategy proposed by Lee and Thompson (2008) within a Bayesian framework specifies the distribution of the risk measure through skewed extensions of the Normal and the $t$ distributions belonging to the Fernandez and Steel (1998) family. The main drawback is the difficult interpretation of the parameters in the distributions and the discontinuity of the Fernandez and Steel family derivatives makes standard likelihood inference not applicable. Guolo (2013) uses a Skew-normal distribution (Azzalini, 1985) in order to prevent deviations from normality due to skewness. The price to pay is a computational complexity of the approach which requires the evaluation of the likelihood function through numerical procedures.

#### 22.2.2.2 Functional Approaches

Only a few solutions have been developed in the literature to face the measurement error problem while avoiding the specification of a distribution for the unobserved risk measure $X_i$. When $x_1, \ldots, x_n$ are considered as nuisance parameters to be estimated, the gain in robustness to misspecification of the control risk distribution is paid in terms of efficiency of the inferential conclusions. As the dimensionality of the parameter space increases, in fact, a fully parametric approach becomes less efficient and may lead to inconsistent estimators (e.g., Ghidey et al., 2013). See also the criticism in van Houwelingen and Senn (1999) and Arends et al. (2000) about a similar approach performed in Thompson et al. (1997) within a Bayesian framework with non-informative prior on $x_1, \ldots, x_n$. Recently, Ghidey et al. (2013) solve the inconsistency problem by focusing on the *corrected score approach* and the *conditional score approach*. The corrected score estimator is derived as the solution of a set of unbiased estimating equations, with a sandwich estimate of the standard error. The conditional score equations are obtained by conditioning on the sufficient statistic for $X_i$. The variability of the resulting estimator is still evaluated through the sandwich formula. While empirical results show that the estimators agree in case of small measurement error, the conditional score estimator is more efficient for large measurement error and small sample size. The main drawback of the conditional score approach, however, is related to the presence of multiple roots, not all guaranteed to be consistent (Stefanski and Carroll, 1987; Tsiatis and Davidian, 2001).

Guolo (2014) investigates the use of SIMEX (Stefanski and Carroll, 1995; Carroll et al., 2006, Chapter 5) to correct for measurement error without specifying a distribution for the control risk. The attention is paid to the approximate measurement error structure. SIMEX performance is comparable to a fully likelihood approach when the normality assumption for $X_i$ holds. Under departures from the normality assumption, a substantial improvement of inferential results using SIMEX over fully parametric alternatives is experienced, especially in the estimation of the between-study variance component $\tau^2$. From a practical point of view, numerical instabilities of the likelihood approach in case of small sample size or small values of the variance components have not been experienced with SIMEX. Disadvantages of SIMEX include a possible increase of the computational burden when extending the model (22.2) in order to include additional study-specific covariates.

### 22.2.3 Software

At the time of writing, only some of the approaches developed for measurement error correction are accompanied by the code necessary for a user-friendly implementation, while no dedicated packages are available yet in the common statistical softwares. Code in the `R` programming language (R Core Team, 2018) is available to reproduce the methods described in Arends et al. (2000),

Ghidey et al. (2013), Guolo (2013, 2014). BUGS code is available in the Appendix of Sharp and Thompson (2000) to reproduce the hierarchical approaches in McIntosh (1996) and Thompson et al. (1997), among others. It is worth mentioning the extension of the approach in Arends et al. (2000) to network meta-analysis provided by Achana et al. (2013), who made available the WinBUGS code in the Appendix of the paper.

## 22.3 Meta-analysis of Diagnostic Tests

Control risk regression represents an instance of the bivariate meta-analysis, as discussed in van Houwelingen et al. (2002), among others, where the risk of measurement error in affecting inferential results is known. Within a similar bivariate context, meta-analysis of diagnostic test accuracy represents an additional framework where measurement errors easily occur. With reference to the medical literature, where diagnostic instruments are routinely used, we consider a test as an instrument to classify patients with a certain disease state of interest and patients without the disease. For simplicity, the attention will be paid to a dichotomous test, that is, a single threshold test distinguishing diseased and not diseased subjects. This is by far the most common situation in practice as well as the one receiving most of the attention in the literature. Extensions to multiple responses diagnostic tests will be discussed later.

Meta-analysis for assessing the accuracy of diagnostic tests differ from meta-analysis of treatment effectiveness, mainly because the information available from each study is not a single summary statistic but a pair of related statistics, typically the sensitivity and the specificity of the diagnostic test. Accordingly, different strategies are needed to properly pooling the study information, accounting for between-study heterogeneity and correcting for possible measurement errors. Results are commonly provided in terms of receiver operating characteristic (ROC) curves, in order to depict the pattern of sensitivities and specificities when the test is performed at different thresholds.

### 22.3.1 Background

Suppose that the studies included in the meta-analysis provide information about a continuous diagnostic (bio)marker. Values of the marker under or above a threshold provide the results of the dichotomous diagnostic test. A diagnostic study is commonly evaluated in terms of *sensitivity* $SE$, the conditional probability of testing positive in diseased subjects, and *specificity* $SP$, the conditional probability of testing negative in nondiseased subjects. Changes in the threshold provide different pairs of sensitivity and specificity, represented by the ROC curve.

The first approach to estimate the ROC curve, called Summary ROC (SROC), is due to Littenberg and Moses (1993). See also Arends et al. (2008). The underlying model considers a transformation from the marker to the test $M$ such that

$$P(M < m|nondiseased) = \frac{e^m}{1+e^m}$$

and

$$P(M < m|diseased) = \frac{e^{-\beta_0+\beta_x m}}{1+e^{-\beta_0+\beta_x m}},$$

for some $\beta_0 \geq 0$ and $\beta_x > 0$. By such a specification, the difference between the mean value in the diseased and nondiseased subjects is $\beta_0/\beta_x$, with a standard deviation equal to $1/\beta_x$. Let $\lambda$ denote the threshold at which the result of the test $M$ is considered positive. Then, the specificity is

$$SP = P(M \leq \lambda|nondiseased) = e^{\lambda}/(1+e^{\lambda}).$$

Littenberg and Moses (1993) focus on the false positive rate defined as the complementary to the specificity, such that $X = \text{logit}(1-SP) = \lambda$. Similarly, the true positive rate or the sensitivity is

$$SE = P(M \geq \lambda|diseased) = \frac{1}{1+e^{-\beta_0+\beta_x\lambda}},$$

so that $Y = \text{logit}(SE) = \beta_0 - \beta_x\lambda$. Accordingly, the linear relationship

$$Y = \beta_0 + \beta_x X, \tag{22.6}$$

summarizes the ROC curve, with $\beta_x$ equal to 1 corresponding to the symmetric ROC curve.

Consider the data from study $i$ in the meta-analysis represented by a two-by-two table as the one reported in Table 22.1, including the number of diseased patients with a positive test result (true positives, $n_{11i}$) or a negative result (false positives, $n_{01i}$), and the number of healthy subjects with a positive test result (false negatives, $n_{10i}$) or a negative test result(true negatives, $n_{00i}$). In order to judge the diagnostic test, the benchmark in identifying the patients is represented by the reference test, also known as *gold standard.*
Let $n_{1i} = n_{11i} + n_{10i}$ be the number of total positives and $n_{0i} = n_{00i} + n_{01i}$ the number of total negatives. Then, the estimate of the sensitivity in study $i$ is given by $n_{11i}/n_{1i}$ and the estimate of the specificity in study $i$ is given by $n_{00i}/n_{0i}$.

In order to obtain an estimation of the ROC curve for a diagnostic marker, Littenberg and Moses (1993) write relationship (22.6) in terms of the difference between (logit of) sensitivity and (logit of) 1-specificity and their sum, namely,

$$D = \beta_0' + \beta_x' S,$$

**TABLE 22.1**
True positives, false positives, true negatives, false negatives from a diagnostic test compared to the reference test.

| | Reference test | |
|---|---|---|
| Diagnostic test | Positive | Negative |
| Positive | $n_{11i}$ | $n_{01i}$ |
| Negative | $n_{10i}$ | $n_{00i}$ |
| | $n_{1i}$ | $n_{0i}$ |

with $D = Y - X$, $S = Y + X$, $\beta_0' = 2\beta_0/(\beta_x + 1)$, $\beta_0' \geq 0$, and $\beta_x' = (\beta_x - 1)/(\beta_x + 1)$, $-1 < \beta_x' < 1$. Quantity $D$ is often referred to as the *diagnostic odds ratio*, the log-odds ratio of a positive test result for diseased patients relative to nondiseased patients ad it represents a single overall indicator of the diagnostic accuracy of a test. Quantity $S$ is related to the threshold of the test, as it is a measure of how often the test is positive. Parameters $\beta_0'$ and $\beta_x'$ are obtained through the least squares regression on the sample based versions of $D$ and $S$ for study $i$, namely $D_i = Y_i - X_i$ and $S_i = Y_i + X_i$, given by $D_i^*$ and $S_i^*$ respectively,

$$D_i^* = \beta_0' + \beta_x' S_i^* + \varepsilon_i, \tag{22.7}$$

where $\varepsilon_i$ is a random error and $D_i^*$ and $S_i^*$ are estimated as

$$d_i^* = y_i^* - x_i^* = \text{logit}(n_{11i}/n_{1i}) - \text{logit}(n_{01i}/n_{0i})$$

and

$$s_i^* = y_i^* + x_i^* = \text{logit}(n_{11i}/n_{1i}) + \text{logit}(n_{01i}/n_{0i}),$$

where $y_i^*$ and $x_i^*$ are the measures of $Y_i$ and $X_i$ from study $i$ and $\text{logit}(p) = \ln\{p/(1-p)\}$.

The SROC is obtained by transforming the estimate of the relationship between $D_i$ and $S_i$ to the ROC space. The SROC model assumes that the differences across the studies result from different thresholds for test positivity. When $\beta_x' = 0$, the curve is symmetric and the log-odds ratio is constant across the studies.

The proposal in Littenberg and Moses (1993) represents a step ahead with respect to preliminary approaches, still diffuse in medical investigations, based on separate univariate meta-analyses for sensitivity and specificity of diagnostic tests, carried out ignoring their positive correlation. Nevertheless, the SROC method has been largely criticised in the literature as a source of unreliable inferential conclusions (e.g., Rutter and Gatsonis, 2001; Arends et al., 2008). First, the approach has a fixed-effects structure, as variability is due only to within-study sampling and threshold effect. Possible sources of between-study heterogeneity, such as study setting and patients' characteristics, are not taken into account. A second substantial drawback is related to the measurement error problem. The independent variable $S_i^*$ in the regression model (22.7) is a summary measure derived from each study included in the meta-analysis and, thus, it is prone to measurement error (e.g., Thompson, 1994). Ignoring it leads to a serious bias of the slope of relationship (22.7), as a consequence of the regression to the mean effect.

The measurement error framework in meta-analysis of diagnostic test accuracy has some similarities as well as interesting differences with respect to control risk regression. The measurement error in $S_i^*$ is the consequence of the measurement error in the observed version of $X_i$ and $Y_i$. Both the error prone variables $X_i^*$ and $Y_i^*$ from study $i$, although different in meaning from the variables in control risk regression, are subjected to measurement error as they represent summary information about the (logit of) sensitivity ad specificity in the source population. The role played by the variables in control risk regression and in meta-analysis of diagnostic accuracy studies is substantially different. In control risk regression, in fact, $Y_i$ represents the response variable, to be related to the measure of risk in the control condition, $X_i$. When dealing with diagnostic accuracy studies, there is not an undoubtedly defined response variable or covariate, as $Y_i$ and $X_i$ can alternatively play one of the roles in order to characterize different summary ROC curves. For example, the regression of $Y_i$ on $X_i$ results in a SROC curve giving the median sensitivity for a certain value of the specificity. Again, the regression of $D_i$ on $S_i$ turns out in the Littenberg and Moses SROC curve. See Arends et al. (2008) for a detailed description of the possibles choices of summary ROC curves available from $(X_i, Y_i)$. Only when a specific regression model is chosen in order to obtain a particular SROC curve, then the role of response and covariate is clearly identified.

### 22.3.2 Measurement Error Correction Methods

#### 22.3.2.1 Bivariate Approach

In order to overcome many of the drawbacks related to the SROC approach, a category of methods based on bivariate mixed-effects models for relating sensitivity and specificity simultaneously has been proposed, e.g., Reitsma et al. (2005), Chu and Cole (2006), Arends et al. (2008), Chu et al. (2012). Following Reitsma et al. (2005) and Arends et al. (2008), the bivariate mixed-effects model has a hierarchical structure with a *between-study model* relating the random effects $Y_i$ and $X_i$ via the bivariate Normal distribution

$$\begin{pmatrix} Y_i \\ X_i \end{pmatrix} \sim \text{Normal}_2\left(\begin{pmatrix} \overline{y} \\ \overline{x} \end{pmatrix}, \begin{pmatrix} \sigma_y^2 & \rho\sigma_y\sigma_x \\ \rho\sigma_y\sigma_x & \sigma_x^2 \end{pmatrix}\right), \tag{22.8}$$

where $\overline{y}$ and $\overline{x}$ represent the means over the studies, $\sigma_y^2$ and $\sigma_x^2$ denote the between-study variances of $Y_i$ and $X_i$, respectively, and $\rho$ is the correlation coefficient. As sensitivity and specificity of a test tend to be negatively correlated, then $Y_i$ and $X_i$ tend to be positively correlated, so that $\rho > 0$.

The *within-study model* takes account of the measurement error in the sample versions of $Y_i$ and $X_i$ given by $Y_i^*$ and $X_i^*$. A common choice is an *approximation of the measurement error distribution* using a bivariate Normal specification for $(Y_i^*, X_i^*)^{\mathrm{T}}$ given $(Y_i = y_i, X_i = x_i)^{\mathrm{T}}$,

$$\begin{pmatrix} Y_i^* \\ X_i^* \end{pmatrix} \sim \text{Normal}_2\left(\begin{pmatrix} y_i \\ x_i \end{pmatrix}, \begin{pmatrix} n_{1i}^{-1} + (n_{1i} - n_{11i})^{-1} & 0 \\ 0 & n_{0i}^{-1} + (n_{0i} - n_{00i})^{-1} \end{pmatrix}\right). \tag{22.9}$$

The within-study variance/covariance matrix in (22.9) is diagonal as sensitivity and specificity are measured on different subjects within each study, implying their covariance being null. The non-zero entries in the matrix are the within-study estimated variances for the logit sensitivity and specificity. See, for example, Arends et al. (2008).

Models (22.8)–(22.9) allow to specify the marginal distribution for $(Y_i, X_i)^{\mathrm{T}}$ as a bivariate Normal distribution with components

$$\begin{pmatrix} Y_i \\ X_i \end{pmatrix} \sim \text{Normal}_2\left(\begin{pmatrix} \overline{y} \\ \overline{x} \end{pmatrix}, \Sigma_i\right),$$

where

$$\Sigma_i = \begin{pmatrix} \sigma_y^2 + n_{1i}^{-1} + (n_{1i} - n_{11i})^{-1} & \rho\sigma_y\sigma_x \\ \rho\sigma_y\sigma_x & \sigma_x^2 + n_{0i}^{-1} + (n_{0i} - n_{00i})^{-1} \end{pmatrix}.$$

Compared to the approach in Littenberg and Moses (1992), the bivariate Normal model, commonly termed Normal-Normal model, takes into account the measurement error problem via a structural approach, by modeling the uncertainty in measuring $X_i$ via $X_i^*$. From a practical point of view, the fit of the resulting approximate model with respect to the parameter vector $\theta = \left(\overline{y}, \overline{x}, \sigma_y^2, \sigma_x^2, \rho\right)^{\mathrm{T}}$ has no computational difficulties. Despite such advantages, criticism towards the Normal-Normal model has arisen. First of all, the approach needs an ad hoc correction that adds 0.5 to the two-by-two table cells equal to zero, in order to avoid unreliable estimates of terms in $\Sigma_i$. Moreover, the risk of biased inferential conclusions is substantial in case of small sample size, when the approximation to the Normal does not hold (Chu and Cole, 2006; Hamza et al., 2008a; Guolo, 2017).

The Normal-Normal model has an interesting interpretation in terms of the model previously suggested by Rutter and Gatsonis (2001) within a Bayesian framework (Harbord et al., 2007). The model in Rutter and Gatsonis (2001) solves many of the drawbacks of the SROC approach, the measurement error included, at the price of more involved parameterization and implementation, which reduce its appealing in routine practice.

The *exact measurement error model* considers that the number of true positives and false positives observed within each study are realizations of

Binomial variables (Chu and Cole, 2006; Arends et al., 2008),

$$n_{11i} \sim \text{Binomial}\left(n_{1i}, (1+e^{-y_i})^{-1}\right) \tag{22.10}$$

and

$$n_{10i} \sim \text{Binomial}\left(n_{0i}, (1+e^{-x_i})^{-1}\right). \tag{22.11}$$

The resulting generalized model specified by (22.8) with error model expressed as in (22.10)–(22.11), commonly termed Binomial-Normal model, avoids the ad hoc correction needed by the approximated solution, but it does not provide a likelihood function for $\theta$ in closed-form. Accordingly, standard software cannot be used for inference and numerical integration is needed. Several authors warn against the risk of convergence problems of optimization algorithms applied to the Binomial-Normal model in terms of non-positive definite variance/covariance matrix and values of the variance components on the boundary of the parameter space (e.g., Hamza et al., 2008b; Chen et al., 2017; Takwoingi et al., 2017; Guolo, 2017). High failure rate occurs when the sample size is small or under departures from the normality assumption for the random effects. See, for example, the simulation experiments in Chen et al. (2017) and in Guolo (2017), highlighting failure rates larger than the Normal-Normal model under $t$ or Skew-normal random-effects distributions. A step ahead towards the avoidance of nonconvergence problems and retrieval of some computational simplicity is the composite likelihood approach in Chen et al. (2017), who modify the Binomial-Normal model using an independent working assumption between sensitivity and specificity, that is, by fixing the between-study correlation equal to zero.

Once the maximum likelihood estimate of $\theta$ is obtained, with either the approximate or the exact within-study model, the construction of a summary ROC curve can be obtained as a characterization of the estimated bivariate model (22.8), see Arends et al. (2008). A common example is the regression line of $y_i$ on $x_i$ given by $y_i = \overline{y} + \frac{\sigma_{yx}}{\sigma_x^2}(x_i - \overline{x})$ to estimate the median sensitivity for a given value of 1-specificity when transformed to the ROC space.

#### 22.3.2.2 Alternative Approaches

A recent literature has focused on extensions and modifications of the bivariate model introduced in the previous section.

A Bayesian version is implemented in Verde (2010), who specifies a bivariate Normal between-study model based on differences and sums of appropriate modifications of the true positive rate and the false positive rate for each study included in the meta-analysis. The Bayesian approach in Paul et al. (2010) considers integrated nested Laplace approximations for inference according to the Binomial-Normal model formulation, with the main aim of reducing the numerical drawbacks of the likelihood approach, especially in case of small sample size. Guo et al. (2017) extend the methodology in Paul et al. (2010) by investigating the penalized complexity prior framework (Simpson et al.,

2017) for selecting informative priors for the variance parameters and the correlation parameter.

A different part of the recent literature has considered the use of copula representation. Although the attention is not directly focused on the measurement error problem, the issue is implicitly taken into account. Kuss et al. (2014) modify the Binomial-Normal model by describing the sensitivity and the specificity for each study included in the meta-analysis on their original scale through Beta distributions, instead of modeling the distribution of their logits $Y_i$ and $X_i$. The correlation between the number of true positives and true negatives is taken into account by a bivariate copula. The resulting model is a bivariate logistic regression model, as for the Binomial-Normal approach, but with the likelihood function in closed-form. Nikoloulopoulos (2015) generalizes the Binomial-Normal model using a copula representation of the random-effects distribution with Normal margins and suggests a copula mixed model for sensitivity and specificity on the original scale with Beta margins. With respect to this, the approach in Kuss et al. (2014) is an approximation as they use a copula model for the true positives and true negatives that have Beta-Binomial margins.

Chen et al. (2016b) propose a Beta-Binomial model in the same spirit of Kuss et al. (2014), although with no use of copula representation. They refer to the bivariate Sarmanov distribution family to describe the sensitivity and the specificity for each study following Chu et al. (2012) and then rely on a composite likelihood approach for inference in line with Chen et al. (2017). See also Nikoloulopoulos (2017) for a comparison of the composite likelihood method in Chen et al. (2016b) and the copula random-effects model in Nikoloulopoulos (2015).

Eusebi et al. (2014) extend the Binomial-Normal model with a discrete latent variable in order to cluster the studies and provide a different between-study correlation between sensitivity and specificity per latent class.

Recently, Guolo (2017) suggested the use of SIMEX as a *functional approach* to correct for measurement error in meta-analysis of diagnostic accuracy studies. As measurement error affects both the response and the covariate, whichever the role played by $Y_i$ and $X_i$, the reference is to the double SIMEX introduced by Holcomb (1999). The performance of SIMEX is comparable to likelihood-based solutions, in either the Normal-Normal model or the Binomial-Normal model, when the normality assumption for the random-effects holds, and superior in case of low to high skewness in the random-effects distribution. From a computational point of view, SIMEX does not experience convergence problems neither under departures from the normality assumption nor in case of small sample size or increasing correlation between (logits of) sensitivity and specificity.

The use of a logit transformation for modeling the distribution of the sensitivity and the specificity is the most common choice in applications. Some alternatives, as the probit transformation or the complementary log-log transformation, have been discussed within the bivariate modeling approach in Chu et al. (2010) and in Doebler et al. (2012) and evaluated in scenarios including small sample size or skewed distributions. A recent alternative is suggested by Negeri et al. (2018) with reference to the Normal-Normal model. The Authors investigate the use of two variance-stabilizing transformations, namely, the arcsine square and the Freeman-Tukey double arcsine transformation (Freeman and Tukey, 1950) to better approximate normality. Advantages over the Normal-Normal model based of logits include no convergence issues neither an ad hoc continuity correction in case of sparse data.

#### 22.3.2.3 Multiple Thresholds

Often, the performance of a diagnostic test is evaluated at multiple thresholds representing, for example, increasing levels of severity of a pathology. Correspondingly, each study included in a meta-analysis identifies diseased and nondiseased patients provided by the test at different thresholds, thus resulting in a couple of sensitivity and specificity for each threshold. Accounting for multiple outcomes per study makes the problem of diagnostic test accuracy belonging to the so-called *multivariate meta-analysis*. Within this framework, several proposals in the literature extend the bivariate approach developed for the single threshold case, although with no explicit reference to the measurement error framework.

Hamza et al. (2009) extend the Binomial-Normal model in Arends et al. (2008) to handle meta-analysis of diagnostic accuracy studies with multiple, possibly different, thresholds per study. The presence of multiple information from each single study included in the meta-analysis complicates the within-study model, in this way making the likelihood evaluation more troublesome. One of the main limits of the approach, in fact, is related to convergence problems and the unreliability of likelihood-based solutions for large number of thresholds which implies a substantial increase of the parameter dimension. Riley et al. (2014) aim at reducing the complexity and the computational limits of the approach in Hamza et al. (2009) at the price of relying on the approximate Normal model in place of the exact distribution for the within-study components. Such an approximation is questionable in case of small sample study. Alternative approaches include the random-effects approach for ordinal models in Bipat and Zwinderman (2010), the Poisson-correlated gamma frailty model in Putter et al. (2010), the linear random-effects model for describing the distribution function of the biomarkers for diseased and nondiseased patients in Steinhauser et al. (2016).

### 22.3.3 Software

Much of the software developed to implement measurement error correction approaches is made available by the authors through the supplementary material accompanying their published papers. Arends et al. (2008) made available the SAS code needed to reproduce the data analysis, Hamza et al. (2008)

made available the SAS code needed to fit the Binomial-Normal model, Eusebi et al. (2014) made available the LATENT GOLD code to implement the latent class bivariate model, while Guolo (2017) made available the `R` code to implement the double SIMEX approach. Details about the `R` code useful to implement the integrated nested Laplace approximations in the bivariate model are reported in Paul et al. (2010, Appendix). The Winbugs code to implement the method in Bipat and Zwinderman (2010) is available in the appendix of the paper. The `R` code to reproduce the analyses in Steinhauser et al. (2016) and in Negeri et al. (2018) is available as supporting information of the papers.

In some cases, the software is made available as `R` package. The copula random-effects model developed by Nikoloulopoulos (2015) is implemented in the `R` package `CopulaREMADA` (Nikoloulopoulos, 2016). The composite likelihood approach in Chen et al. (2016b, 2017) is implemented in the `R` package `xmeta` (Chen et al., 2016a). The model in Reitsma et al. (2005) is implemented in the `R` packages `Metatron` (Huang, 2014) and `mada` (Doebler, 2017). The Bayesian approach in Verde (2010) is implemented in the `R` package `bamdit` (Verde, 2017). The Bayesian bivariate meta-analysis based on the integrated nested Laplace approximations, also supporting the penalized complexity prior framework as described in Guo et al. (2017), is implemented in the `R` package `meta4diag` (Guo and Riebler, 2018).

## Bibliography

Achana, F. A., Cooper, N. J., Dias, S., Lu, G., Rice, S. J. C., Kendrick, D., and Sutton, A. (2013). Extending methods for investigating the relationship between treatment effect and baseline risk from pairwise meta-analysis to network meta-analysis. *Statistics in Medicine*, 32, 752-771.

Arends, L. R., Hamza, T. H., van Houwelingen, H. C., Heijenbrok-Kal, M. H., Hunink, M. G. M., and Stijnen, T. (2008). Bivariate random effects meta-analysis of ROC curves. *Medical Decision Making*, 28, 621-638.

Arends, L. R., Hoes, A. W., Lubsen, J., Grobbee, D. E., and Stijnen, T. (2000). Baseline risk as predictor of treatment benefit: three clinical meta-re-analyses. *Statistics in Medicine*, 19, 3497-3518.

Azzalini, A. (1985). A class of distributions which includes the normal ones. *Scandinavian Journal of Statistics*, 12, 171-178.

Bipat, S. and Zwinderman, A. H. (2010). Multivariate fixed- and random-effects models for summarizing ordinal data in meta-analysis of diagnostic staging studies. *Research Synthesis Methods*, 1, 136-148.

Brand, R. and Kragt, H. (1992). Importance of trends in the interpretation of an overall odds ratio in the meta-analysis of clinical trials. *Statistics in Medicine*, 11, 2077-2082.

Carroll, R. J., Ruppert, D., Stefanski, L. A., and Crainiceanu, C. (2006). *Measurement Error in Nonlinear Models: A Modern Perspective.* Chapman & Hall, CRC Press, Boca Raton.

Chen, Y., Hong, C., Chu, H., and Liu, Y. (2016a). xmeta: A Toolbox for Multivariate Meta-Analysis. *R package* version 1.1-4. https://CRAN.R-project.org/package=xmeta

Chen, Y., Hong, C., Ning, Y., and Su, X. (2016b). Meta-analysis of studies with bivariate binary outcomes: a marginal beta-binomial model approach. *Statistics in Medicine*, 35, 21-40.

Chen, Y., Liu, Y., Ning, J., Nie, L., Zhu, H., and Chu, H. (2017). A composite likelihood method for bivariate meta-analysis in diagnostic systematic reviews. *Statistical Methods in Medical Research*, 26, 914-930.

Chu, H. and Cole, S.R. (2006). Bivariate meta-analysis of sensitivity and specificity with sparse data: a generalized linear mixed model approach. *Journal of Clinical Epidemiology*, 59, 1331-1333.

Chu, H., Guo, H. and Zhou, Y. (2010). Bivariate random effects meta-analysis of diagnostic studies using generalized linear mixed models. *Medical Decision Making*, 30, 499-508.

Chu, H., Nie, L., Chen, Y., Huang, Y., and Sun, W. (2012). Bivariate random effects models for meta-analysis of comparative studies with binary outcomes: methods for the absolute risk difference and relative risk. *Statistical Methods in Medical Research*, 21, 621-633.

DerSimonian, R. and Laird, N. (1986). Meta-analysis in clinical trials. *Controlled Clinical Trials*, 7, 177-188.

Doebler P. (2017). mada: Meta-analysis of diagnostic accuracy. *R package* version 0.5.8. https://CRAN.R-project.org/package=mada

Doebler, P., Holling, H., and Böhning, D. (2012). A mixed model approach to meta-analysis of diagnostic studies with binary test outcome. *Psychological Methods*, 17, 418-436.

Eusebi, P., Reitsma, J. B., and Vermunt, J. K. (2014). Latent class bivariate model for the meta-analysis of diagnostic test accuracy studies. *BMC Medical Research Methodology*, 14, 88.

Fernandez, C. and Steel, M. F. J. (1998). On Bayesian modelling of fat tails and skewness. *Journal of American Statistical Association*, 93, 359-371.

Freeman, M. F. and Tukey, J. W. (1950). Transformations related to the angular and the square root. *Annals of Mathematical Statistics*, 21, 607-611.

Ghidey, W., Lesaffre, E., and Stijnen, T. (2007). Semi-parametric modelling of the distribution of the baseline risk in meta-analysis. *Statistics in Medicine*, 26, 5434-5444.

Ghidey, W., Stijnen, T., and van Houwelingen, H. C. (2013). Modelling the effect of baseline risk in meta-analysis: A review from the perspective of errors-in-variables regression. *Statistical Methods in Medical Research*, 22, 307-323.

Guo, J. and Riebler, A. (2018). meta4diag: Bayesian bivariate meta-analysis of diagnostic test studies for routine practice. *Journal of Statistical Software*, 83, 1-31.

Guo, J., Riebler, A., and Rue, H. (2017). Bayesian bivariate meta-analysis of diagnostic test studies with interpretable priors. *Statistics in Medicine*, 36, 3039-3058.

Guolo, A. (2008). A flexible approach to measurement error correction in case-control studies. *Biometrics*, 64, 1207-1214.

Guolo, A. (2013). Flexibly modeling the baseline risk in meta-analysis. *Statistics in Medicine*, 32, 40-50.

Guolo, A. (2014). The SIMEX approach to measurement error correction in meta-analysis with baseline risk as covariate. *Statistics in Medicine*, 33, 2062-2076.

Guolo, A. (2017). A double SIMEX approach for bivariate random-effects meta-analysis of diagnostic accuracy studies. *BMC Medical Research Methodology*, 17, 6.

Gurevitch, J., Koricheva, J., Nakagawa, S., and Stewart, G. (2018). Meta-analysis and the science of research synthesis. *Nature*, 555, 175-182.

Hamza, T. H., Arends, L. R., van Houwelingen, H. C., and Stijnen, T. (2009). Multivariate random effects meta-analysis of diagnostic tests with multiple thresholds. *BMC Medical Research Methodology*, 10, 73.

Hamza, T. H., van Houwelingen, H. C., and Stijnen, T. (2008a). The binomial distribution of meta-analysis was preferred to model within-study variability. *Journal of Clinical Epidemiology*, 61, 41-51.

Hamza, T. H., Reitsma, J. B., and Stijnen, T. (2008b). Meta-analysis of diagnostic studies: A comparison of random intercept, normal-normal, and binomial-normal bivariate summary ROC approaches. *Medical Decision Making*, 28, 639-649.

Harbord, R. M., Deeks, J. J., Egger, M., Whiting, P., and Sterne, J.A. (2007). A unification of models for meta-analysis of diagnostic accuracy studies. *Biostatistics*, 8, 239-251.

Ho, K. M. and Sheridan, D. J. (2006). Meta-analysis of frusemide to prevent or treat acute renal failure. *British Medical Journal*, 333, 420-423.

Hoaglin, D. C. (2015). We know less than we should about methods of meta-analysis. *Research Synthesis Methods*, 6, 287-289.

Holcomb, J. (1999). Regression with covariates and outcome calculated from a common set of variables measured with error: Estimation using the SIMEX method. *Statistics in Medicine*, 18, 2847-2862.

van Houwelingen, H. C., Arends, L. R., and Stijnen, T. (2002). Advanced methods in meta-analysis: multivariate approach and meta-regression. *Statistics in Medicine*, 21, 589-624.

van Houwelingen, H. C. and Senn, S. (1999). Investigating underlying risk as a source of heterogeneity in meta-analysis (letter). *Statistics in Medicine*, 18, 107-113.

Huang, H. (2014). Metatron: Meta-analysis for Classification Data and Correction to Imperfect Reference. R package version 0.1-1. https://CRAN.R-project.org/package=Metatron

Koricheva, J., Gurevitch, J., and Mengersen, K. (Eds.). (2013). *Handbook of Meta-analysis in Ecology and Evolution.* Princeton University Press.

Kuss, O., Hoyer, A., and Solms, A. (2014). Meta-analysis for diagnostic accuracy studies: a new statistical model using beta-binomial distributions and bivariate copulas. *Statistics in Medicine*, 33, 17-30.

Lee, J. L. and Thompson, S. G. (2008). Flexible parametric models for random-effects distributions. *Statistics in Medicine*, 27, 418-434.

Littenberg, B. and Moses, L. E. (1993). Estimating diagnostic-accuracy from multiple conflicting reports: a new meta-analytic method. *Medical Decision Making*, 13, 313-321.

McIntosh, M. W. (1996). The population risk as an explanatory variable in research synthesis of clinical trials. *Statistics in Medicine*, 15, 1713-1728.

Negeri, Z. F., Shaikh, M., and Beyene, J. (2018). Bivariate random-effects meta-analysis models for diagnostic test accuracy studies using arcsine-based transformations. *Biometrical Journal*, 60, 827-844.

Nikoloulopoulos, A. K. (2015). A mixed effect model for bivariate meta-analysis of diagnostic test accuracy studies using a copula representation of the random effects distribution. *Statistics in Medicine*, 34, 3842-3865.

Nikoloulopoulos, A. K. (2016). CopulaREMADA: Copula Mixed Effect Models for Bivariate and Trivariate Meta-Analysis of Diagnostic Test Accuracy Studies. *R package* version 1.0. https://CRAN.R-project.org/package=CopulaREMADA

Nikoloulopoulos, A. K. (2018). On composite likelihood in bivariate meta-analysis of diagnostic test accuracy studies. *AStA Advances in Statistical Analysis*, 102, 211-227.

Paul, M., Riebler, A., Bachmann, L. M., Ruem H., and Held, L. (2010). Bayesian bivariate meta-analysis of diagnostic test studies using integrated nested Laplace approximations. *Statistics in Medicine*, 29, 1325-1339.

Putter, H., Fiocco, M., and Stijnen T. (2010). Meta-analysis of diagnostic test accuracy studies with multiple thresholds using survival methods. *Biometrical Journal*, 1, 95-110.

R Core Team (2018). *R: A Language and Environment for Statistical Computing.* R Foundation for Statistical Computing, Vienna, Austria. URL https://www.R-project.org/.

Reitsma, J. B., Glas, A. S., Rutjes, A. W. S., Scholten, R. J., Bossuyt, P. M., and Zwinderman, A. H. (2005). Bivariate analysis of sensitivity and specificity produces informative summary measures in diagnostic reviews. *Journal of Clinical Epidemiology*, 58, 982-990.

Riley, R. D., Takwoingi, Y., Trikalinos, T., Guha, A., Biswas, A., Ensor, J., Morris, R. K., and Deeks, J. J. (2014). Meta-analysis of test accuracy studies with multiple and missing thresholds: A multivariate-normal model. *Journal of Biometrics & Biostatistics*, 5, 3.

Roberts, C. J. (2005). Issues in meta-regression analysis: an overview. *Journal of Economics Surveys*, 19, 295-298.

Rutter, C. M. and Gatsonis, C. A. (2001). A hierarchical regression approach to meta-analysis of diagnostic test accuracy evaluations. *Statistics in Medicine*, 20, 2865-2884.

Schmid, C. H., Lau, J., McIntosh, M. W., and Cappelleri, J. C. (1998). An empirical study of the effect of the control rate as a predictor of treatment efficacy in meta-analysis of clinical trials. *Statistics in Medicine*, 17, 1923-1942.

Schmid, C. H., Stark, P. C., Berlin, J. A., Landais, P., and Lau, J. (2004). Meta-regression detected associations between heterogeneous treatment effects and study-level, but not patient-level, factors. *Journal of Clinical Epidemiology*, 57, 683-697.

Senn, S. (1994). Importance of trends in the interpretation of an overall odds ratio in the meta-analysis of clinical trials. Letters to the editor (with author's reply). *Statistics in Medicine*, 13, 293-296.

Sharp, S. J. and Thompson, S. G. (2000). Analysing the relationship between treatment effect and underlying risk in meta-analysis: comparison and development of approaches. *Statistics in Medicine*, 19, 3251-3274.

Sharp, S. J., Thompson, S. G., and Altman, D. G. (1996). The relation between treatment benefit and underlying risk in meta-analysis. *British Medical Journal*, 313, 735-738.

Simpson, D., Rue, H., Riebler, A., Martins, T. G., and Sørbye, S. H. (2017). Penalising model component complexity: A principled, practical approach to constructing priors. *Statistical Science*, 32, 1-28.

Stefanski, L. A. and Carroll, R. J. (1987). Conditional scores and optimal scores for generalized linear measurement-error models. *Biometrika*, 74, 703-716.

Stefanski, L. A. and Cook J. R. (1995). Simulation-extrapolation: The measurement error jackknife. *Journal of the American Statistical Association*, 90, 1247-1256.

Steinhauser, S., Schumacher, M., and Rücker, G. (2016). Modelling multiple thresholds in meta-analysis of diagnostic test accuracy studies. *BMC Medical Research Methodology*, 16, 97.

Sutton, A. J. and Higgins, J. P. T. (2008). Recent developments in meta-analysis. *Statistics in Medicine*, 27, 625-650.

Takwoingi, Y., Guo, B., Riley, R. D., and Deeks, J. J. (2017). Performance of methods for meta-analysis of diagnostic test accuracy with few studies or sparse data. *Statistical Methods in Medical Research*, 26, 1896-1911.

Thompson, S. G. (1994). Why sources of heterogeneity in meta-analysis should be investigated. *British Medical Journal*, 309, 1351-1355.

Thompson, S. G., Smith, T. C., and Sharp, S. J. (1997). Investigating underlying risk as a source of heterogeneity in meta-analysis. *Statistics in Medicine*, 16, 2741-2758.

Tsiatis, A. A. and Davidian, M. (2001). A semiparametric estimator for the proportional hazards model with longitudinal covariates measured with error. *Biometrika*, 88, 447-458.

Verbeke, G. and Lesaffre, E. (1997). The effect of misspecifying the random effects distribution in linear models for longitudinal data. *Computational Statistics and Data Analysis*, 23, 541-556.

Verde, P. E. (2010). Meta-analysis of diagnostic test data: A bivariate Bayesian modeling approach. *Statistics in Medicine*, 29, 3088-3102.

Verde, P. E. (2017). bamdit: Bayesian Meta-Analysis of Diagnostic Test Data. R package version 3.1.0. https://CRAN.R-project.org/package=bamdit

Viechtbauer, W. (2007a). Confidence intervals for the amount of heterogeneity in meta-analysis. *Statistics in Medicine*, 26, 37-52.

Viechtbauer, W. (2007b). Hypothesis tests for population heterogeneity in meta- analysis. *British Journal of Mathematical and Statistical Psychology*, 60, 29-60.

Wang, H., Boissel, J. -P., and Nony, P. (2009). Revisiting the relationship between baseline risk and risk under treatment. *Emerging Themes in Epidemiology*, 6, 1.

Zeng, D. and Lin, D. Y. (2015). On random-effects meta-analysis. *Biometrika*, 102, 281-294.

Zhang, D. and Davidian, M. (2001). Linear mixed models with flexible distributions of random effects for longitudinal data. *Biometrics*, 57, 795-802.

# Part VII

# Bayesian Analysis

# 23

# *Bayesian Adjustment for Misclassification*

**James D. Stamey and John W. Seaman Jr.**

## CONTENTS



## 23.1 Introduction

Misclassification in binary variables is a common problem that is particularly prevalent in areas such as public health, epidemiology, and quality control. Frequentist approaches to accounting for misclassification have a long history dating back to at least Bross (1954) and the highly influential paper by Tenenbein (1970). The latter introduced the *double sampling scheme*, in which a subset of the fallibly classified subjects is re-examined with an infallible instrument—a *gold standard*—producing a *validation data set.*

Early frequentist approaches are generally based on one of two assumptions. One is that the diagnostic test has known properties. Specifically, the probability of a true positive, or *sensitivity*, $S$, and the the probability of a true negative, or *specificity*, $C$, are assumed known. If $S$ and $C$ are not known, then early approaches assumed that the binary variable could be measured twice, first with a cheap, fallible instrument and then again with a more expensive, infallible instrument, leading to the double sampling scheme.

Of course, an infallible classifier may not be available. Hui and Walter (1980) demonstrate that, for samples from two distinct populations with

DOI: 10.1201/9781315101279-23 

sufficiently distinct prevalences, two conditionally independent, fallible classifiers can render all the unknown parameters estimable. Most of these methods require the usual large-sample approximations for the construction of interval estimates or testing of hypotheses.

Early Bayesian approaches to the problem of binary misclassification often extended the double sampling method of Tenenbein and assumed the availability of validation data, that is, where both a fallible and infallible classifier are used. Prescott and Garthwaite (2002) provide excellent examples of this, based on well known cervical cancer and sudden infant death syndrome data sets.

Again, a gold standard may not be available, precluding the use of double sampling. In that context, Joseph et al. (1995) consider Bayesian analyses of a single binomial proportion while Gustafson et al. (2001) consider the comparison of two proportions where expert elicited informative priors are used in order to adjust for misclassification. The result of such efforts are partially identified models (Gustafson, 2015) that have the virtue of avoiding the fixing of $S$ and $C$ without ignoring misclassification. Bayesian methods for binary misclassification problems have been extended to regression models with covariate misclassification Beavers and Stamey (2012), and binary regression models with misclassification in the response (McInturff et al., 2004; Prescott and Garthwaite, 2002).

The use of a joint prior on $S$ and $C$ can be thought of as part of an integral sensitivity analysis (Greenland, 2009). The joint prior for the diagnostic test parameters simultaneously accounts for a range of values for sensitivity and specificity instead of a sequence of fixed values as would be used in a frequentist Monte Carlo sensitivity analysis (Lash and Silliman, 2000). The Bayesian approach has the advantage that it is part of the overall analysis and not a separate step; that is, when sensitivity and specificity are unknown but are provided with a joint prior, a sensitivity analysis is implicit in the formulation of the posterior.

Accounting for misclassification, or other forms of non-sampling bias such as unmeasured confounding and measurement error in continuous covariates, generally adds more parameters to the model than can be estimated by the sample alone. In this chapter we focus on three approaches to correct for misclassification that directly address this lack of sufficient information. These methods are informative priors, validation data, and multiple diagnostic tests. Validation data and multiple testing are also commonly used by frequentists. The use of informative priors is the most distinctively Bayesian approach of the three and has been applied in many situations where identifiability is an issue. Eberly and Carlin (2000) demonstrate how multiple random effects in spatial models can yield non-identifiable models and posterior inference is dependent upon informative priors. McCandless et al. (2007) address unmeasured confounding by use of priors in a Bayesian context. Greenland (2009) provides an overview of Bayesian correction for selection bias, unmeasured confounding, and covariate misclassification.

This chapter is organized as follows. We first review the three approaches of misclassification correction discussed above, using the single-proportion case for illustration. We next consider multiple population cases including logistic regression with response misclassification. Following this we discuss alternative prior configurations besides the generally considered conjugate forms. We close with a discussion about other areas of application and software.

## 23.2 Methods of Adjusting for Misclassification

We begin by describing three common methods for adjusting for misclassification: using validation data, using multiple fallible assessments, and using expert elicited priors. Only the latter is exclusively Bayesian. However, the other two approaches have advantages within a Bayesian framework they need not have in the frequentist paradigm.

### 23.2.1 Using Validation Data: A Bayesian Two-Stage Method

Early frequentist approaches such as Tenenbien (1970) assumed the availability of an expensive gold standard for a (usually small) fraction of the data. Thus the data are split into two independent samples we refer to as the *validation study data*, where both the fallible and infallible classifier are applied, and the *main study data*, where only the fallible test is applied. In a validation study of size $n_v$, we denote the true count as $Y_v$, the fallible count as $Y_v^*$, the number of true positives as $Y_{1v}$, and number of false negatives as $Y_{2v}$. Thus $Y_v = Y_{1v} + Y_{2v}$. Let the sensitivity and specificity be denoted by $S$ and $C$, respectively. Suppose we observe $\mathbf{Y}_v \equiv (Y_{1v}, Y_{2v}, Y_v^*)$ yielding $\mathbf{y}_v \equiv (y_{1v}, y_{2v}, y_v^*)$. Then the likelihood from the validation sample is

$$l(\theta, S, C|\mathbf{y}_v) = \theta^{y_{1v}+y_{2v}}(1-\theta)^{n_v-y_{1v}-y_{2v}} S^{y_{1v}}(1-S)^{y_{2v}} \times C^{n_v-y_v^*-y_{2v}}(1-C)^{y_v^*-y_{1v}}. \quad (23.1)$$

The validation data can form the basis of informative priors for $\theta, S$, and $C$ by putting uniform, i.e., Beta(1, 1), priors on each of the parameters and combining with the validation data.[1] This first stage of the method yields the following posteriors based on the validation data:

$$\begin{aligned} \theta|\mathbf{y}_v &\sim \text{Beta}(y_{1v} + y_{2v} + 1, n_v - y_{1v} - y_{2v} + 1), \\ S|\mathbf{y}_v &\sim \text{Beta}(y_{1v} + 1, y_{2v} + 1), \end{aligned} \quad (23.2)$$

[1] Beta$(a, b)$ denotes a beta distribution with shape parameters $a$ and $b$.

and

$$C|\mathbf{y}_v \sim \text{Beta}(n_v - y_v^* - y_{2v} + 1, y_v^* - y_{1v} + 1).$$

These posterior distributions become the priors for the main study data, consisting of $n$ Bernoulli events yielding the count $Y^*$, where

$$Y^* \sim \text{Binomial}(n, \theta^*)$$

and $\theta^* = \theta S + (1-\theta)(1-C)$. If we observe $Y^* = y^*$, this yields the joint posterior

$$\begin{aligned}\pi(\theta, S, C|\mathbf{y}_v, y^*) \propto\ & (\theta S + (1-\theta)(1-C))^{y^*} (\theta(1-S) + (1-\theta)C)^{n-y^*} \\ & \times \theta^{y_{1v}+y_{2v}}(1-\theta)^{n_v - y_{1v} - y_{2v}} S^{y_{1v}}(1-S)^{y_{2v}} \\ & \times C^{n_v - y_v^* - y_{2v}}(1-C)^{y_v^* - y_{1v}},\end{aligned} \tag{23.3}$$

thus completing the second stage of the analysis. There is no convenient closed form for the marginal posterior distribution of any of the parameters. MCMC methods (Christensen et al., 2011) are generally used to perform inference on misclassification models. We discuss commonly used packages in Section 23.5.

A variation on this two-stage method treats the missing true positives and false negatives as missing data. Called the *latent class model*, it makes sampling from the posterior distribution in the second stage considerably simpler. Partition the unobserved true count $Y$ into $Y = Y_1 + Y_2$, the sum of true positives and false negatives, as we did with the validation data likelihood. Then, again using the priors based on (23.2), the joint posterior is

$$\begin{aligned}\pi(\theta, S, C, Y_1, Y_2|\mathbf{y}_v, y^*) =\ & \theta^{Y_1+Y_2+y_{1v}+y_{2v}}(1-\theta)^{n-Y_1-Y_2+n_v-y_{1v}-y_{2v}} \\ & \times S^{Y_1+y_{2v}}(1-S)^{Y_2+y_{2v}} \\ & \times C^{n-y^*-Y_2+n_v-y_v^*-y_{2v}}(1-C)^{y^*-Y_1+y_v^*-y_{1v}}.\end{aligned} \tag{23.4}$$

This joint posterior has full conditional distributions that facilitate sampling. Specifically, the full conditionals are beta distributions for $\theta, S$, and $C$. The true positives, $Y_1$, and false negatives, $Y_2$, each have binomial full conditionals. For more details see Joseph et al. (1995).

If validation data is used with Beta$(1, 1)$ priors leading to (23.2) as discussed above, then the marginal posterior distributions from (23.3) or (23.4) will be centered approximately at the corresponding maximum likelihood estimates (MLE) thus yielding very similar Bayesian point estimates. The similarity ends there, however, as the Bayesian method does not need large sample approximations to provide corresponding interval estimates or hypotheses tests. This is a major advantage of the Bayesian approach to inference in general. Furthermore, the Bayesian procedure affords straightforward combination of multiple validation data sets, if available, into one coherent analysis. For instance, there may be previous studies of sensitivity using only disease-positive subjects. The Bayesian approach can utilize this additional information about $S$ in the joint prior distribution.

As an example of this Bayesian two-stage method, we consider the well-known case-control data set found in Prescott and Garthwaite (2002). The data concern a potential link between exposure to herpes simplex virus (HSV) and invasive cervical cancer. Exposure to HSV was tested in $n = 693$ cases using a relatively inaccurate measure. A random sample of 39 of the cases were also tested for HSV exposure using a gold-standard method. See Prescott and Garthwaite (2002) for more detail. In the validation data of size $n_v = 39$, there were $Y_{1v} = 18$ true positives, $Y_{2v} = 5$ false negatives, and $Y_v^* = 21$ apparent positives from the fallible classifier. Using (23.2) to form priors for the second stage, we have

$$\begin{aligned} \theta &\sim \text{Beta}(24, 17), \\ S &\sim \text{Beta}(19, 6), \\ \text{and} \qquad C &\sim \text{Beta}(14, 4). \end{aligned} \tag{23.5}$$

Prescott and Garthwaite (2002) begin with initial Beta(0, 0) priors instead of the uniform priors we used to arrive at the stage-one posteriors (23.2).[2] While the Beta(0, 0) prior has the nice property that each first-stage posterior has the same mean as the sample proportions from the validation data, these validation studies are often quite small. Consequently, having 0 counts in one or more cells is not unusual and a Beta(0, 0) initial prior would then result in a degenerate prior for the main study data. Therefore we recommend at minimum using Beta(0.1, 0.1) priors. Of course, ideally, there will be expert information about the parameters that can be incorporated along with the validation data.

The main study data is a sample of $n = 693$ with $Y^* = 375$. If we ignore misclassification, treating $Y^*$ as if it were measured without error, and use a Beta(1, 1) prior on $\theta^*$, the resulting posterior is a Beta(376, 319) which has a posterior mean of 0.541 and a 95% credible interval of (0.504, 0.578). Accounting for the misclassification using the validation data in a two-stage Bayesian model, we obtain a posterior on $\theta$ with mean 0.588 and a 95% credible interval of (0.461, 0.712). These two posteriors are graphed in Figure 23.1. The contrast is stark. The Bayesian correction yields a posterior mean that is outside the uncorrected 95% interval. The posterior for the corrected model has considerably more variability, reflecting the greater uncertainty inherent in acknowledging misclassfication. This illustrates a general truth about the impact of ignoring misclassification and the characteristics of the corrected estimators. Ignoring misclassification not only yields biased estimators, but the associated interval lengths are artificially attenuated and have sub-nominal coverage. The corrected estimators usually have lower bias albeit at the expense of higher posterior uncertainty.

[2]Here, Beta(0, 0) denotes the improper prior obtained by taking $a \to 0$ and $b \to 0$ in a Beta($a, b$) prior. This is known as the Haldane prior, after J.B.S. Haldane (1948). For binomial data, the posterior will be proper as long as at least one "success" is observed.

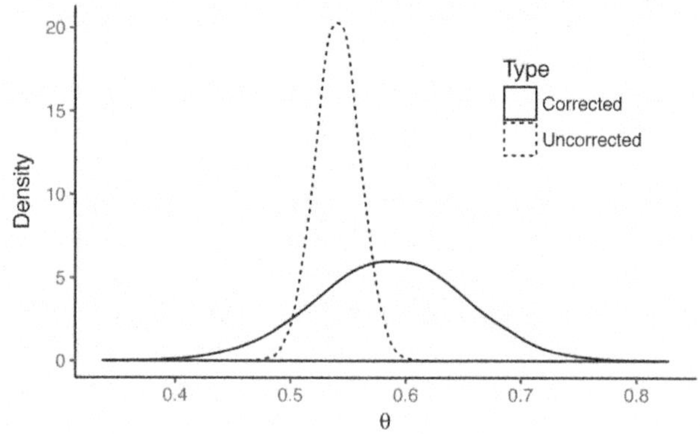


**FIGURE 23.1**
Comparison of posterior densities for $\theta$ with correction for misclassification and without.

### 23.2.2 When No Validation Data Is Available

If no gold standard test is available, the two-stage approach is not possible, and one must accommodate inevitable identifiability issues if $S$ and $C$ are to remain unspecified. As noted in Rahme and Joseph (1998), there is only one degree of freedom in the data with three parameters to estimate. Thus, a likelihood-based procedure would require two of the parameters—typically $S$ and $C$—to be replaced with fixed values. A sensitivity analysis can proceed by considering various combinations of $S$ and $C$.

Similarly, a Bayesian approach that uses Beta(1, 1) priors for all three parameters is not-identified. However, a Bayesian model that has informative priors for $S$ and $C$ yields posterior distributions that are partially identified Gustafson (2015). Denote such informative priors by

$$\begin{aligned} \theta &\sim \text{Beta}(a_\theta, b_\theta), \\ S &\sim \text{Beta}(a_S, b_S), \end{aligned} \tag{23.6}$$

and

$$C \sim \text{Beta}(a_C, b_C).$$

There is a considerable literature on how to elicit beta distributions from single and multiple experts (O'Hagan et al., 2006). A commonly used method requires the specification of a mode and a percentile. This is implemented, for example, in the R function beta buster in the epiR package (Stevenson et al., 2015).

For binomial data with misclassification and the prior structure (23.6), the joint posterior is similar to the validation data model with expert elicited values taking the place of the validation data. If we observe $Y^* = y^*$ the posterior is

$$\pi(\theta, S, C|y^*) = \left[\theta S + (1-\theta)(1-C)\right]^{y^*} \left[\theta(1-S) + (1-\theta)C\right]^{n-y^*} \times \theta^{a_\theta - 1}(1-\theta)^{b_\theta - 1} S^{a_S - 1}(1-S)^{b_S - 1} C^{a_C - 1}(1-C)^{b_C - 1}. \quad (23.7)$$

To illustrate the one-sample case we consider the data in Joseph et al. (1995). The parameter of interest is the proportion of Cambodian refugees infected with *Strongyloides stercoralis*, a human pathogenic parasitic roundworm which causes the disease strongyloidiasis. Using a stool examination, $Y^* = 40$ of $n = 162$ of the subjects tested positive. Consulting with a panel of experts, priors on the sensitivity and specificity were determined to be $S \sim \text{Beta}(4.44, 13.31)$ and $C \sim \text{Beta}(71.25, 3.75)$, respectively. Using (23.7) yielded a posterior mean for $\theta$ of 0.7402 with standard deviation 0.1677 and 95% credible set $[0.391, 0.988]$.

We have plotted the priors and posteriors for each of the three parameters in Figure 23.2. Comparing the prior for each parameter with its posterior reveals little updating from the data. Indeed, the prior and posterior for $S$ are almost identical while there is some updating for $\theta$ and $C$. This is the result of the lack of an identifiable model.

The first casualty of unidentifiability is consistency in estimation (Gustafson, 2015). Therefore it is unsurprising that this model is not rendered identifiable by increasing the sample size, the use of informative priors

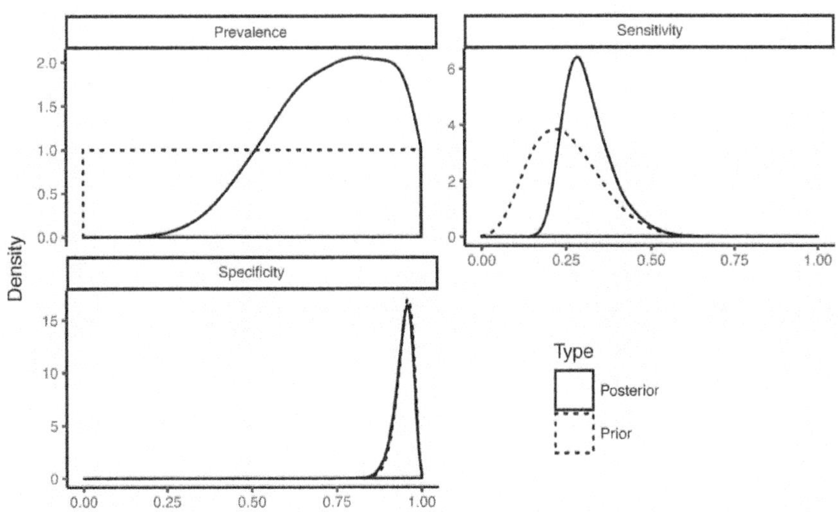


**FIGURE 23.2**
Prior and posterior densities for the *Strongyloides stercoralis* model.

**TABLE 23.1**
Posterior mean and standard deviation for $\theta$ using the *Strongyloides* data for three sample sizes.

| Sample Size | Mean | Standard Deviation |
|---|---|---|
| 162 | 0.740 | 0.167 |
| 1620 | 0.758 | 0.155 |
| 16200 | 0.756 | 0.151 |

notwithstanding: as the sample size increases, the posterior variability does not go to 0. To illustrate, we re-fit the model in (23.7) for two larger sample sizes. Specifically, we multiplied the sample by 10 and 100, preserving the proportion of positive disease tests and using the same prior distributions. The means and standard deviations for the posterior of $\theta$ are provided in Table 23.1. Increasing the sample size results in only limited reduction in the posterior standard deviation. See the text by Gustafson (2015) for more details on determining the asymptotic limit of partially identified models such as this one.

### 23.2.3 Multiple Diagnostic Tests

Using multiple tests in order to overcome unidentifiability in misclassification models is not an exclusively Bayesian idea. It dates back at least to Hui and Walter (1980) who find MLE's assuming two conditionally independent tests and two distinct populations. However, in many cases, even with more than one diagnostic test, the model is still unidentified and, in a Bayesian approach, requires informative priors on some parameters. Joseph et al. (1995) note that adding a second, conditionally independent test raises the degrees of freedom from 1 to 3. However, this also adds two additional parameters, still yielding an unidentified model. Let $Y_{11}^*$ be the number of subjects who test positive on both tests, $Y_{10}^*$ the number of subjects who test positive on the first test and negative on the second, etc. If we observe $Y_{ij}^* = y_{ij}^*$ for $i, j = 0, 1$, then the likelihood for this model is

$$
\begin{aligned}
l(\theta, S_1, C_1, S_2, C_2 | y_{11}^*, y_{10}^*, y_{01}^*, y_{00}^*) \propto & \qquad (23.8) \\
& \left[\theta S_1 S_2 + (1-\theta)(1-C_1)(1-C_2)\right]^{y_{11}^*} \\
& \times \left[\theta S_1 (1-S_2) + (1-\theta)(1-C_1)C_2\right]^{y_{10}^*} \\
& \times \left[\theta (1-S_1) S_2 + (1-\theta)C_1(1-C_2)\right]^{y_{01}^*} \\
& \times \left[\theta (1-S_1)(1-S_2) + (1-\theta)C_1 C_2\right]^{y_{00}^*}.
\end{aligned}
$$

For a Bayesian analysis, informative priors are required for at least two parameters. Typically, some information is available on the sensitivities and specificities of both tests.

Dendukuri and Joseph (2001) extend the conditionally independent two-test model to allow for correlated tests. This model is more realistic at the cost of an additional two parameters: there are still just 3 degrees of freedom and now there are 7 unknown parameters. In this formulation, the probability of two positive tests given a true positive is $S_1S_2 + \gamma_S$. Similarly, the probability of positive result and a negative result given a true positive is $S_1(1-S_2) - \gamma_C$. Here, $\gamma_S$ and $\gamma_C$ are typically positive but, in general, it can be shown that

$$(S_1 - 1)(1 - S_2) \le \gamma_S \le \min\{S_1, S_2\} - S_1S_2, \tag{23.9}$$

and

$$(C_1 - 1)(1 - C_2) \le \gamma_C \le \min\{C_1, C_2\} - C_1C_2. \tag{23.10}$$

The resulting likelihood is

$$\begin{aligned} l(\theta, S_1, C_1, S_2, C_2, \gamma_S, \gamma_C | y^*_{11}, y^*_{10}, y^*_{01}, y^*_{00}) \propto & \qquad (23.11) \\ \{\theta(S_1S_2 + \gamma_S) + (1-\theta)[(1-C_1)(1-C_2) + \gamma_C]\}^{y^*_{11}} & \\ \times\{[\theta S_1(1-S_2) - \gamma_S] + (1-\theta)[(1-C_1)C_2 - \gamma_C]\}^{y^*_{10}} & \\ \times\{\theta[(1-S_1)S_2 - \gamma_S] + (1-\theta)[C_1(1-C_2) - \gamma_C]\}^{y^*_{01}} & \\ \times\{\theta[(1-S_1)(1-S_2) + \gamma_S] + (1-\theta)[C_1C_2 + \gamma_C]\}^{y^*_{00}}. & \end{aligned}$$

The conditional independence model (23.8) results when $\gamma_S = \gamma_C = 0$.

Latent class models that bring in unobserved true counts allow for simpler full conditionals, similar to the one sample case, but this is not required in commonly used software such as JAGS (Plummer, 2003) and Stan (2016).

Uniform priors are generally used for $\gamma_S$ and $\gamma_C$, with support given by (23.9) and (23.10), respectively. Often, the tests are thought to be positively correlated, in which case the lower bound in both (23.9) and (23.10) is taken to be 0, forcing a positive relationship between the two tests. An important issue is determining whether the conditional independence or the correlated model should be used.

As an illustration, we return to the *Strongyloides* example introduced in Section 23.2.2, which is also examined in Dendukuri and Joseph (2001). Again, we have $n = 162$ yielding the counts $Y^*_{11} = 38, Y^*_{10} = 2, Y^*_{01} = 87$, and $Y^*_{00} = 33$. We will fit three models to this data. First, we assume conditional independence of the tests, using (23.8). Then we use the dependence data model (23.11) with uniform priors and lower bounds of 0 for $\gamma_S$ and $\gamma_C$. Finally, again using (23.11), we construct priors permitting negative values for $\gamma_S$ and $\gamma_C$. The results are given in Tables 23.2, 23.3, and 23.4. The conditional independence model yields a posterior for the prevalence, $\theta$, with a smaller standard deviation and substantially smaller mean than the two dependency models.

**TABLE 23.2**

Posterior summary for the model assuming conditionally independent tests using (23.8) and uniform priors. Lower and upper bounds are for 95% equal-tailed intervals.

| | mean | sd | lower | upper |
|---|---|---|---|---|
| $C_1$ | 0.957 | 0.021 | 0.907 | 0.988 |
| $C_2$ | 0.682 | 0.160 | 0.368 | 0.953 |
| $S_1$ | 0.311 | 0.052 | 0.223 | 0.431 |
| $S_2$ | 0.884 | 0.041 | 0.793 | 0.952 |
| $\theta$ | 0.755 | 0.101 | 0.517 | 0.922 |

The latter, however, suggest that the covariance terms are quite small (in the positive case, Table 23.3) or possibly zero (in the general case, Table 23.4).

The results above seem to suggest that the conditional independence model is the "correct" model. While this is reasonable, we suggest caution when using posterior intervals for $\gamma_S$ and $\gamma_C$ to decide whether or not the conditional dependence model is correct. Since these models are only partially identifiable, there is considerable posterior uncertainty. The consequent wide interval estimates make dependence plausible even if zero is contained in them. Because of this, we recommend choosing between (23.8) and (23.11) using technical knowledge about the tests. If, for example, similar mechanisms are being used, then the dependence model should be used.

Hui and Walter (1980) addressed the identifiability issue in the case of two diagnostic tests by expanding the model to include a second, distinct, population. Counterintuitively, by adding a sixth parameter, an identifiable model obtains because the data can now be summarized in two independent $2 \times 2$ tables, each with three degrees of freedom. The likelihood contribution from each population has the form (23.8), with the complete likelihood being the product of both. The corresponding likelihood equations

**TABLE 23.3**

Posterior summary for the model assuming conditionally independent tests using (23.11) and uniform priors for positive $\gamma_S$ and $\gamma_C$. Lower and upper bounds are for 95% equal-tailed intervals.

| | mean | sd | lower | upper |
|---|---|---|---|---|
| $C_1$ | 0.949 | 0.024 | 0.891 | 0.986 |
| $C_2$ | 0.646 | 0.183 | 0.284 | 0.950 |
| $S_1$ | 0.285 | 0.050 | 0.205 | 0.402 |
| $S_2$ | 0.838 | 0.049 | 0.744 | 0.930 |
| $\gamma_C$ | 0.016 | 0.014 | 0.000 | 0.051 |
| $\gamma_S$ | 0.028 | 0.014 | 0.003 | 0.057 |
| $\theta$ | 0.822 | 0.116 | 0.534 | 0.988 |

**TABLE 23.4**
Posterior summary for the model assuming conditionally independent tests using (23.11) and uniform priors for arbitrary $\gamma_S$ and $\gamma_C$. Lower and upper bounds are for 95% equal-tailed intervals.

| | mean | sd | lower | upper |
|---|---|---|---|---|
| $C_1$ | 0.951 | 0.024 | 0.894 | 0.987 |
| $C_2$ | 0.651 | 0.181 | 0.297 | 0.953 |
| $S_1$ | 0.294 | 0.052 | 0.211 | 0.417 |
| $S_2$ | 0.844 | 0.051 | 0.747 | 0.940 |
| $\gamma_C$ | 0.008 | 0.017 | −0.022 | 0.050 |
| $\gamma_S$ | 0.026 | 0.017 | −0.010 | 0.059 |
| $\theta$ | 0.814 | 0.117 | 0.532 | 0.987 |

have two distinct solutions. If $(\widehat{\theta}_1, \widehat{\theta}_2, \widehat{S}_1, \widehat{S}_2, \widehat{C}_1, \widehat{C}_2)$ is one then, necessarily, $(1-\widehat{\theta}_1, 1-\widehat{\theta}_2, 1-\widehat{S}_1, 1-\widehat{S}_2, 1-\widehat{C}_1, 1-\widehat{C}_2)$ will be another (Hui and Walter, 1980). For such a model Johnson et al. (2001) consider a Bayesian approach. Unlike the case with one population, uniform priors for all parameters can be used, but, care must be taken. For example, if one chooses starting values at 0.5 for the probability parameters, the MCMC approximations of the posterior distribution may have trouble converging, being attracted to the vicinity of both MLE's, or will be centered at either of these locations—and not necessarily the "true" value. Thus, starting values for chains should be judiciously chosen and available information should be incorporated in the priors if possible. If the tests are dependent, we again arrive at an overparameterized model requiring informative priors for at least two parameters.

To illustrate the effect of adding a second test, we augment the *Strongyloides* data by adding a second population with a lower prevalence. Specifically, we generated a data set with a prevalence of 0.2 yielding the counts $Y^*_{112} = 14, Y^*_{102} = 5, Y^*_{012} = 86$, and $Y^*_{002} = 57$. The third subscript indicates this is a second population. We first illustrate the importance of starting values for the MCMC chains. In Table 23.5 we provide the posterior means and 95% intervals for the case where the starting values for all the parameters are set to be 0.5. In Table 23.6 posterior summaries are provided for starting values on sensitivities and specificities centered at the prior means from Joseph et al. (1995). Note the vastly different results. This is the exact situation that, in the frequentist context, Hui and Walter warn that the likelihood is maximized at two places. Interestingly, this sensitivity to starting values appears to diminish if informative priors are used on some of the parameters. For example, if we use the priors from Joseph et al. (1995) then, even with starting values of 0.5 for all parameters, the posteriors of all the parameters are on the "correct" side of 0.5.

The main advantage of the two population case is the increase of marginal benefit of an increased sample size. For instance, when we multiply counts

**TABLE 23.5**
Posterior summary resulting from bad starting values. Lower and upper bounds are for 95% equal-tailed intervals.

| | mean | sd | lower | upper |
|---|---|---|---|---|
| $C_1$ | 0.571 | 0.128 | 0.231 | 0.753 |
| $C_2$ | 0.065 | 0.050 | 0.002 | 0.190 |
| $S_1$ | 0.063 | 0.029 | 0.010 | 0.124 |
| $S_2$ | 0.547 | 0.076 | 0.363 | 0.661 |
| $\theta_1$ | 0.461 | 0.140 | 0.184 | 0.739 |
| $\theta_2$ | 0.830 | 0.113 | 0.540 | 0.985 |

in the original data set by 10, the posterior standard deviation of $\theta$ is approximately 0.07, while for the two-population case, the posterior standard deviation of $\theta$ is approximately 0.04. As Johnson et al. (2001) show, the posterior variability continues to decrease as the sample size increases for the two-population case but does not for the partially identified one-population case.

The model incorporating two tests discussed in the last section can be extended to as many tests as are available. For three conditionally independent tests, an identifiable model results, even with non-informative priors on all parameters. From a frequentist standpoint, Pouillot et al. (2002) give an overview of the multiple test approach and provide software for computing MLE's, interval estimates, and, when there are enough degrees of freedom, a goodness of fit test. The goodness of fit test is to determine if the conditional independence between tests is reasonable. From a Bayesian perspective, Dendukuri et al. (2010) demonstrate the difference in required sample sizes for the three-test case versus two tests, also illustrating the value of informative priors. They provide software to implement their methodology. Although the cost for having more tests is greater per subject, the result can be fewer subjects overall.

**TABLE 23.6**
Posterior results resulting from good starting values. Lower and upper bounds are for 95% equal-tailed intervals.

| | mean | sd | lower | upper |
|---|---|---|---|---|
| $C_1$ | 0.936 | 0.029 | 0.876 | 0.989 |
| $C_2$ | 0.451 | 0.075 | 0.339 | 0.634 |
| $S_1$ | 0.428 | 0.125 | 0.249 | 0.755 |
| $S_2$ | 0.933 | 0.050 | 0.810 | 0.997 |
| $\theta_1$ | 0.539 | 0.138 | 0.269 | 0.811 |
| $\theta_2$ | 0.167 | 0.110 | 0.016 | 0.442 |

## 23.3 Regression Models

Misclassification can impact regression in both the form of misclassified covariates and misclassified response. Commonly used approaches to adjust for misclassification in regression models are as discussed earlier: validation data, expert elicited priors, multiple diagnostic tests, or some combination of the three. There are numerous examples of Bayesian approaches to correct for misclassification in a binary covariate. Prescott and Garthwaite (2002) use validation data in order to obtain informative priors for a regression with a misclassified risk factor. Ren and Stone (2007) consider the case of multiple diagnostic tests for a logistic regression with misclassification. Beavers and Stamey (2012) extend this to determine the sample size required to obtain a desired interval width or power. Gustafson (2003) has a wealth of examples of using informative priors and multiple diagnostic tests to correct for misclassified variables in case-control studies and other regression models.

We illustrate an example with misclassification in the response similar to that of McInturrf et al. (2004) and Paulino et al. (2003). Assuming covariates are not measured with error, the model is, for $i = 1, \ldots, n$,

$$Y_i \sim \text{Bernoulli}(\theta_i)$$

where

$$\text{logit}(\theta_i) = \beta_0 + \beta_1 x_{1i} + \cdots + \beta_p x_{pi}.$$

As in the previous models, the imperfect $Y_i^*$ is observed instead of $Y_i$. Instead of a single apparent prevalence, $\theta^*$, we have

$$\theta_i^* = \theta_i S + (1 - \theta_i)(1 - C).$$

The model can be extended to allow $S$ and $C$ to also depend on covariates, but this requires either validation data or considerable effort at eliciting priors via a method like conditional means priors where priors are elicited for $S$ and $C$ across a judiciously selected range of covariate values (Bedrick et al., 1996).

For our example, we assume a single $S$ and $C$. We consider the data in Paulino et al. (2003) where the observed response is a positive test for HPV and the covariates are history of vulvar warts, denoted $X_1$, new sexual partners in the previous two months, denoted $X_2$, and a history of herpes simplex, denoted $X_3$. Paulino et al. assumed the misclassification was not related to the covariates. The authors elicited expert opinion on misclassification rates based on known samples. The resulting priors were $S \sim \text{Beta}(37.65, 3.14)$ and $C \sim \text{Beta}(153.3, 8.39)$. The original analysis was actually in terms of the false negative rate, $1 - S$, and false positive rate, $1 - C$, but we use $S$ and $C$ to be consistent with our previous examples.

**TABLE 23.7**
Posterior summaries for the model accounting for misclassification. Lower and upper bounds are for 95% equal-tailed intervals.

| | mean | sd | lower | upper |
|---|---|---|---|---|
| $C$ | 0.947 | 0.017 | 0.907 | 0.976 |
| $S$ | 0.904 | 0.047 | 0.793 | 0.977 |
| $\beta_0$ | −0.309 | 0.187 | −0.653 | 0.085 |
| $\beta_1$ | 0.780 | 0.195 | 0.423 | 1.195 |
| $\beta_2$ | −0.239 | 0.175 | −0.591 | 0.095 |
| $\beta_3$ | 1.770 | 0.436 | 1.259 | 2.762 |

For the covariates we consider normal priors with means of 0 and variances of 10. While the "default" prior used in packages such as JAGS (Plummer, 2003) and OpenBUGS (Spiegelhalter et al., 2006) for regression parameters is often normal with standard deviations of 1000, we recommend against using such large values. In our experience, convergence of the Markov chains can be poor when extremely large (and interpretationally absurd) values are used for variances. The magnitude of logistic regression parameters rarely exceeds 10. For instance, for a regression coefficient, a normal prior with standard deviation of 2 has a 95% prior interval of (0.02, 54.60) for the odds ratio. Just as work and careful thought is required to construct priors on sensitivity and specificity, priors for the regression coefficients demand rational effort.

We analyzed the HPV data twice. First, accounting for misclassification with the informative priors for the sensitivity and specificity and, next, ignoring the misclassification. The results are provided in Tables 23.7 and 23.8. In Figure 23.3 we provide the posterior densities of $\beta_1$ for both models. These results demonstrate that regression models are affected similarly to the one- and two-population models we previously considered. That is, correcting for misclassification shifts the mean and tends to increase variability.

**TABLE 23.8**
Posterior summaries for the model ignoring misclassification. Lower and upper bounds are for 95% equal-tailed intervals.

| | mean | sd | lower | upper |
|---|---|---|---|---|
| $\beta_0$ | −0.334 | 0.122 | −0.575 | −0.092 |
| $\beta_1$ | 0.618 | 0.138 | 0.347 | 0.892 |
| $\beta_2$ | −0.209 | 0.137 | −0.481 | 0.058 |
| $\beta_3$ | 1.345 | 0.142 | 1.066 | 1.629 |

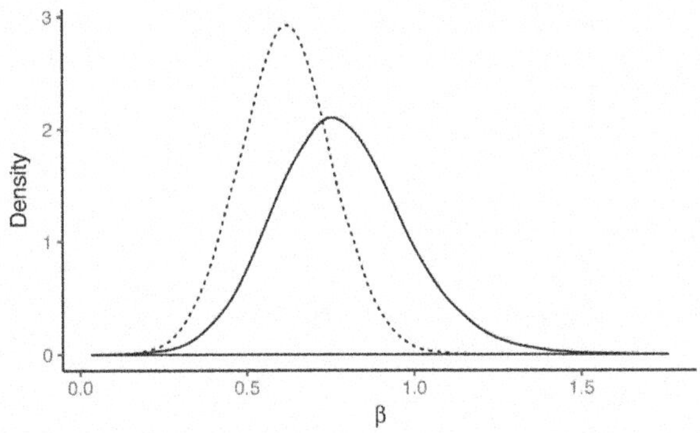


**FIGURE 23.3**
Prior (dashed) and posterior (solid) densities for $\beta_1$ for the HPV data with and without correction for misclassification.

## 23.4 Alternative Prior Structures

We have focused on the case of independent beta priors for the sensitivity and specificity. There are many advantages to this structure. First, it allows for considering each parameter separately in the prior elicitation process, whether the information comes from experts or validation data. For example, if there are multiple data sources, some of which only have information about the sensitivity, then having independent priors allows for straightforward use of the prior data/expert information. Second, when coding the MCMC algorithm, having independent priors leads to full conditional distributions that are easily sampled.

Other prior structures may be appropriate in some situations. A common restriction implemented in misclassification models is that $S + C > 1$. If this were not the case then the test would be worse than guessing and the strategy would be to switch what is a positive and what is a negative and then $S + C > 1$. The requirement that $S + C > 1$ is equivalent to $FN + FP < 1$ where $FN$ denotes the probability of a false negative and $FP$ denotes the probability of a false positive. This requirement allows for a Dirichlet prior to be placed jointly on the false positive and false negative probabilities. That is

$$p(FP, FN) \propto FP^{a_1-1} FN^{a_2-1} (1 - FP - FN)^{a_3-1},$$

where $a_1$, $a_2$, and $a_3$ are elicited from expert information or determined from validation data. The restriction in the Dirichlet induces a very strong negative correlation between the two parameters: as one of the parameters increases, the other is likely to decrease. While it is true that tests with high sensitivity often have lower specificity (and vice versa), this need not be the case. Furthermore, eliciting a prior for this very specific condition can be difficult.

Another way to allow for correlation between the sensitivity and specificity is to consider a bivariate normal prior for the logits. That is, define $\theta_1 = \text{logit}(S)$ and $\theta_2 = \text{logit}(C)$. We then assign a bivariate normal prior for $\theta_1$ and $\theta_2$ with mean vector $(\mu_1, \mu_2)'$ and covariance matrix

$$\begin{bmatrix} \sigma_1^2 & \rho\sigma_1\sigma_2 \\ \rho\sigma_1\sigma_2 & \sigma_2^2 \end{bmatrix}.$$

Contrasted with the Dirichlet prior, the bivariate normal allows for both positive and negative correlation. There is considerable literature on how to elicit normal priors. A potential drawback is that, unlike with the beta priors where prior data could easily be incorporated into the prior, the bivariate normal for the logits is not conjugate.

## 23.5 Software

Early Bayesian approaches to correct for misclassification required the researcher to write their own code, often in languages such as FORTRAN and C++. As we saw with the model (23.4), augmenting the data with the latent true counts and using conjugate independent beta priors yields a model with full conditionals that are easily sampled using a Gibbs sampler. However, for hierarchical and more complicated regression models, more sophisticated methods such as Metropolis-Hastings are required. With the advent of more user friendly software such as OpenBUGS (Spiegelhalter et al., 2006), JAGS (Plummer, 2003), and Stan (2016), it is relatively straight forward to program all the models discussed in this chapter. Many of the papers referenced include the code either as appendices or link to websites with the code. Chapter 14 of Christensen et al. (2011) is an excellent starting place to see how to implement these models in OpenBUGS. For all the examples considered in this chapter, we have used OpenBUGS. Each posterior is approximated after a 10,000 iteration burn-in. Two chains with different starting values were run for another 10,000 iterations making 20,000 iterations used for inference. Convergence was checked by analyzing history plots, autocorrelation plots, and the Gelman-Rubin-Brooks diagnostic (Brooks and Gelman, 1996).

## 23.6 Conclusion

In this Chapter we have provided an overview of correcting for misclassification of a binary variable via Bayesian methods. We focused on three approaches for performing the correction: Informative priors, validation data, and multiple diagnostic tests. We considered both single and multiple population situations. Areas of recent development that we did not consider here include hierarchical models and sample size determination (Branscum, 2006). Veterinary epidemiology often has need for misclassification models as the diagnostic tests used in the field are rarely 100% accurate. Since it is common to sample from multiple herds, Bayesian hierarchical models are applied. Hanson et al. (Hanson et al., 2003) and Norton et al. (2010) provide excellent examples of applications of the methods discussed here in fully Bayesian hierarchical models for modeling disease rates without a gold standard. As detailed in Gustafson (2015), for many of the models we have discussed, an infinite sample size does not guarantee a specified precision for estimators. Thus there is considerable interest in determining what level of precision is possible in scenarios with fixed resources. Work by Dendukuri et al. (2010) and Stamey et al. (2005) provide examples of how to determine the sample size required for one and two sample models when the response is misclassified. They both illustrate that multiple tests require smaller sample sizes than single tests.

## Bibliography

Beavers, D. P. and Stamey, J. D. (2012). Bayesian sample size determination for binary regression with a misclassified covariate and no gold standard. *Computational Statistics and Data Analysis*, 56, 2574-2582.

Bedrick, E., Christensen, R., and Johnson, W. (1996). Bayesian binomial regression: Predicting survival at a trauma center. *Journal of the American Statistical Association*, 51, 211–218.

Branscum, A., Johnson, W., and Gardner, I. (2006). Sample size calculations for disease freedom and prevalence estimation surveys. *Statistics in Medicine*, 25, 2658-2674.

Brooks, S. and Gelman, A. (1996). General methods for monitoring convergence of iterative simulations. *Journal of Computational and Graphical Statistics*, 7, 434-455.

Bross, I. (1954). Misclassification in 2 x 2 tables. *Biometrics*, 10, 478-486.

Christensen, R., Johnson, W., Branscum, A., and Hanson, T. E. (2011). *Bayesian Ideas and Data Analysis: An Introduction for Scientists and Statisticians.* CRC Press, Boca Raton, USA.

Dendukuri, N., Blisle, P., and Joseph, L. (2010). Bayesian sample size for diagnostic test studies in the absence of a gold standard: Comparing identifiable with nonidentifiable models. *Statistics in Medicine*, 29, 2688-2697.

Dendukuri, N. and Joseph, L. (2001). Bayesian approaches to modeling the conditional dependence between multiple diagnostic tests. *Biometrics*, 57, 158-167.

Eberly, L. E. and Carlin, B. P. (2000). Identifiability and convergence issues for Markov chain Monte Carlo fitting of spatial models. *Statistics in Medicine*, 19, 158-167.

Greenland, S. (2009). Bayesian perspectives for epidemiologic research: III. Bias analysis via missing-data methods. *International Journal of Epidemiology*, 38, 1662-1673.

Gustafson, P. (2003). *Measurement Error and Misclassification in Statistics and Epidemiology: Impacts and Bayesian Adjustments.* CRC Press, Boca Raton, USA.

Gustafson, P. (2015). *Bayesian Inference for Partially Identified Models: Exploring the Limits of Limited Data.* CRC Press, Boca Raton, USA.

Gustafson, P., Le, N. D., and Saskin, R. (2001). Casecontrol analysis with partial knowledge of exposure misclassification probabilities. *Biometrics*, 57, 598-609.

Haldane, J. (1948). The precision of observed values of small frequencies. *Biometrika*, 35, 297-303.

Hanson, T., Johnson, W. O., and Gardner, I. A. (2003). Hierarchical models for estimating herd prevalence and test accuracy in the absence of a gold standard. *Journal of Agricultural, Biological, and Environmental Statistics*, 8, 223-239.

Hui, S. L. and Walter, S. D. (1980). Estimating the error rates of diagnostic tests. *Biometrics*, 36, 167-171.

Johnson, W. O., Gastwirth, J. L., and Pearson, L. M. (2001). Screening without a "gold standard": the Hui-Walter paradigm revisited. *American Journal of Epidemiology*, 153, 263-272.

Joseph, L., Gyorkos, T. W., and Coupal, L. (1995). Bayesian estimation of disease prevalence and the parameters of diagnostic tests in the absence of a gold standard. *American Journal of Epidemiology*, 141, 921-924.

Lash, T. L. and Silliman, R. A. (2000). A sensitivity anslysis to separate bias due to confounding from bias due to predicting misclassification by a variable that does both. *Epidemiology*, 11, 544-549.

McCandless, L. C., Gustafson, P., and Levy, A. (2007). Bayesian sensitivity analysis for unmeasured confounding in observational studies. *Statistics in Medicine*, 26, 2331-2347.

McInturff, P., Johnson, W. O., Cowling, D., and Gardner, I. A. (2004). Modelling risk when binary outcomes are subject to error. *Statistics in Medicine*, 23, 1095-1109.

O'Hagan, A., Buck, C., Daneshkhah, A., Eiser, J., Garthwaite, P., Jenkinson, D., Oakley, J., and Rakow, T. (2006). *Uncertain Judgements.* John Wiley and Sons, New York.

Paulino, C., Soares, P., and Neuhaus, J. (2003). Binomial regression with misclassification. *Biometrics*, 59, 670-675.

Plummer, M. (2003). *Jags: A Program for Analysis of Bayesian Graphical Models using Gibbs Sampling. Proceedings of the 3rd international workshop on distributed statistical computing.* Vol. 124. No. 125.10. 2003.

Pouillot, R., Gerbier, G., and Gardner, I. A. (2002). "TAGS", a program for the evaluation of test accuracy in the absence of a gold standard. *Preventive Veterinary Medicine*, 53, 67-81.

Prescott, G. J. and Garthwaite, P. H. (2002). A simple Bayesian analysis of misclassified binary data with a validation substudy. *Biometrics*, 58, 454-458.

Rahme, E. and Joseph, L. (1998). Estimating the prevalence of a rare disease: adjusted maximum likelihood. *Journal of the Royal Statistical Society, Series D*, 47, 149-158.

Ren, D. and Stone, R. A. (2007). A Bayesian adjustment for covariate misclassification with correlated binary outcome data. *Journal of Applied Statistics*, 34, 1019-1034.

Spiegelhalter, D., Best, N., and Lunn, D. (2006). Open Bugs User Manual, version 2.20; Cambridge, uk: Mrc biostatistics unit.

Stamey, J. D., Seaman, Jr., J. W., and Young, D. M. (2005). Bayesian samplesize determination for inference on two binomial populations with no gold standard classifier. *Statistics in Medicine*, 24, 2963-2976.

Stan Development Team. (2016). RStan: the R interface to Stan, 2016. R package version 2.14.1.

Stevenson, M., Nunes, T., Heuer, C., Marshall, J., Sanchez, J., Thornton, R., Reiczigel, J., Robison-Cox, J., Sebastiani, P., Solymos, P., Yoshida, K., and Firestone, S. (2015). *epiR: An R package for the analysis of epidemiological data. R package version 0.9-69.*

Tenenbein, A. (1970). A double sampling scheme for estimating from binomial data with misclassifications. *Journal of the American Statistical Association*, 65, 1350-1361.

Tenenbein, A. (1970). A double sampling scheme for estimating from misclassified multinomial data with applications to sampling inspection. *Journal of the American Statistical Association*, 14, 187-202.

# 24

# *Bayesian Approaches for Handling Covariate Measurement Error*

**Samiran Sinha**

## CONTENTS



## 24.1 Introduction

Errors in covariates or covariate measurement error arises when the observed covariate values are not the exact measurement of the targeted continuous covariate, rather they are a convoluted version of the true value of the covariate and a noise, called measurement error. The measurement error issue is widespread in observational studies (Lee and Burstyn, 2016), laboratory measurements (Asirvatham et al., 2013; Lachin, 2004), and in survey sampling (Biemer et al., 2004). Regression analysis in the presence of a covariate measured with errors leads to biased parameter estimators. The questions are, how do we prevent that bias and what are the proper ways of analyzing such data. There are numerous choices, depending on the model we want to fit to the data, and the nature of the available data. We shall focus our attention to the Bayesian inference that has a number of advantages over some classical approaches (Bartlett and Keogh, 2017).

For a standard Bayesian inference one needs to specify the likelihood function and the prior distribution of the unknown parameters. We introduce some general notations that will be used throughout the chapter. We shall use $Y$, $X$, and $\boldsymbol{Z}$ to denote the response, the underlying latent covariate, and a vector

DOI: 10.1201/9781315101279-24

of error-free covariates, respectively. The surrogate variable for $X$ will be denoted by $X^*$, and it is assumed that conditional on $X$, $X^*$ is independent of $Y$ and $\boldsymbol{Z}$ (Richardson and Gilks, 1993). Usually observed data are $(Y, X^*, \boldsymbol{Z})$, this is often referred to as the main data. The likelihood function contains a) a model for the response $Y$ given the covariates $X, \boldsymbol{Z}$, $f_y(Y|X, \boldsymbol{Z}; \boldsymbol{\theta})$, b) a model for the latent covariate $X$ given all other error-free covariates $\boldsymbol{Z}$, $f_x(X|\boldsymbol{Z}; \boldsymbol{\gamma})$, and c) a model for the surrogate $X^*$ given $X$, $f_u(X^*|X, \boldsymbol{\phi})$ (also can be denoted as $f_{x^*|x}(X^*|X, \boldsymbol{\phi})$). The third component given in c) is the measurement error's distribution. In this chapter, the measurement error's distribution is assumed to be independent of $Y$ and $\boldsymbol{Z}$ conditional on $X$. For the inference of the conditional model for $Y$ given $X$ and $\boldsymbol{Z}$, we do not need a model for $\boldsymbol{Z}$. In the next step, the prior distribution $\pi(\boldsymbol{\theta}, \boldsymbol{\gamma}, \boldsymbol{\phi})$ for $\boldsymbol{\theta}$, $\boldsymbol{\gamma}$, and $\boldsymbol{\phi}$ is specified. The ultimate goal is to make inference on $\boldsymbol{\theta}$ and its functionals, and the statistical inference on the model parameters is based on the posterior distribution

$$\pi(\boldsymbol{\theta}, \boldsymbol{\gamma}, \boldsymbol{\phi}|\text{Data}) \propto \mathcal{L}(\boldsymbol{\theta}, \boldsymbol{\gamma}, \boldsymbol{\phi}|\text{Data})\pi(\boldsymbol{\theta}, \boldsymbol{\gamma}, \boldsymbol{\phi}),$$

where $\mathcal{L}(\boldsymbol{\theta}, \boldsymbol{\gamma}, \boldsymbol{\phi}|\text{Data})$ denotes the likelihood function of the parameters given the observed data. The likelihood function takes different forms based on the nature of the available data, and the assumptions we make on the likelihood components a), b), c).

The likelihood function $\mathcal{L}(\boldsymbol{\theta}, \boldsymbol{\gamma}, \boldsymbol{\phi}|\text{Data})$ is obtained after integrating out the latent $X$ with respect to its conditional distribution, $f_{x|x^*,z}(X|X^*, \boldsymbol{Z})$. Note that the conditional distribution $f_{x|x^*,z}(X|X^*, \boldsymbol{Z}) \propto f_x(X|\boldsymbol{Z}, \boldsymbol{\gamma}) f_u(X^*|X, \boldsymbol{\phi})$. As opposed to this classical measurement error scenario, in the *Berkson error model* $f_{x|x^*,z}(X|X^*, Z)$ is directly modeled using validation data (Mallick and Gelfand, 1996). Although, for both models we eventually need $f_{x|x^*,z}(X|X^*, \boldsymbol{Z})$, decision on which of classical measurement error or the Berkson error model to be used should be made judiciously depending on the data generating process. Importantly, for the unbiased Berkson error model where $X = X^* + U$, the naive regression parameter estimates are consistent. On the contrary, for the classical measurement error model where $X^* = X + U$, the naive regression parameter estimates are inconsistent. Importantly, in both cases, the mean of the measurement error $U$ is assumed to be zero.

In order to obtain the induced model $f_{y|x^*,z}(Y|X^*, \boldsymbol{Z})$ we need $f_{x|x^*,z}(X|X^*, \boldsymbol{Z})$ that must be estimated from validation data. Although there could be different kinds of validation data (Richardson and Gilks, 1993), we shall discuss mainly two scenarios. In the first scenario, along with the main data, the gold standard $X$ is observed on a set of subjects, and these subjects could be either a part of the main data or independent of the main data. The former is called internal validation data while the later is called external validation data. Other than $X$, the validation data also contain $X^*$ and $\boldsymbol{Z}$, that help to assess the distributions $f_x(X|\boldsymbol{Z}, \boldsymbol{\gamma})$ and $f_u(X^*|X, \boldsymbol{\phi})$. The motivating data example from the Nurses Health Study discussed in Richardson and

Gilks (1993) is of this kind. In the second scenario $X$ is never observed, instead replicated measurements on $X^*$ are observed for all subjects of the main data, or on a subset of the main study. The dataset considered in Sinha and Wang (2017) is of this kind. Also, the dataset of Sinha et al. (2010) was of the second kind because $X$ was never observed in any subset of the data. Because $X$ is never observed, it is difficult to assess the goodness-of-fit of the assumed model $f_x(X|\boldsymbol{Z}, \gamma)$. On the other hand, an incorrect model for $X$ will result in biased estimates. Motivated by this fact researchers have considered a non-parametric model for $f_x(X|\boldsymbol{Z}, \gamma)$ by using a non-parametric Bayesian approach. In principle, misspecification of the the measurement error distribution $f_u(X^*|X, \phi)$ can also lead to biased estimates. However, the measurement error is usually modelled via a parametric distribution that is symmetric around zero, such as mean-zero Normal distribution. So, as long as the true model for the measurement error belongs to a family of symmetric distributions, misspecification bias due to the measurement error distribution is relatively less than the bias due to an incorrect model for $X$.

Rather than modelling $X$ given $\boldsymbol{Z}$ by a known parametric distribution $f_x(X|\boldsymbol{Z}, \gamma)$ with unknown parameter $\gamma$, in the non-parametric Bayesian set-up the distribution of $X$ given $\boldsymbol{Z}$ is assumed to be random in a class of probability distributions. Then a prior distribution is assigned on the random distribution over the class of distributions. Any distribution on the class of probability distributions is known as a process, and in principle, Bayesian nonparametric methods can be performed with the Gaussian process, Dirichlet process (Neal, 2000), Dirichlet diffusion trees (Neal, 2003), Indian Buffet process (Griffiths and Ghahramani, 2011), Stick-breaking process (Ishwaran and James, 2001), just to name a few. The advent of the MCMC method enabled us to use the Bayesian method in this situation of uncertain covariate values.

Although there has been a plethora of articles on Bayesian approaches for analyzing data in the presence of covariate measurement error, due to limited space we shall review a handful of papers with a continuous response $Y$ (Section 2), a binary response (Section 3), and when the response is right censored time-to-event data (Section 4). Concluding remarks and some directions of future research are given in Section 5. For an in-depth Bayesian treatment of the misclassification and covariate measurement error in statistics and epidemiology, readers should consult with Gustafson (2004).

## 24.2 Continuous Response Scenario

Suppose that the observed data $(Y_i, X_i^*)$, $i = 1, \ldots, n$ is a random sample from a target population. Our interest is in estimating the regression parameter $\boldsymbol{\theta} = (\theta_0, \theta_1)^T$ of the linear model

$$Y_i = \theta_0 + \theta_1 X_i + e_i,$$

where $e_i$ is assumed to be iid Normal$(0, \sigma_e^2)$. The likelihood of the data is

$$\mathcal{L} = \prod_{i=1}^{n} f_{y|x^*}(Y_i|X_i^*) = \prod_{i=1}^{n} \int \frac{1}{\sqrt{2\pi\sigma_e^2}} \exp\Big\{-\frac{(Y_i - \theta_0 - \theta_1 X_i)^2}{2\sigma_e^2}\Big\}$$
$$f_{x|x^*}(X_i|X_i^*)dX_i,$$

where $f_{x|x^*}(X_i|X_i^*)$ denotes the density of the unobserved $X$ given the observed surrogate $X^*$. Suppose that $f_{x|x^*}(X_i|X_i^*)$ is known. Bayesian inference of $\boldsymbol{\theta}$ and $\sigma_e^2$ proceeds by specifying prior distribution on these parameters. Although a normal and inverse-gamma priors are generally used for these parameters, other priors can also be used. The integral in $\mathcal{L}$ may not have an analytic form. In that case, to avoid the integration, in the MCMC method, along with the parameters, the latent $X_1, \ldots, X_n$ are also sampled. As opposed to the inconsistent naive method where one regresses $Y$ on $X^*$, this likelihood based method yields consistent parameter estimates for $\boldsymbol{\theta}$ and $\sigma_e^2$ provided $f_{x|x^*}$ is correctly specified. Note that if $f_{x|x^*}(X_i|X_i^*)$ is assumed to follow Normal$(\gamma_0 + \gamma_1 X_i^*, \sigma_{x|x^*}^2)$ with unknown $\gamma_0, \gamma_1, \sigma_{x|x^*}^2$, then parameters are not identifiable in the classical sense. In essence, the data $(Y, X^*)$ do not have information to estimate $f_{x|x^*}(X|X^*)$, and to estimate it we need a validation dataset. Secondly, rather than working with $\prod_{i=1}^{n} f_{y|x^*}(Y_i|X_i^*)$, statistical inference can also be based on the joint distribution of $Y$ and $X^*$, $\prod_{i=1}^{n} f_{y,x^*}(Y_i, X_i^*)$. Kelly (2007) discussed applications of Bayesian methods for the linear regression in the astronomical data through various methods of modelling $f_{x|x^*}(X_i|X_i^*)$ in terms of the model of the latent variable $f_x(X)$ and the model for the measurement error $f_{x^*|x}(X^*|X)$.

Dellaportas and Stephens (1995) considered classical measurement error and Berkson error problem in a multi-level regression problem, and we present their classical measurement error problem here. The motivating data for their research came in the form of average weight of fish recorded over a time period from a pisciculture study. Let $Y_{i,j}$ be the average weight of fish from the $i$th tank at the end of the $(j+1)$th week, $i = 1, \ldots, 6$, and $j = 1, 2, \ldots, 8$. Here $j = 1$ denotes the baseline measurement. All tanks were kept in the same temperature, and the fish were of the same age. Biological phenomena dictated a linear model for the average weight with a varying slope

$$Y_{i,j} = \beta_0 + \beta_{1,i} t_j + \epsilon_{i,j},$$

where $t_j$ denotes the number of days from the beginning of the study till the end of the $(j+1)$th week. The slope was modeled in terms of the mean oxygen content $X_i$ for the $i$th tank over the weeks,

$$\beta_{1,i} = \frac{X_i - \phi_1}{X_i \phi_2^{-1} - \phi_3} + e_i, \tag{1}$$

and this three-parameter model for $\beta_{1,i}$ met biologist's belief that the slope must be constant $(= \phi_2)$ for high oxygen content, and should be close to zero for low oxygen content. The interest was in estimation of the slope parameters. Although $X_i$ was unobserved, daily oxygen content $X^*_{i,k}$ over the 7 weeks (49 days) was measured for each tank, and the classical additive measurement error model was adopted:

$$X^*_{i,k} = X_i + U_{i,k},\ i = 1, \dots, 6,\ k = 1, \dots, 49.$$

It was also assumed that $\epsilon_{i,j} \overset{iid}{\sim} \text{Normal}(0, \sigma^2_\epsilon)$, $e_i \overset{iid}{\sim} \text{Normal}(0, \sigma^2_e)$, $U_{i,k} \overset{iid}{\sim} \text{Normal}(0, \sigma^2_u)$. Furthermore, an improper probability model for $X$, $f_x(X_i) \propto 1$, and proper priors on $\gamma = (\beta_0, \phi_1, \phi_2, \phi_3, \sigma^2_e, \sigma^2_\epsilon, \sigma^2_u)^T$ were used. Suppose that $\pi(\gamma)$ denotes the prior on $\gamma$, then the following joint posterior was used to make inference on $\psi = (X_1, \dots, X_6, \beta_{1,1}, \cdots, \beta_{1,6}, \gamma^T)^T$:

$$\begin{aligned}
\pi(\psi|\text{data}) \propto & \prod_{i=1}^{6}\prod_{j=0}^{7} \frac{1}{(\sigma^2_\epsilon)^{1/2}} \exp\left\{-\frac{(Y_{i,j} - \beta_0 - \beta_{1,i} t_j)^2}{2\sigma^2_\epsilon}\right\} \times \frac{1}{(\sigma^2_u)^{49/2}} \\
& \times \exp\left\{-\sum_{k=1}^{49} \frac{(X^*_{i,k} - X_i)^2}{2\sigma^2_u}\right\} \\
& \times \frac{1}{(\sigma^2_e)^{1/2}} \exp\left\{-\frac{1}{2\sigma^2_e}\left(\beta_{1,i} - \frac{X_i - \phi_1}{X_i\phi_2^{-1} - \phi_3}\right)^2\right\} \times \pi(\gamma).
\end{aligned}$$

Finally, they proposed a Gibbs sampling algorithm to sample $\psi$ from its posterior distribution $\pi(\psi|\text{data})$. Some of the full conditional distributions were non-standard, such as the conditional distribution of $X_i$ was

$$\pi_{\text{fc}}(X_i) \propto \exp\left\{-\sum_{k=1}^{49} \frac{(X^*_{i,k} - X_i)^2}{2\sigma^2_u} - \frac{1}{2\sigma^2_e}\left(\beta_{1,i} - \frac{X_i - \phi_1}{X_i\phi_2^{-1} - \phi_3}\right)^2\right\}.$$

For sampling from such non-standard distributions, the authors proposed to use Metropolis-Hastings algorithm. As opposed to this Bayesian approach, in a naive method one would replace $X_i$ by $\overline{X}^*_i = \sum_{j=1}^{49} X^*_{i,j}/49$ in model (1).

Next we discuss the measurement error issue in a nonparametric regression model, where the model for the response $Y$ is $Y = m(X) + e$, with $E(e|X)$ is assumed to be zero and $\text{var}(e|X) < \infty$. The interest is in estimation and statistical inference of the unknown regression function $m$ over a compact interval $[a, b]$. When $X$ is observed, the optimal mean-squared convergence rate is $O(n^{-2/5})$. However, the convergence rate is much slower than $O(n^{-2/5})$ when $X$ is measured with error (Fan and Truong, 1993; Schennach, 2004). The slower rate of convergence happens due to the deconvolution procedure to obtain the true underlying density for $X$ using the data on its surrogate variable $X^*$. Particularly, for a given smoothness of the function $m$, the mean-squared convergence rate depends on the degree of *smoothness* of the measurement error density. To circumvent the relatively high bias and low efficiency issue of the classical approaches, Berry et al. (2002) proposed a Bayesian solution to this important problem. Advantage of the Bayesian method stems mainly from a) natural way of estimating the smoothing parameters, b) modelling the regression function using almost orthogonal $B$ spline basis functions, and c) learning of $X$ through an assumed model for $X$, observed surrogate variable for $X$ and the measurement error model.

For the sake of simplicity assume that the observed data are $(Y_i, X^*_{i,1}, \ldots, X^*_{i,r})$, $i = 1, \ldots, n$, where $X^*_{i,1}, \ldots, X^*_{i,r}$ denote replicated measurements on the surrogate variable $X^*$. However, the proposed method of Berry et al. (2002) can handle the case where the number of replications $r_i$ varies with $i$. They assumed that $e \sim \text{Normal}(0, \sigma_e^2)$, $X^*_{i,j} = X_i + U_{i,j}$, and $U_{i,j} \sim \text{Normal}(0, \sigma_u^2)$. One of their proposals was to estimate $m$ via smoothing splines $\boldsymbol{g} = (g(X_1), \ldots, g(X_n))^T$ that places a knot at every value of $X$. They showed that estimation of the smoothing spline via penalizing the integrated squared curvature is equivalent to estimating $\boldsymbol{g}$ with prior distribution $\pi(\boldsymbol{g}) \propto (\alpha/\sigma_e^2)^{n/2-1} \exp\{-(\alpha/2\sigma_e^2)\boldsymbol{g}^T K \boldsymbol{g}\}$, where the expression of $K$ is given in Eubank (1999). Under the assumption that the latent $X$ follows $\text{Normal}(\mu_x, \sigma_x^2)$, the likelihood involving all the parameters and the latent variables is

$$\mathcal{L} = \prod_{i=1}^{n} \frac{1}{\sqrt{\sigma_e^2 \sigma_x^2 \sigma_u^{2r}}} \exp\left[-\frac{\{Y_i - g(X_i)\}^2}{2\sigma_e^2} - \sum_{j=1}^{r} \frac{(X^*_{i,j} - X_i)^2}{2\sigma_u^2} - \frac{(X_i - \mu_x)^2}{2\sigma_x^2}\right].$$

In their fully Bayesian approach, inverse-gamma prior for the variance components, $\sigma_e^2$, $\sigma_u^2$ and $\sigma_x^2$, a normal prior distribution for $\mu_x$, and a gamma prior for $(\alpha/\sigma_e^2)$ were adopted. Then model parameters were sampled from their joint posterior distribution through Gibbs sampling. For a large $n$, a more practical approach was proposed where $m(x)$ was approximated by regression spline $\boldsymbol{B}(x)^T \boldsymbol{\beta}$ with $\boldsymbol{B}(x) = (B_1(x), \ldots, B_p(X))^T$ denoting the vector of spline basis functions. For B-splines, one needs to specify the degree of the function, such as 1, 2, 3 etc, and a set of interior knots. The number of spline basis functions $p$ =the number of interior knots+degree of the spline+1, and $p$ should be much smaller than $n$. Importantly, results differ with the location of knots. To get a robust estimates, a large number of knots were chosen over the domain of interest, then parameters, such as $\boldsymbol{\beta}$'s were estimated by penalizing overfitting. In the Bayesian context, $\boldsymbol{\beta}$'s were estimated with the prior $\pi(\boldsymbol{\beta}) \propto \exp(-\alpha \boldsymbol{\beta}^T \boldsymbol{D} \boldsymbol{\beta})$, usually $\boldsymbol{D}$ is chosen such that $\boldsymbol{\beta}^T \boldsymbol{D} \boldsymbol{\beta} = \sum_{k=3}^{p} (\Delta_2 \beta_k)^2$ and $\Delta_2 \beta_k = (\beta_k - 2\beta_{k-1} + \beta_{k-2})$. In essence, $\boldsymbol{\beta}^T \boldsymbol{D} \boldsymbol{\beta}$ is an approximate measure of the curvature of the regression function and $\alpha$ regulates the smoothness of the function.

The performance of the proposed method was judged in extensive simulation studies, and compared with the naive smoothing spline approach. One advantage of the Bayesian method in the nonparametric regression is the automatic selection of the smoothing parameter. Furthermore, the latent $X_i$'s are sampled from their predictive distributions that make use of all available information through all observed variables $Y$'s and $X^*$'s. A more flexible model for the distribution of $X$ would certainly provide more robust results. Secondly, the Gibbs sampling method potentially yields highly correlated observations resulting in a slower rate of convergence. It is worth investigating how the use of a collapsed Gibbs sampling method (Teh et al., 2007) or Hamiltonian Monte Carlo (Neal, 2011) improves the convergence.

Next we discuss the measurement error issue in the multilevel item response model that has received less attention from statisticians. We start with the following example from Fox and Glass (2003) on education research, where mathematics test score on $n = 3,713$ 4th grade students from $J = 198$ regular primary schools are available. The interest was in finding association between the mathematics achievement, educational provisions at the school level and adaptive instruction by teachers. Here each school represents a cluster, and students are nested within schools, and we shall use $i(j)$ to denote index $i$ nested within cluster $j$. The assumed model for the test response for the $i$th subject in the $j$th school was

$$Y_{i(j)} = \beta_{0(j)} + \beta_{1(j)} IQ_{i(j)} + e_{i(j)},$$

where $e_{i(j)}$ assumed to follow Normal$(0, \sigma_e^2)$, and $IQ_{i(j)}$ denotes the true intelligence of the subject. Importantly, conditional on the predictor $IQ$ and the regression coefficients, the responses were assumed to be independent. In the second level, the regression coefficients $(\beta_{0(j)}, \beta_{1(j)})$ were modeled in terms of school-level predictor, $AI$, the willingness and capability to introduce adaptive instruction,

$$\begin{aligned} \beta_{0(j)} &= \gamma_{0,0} + \gamma_{0,1} AI_j + u_j, \\ \beta_{1(j)} &= \gamma_{1,0}, \end{aligned}$$

where $u_j$'s were assumed to be iid Normal$(0, \sigma_u^2)$. Although in this particular example $\beta_{1,j}$ was assumed to be fixed across the schools, in a general model one may allow it to vary across the schools, and may allow it to depend on level-2 predictors. Importantly, if one of level-1 ($IQ$) and level-2 ($AI$) predictor is observed with errors, then it requires a careful latent variable modelling to take into account the measurement error issue. For instance, in this education research example, $IQ$ was measured via an intelligence test of $m^{(1)} = 37$ items, and $AI$ was measured via a test consisted of $m^{(2)} = 23$ dichotomous (yes/no) scored items taken by teachers, so the true $IQ$ and $AI$ were never actually observed.

For the ease of presentation, we shall denote the level-1 and level-2 predictors, $IQ_{i(j)}$ and $AI_j$ by $X_{i(j)}^{(1)}$ and $X_j^{(2)}$, respectively. In the item response theory, the true predictors are connected with the binary responses of the corresponding test through the normal ogive model, where

$$\begin{aligned} \text{pr}(X_{i(j),k}^{*,(1)} = 1 | X_{i(j)}^{(1)}, a_k^{(1)}, b_k^{(1)}) &= \Phi(X_{i(j)}^{(1)} a_k^{(1)} - b_k^{(1)}), \quad (2) \\ \text{pr}(X_{j,r}^{*,(2)} = 1 | X_j^{(2)}, a_k^{(2)}, b_k^{(2)}) &= \Phi(X_j^{(2)} a_r^{(2)} - b_r^{(2)}), \quad (3) \end{aligned}$$

$X_{i(j),k}^{*,(1)} (X_{j,r}^{*,(2)})$ is the response for the $k$th ($r$th) item for the test measuring

$X_{i(j)}^{(1)}(X_j^{(2)})$, $\Phi$ is the CDF of standard normal variable, and $a_k^{(1)}$ $(a_r^{(2)})$ and $b_k^{(1)}$ $(b_r^{(2)})$ are the discrimination and difficulty parameter of item $k$ $(r)$ for the test to measure the level-1 (level-2) predictor. For estimating all these model parameters, the Bayesian approach is the most sensible one that can incorporate information from different levels in a natural way. Fox and Glass (2003) then proposed to estimate the model parameters by the MCMC method where they sampled each of the parameters from their full conditional distribution. To avoid sampling from a non-standard distribution, they expressed (2) and (3) in terms integrals of latent variables, $Z_{i(j),k}^{(1)}$ and $Z_{j,r}^{(2)}$, and their likelihood was

$$
\begin{aligned}
\mathcal{L} &= \prod_{i(j)=1}^{n}\prod_{j=1}^{J}\frac{1}{2\sigma_e^2}\exp\Big\{-\frac{(Y_{i(j)}-\beta_{0(j)}-\gamma_{1,0}X_{i(j)}^{(1)})^2}{2\sigma_e^2}\Big\}\\
&\quad\times\frac{1}{2\sigma_u^2}\exp\Big\{-\frac{(\beta_{0(j)}-\gamma_{0,0}-\gamma_{0,1}X_j^{(2)})^2}{2\sigma_u^2}\Big\}\\
&\quad\times\prod_{k=1}^{m^{(1)}}\{\int I(Z_{i(j),k}^{(1)}>0)\phi(Z_{i(j),k}^{(1)},X_{i(j)}^{(1)}a_k^{(1)}-b_k^{(1)},1)dZ_{i(j),k}^{(1)}\}^{X_{i(j),k}^{*,(1)}}\\
&\quad\times\{\int I(Z_{i(j),k}^{(1)}<0)\phi(Z_{i(j),k}^{(1)},X_{i(j)}^{(1)}a_k^{(1)}-b_k^{(1)},1)dZ_{i(j),k}^{(1)}\}^{1-X_{i(j),k}^{*,(1)}}\\
&\quad\times\prod_{r=1}^{m^{(2)}}\{\int I(Z_{j,r}^{(2)}>0)\phi(Z_{j,r}^{(2)},X_j^{(2)}a_r^{(2)}-b_r^{(2)},1)dZ_{j,r}^{(2)}\}^{X_{j,r}^{*,(2)}}\\
&\quad\times\{\int I(Z_{j,r}^{(2)}<0)\phi(Z_{j,r}^{(2)},X_j^{(2)}a_r^{(2)}-b_r^{(2)},1)dZ_{j,r}^{(2)}\}^{1-X_{j,r}^{*,(2)}},
\end{aligned}
$$

where $\phi(\cdot,\mu,\sigma) = \exp\{-(\cdot-\mu)^2/2\sigma^2\}/\sqrt{2\pi\sigma^2}$, the density function of Normal$(\mu,\sigma^2)$ distribution. The authors estimated the parameters under non-informative priors for all the parameters. In the MCMC computation all parameters and the latent variables, $X_{i(j)}^{(1)}$, $X_{(j)}^{(2)}$, and $Z_{i(j),k}^{(1)}$ and $Z_{j,r}^{(2)}$ were sampled from their respective conditional distributions. Note that the latent variable $Z_{i(j),k}^{(1)}$ was sampled from $\phi(v,X_{i(j)}^{(1)}a_k^{(1)}-b_k^{(1)},1)I(v>0)$ when $X_{i(j),k}^{*,(1)}=1$ and from $\phi(v,X_{i(j)}^{(1)}a_k^{(1)}-b_k^{(1)},1)I(v<0)$ when $X_{i(j),k}^{*,(1)}=0$, for $k=1,\ldots,m^{(1)}$, and $Z_{j,r}^{(2)}$ was sampled from $\phi(v,X_j^{(2)}a_r^{(2)}-b_r^{(2)},1)I(v>0)$ when $X_{j,r}^{*,(2)}=1$ and from $\phi(v,X_j^{(2)}a_r^{(2)}-b_r^{(2)},1)I(v<0)$ when $X_{j,r}^{*,(2)}=0$ , for $r=1,\ldots,m^{(2)}$. Then the authors showed effectiveness of the proposed method through simulation studies and applied the method to analyze this education research dataset. The authors also considered the general case with multiple level-1 and level-2 predictors, and a subset of them were measured with errors while some predictors were observed without any error. Obviously this multilevel problem has a lot of potential in social sciences, and there is room to improve the methodology by using 1) a flexible distribution in modelling the regression coefficients at level-2, and 2) fast and scalable Bayesian computational algorithm for handling *tall* datasets that arise in education surveys.

Next we shall discuss a Bayesian method that was considered by Boonstra et al. (2013) for improved prediction using auxiliary variable information. Their problem was motivated by the gene-expression data for predicting survival of lung cancer patients. They denoted the survival time by $Y$, while $\boldsymbol{X}$ was used to denote the main covariate that was related with $Y$ and $\boldsymbol{X}^*$ was an auxiliary variable. Here $\boldsymbol{X}^*$ and $\boldsymbol{X}$ denote the gene-expression of 91 genes on the log-scale using Affymetric microarray and qRT-PCR measurements, respectively. For 439 tumors $(Y, \boldsymbol{X}^*)$ were available, and among them only 47 tumors had measurements on all three variables, $(Y, \boldsymbol{X}, \boldsymbol{X}^*)$. The qRT-PCR method is more expensive and provides a more accurate gene expression level. Their model was

$$Y = \alpha_0 + \boldsymbol{\alpha}^T \boldsymbol{X} + e,\ e \sim \text{Normal}(0, \sigma_e^2).$$

The goal was prediction of $Y^\dagger$ for a new subject with $\boldsymbol{X} = \boldsymbol{X}^\dagger$. The predictor is $\widehat{\alpha}_0 + \widehat{\boldsymbol{\alpha}}^T \boldsymbol{X}^\dagger$, and the mean-squared prediction error is measured via MSE $E\{Y^\dagger - \widehat{\alpha}_0 - \widehat{\boldsymbol{\alpha}}^T \boldsymbol{X}^\dagger\}^2$. However, the concern is that the dimension of $\boldsymbol{\alpha}$ is larger than the number of available observations where both $Y$ and $\boldsymbol{X}$ were observed. Therefore, the authors considered several penalized regression methods and a Bayesian method. Here we present their Bayesian method that is more relevant in our context. They assumed that the auxiliary variable $\boldsymbol{X}^*$ is related with $\boldsymbol{X}$ by

$$\boldsymbol{X}^* = \psi J_p + \nu \boldsymbol{X} + \boldsymbol{u},\ \boldsymbol{u} \sim \text{Normal}_p(0, \sigma_u^2 I_p),$$

where $p = 91$ and $J_p = (1, \ldots, 1)^T$ denotes a vector of $p$ ones, and $I_p$ denotes the identity matrix order $p$. Furthermore, they assumed that $\boldsymbol{X} \sim \text{Normal}(\boldsymbol{\mu}_x, \Sigma_x)$. Suppose that $\delta_i = 1$ denotes the cases where $(Y, \boldsymbol{X}^*, \boldsymbol{X})$ are observed and zero otherwise. Then their likelihood is

$$\begin{aligned}
\mathcal{L} \;=\; & \prod_{i:\delta_i=1} \frac{1}{(\sigma_e^2)^{1/2}} \exp\left\{-\frac{(Y_i - \alpha_0 - \boldsymbol{\alpha}^T \boldsymbol{X}_i)^2}{2\sigma_e^2}\right\} \frac{1}{(\sigma_u^2)^{p/2}} \\
& \times \exp\left\{-\frac{(\boldsymbol{X}_i^* - \psi J_p - \nu \boldsymbol{X}_i)^{\otimes 2}}{2\sigma_u^2}\right\} \\
& \times \frac{1}{|\Sigma_x|^{1/2}} \exp\left\{-\frac{(\boldsymbol{X}_i - \mu_x)^T \Sigma_x^{-1} (\boldsymbol{X}_i - \mu_x)}{2}\right\} \\
& \prod_{i:\delta_i=0} \int \frac{1}{(\sigma_e^2)^{1/2}} \exp\left\{-\frac{(Y_i - \alpha_0 - \boldsymbol{\alpha}^T \boldsymbol{X}_i)^2}{2\sigma_e^2}\right\} \frac{1}{(\sigma_u^2)^{p/2}} \\
& \times \exp\left\{-\frac{(\boldsymbol{X}_i^* - \psi J_p - \nu \boldsymbol{X}_i)^{\otimes 2}}{2\sigma_u^2}\right\} \\
& \frac{1}{|\Sigma_x|^{1/2}} \exp\left\{-\frac{(\boldsymbol{X}_i - \mu_x)^T \Sigma_x^{-1} (\boldsymbol{X}_i - \mu_x)}{2}\right\} d\boldsymbol{X}_i,
\end{aligned}$$

where $a^{\otimes 2} = a^T a$. The authors then used Normal$_p\{0, (\sigma_e^2/\lambda)I_p\}$ prior on $\boldsymbol{\alpha}$ and Wishart prior with degrees of freedom $3p$ and scale $(2p-1)^{-1}\Omega_x^{-1}$ on $\Sigma_x^{-1}$, where $\Omega_x = \text{diag}\{\sum_{i:\delta_i=1} \boldsymbol{X}_i \boldsymbol{X}_i^T / \sum_i I(\delta_i = 1)\}$. On the other parameters, $(\alpha_0, \log(\sigma_e^2), \psi, \nu, \log(\sigma_u^2), \boldsymbol{\mu}_x, \lambda)$, Jeffrey's prior was used. The posterior mean of $\boldsymbol{\alpha}$ was considered as the estimator $\widehat{\boldsymbol{\alpha}}$. Through extensive simulation studies they investigated prediction performance (MSE) of different methods with varying $p$, $\rho$, the correlation between $\boldsymbol{X}$ and $\boldsymbol{X}^*$, $n_A = \sum_i I(\delta_i = 1)$ and $n_B = \sum_i I(\delta_i = 0)$, and $R^2$, the coefficient of determination of the linear regression of $Y$ on $\boldsymbol{X}$. Their results indicated the performance of the Bayesian method was quite satisfactory compared to other approaches. Finally, they had applied their methods on a test dataset on lung cancer to predict the survival time.

## 24.3 Binary Case

Schmid and Rosner (1993) were the first to formally consider a Bayesian approach for solving measurement error issue in the logistic model that is widely used in medical and social sciences. Their methodology was described in the context of a dataset from the Nurses Health Study, a prospective cohort study. The main data consist of demographics, cancer outcome $Y$ over a follow-up period, and information on food and beverage intake collected through food frequency questionnaire (FFQ) from thousands of registered nurses in the United States. The interest was in finding association between the risk of breast cancer and the long-term average daily alcohol consumption $X$, adjusted with age $Z$. For the sake of simplicity, here we present only the logistic model. However, their general methodology is applicable to other types of models for $Y$ given $X$ and $Z$. They assumed

$$\text{pr}(Y = 1|X, Z) = H(\beta_0 + \beta_1 X + \beta_2 Z),$$

where $H(u) = 1/\{1 + \exp(-u)\}$. The goal was consistent estimation of $\boldsymbol{\beta} = (\beta_0, \beta_1, \beta_2)^T$. However, the long-term average daily alcohol consumption derived from FFQ is considered as proxy $X^*$ for the true intake $X$. To assess the accuracy of the questionnaire response $X^*$, a detailed diet history was collected from a subsample of 173 nurses during four one-week periods at three-month intervals in the year following the completion of the questionnaire. This long-period diet history allowed researchers to assess seasonal and day-to-day variations in the diet. Finally this detailed diet history and the response to FFQ constitute a validation study to estimate any random and systematic measurement error.

Denote the main data and validation data by $\boldsymbol{D} = (Y_i, X_i^*, Z_i, i = 1, \ldots, n)$ and $\boldsymbol{V} = (Y_j, X_j^*, X_j, Z_j, j = 1, \ldots, n_v)$, respectively. Importantly, the set of subjects in the validation data $\boldsymbol{V}$ was a subset of the subjects included in $\boldsymbol{D}$. Assume that $X^*$, $Z$, $X$ are centered at zero. Next $X$ was modeled parametrically in terms of $X^*$ and $Z$ as

$$X = h(X^*, Z, \gamma) + e,$$

where $h$ is a function that is known up to a finite dimensional parameter $\gamma$, and $e \sim \text{Normal}(0, \sigma^2)$. Define $\boldsymbol{\psi} = (\gamma^T, \sigma^2)^T$, and let $\pi(\boldsymbol{\psi})$ be the prior distribution for $\boldsymbol{\psi}$. Next, the induced model for $Y$ given $X^*$ and $Z$ is

$$\begin{aligned}\text{pr}(Y = 1|X^*, Z, \boldsymbol{\beta}, \boldsymbol{\psi}) &= \int \text{pr}(Y = 1|X, Z, \boldsymbol{\beta}) f_{x|x^*,z}(X|X^*, Z, \boldsymbol{\psi}) dX \\ &= \int H(\beta_0 + \beta_1 X + \beta_2 Z) \times \frac{1}{\sqrt{2\pi\sigma^2}} \\ &\quad \times \exp\left[-\frac{\{X - h(X^*, Z, \gamma)\}^2}{2\sigma^2}\right] dX,\end{aligned}$$

and Schmid and Rosner (1993) used this to obtain the likelihood for the main dataset,

$$\mathcal{L}(\boldsymbol{\beta}|\boldsymbol{\psi}) = \prod_{i=1}^{n} \{\text{pr}(Y = 1|X_i^*, Z_i, \boldsymbol{\beta}, \boldsymbol{\psi})\}^{Y_i} \{1 - \text{pr}(Y = 1|X_i^*, Z_i, \boldsymbol{\beta}, \boldsymbol{\psi})\}^{1-Y_i}.$$

Let $\pi(\boldsymbol{\beta})$ and $\pi(\boldsymbol{\psi})$ be the prior for $\boldsymbol{\beta}$ and $\boldsymbol{\psi}$, respectively, then the posterior distribution conditional on $\boldsymbol{\psi}$ is proportional to $\pi(\boldsymbol{\beta}|\boldsymbol{D}, \boldsymbol{\psi}) \propto \pi(\boldsymbol{\beta})\mathcal{L}(\boldsymbol{\beta}|\boldsymbol{\psi})$. Suppose that interest is in calculating the posterior mean of a function $g$ of $\boldsymbol{\beta}$. For instance $g(\boldsymbol{\beta}) = \beta_1$, $g(\boldsymbol{\beta}) = \beta_1^2$, or $g(\boldsymbol{\beta}) = \text{pr}(Y = 1|X_{Q_3}, Z_{\text{med}}) - \text{pr}(Y = 1|X_{Q_1}, Z_{\text{med}})$, the effect of changing the alcohol consumption from the first quartile $X_{Q_1}$ to the third quartile $X_{Q_3}$ while the age is fixed to the median age $Z_{\text{med}}$ of the cohort. In general one can obtain

$$E\{g(\boldsymbol{\beta})|\boldsymbol{\psi}\} = \frac{\int g(\boldsymbol{\beta})\pi(\boldsymbol{\beta})L(\boldsymbol{\beta}|\boldsymbol{\psi})d\boldsymbol{\beta}}{\int \pi(\boldsymbol{\beta})L(\boldsymbol{\beta}|\boldsymbol{\psi})d\boldsymbol{\beta}}.$$

Define $\widehat{g}_k = E\{g(\boldsymbol{\beta})|\boldsymbol{\psi} = \boldsymbol{\psi}_k\}$, where $\boldsymbol{\psi}_k$ is a random draw from its posterior distribution

$$\pi(\boldsymbol{\psi}|\boldsymbol{V}) \propto \pi(\boldsymbol{\psi}) \times \prod_{j=1}^{n_v} f_{x|x^*,z}(X_j|X_j^*, Z_j, \boldsymbol{\psi}).$$

The authors recommended to use MCMC samples to draw random numbers from $\pi(\boldsymbol{\beta}|\boldsymbol{D}, \boldsymbol{\psi} = \boldsymbol{\psi}_k)$, and use them to obtain the Monte Carlo average $\sum_{k=1}^{K} \widehat{g}_k/K$ to estimate $E\{g(\boldsymbol{\beta})\}$, where $(\widehat{g}_1, \ldots, \widehat{g}_K)^T$ correspond to $K$ random draws $(\boldsymbol{\psi}_1, \ldots, \boldsymbol{\psi}_K)^T$. A special case of linear $h$ was considered for illustration. The authors proposed an extension of the methodology 1) when $X$ and $Z$ are multivariate and 2) when $X$ given $X^*$ and $Z$ follows a mixture of distributions. Some key issues of the proposed approach warrant a discussion.

Rather than assuming an additive measurement error accompanied by 1) a model assumption on the measurement error, and 2) a model assumption on the latent $X$, the authors directly modeled the distribution of $X$ in terms of $X^*$ and $Z$. This sort of model is known as the Berkson-error model. The proposed estimation was a two-step procedure, first $\boldsymbol{\psi}$ was estimated from the validation data and then conditional on $\boldsymbol{\psi}$, $\boldsymbol{\beta}$ was estimated. Alternatively, a more efficient approach would be to estimate all model parameters together taking into account the fact that the validation data is a subset of the main data instead of treating the two datasets independently.

Next we discuss the measurement error issue in a partly generalized linear model. Motivated by the NIH-AARP Diet and Health Study, a large prospective study to find association between diet and different cancers, Sinha et al. (2010) proposed a solution of a general non-linear nonparametric regression problem. This work involved considerable generalization of the measurement error issue in the logistic model. Suppose that $X$, $\boldsymbol{Z}$ and $Y$ denote the usual nutrient intake, a set of error-free covariates, and health indicator (e.g., diagnosed with breast cancer or not during the follow-up period). The model was

$$\text{pr}(Y = 1|X, Z) = H(g_{\text{risk}}(X) + \boldsymbol{\beta}_{\text{risk}}^T \boldsymbol{Z}),$$

where $g_{\text{risk}}(X)$ is assumed to be sufficiently smooth but an unknown function. The interest was in estimating and making inference on the risk function $g_{\text{risk}}(X)$ for $X \in [a, b]$ and the regression parameter $\boldsymbol{\beta}_{\text{risk}}$. As mentioned before, estimation of the nonparametric regression function is a difficult problem in practice as it requires a deconvolution technique to obtain the density function of $X$, and more so when the response variable is binary. In their motivating example, $(Y_i, Q_i, \boldsymbol{Z}_i)$, $i = 1, \ldots, n$ were obtained from $n$ independent subjects, where $Q_i$ denotes the nutrient intake collected through food frequency questionnaire. Independent of the main study, in a validation dataset $Q_i$, $\boldsymbol{Z}_i$, and $X_{i,1}^*, X_{i,2}^*$, the two 24-hr recalls on the nutrient intake were collected from $m$ individuals, $(Q_i, X_{i,1}^*, X_{i,2}^*, \boldsymbol{Z}_i)\ i = 1, \ldots, m$. The combined dataset had $n+m$ subjects, and indicator $R_i$ takes on 1 or 0 depending on if the $i$th subject is in the validation data or main study.

Although $X$, the usual intake, was never observed, two 24-hr recalls were considered unbiased surrogate for $X$, that means they assumed $X_{i,j}^* = X_i + U_{i,j}$, and intake measured via FFQ was modeled as

$$Q_i = g_{\text{cal}}(X_i) + \boldsymbol{\beta}_{\text{cal}}^T \boldsymbol{Z}_i + U_{i,\text{cal}},$$

where $U_{i,j}$ and $U_{i,\text{cal}}$ were assumed to follow iid Normal$(0, \sigma_u^2)$ and Normal$(0, \sigma_{\text{cal}}^2)$, respectively. This nonparametric modelling of $Q_i$ in terms of $X_i$ makes the work distinct from other previous work on measurement error in the binary regression model. For identifiability of $X$, and $g_{\text{risk}}$ function, monotonicity constraint on $g_{\text{cal}}$ was imposed. Then under the assumption that both $g_{\text{risk}}$ and $g_{\text{cal}}$ belong to the 3-rd order Sobolev space, they modelled these nonparametric functions using cubic B-spline basis functions. Assuming that $\tau_{1,r} < \cdots < \tau_{n_r,r}$ are the inner knot points over the set $[a, b]$, $g_{\text{risk}}(X)$ was approximated as

$$\sum_{l=1}^{n_r+4} B_{l,r}(X)\gamma_{l,\text{risk}}.$$

Here $B_{1,r}(X), \ldots, B_{n_r+4,r}(X)$ denote B-spline basis functions. They recommended taking a fairly large number of knot points, and to avoid overfitting, they proposed estimating $\boldsymbol{\gamma}_{\text{risk}} = (\gamma_{1,\text{risk}}, \cdots, \gamma_{n_r+4,\text{risk}})^T$ by penalizing a large curvature. This penalization comes naturally in a Bayesian set-up through an appropriate choice of the prior distribution on the parameters, such as, taking $\pi(\boldsymbol{\gamma}_{\text{risk}}) \propto \delta_{\text{risk}}^{(n_r+4)/2} \exp\{-(\delta_{\text{risk}}/2)\sum_{l=3}^{n_r+4}(\gamma_{l,\text{risk}} - 2\gamma_{l-1,\text{risk}} + \gamma_{l-2,\text{risk}})^2 - (\delta_{\text{risk}}/2V)\boldsymbol{\gamma}_{\text{risk}}^T\boldsymbol{\gamma}_{\text{risk}}\}$. The first term in the exponent is the square of the 2nd order finite difference of the spline coefficients, that measures the square of the curvature of the function. However, this quadratic term is not of full rank. Therefore, they added the second term in the exponent to make the prior on $\boldsymbol{\gamma}_{\text{risk}}$ proper. Here $V$ was set to a very large number, and authors took $V = 10^8$. Following the similar idea, $g_{\text{cal}}(X)$ was approximated by

$$\sum_{l=1}^{n_c+4} B_{l,c}(X)\gamma_{l,\text{cal}},$$

where $B_{1,c}(X), \ldots, B_{n_c+4,c}(X)$ denote B-spline basis functions for inner knot points $\tau_{1,c} < \cdots < \tau_{n_c,c}$. They put a restriction that $\gamma_{1,\text{cal}} \leq \cdots \leq \gamma_{n_c+4,\text{cal}}$ to impose the monotonicity constraint.

For a flexible modelling of the distribution of $X$ given $\boldsymbol{Z}$, they assumed that conditional on $\mu_x, \sigma_x^2, \zeta_x$, $X|\boldsymbol{Z} \sim \text{Normal}(\theta_1 + \boldsymbol{\zeta}_x^T\boldsymbol{Z}, \theta_2)$, and assumed that $\boldsymbol{\theta} = (\theta_1, \theta_2)$ followed a random distribution defined on the Borel $\sigma$-algebra constructed out of $(-\infty, \infty) \times (0, \infty)$, and assumed that the random probability measure followed the Dirichlet process with precision parameter $\alpha$ and the base probability measure $\mathcal{G}$. In notation, $\boldsymbol{\theta} \sim G$, $G \sim DP(\alpha, \mathcal{G})$. This model assumption implies that the conditional density of $X$ given $\boldsymbol{Z}$ is an infinite mixture of normal distributions where the mixing weights and mass points are random, that means, a priori,

$$f(X|\boldsymbol{Z}_i) = \sum_{l=1}^{\infty} \omega_l(v)\frac{1}{\sqrt{2\pi\theta_{i,2}}}\exp\left\{-\frac{1}{2\theta_{i,2}}(X - \theta_{i,1} - \boldsymbol{\zeta}_x^T\boldsymbol{Z}_i)^2\right\}I(\boldsymbol{\theta}_i = \boldsymbol{\vartheta}_l),$$

where $\boldsymbol{\vartheta}_1, \boldsymbol{\vartheta}_2, \ldots, \overset{iid}{\sim} \mathcal{G}$ and $\omega_l(v) = v_l\prod_{r=1}^{l-1}(1 - v_r)$, and $v_1, v_2, \ldots, \sim$ Beta$(1, \alpha)$ distribution. The above stick-breaking structure clearly implies that the parameter $\boldsymbol{\theta}$ could take one of $(\boldsymbol{\vartheta}_1, \boldsymbol{\vartheta}_2, \ldots,)$ with probability $(\omega_1(v), \omega_2(v), \ldots)$. With $\boldsymbol{\psi} = \left(\boldsymbol{\beta}_{\text{cal}}^T, \boldsymbol{\beta}_{\text{risk}}^T, \boldsymbol{\gamma}_{\text{cal}}^T, \boldsymbol{\gamma}_{\text{risk}}^T, \boldsymbol{\zeta}_x^T, \sigma_{\text{cal}}^2, \sigma_u^2\right)^T$, the observed data likelihood function was

$$\mathcal{L}_o = \int \prod_{i=1}^{n+m} \left\{ f^{1-R_i}(Y_i, Q_i|\boldsymbol{Z}_i, \boldsymbol{\theta}, \boldsymbol{\psi}) f^{R_i}(Q_i, X^*_{i,j}, j = 1, \cdots, J|\boldsymbol{Z}_i, \boldsymbol{\theta}, \boldsymbol{\psi}) \right\}$$

$dG(\boldsymbol{\theta})$,
where

$$\begin{aligned}
& f(Y_i, Q_i|\boldsymbol{Z}_i, \boldsymbol{\theta}, \boldsymbol{\psi}) \\
&= \int \mathrm{pr}^{Y_i}(Y = 1|X_i, \boldsymbol{Z}_i, \boldsymbol{\psi}) \mathrm{pr}^{1-Y_i}(Y = 0|X_i, \boldsymbol{Z}_i, \boldsymbol{\psi}) f(Q_i|X_i, \boldsymbol{Z}_i, \boldsymbol{\theta}) \\
& \quad \times f(X_i|\boldsymbol{Z}_i, \boldsymbol{\theta}, \boldsymbol{\psi}) dX_i \\
&= \int \frac{\exp[Y_i\{g_{\text{risk}}(X_i) + \boldsymbol{Z}_i^T \boldsymbol{\beta}_{\text{risk}}\}]}{1 + \exp\{g_{\text{risk}}(X_i) + \boldsymbol{Z}_i^T \boldsymbol{\beta}_{\text{risk}}\}} \frac{1}{(\sigma^2_{\text{cal}})^{1/2}} \\
& \quad \exp\left[ -\frac{1}{2\sigma^2_{\text{cal}}} \{Q_i - g_{\text{cal}}(X_i) - \boldsymbol{Z}_i^T \boldsymbol{\beta}_{\text{cal}}\}^2 \right] \\
& \qquad \times \frac{1}{\sqrt{\theta_{i,2}}} \exp\left\{ -\frac{1}{2\theta_{i,2}} (X_i - \theta_{i,1} - \boldsymbol{Z}_i^T \boldsymbol{\zeta}_x)^2 \right\} dX_i, \\
& f(Q_i, X^*_{i,1}, \ldots, X^*_{i,J}|\boldsymbol{Z}_i, \boldsymbol{\theta}, \boldsymbol{\psi}) \\
&= \int f(Q_i, X^*_{i,1}, \ldots, X^*_{i,J}, X_i|\boldsymbol{Z}_i, \boldsymbol{\theta}, \boldsymbol{\psi}) dX_i \\
&= \int \frac{1}{(\sigma^2_{\text{cal}})^{1/2}} \exp\left[ -\frac{1}{2\sigma^2_{\text{cal}}} \{Q_i - g_{\text{cal}}(X_i) - \boldsymbol{Z}_i^T \boldsymbol{\beta}_{\text{cal}}\}^2 \right] \\
& \quad \times \frac{1}{(\sigma^2_u)^{J/2}} \exp\left\{ -\frac{1}{2\sigma^2_u} \sum_{j=1}^{J} (X^*_{i,j} - X_i)^2 \right\} \\
& \qquad \times \frac{1}{\sqrt{\theta_{i,2}}} \exp\left\{ -\frac{1}{2\theta_{i,2}} (X_i - \theta_{i,1} - \boldsymbol{Z}_i^T \boldsymbol{\zeta}_x)^2 \right\} dX_i.
\end{aligned}$$

The MCMC method was used to sample from the posterior distribution. Particularly, rather than using a prior distribution on the precision parameter $\alpha$ of the Dirichlet process, using a characterization of the average number of clusters, they estimated $\alpha$ by solving an equation in each MCMC iteration. Through extensive simulation studies they showed how effective the Bayesian method was in estimating the parametric and nonparametric component of the risk model, and compared its performance with the existing approaches.

Next we turn our attention to case-control studies where data are collected retrospectively, and sampling is no longer random from the underlying population. Instead, sampling depends on the outcome variable. To be specific, suppose that a population has $N_1$ subjects with response variable $Y = 1$, and $N_0$ subjects with response $Y = 0$. Subjects with $Y = 1$ and $Y = 0$ are called cases and controls, respectively. The sample data consists of $n_0$ controls sampled from $N_0$ subjects, and $n_1$ cases sampled out of $N_1$ cases. For the $n = n_0 + n_1$ sampled subjects, exposure or covariate information is collected retrospectively. Müller and Roeder (1997) were the first to consider a Bayesian approach for handling measurement error in covariates in a case-control study. The goal was estimation of the regression parameters of the logistic model $\text{pr}(Y = 1|X, \boldsymbol{Z}) = H(\beta_0 + \beta_1 X + \boldsymbol{\beta}_2^T \boldsymbol{Z})$ based on case-control data on $n$ subjects. Following Prentice and Pike (1979), Müller and Roeder (1997) showed that the case-control data do not provide information on $\beta_0$, and in the Bayesian context one can make correct posterior inference on the regression parameters $(\beta_1, \boldsymbol{\beta}_2)$, if $\beta_0$ and $(\beta_1, \boldsymbol{\beta}_2)$ are a priori independent. The observed data for case-control study can be denoted by $(Y_i, X_i^*, \boldsymbol{Z}_i)$ for $i = 1, \ldots, n$, where $X_i^*$ is a surrogate measurement for $X_i$. It was assumed that $X_i$ was observed only for a set of the subjects that were included in the main study. Therefore, the validation data were $(Y_i, X_i, X_i^*, \boldsymbol{Z}_i)$ for $i \in V$, and the main study was $(Y_i, X_i^*, \boldsymbol{Z}_i)$ for $i \in V^c$, and $|V \cup V^c| = n$. Müller and Roeder (1997) proposed a general solution in the sense that they did not adopt the classical additive measurement error assumption between the surrogate $X^*$ and the latent $X$, instead they modeled the joint distribution of $\widetilde{\boldsymbol{X}} = (X, X^*, \boldsymbol{Z}^T)^T$ using a Dirichlet process (DP) mixture of multivariate normal distributions, that means the model was

$$
\begin{aligned}
f(\widetilde{\boldsymbol{X}}_i|\boldsymbol{\theta}_i, \Sigma_i) &\propto \exp\{-\frac{1}{2}(\widetilde{\boldsymbol{X}}_i - \boldsymbol{\theta}_i)^T \Sigma_i^{-1} (\widetilde{\boldsymbol{X}}_i - \boldsymbol{\theta}_i)\}; \\
(\boldsymbol{\theta}_i, \Sigma_i) &\propto G(\text{a random distribution}); \\
G &\sim DP(\alpha \mathcal{G}).
\end{aligned}
$$

Suppose $\boldsymbol{\psi}$ denotes all $\boldsymbol{\theta}_i$ and $\Sigma_i$ parameters. Then the likelihood of the observed data is

$$
\mathcal{L}(\boldsymbol{\beta}, \boldsymbol{\psi}) \propto \prod_{i \in V} f(X_i, X_i^*, \boldsymbol{Z}_i|Y_i, \boldsymbol{\beta}, \boldsymbol{\psi}) \prod_{i \in V^c} f(X_i^*, \boldsymbol{Z}_i|Y_i, \boldsymbol{\beta}, \boldsymbol{\psi}),
$$

and the terms of the likelihood conditional on the response $Y$ are

$$
\begin{aligned}
& f(X_i, X_i^*, \boldsymbol{Z}_i|Y_i, \boldsymbol{\beta}, \boldsymbol{\psi}) \\
&= \frac{\text{pr}^{Y_i}(Y = 1|X_i, \boldsymbol{Z}_i)\text{pr}^{1-Y_i}(Y = 0|X_i, \boldsymbol{Z}_i) f(X_i, X_i^*, \boldsymbol{Z}_i)}{\int \text{pr}^{Y_i}(Y = 1|X_i, \boldsymbol{Z}_i)\text{pr}^{1-Y_i}(Y = 0|X_i, \boldsymbol{Z}_i) f(X_i, X_i^*, \boldsymbol{Z}_i) d(X_i, X_i^*, \boldsymbol{Z}_i)}; \\
& f(X_i^*, \boldsymbol{Z}_i|Y_i, \boldsymbol{\beta}, \boldsymbol{\psi}) \\
&= \frac{\int \text{pr}^{Y_i}(Y = 1|X_i, \boldsymbol{Z}_i)\text{pr}^{1-Y_i}(Y = 0|X_i, \boldsymbol{Z}_i) f(X_i, X_i^*, \boldsymbol{Z}_i) dX_i}{\int \text{pr}^{Y_i}(Y = 1|X_i, \boldsymbol{Z}_i)\text{pr}^{1-Y_i}(Y = 0|X_i, \boldsymbol{Z}_i) f(X_i, X_i^*, \boldsymbol{Z}_i) d(X_i, X_i^*, \boldsymbol{Z}_i)}.
\end{aligned}
$$

Posterior samples were drawn using the MCMC method. They used prior distribution on all the parameters including the precision parameter $\alpha$ of the Dirichlet process prior, and for updating the Dirichlet process related parameters, they adopted Escobar and West's (1995) algorithm. Müller and Roeder (1997) recommended to use a log-linear model when $\boldsymbol{Z}$ contains a binary or categorical component.

Although the method was quite general and robust due to nonparametric modelling of the covariate distribution, the MCMC computation involving the Dirichlet process is not straightforward that anyone can use. To overcome this issue Gustafson et al. (2002) proposed an alternative approach. Exploiting the structure of the logistic model for the response $Y$ given $X$, they established that $f(X|Y=1) = f(X|Y=0)\exp(\beta_0^\dagger + \beta_1 X)$, where $\beta_0^\dagger = \beta_0 - \log\{\text{pr}(Y = 1)/\text{pr}(Y=0)\}$. Note that $\text{pr}(Y=1)$ or $\text{pr}(Y=0)$ cannot be estimated from the case-control sample, so is $\beta_0$. Because $f(X|Y=1)$ is a density function, $1 = \int f(X|Y=1)dX = \int f(X|Y=0)\exp(\beta_0^\dagger + \beta_1 X)dX$. Thus, $\beta_0^\dagger$ is a function of $\beta_1$ and $f_0(X) = f(X|Y=0)$, that means, $\beta_0^\dagger = \beta_0^\dagger(\beta_1, f_0)$. Under the assumption that $f_u(X^*|X)$, the conditional distribution of $X^*$ given $X$, is completely known, the likelihood of the case-control sample $(Y_i, X_i^*)$, $i = 1, \ldots, n = (n_0 + n_1)$ is

$$\begin{aligned}
\mathcal{L} &= \prod_{i=1}^{n} \int f_u(X_i^*|X_i, Y_i) f(X_i|Y_i) dX_i \\
&= \prod_{i=1}^{n} \int f_u(X_i^*|X_i, Y_i) f_0(X_i) \exp[Y_i\{\beta_0^\dagger(\beta_1, f_0) + \beta_1 X\}] dX_i.
\end{aligned}$$

The likelihood $\mathcal{L}$ contains two unknown parameters, finite-dimensional $\beta_1$ and infinite-dimensional $f_0(X_i)$. Rather than estimating the infinite-dimensional parameter $f_0$ as it is, after some reparametrization, they proposed to estimate the mass points of the reparametrized density over a set of grid points in the range of $X$. Along with the prior for the other parameters, they used a Dirichlet prior for the probability masses at the grid values. By approximating the infinite-dimensional parameter by a finite-dimensional parameter, they achieved a greater computational efficiency that is useful for analyzing a large dataset. A somewhat similar idea, known as the nonparametric maximum likelihood method in the classical literature, was used by Rabe-Heketh et al. (2003) for reducing the measurement error bias in the logistic regression model, where the number of such grid points was allowed to increase with the sample size.

## 24.4 Time-to-Event Models

Now we consider the covariate measurement error issue in survival models. Here we discuss the models exclusively for right-censored data where censoring time and the actual time-to-event are assumed to be independent. Note that usual right censored time-to-event data consists of $(V_i, \Delta_i, X_i, \boldsymbol{Z}_i), i = 1, \ldots, n$, where $V_i = \min(T_i, C_i)$ denotes the minimum of the time-to-event $T_i$ and the censoring time $C_i$, $\Delta_i = I(T_i \le C_i)$ denotes the right censoring indicator, and $X_i$ and $\boldsymbol{Z}_i$ are covariates. In the errors-in-covariate scenario, instead of $X_i$, a surrogate variable $X_i^*$ is observed. There are two possibilities, either an external or internal validation dataset is observed. The validation data help us to identify the conditional distribution of $X_i$ given $X_i^*$ and $\boldsymbol{Z}_i$. For modelling the time-to-event in terms of covariates, often researchers consider the hazard function $h(t; X, \boldsymbol{Z})$ defined in terms of covariates. Suppose that from some source, $f_{x|x^*,z}(X|X^*, \boldsymbol{Z})$ is known. Then the likelihood function based on the data $(V_i, \Delta_i, X_i^*, \boldsymbol{Z}_i)$, $i = 1, \ldots, n$ is

$$\mathcal{L} = \prod_{i=1}^{n} \int \{h(V_i, X_i, \boldsymbol{Z}_i)\}^{\Delta_i} \exp\{-\int_0^{V_i} h(u, X_i, \boldsymbol{Z}_i)du\} f(X_i|X_i^*, \boldsymbol{Z}_i)dX_i.$$

In the proportional proportional hazard model,

$$h(t; X, \boldsymbol{Z}) = h_0(t) \exp(X\beta_1 + \boldsymbol{Z}^T \boldsymbol{\beta}_2),$$

where $h_0(t)$ is the baseline hazard function while $\beta_1$ and $\boldsymbol{\beta}_2$ are interpreted as the log-hazard risk parameters for $X$ and $\boldsymbol{Z}$, and the corresponding likelihood function is

$$\begin{aligned}\mathcal{L} &= \prod_{i=1}^{n} \int \{h_0(V_i) \exp(\beta_1 X_i + \boldsymbol{\beta}_2^T \boldsymbol{Z}_i)\}^{\Delta_i} \\ &\quad \times \exp\{-\exp(\beta_1 X_i + \boldsymbol{\beta}_2^T \boldsymbol{Z}_i) \int_0^{V_i} h_0(u)du\} f(X_i|X_i^*, \boldsymbol{Z}_i)dX_i.\end{aligned}$$

If a parametric model is adopted for $h_0(t)$, such as $h_0(t) = \gamma t^{\eta-1}$, then the entire problem becomes parametric, and one can then put a proper prior distribution on the parameters, and carry out Bayesian inference. If $h_0(t)$ is left unspecified, then one can put Gamma process prior with independent increment on the cumulative baseline hazard, $H_0(t) = \int_0^t h_0(u)du$ (Sinha et al., 2015). A general nonparametric Bayesian treatment of the survival function using neutral to the right (NTR) processes can be found in Hjort (1990).

One particular interest was when the effect of $X$ was left unspecified. This is a problem of nonparametric regression and has a lot of applications in the medical field where the interest is in understanding the pattern of association. Cheng and Crainiceanu (2009) considered this nonparametric regression problem in survival analysis in the presence of covariate measurement error. They were motivated by the ARIC study, a multi-purpose large epidemiologic study, where one of the goals was to find association between the time to chronic kidney disease (CKD) and the true glomerular filtration rate (GFR) of the kidney. The true GFR was never observed, rather eGFR was observed that was treated as the proxy for GFR. So, they considered the following hazard function,

$$h(t; X, \boldsymbol{Z}) = h_0(t) \exp\{g(X) + \boldsymbol{Z}^T \boldsymbol{\beta}_2\},$$

where $g$ was assumed to be a sufficiently smooth function, and the goal was estimation of $g$ and $\boldsymbol{\beta}_2$. They had assumed that $X_i^* = X_i + U_i$, where $U_i \sim$ Normal$(0, \sigma_u^2)$, and the value of $\sigma_u^2$ was assumed to be known. In fact, the error variability $\sigma_u^2$ was estimated separately based on replicated measurements of eGFR in the third National Health and Nutrition Examination Survey (NHANES III). They approximated $g(X)$ by

$$g_a(X) = \sum_{r=1}^{K_1} B_r(X)\beta_{x,r},$$

where $B_1(X), \ldots, B_{K_1}(X)$ are $K_1$ B-spline basis functions based on a given set of knot points chosen by practitioners, and $\boldsymbol{\beta}_x = (\beta_{x,1}, \ldots, \beta_{x,K_1})^T$ are the corresponding coefficients that need to be estimated from the data. Particularly, they assumed a priori

$$\begin{aligned}&\beta_{x,r} \sim \text{Normal}(2\beta_{x,r-1} - \beta_{x,r-2}, \lambda_\beta^2) \text{ for } r = 3, \ldots, K_1;\\&\beta_{x,2} \sim \text{Normal}(0, \lambda_{b0}^2),\ \beta_{x,1} \sim \text{Normal}(0, \lambda_{b0}^2),\end{aligned}$$

where $\lambda_{b0}^2$ was set to a very large number so that prior distribution of $\beta_{x,1}$ and $\beta_{x,2}$ are effectively noninformative while the prior for $\boldsymbol{\beta}_x$ is proper. Here $\lambda_\beta^2$ acts as the smoothing parameter, and they have used an inverse-gamma prior on this parameter. They approximated the logarithm of the baseline hazard using splines

$$\log\{h_0(t)\} \approx \sum_{r=1}^{K_2} B_r(t)\gamma_r,$$

where $B_1(t), \ldots, B_{K_2}(t)$ denote the spline basis functions based on a given set of knot points on the time interval $[0, \tau]$. For estimating the logarithm of baseline hazard by penalizing a *large* change (that is measured via the first derivative), authors proposed the following prior on the coefficients $\boldsymbol{\gamma} = (\gamma_1, \ldots, \gamma_{K_2})^T$:

$$\gamma_r \sim \text{Normal}(\gamma_{r-1}, \lambda_\gamma^2) \text{ for } r = 2, \ldots, K_2,\ \gamma_1 \sim \text{Normal}(0, \lambda_{g0}^2).$$

Following the above arguments related to $\boldsymbol{\beta}_x$, $\lambda_{g0}^2$ was also set to a very large number, and an inverse-gamma prior was used on the smoothing parameter $\lambda_\gamma^2$. Under the assumption that the latent $X$ given $\boldsymbol{Z}$ follows Normal$(\mu_0 + \boldsymbol{\mu}_1^T\boldsymbol{Z}, \sigma_x^2)$, their likelihood becomes

$$\begin{aligned}\mathcal{L} &= \prod_{i=1}^{n}\int \exp\{\sum_{r=1}^{K_2} B_r(V_i)\gamma_r + \sum_{r=1}^{K_1} B_r(X)\beta_{x,r} + \boldsymbol{\beta}_2^T\boldsymbol{Z}_i\}\\&\quad\times \exp\left[-\exp\{\sum_{r=1}^{K_1} B_r(X)\beta_{x,r} + \boldsymbol{\beta}_2^T\boldsymbol{Z}_i\}\int_0^{V_i}\exp\{\sum_{r=1}^{K_2} B_r(u)\gamma_r\}du\right]\\&\quad\times \exp\left\{-\frac{(X_i^* - X)^2}{2\sigma_u^2}\right\}\times\frac{1}{\sqrt{2\pi\sigma_x^2}}\exp\left\{-\frac{(X - \mu_0 - \boldsymbol{\mu}_1^T\boldsymbol{Z}_i)^2}{2\sigma_x^2}\right\}dX.\end{aligned}$$

Then they used normal prior on $\boldsymbol{\beta}_2$, $\mu_0$, $\boldsymbol{\mu}_1$, and an inverse-gamma prior on $\sigma_x^2$. Finally, Gibbs sampling technique was used to sample all the parameters and the latent $X_i, i = 1, \ldots, n$. Numerically they assessed the sensitivity of their approach towards the number of knot points through the average mean squared error of estimation of the nonparametric curves.

Next we consider the accelerated failure time model, where logarithm of the actual time-to-event $T$ is modeled as a linear function of the covariates. The model is

$$\log(T) = \beta_1 X + \boldsymbol{\beta}_2^T \boldsymbol{Z} + e,$$

where $e$ denotes the residual error, and $\beta_1$ and $\boldsymbol{\beta}_2$ are the regression parameters. Compared to the instantaneous hazard interpretation of parameters of the Cox model, here $\beta_1$ and $\boldsymbol{\beta}_2$ can simply be interpreted as the regression parameters associated with $X$ and $\boldsymbol{Z}$ for the mean of $\log(T)$. If a *regular* parametric distribution is assumed for $e$, then the problem becomes a parametric model, and the model parameters can be estimated by maximizing the parametric likelihood. However, any misspecification in the distribution of $e$ will result in biased regression parameter estimates. Therefore, researchers have developed methods where $e$ is assumed to follow an arbitrary distribution independent of $X$ and $\boldsymbol{Z}$ (Christensen and Johnson, 1988; Walker and Mallick, 1999). Estimation of $\boldsymbol{\beta}$ while $e$ is left unspecified is difficult due to the fact that the residual is unobserved and more over for censored subjects available information is sparse. Without any doubt the analysis becomes more complex when covariate $X$ is measured with uncertainties. Sinha and Wang (2017) proposed a Bayesian method for estimating the regression parameter when the observed data are $(V_i, \Delta_i, X_{i,1}^*, \ldots, X_{i,m}^*, \boldsymbol{Z}_i)$, where $X_{i,j}^*$ are assumed to be unbiased surrogates for the latent $X_i$. This is a significant work because three latent components, the distribution of measurement error, the distribution of the unobserved $X$, and the distribution of the residual error $e$, were modelled nonparametricaly to make the method completely robust. They assumed classical additive measurement error model, $X_{i,j}^* = X_i + U_{i,j}$, where the measurement errors $U_{i,j} \overset{iid}{\sim} F_u$. Other than assuming mean zero and finite variance, no other restriction was used on $F_u$. The corresponding density $f_u(\cdot) = dF_u(\cdot)/du$ was modeled using a centered Dirichlet process mixture of normal distributions. For scalable computation they restricted the Dirichlet process to a finite but large number of mixing components. In terms of notations, $U_{i,j} = X_{i,j}^* - X_i \sim \text{Normal}(\theta_{1,i,j,u}, \theta_{2,i,j,u})$, and $\boldsymbol{\theta}_{i,j,u} = (\theta_{1,i,j,u}, \theta_{2,i,j,u})^T$ follows a random distribution $P_u$, and $P_u$ is assumed to follow finite-dimensional centered Dirichlet process prior denoted by $CDP_{N_u}(\alpha_{0u}, H_{0u})$, where $\alpha_{0u}$, $H_{0u}$ and $N_u$ denote the precision parameter, the base probability measure, and the number of mixing components, respectively. Note that $\alpha_{0u}$ governs the variability of the random probability $P_u(A)$

around its mean $H_{0u}(A)$. With the above specification they wrote:

$$\begin{aligned} f_u(X^*_{i,j} - X_i) &= \sum_{k=1}^{N_u} \frac{p_{k,u}}{\sqrt{2\pi\theta_{2,i,j,u}}} \exp\Big\{-\frac{(X_i - \theta_{1,i,j,u})^2}{2\theta_{2,i,j,u}}\Big\} I(\boldsymbol{\theta}_{i,j,u} = \boldsymbol{\theta}^*_{k,u}); \\ (p_{1,u}, \ldots, p_{N_u,u}) &\sim \text{Dirichlet}(\alpha_u/N_u, \ldots, \alpha_u/N_u); \\ \boldsymbol{\theta}^*_{k,u} &= \boldsymbol{\theta}^\dagger_{k,u} - \sum_{k=1}^{N_u} p_{k,u}\boldsymbol{\theta}^\dagger_{k,u}; \\ \boldsymbol{\theta}^\dagger_{k,u} &\sim H_{0u}. \end{aligned}$$

The mean zero assumption on the distribution of measurement error is needed for identifying the distribution of $X$ based on the surrogate measurements (Schennach, 2004). Next they modeled the distribution of $X$ given $\boldsymbol{Z}$, and the distribution of $e$ as a finite-dimensional Dirichlet process mixture of normal distributions. They assumed, $X|\boldsymbol{Z} \sim \text{Normal}(\theta_{1,i,x} + \boldsymbol{\mu}_1^T\boldsymbol{Z}, \theta_{2,i,x})$, $\boldsymbol{\theta}_{i,x} = (\theta_{1,i,x}, \theta_{2,i,x}) \sim P_x$, and the random probability measure $P_x$ follows $DP_{N_x}(\alpha_{0x}, H_{0x})$. Next, they assumed, $e_i|\boldsymbol{\theta}_{i,e} = (\theta_{1,i,e}, \theta_{2,i,e}) \sim \text{Normal}(\theta_{1,i,e}, \theta_{2,i,e})$, $\boldsymbol{\theta}_{i,e} \sim P_e$, and $P_e \sim DP_{N_e}(\alpha_{0e}, H_{0e})$. In these cases, one can also write the density of $X$ and $e$ as finite mixture of normals with random mixing weight and random parameters of the normal components. Thus,

$$\begin{aligned} f_x(X_i|\boldsymbol{Z}_i) &= \sum_{k=1}^{N_u} \frac{p_{k,x}}{\sqrt{2\pi\theta_{2,i,x}}} \exp\Big\{-\frac{(X_i - \theta_{1,i,x} - \boldsymbol{\mu}_1^T\boldsymbol{Z}_i)^2}{2\theta_{2,i,x}}\Big\} I(\boldsymbol{\theta}_{i,x} = \boldsymbol{\theta}^*_{k,x}); \\ (p_{1,x}, \ldots, p_{N_x,x}) &\sim \text{Dirichlet}(\alpha_x/N_x, \ldots, \alpha_x/N_x); \\ \boldsymbol{\theta}^*_{k,x} &\sim H_{0x}; \\ f_e(e_i) &= \sum_{k=1}^{N_e} \frac{p_{k,e}}{\sqrt{2\pi\theta_{2,i,e}}} \exp\Big\{-\frac{(e_i - \theta_{1,i,e})^2}{2\theta_{2,i,e}}\Big\} I(\boldsymbol{\theta}_{i,e} = \boldsymbol{\theta}^*_{k,e}); \\ (p_{1,e}, \ldots, p_{N_e,e}) &\sim \text{Dirichlet}(\alpha_e/N_e, \ldots, \alpha_e/N_e); \\ \boldsymbol{\theta}^*_{k,e} &\sim H_{0e}; \end{aligned}$$

and $e_i = \log(T_i) - \beta_1 X_i - \boldsymbol{\beta}_2^T\boldsymbol{Z}_i$. Statistical inference was made based on the likelihood

$$\begin{aligned} \mathcal{L}_{\text{obs}} &= \prod_{i=1}^{n} \int S_e^{1-\Delta_i}(\log(V_i) - \beta_1 X_i - \boldsymbol{\beta}_2^T\boldsymbol{Z}_i) f_e^{\Delta_i}(\log(V_i) - \beta_1 X_i - \boldsymbol{\beta}_2^T\boldsymbol{Z}_i) \\ &\quad \times f_x(X_i|\boldsymbol{Z}_i) \prod_{j=1}^{m} f_u(X^*_{i,j} - X_i) dX_i. \end{aligned}$$

The proposed method proceeded after specifying a prior distribution for all parameters and hyperparameters. Bayesian MCMC mechanism was used to sample from the posterior distribution. Importantly, along with the parameters, in each MCMC iteration unobserved $X_i$, $i = 1 = 1, \ldots, n$ were sampled from their full conditional distributions. To avoid the computation of $S_e(\tau) = \int_{\tau}^{\infty} f_e(\cdot)d\cdot$, for the right censored subjects, the latent time-to-event $T_i$ was sampled from the truncated normal distribution with mean $\beta_1 X_i + \boldsymbol{\beta}_2^T \boldsymbol{Z}_i + \theta_{1,i,e}$ and variance $\theta_{2,i,e}$.

The performance of the proposed method was judged and compared with the naive, regression calibration, and the simulation and extrapolation (SIMEX) approach in extensive simulation studies. They considered different distributions for $e$, $U$, and $X$ given $\boldsymbol{Z}$. Overall the proposed method performed the best compared to the other approaches. They even showed the widely used SIMEX approach can perform worse. Particularly, when $X$ follows a non-normal distribution with variance 1, the measurement error variance is 1, and 25% subjects are right censored, the bias of the proposed method is much smaller than that of the SIMEX approach with comparable variances. Next, they applied their method to analyze a dataset from an AIDS clinical trial, where the interest was to find association between the time to AIDS or death from the time treatment started among HIV positive patients and four treatments and the baseline CD4 count. Note that accurate measurement of CD4 count cannot be made, therefore this measurement uncertainty is assessed through multiple measurements of the CD4 counts at the baseline.

Next we consider high-throughput data in survival analysis. With the advancement of high throughput technology, genetic or molecular level information is becoming abundant, and making a connection between genetic and clinical level information is a desirable research direction. Towards that goal, Tadesse et al. (2005) analyzed a DNA microarray dataset to find association between several genes (more than 12,000 genes) and the time-to-relapse of acute lymphoblastic leukemia after the patients received conventional intensive combination chemotherapy. GeneChip array measures abundance of mRNA corresponding to a gene, and it is measured via 11-20 probe pairs. Each probe pair consists of a perfect match (PM) and a mis-match (MM) probe. The difference between the intensities of PM and MM is the measure of the abundance. Suppose that for a specific gene $g$, $PM_{i,k}$ and $MM_{i,k}$ denote the intensities for the $k$th probe pair for subject $i$, and they were assumed to follow the following model (Li and Wong, 2001),

$$PM_{i,k} = \nu_k + \theta_i \alpha_k + \theta_i \phi_k + \epsilon_{i,k},\ MM_{i,k} = \nu_k + \theta_i \alpha_k + \epsilon^*_{i,k},$$

where $k = 1, \ldots, K$, and $i = 1, \ldots, n$. Note that $K$ is the number of probe pairs, and $n$ denotes the number of subjects in the study. Consequently the model for the observed difference was

$$PM_{i,k} - MM_{i,k} = \theta_i \phi_k + e_{i,k},$$

where random $e_{i,k}$'s ($= \epsilon_{i,k} - \epsilon^*_{i,k}$) were assumed to follow Normal$(0, \sigma_e^2)$. Parameters $\theta_i$ and $\phi_k$ were estimated iteratively with the constraint $\sum_{k=1}^{K} \phi_k^2 = K$. Denote the estimator of $\theta_i$ by $\widehat{\theta}_i$. Tadesse et al. (2005) treated $\widehat{\theta}_i$ as the surrogate for $\theta_i$, and put their relation in the additive measurement error model framework, $\widehat{\theta}_i = \theta_i + U_i$, $U_i \sim \text{Normal}[0, \text{var}(\widehat{\theta}_i)]$, and assumed that the density of $\theta_i$, $f(\theta_i) \propto 1$. Next, they modeled the hazard of the time-to-relapse in terms of $\theta_i$

$$h(t|\theta_i) = h_0(t)\exp(\beta\theta_i),$$

where $\beta$ is the unadjusted effect of gene $g$, while $h_0(t)$ denotes the baseline hazard function. They divided the entire time interval $[0, \tau]$ into $J$ non-overlapping sets, $(0, \tau_1], (\tau_1, \tau_2], \ldots, (\tau_{J-1}, \tau_J]$ $(\tau_J = \tau)$ so that each subinterval contains some failure times. Next they assumed that $h_0(t)$ is $h_j$ in the $j$th interval. Suppose that $d_j$ denotes the number of failures in the $j$th interval, and the observed data are $(V_i, \Delta_i, \widehat{\theta}_i), i = 1, \ldots, n$. That lead them to consider the following likelihood involving the latent variables $\theta_i$'s

$$\begin{aligned}\mathcal{L} \propto & \prod_{j=1}^{J} h_j^{d_j} \exp(\sum_{i=1}^{n} \theta_i\beta\Delta_i) \\ & \times \exp\left[-\sum_{i=1}^{n}\left\{\sum_j h_j I(\tau_{j-1} \le V_i)\exp(\theta_i\beta) + \frac{1}{2\text{var}(\widehat{\theta}_i)}(\widehat{\theta}_i - \theta_i)^2\right\}\right].\end{aligned}$$

They used normal prior on $\beta$ and independent gamma prior on each of the $h_j$ parameters. Then using the Gibbs sampling procedure they sampled $\beta, h_1, \ldots, h_J$, and latent $\theta_1, \ldots, \theta_n$ in each iteration. The main interest was in testing $H_0 : \beta = 0$ versus $H_a : \beta \neq 0$, and for that they computed the posterior probability of the null hypothesis. They calculated the posterior probability of the null hypothesis for each of the 12,625 genes (probe sets) separately.

Usually one would reject the null hypothesis for the $g$th gene, if $\text{pr}(H_{0g}|\text{data})$, the posterior probability of the null hypothesis corresponding to the $g$th gene, is small. However, to control the false discovery rate to $\alpha$, they rejected the null hypothesis for the $g$th gene if $\text{pr}(H_{0g}|\text{data}) < \varepsilon$, where $\varepsilon$ is the largest values such that $C(\varepsilon)/|D(\varepsilon)| \le \alpha$, and $C(\varepsilon) = E(\#\text{false discoveries}|\text{data}) = \sum_{g \in D(\varepsilon)} \text{pr}(H_{0g}|\text{data})$, and $D(\varepsilon) = \{g : \text{pr}(H_{0g}|\text{data}) \le \varepsilon\}$.

With the similar goal, Shen et al. (2008) proposed a method to find the association between a tumor-specific protein expression and a clinical outcome. The protein expression was measured via tissue microarray (TMA). TMA data for a tumor may come from multiple cores, and each core contains up to 1000 tiny biopsy elements. Let $X_i$ be the true expression for the $i$th tumor, and $X^*_{i,j}$ be the observed expression for the $j$th core of the $i$th tumor. They assumed that $X^*_{i,j} = X_i + U_{i,j}$, $j = 1, \ldots, r_i$, and $i = 1, \ldots, n$, and $U_{i,j} \overset{iid}{\sim} \text{Normal}(0, \sigma_u^2)$. The goal was estimation of the parameters of the hazard model of the recurrence time $h(t|X, \boldsymbol{Z}) = h_0(t)\exp(\beta_1 X + \boldsymbol{\beta}_2^T \boldsymbol{Z})$, when $X^*$'s are observed in lieu of $X$. Here $\boldsymbol{Z}$ denotes some clinical covariates. As a first step, they replaced the unobserved $X_i$ by $E(X_i|\boldsymbol{X}^*_i, \boldsymbol{Z}_i)$, where $\boldsymbol{X}^*_i = (X^*_{i,1}, \ldots, X^*_{i,r_i})^T$, and then carried out the model parameter estimation. To compute the above expectation they took both empirical Bayes and full Bayes approaches, and in both cases they modeled

$$X_i = \gamma_0 + \gamma_1^T \boldsymbol{Z}_i + v_i, \tag{4}$$

where $v_i \sim \text{Normal}(0, \sigma_v^2)$. In the second approach, they modeled the number of replications $r_i$ as a Binomial random variable with maximum value $K_i$, denoting the number of cores of TMA, and the success probability was allowed to depend on the covariate $\boldsymbol{Z}$. Then the predicted value of $X_i$ was calculated by $E_{(r_i,K_i)}\{E(X_i|\boldsymbol{X}_i^*, \boldsymbol{Z}_i)\}$, where the outer expectation was on the joint distribution of $r_i$ and $K_i$. Additionally, they considered a joint modelling approach, where the hazard function for the $i$th subject was modelled as $h(t|v_i, \boldsymbol{Z}_i) = h_0(t)\exp(\beta_1 v_i + \boldsymbol{\beta}_2^T \boldsymbol{Z}_i)$, and $v_i$ was the random effect involved in Equation (4). They considered different choices of $h_0(t)$, piecewise constant, and polynomial function of $t$. Their simulation results indicate advantages of the joint modelling approach over the naive method and other two-stage approaches.

## 24.5 Conclusions

Modern computational techniques made Bayesian methods popular everywhere. Consequently, the Bayesian literature on covariate measurement error is growing day-by-day. To cover a broad spectrum of the literature we divided the chapter into several sections, and presented some novel ideas in each section. There could be two types of innovations in any Bayesian approach, one in terms of the model that depends on the available data, and two in terms of computational algorithms. Due to limited space we were not able to discuss all related works. Now, we discuss some areas that require unique Bayesian modelling for handling uncertainties in measured variables.

There are recent attempts at combining different kinds of high-throughput data for better understanding of diseases. There has been some Bayesian work (Cassese et al., 2014; Choi et al., 2010), for finding association between gene expression and the DNA copy number aberration that is believed to hold clues for cancer diseases, and genetic disorders. When the copy number is assessed via comparative genomic hybridization (CGH) array, a measurement error model is needed to make the connection between the surrogate CGH and underlying copy numbers, otherwise the results will be biased. Likewise, for an integrated approach involving next generation sequencing (NGS), microarray, or copy number data, one needs a correct latent variable model that includes the measurement error model as a special case (Blomquist et al., 2015; Nielsen et al., 2011). Particularly, the NGS technology allows us to get huge amounts of RNA-seq data at a low cost. NGS generates millions of short reads, and the main task is to align the reads to a unique genomic location and then quantify the gene expression. Although a majority of the reads are aligned to a unique genomic location, a good proportion of them cannot be aligned to a unique location on the genome. These later groups of reads are aligned to multiple locations, and these reads are called multireads. Instead of ignoring the multireads, a proper method should take into account all the reads and employ an uncertainty model for the multireads (Ji et al., 2011).

Nowadays there is a surge of big data research in engineering, marketing, medical sciences, and social sciences. It would be interesting to see how the measurement error issue takes shape in this emerging field of new research. Specifically, a Bayesian variable selection approach in a high-dimensional or ultra high-dimensional problem with covariate measurement error would be an interesting topic of further research.

A Bayesian approach is a natural choice for dealing with inherent missing values in the causal inference based on observational studies. However, to the best of our knowledge, Bayesian methods have not been much explored in the context of measurement error in the confounding variables, treatment variables, mediation variables - that is commonly encountered in the causal inference (Imai and Yamamoto, 2010; Pearl, 2010).

## Acknowledgment

The author likes to thank Paul Gustafson for his valuable suggestions to improve English in this article.

## References

Asirvatham, J. R., Moses, V., and Bjornson, L. (2013). Errors in potassium measurement: A laboratory perspective for the clinician. *North American Journal of Medical Sciences*, 5, 255-259.

Bartlett, J. W. and Keogh, R. H. (2017). Bayesian correction for covariate measurement error: A frequentist evaluation and comparison with regression calibration. *Statistical Methods in Medical Research.*

Berry, S. M., Carroll, R. J., and Ruppert, D. (2002). Bayesian smoothing and regression splines for measurement error problems. *Journal of the American Statistical Association*, 97, 160-169.

Biemer, P. P., Groves, R. M., Lyberg, L. E., Mathiowetz, N. A., and Sudman, S. (2004). *Measurement errors in surveys.* John Wiley & Sons.

Blomquist, T., Crawford, E. L., Yeo, J., Zhang, X., and Willey, J. C. (2015). Control for stochastic sampling variation and qualitative sequencing error in next generation sequencing. *Biomolecular Detection and Quantification*, 5, 30-33.

Boonstra, P. S., Taylor, J. M. G., and Mukherjee, B. (2013). Incorporating auxiliary information for improved prediction in high-dimensional datasets: An ensemble of shrinkage approaches. *Biostatistics*, 14, 259-272.

Cassese, A., Guindani, M., Tadesse, M. G., Falciani, F., and Vannucci, M. (2014). A hierarchical Bayesian model for inference of copy number variants and their association to gene expression. *Annals of Applied Statistics*, 8, 148-175.

Cheng, Y. J. and Crainiceanu, C. M. (2009). Cox models with smooth functional effect of covariates measured with error. *Journal of the American Statistical Association*, 104, 1144-1154.

Choi, H., Qin, Z., and Ghosh, D. (2010). A double-layered mixture for the joint analysis of DNA copy number and gene expression data. *Journal of Computational Biologyi*, 17, 121-137.

Christensen, R. and Johnson, W. (1988). Modelling accelerated failure time with a Dirichlet process. *Biometrika*, 75, 693-704.

Dellaportas, P. and Stephens, D. A. (1995). Bayesian analysis of errors-in-variables regression models. *Biometrics*, 51, 1085-1095.

Escobar, M. D. and West, M. (1995). Bayesian density estimation and inference using mixtures. *Journal of the American Statistical Association*, 90, 577-588.

Eubank, R. (1999). *Nonparametric Regression and Spline Smoothing.* Marcel Dekker, New York.

Fan, J. and Truong, Y. K. (1993). Nonparametric regression with errors in variables. *The Annals of Statistics*, 21, 1900-1925.

Fox, X. and Glass, X. (2003). Bayesian modelling of measurement error in predictor variables using item response theory. *Psychometrika*, 68, 169-191.

Griffiths, T. L. and Ghahramani, Z. (2011). The Indian Buffet process: An introduction and review. *Journal of Machine Learning Research*, 12, 1185-1224.

Gustafson, P. (2004). *Measurement Error and Misclassification in Statistics and Epidemiology: Impacts and Bayesian Adjustments.* Chapman & Hall.

Gustafson, P., Le, N. D., and Vallée, M. (2002). A Bayesian approach to case-control studies with errors in covariables. *Biostatistics*, 3, 229-243.

Hjort, N. L. (1990). Nonparametric Bayes estimators based on beta processes in models for life history data. *Annal of Statistics*, 18, 1259-1294.

Imai, K. and Yamamoto, T. (2010). Causal inference with differential measurement error: Nonparametric identification and sensitivity analysis. *American Journal of Political Science*, 54, 543-560.

Ishwaran, H. and James, L. F. (2001). Gibbs sampling methods for stick-breaking priors. *Journal of the American Statistical Association*, 96, 161-173.

Ji, Y., Xu, Y., Zhang, Q., Tsui, K. W., Yuan, Y., Norris, C. J., Liang, S., and Liang, H. (2011). BM-map: Bayesian mapping of multireads for next-generation sequencing data. *Biometrics*, 67, 1215-1224.

Kelly, B. C. (2007). Some aspects of measurement error in linear regression of astronomical data. *The Astrophysical Journal*, 665, 1489-1506.

Lachin, J. M. (2004). The role of measurement reliability in clinical trials. *Clinical Trials*, 1, 553-566.

Lee, P. H. and Burstyn, I. (2016). Identification of confounder in epidemiologic data contaminated by measurement error in covariates. *BMC Medical Research Methodology*, 16:54.

Li, C. and Wong, W. H. (2001). Model-based analysis of oligonucleotide arrays: Expression index computation and outlier detection. *Proceedings of the National Academy of Science*, 98, 31-33.

Mallick, B. K. and Gelfand, A. (1996). Semiparametric errors-in-variables models: A Bayesian approach. *Journal of Statistical Planning and Inference*, 52, 307-321.

Müller, P. and Roeder, C. (1997). A Bayesian semiparametric models with covariates measured with error. *Biometrika*, 84, 523-537.

Neal, R. (2011). MCMC using Hamiltonian dynamics. In *Handbook of Markov Chain Monte Carlo.* Chapman and Hall-CRC Press, Boca Raton.

Neal, R. M. (2000). Markov chain sampling methods for Dirichlet process mixture models. *Journal of Computational and Graphical Statistics*, 9, 249-265.

Neal, R. M. (2003). Density modeling and clustering using Dirichlet diffusion trees. *Bayesian Statistics*, 7, 619-629.

Nielsen, R., Paul, J. S., Albrechtsen, A. and Song, Y. S. (2011). Genotype and SNP calling from next-generation sequencing data. *Nature Reviews Genetics*, 12, 443-451.

Pearl, J. (2010). On measurement bias in causal inference. *In Proceedings of the 26th Conference on Uncertaintyand Artificial Intelligence*, Eds. P. Grunwald and P. Spirtes, pp. 425-432. Corvallis, WA: AUAI Press. Available at: http://ftp.cs.ucla.edu/pub/statser/r357.pdf.

Prentice, R. L. and Pike, R. (1979). Logistic disease incidence models and case-control studies. *Biometrika*, 66, 403-411.

Rabe-Hesketh, R., Pickles, A., and Skrondal, A. (2003). Correcting for covariate measurement error in logistic regression using nonparametric maximum likelihood estimation. *Statistical Modelling*, 3, 215-232.

Richardson, S. and Gilks, W. R. (1993). Conditional independence models for epidemiological studies with covariate measurement error. *Statistics in Medicine*, 12, 1703-1722.

Schennach, S. M. (2004). Nonparametric regression in the presence of measurement error. *Econometric Theory*, 20, 1046-1093.

Schmidt, C. H. and Rosner, B. (1993). A Bayesian approach to logistic regression models having measurement error following a mixture distribution. *Statistics in Medicine*, 12, 1141-1153.

Shen, R., Ghosh, D., and Taylor, J. M. G. (2008). Modeling intra-tumor protein expression heterogeneity in tissue microarray experiments. *Statistics in Medicine*, 27, 1944-1959.

Sinha, A., Chi, Z., and Chen, M.-H. (2015). Bayesian inference of hidden Gamma wear process model for survival data with ties. *Statistica Sinica*, 25, 1613-1635.

Sinha, S., Mallick, B. K., Kipnis, V., and Carroll, R. J. (2010). Semiparametric Bayesian analysis of nutritional epidemiology data in the presence of measurement error. *Biometrics*, 66, 444-454.

Sinha, S. and Wang, S. (2017). Semiparametric Bayesian analysis of censored linear regression with errors-in-covariates. *Statistical Methods in Medical Research*, 26, 1389-1415.

Tadesse, M. G., Ibrahim, J. G., Gentleman, R., Chiaretti, S., Ritz, J., and Foa, R. (2005). Bayesian error-in-variable survival model for the analysis of GeneChip arrays. *Biometrics*, 61, 488-497.

Teh, Y. W., Newman, D., and Welling, M. (2007). A collapsed variational Bayesian inference algorithm for latent Dirichlet allocation. *Advances in Neural Information Processing Systems*, 19, 1378-1385.

Walker, S. and Mallick, B. K. (1999). A Bayesian semiparametric accelerated failure time model. *Biometrics*, 55, 477-483.

# Author Index

# *Subject Index*

Note: Locators in *italics* represent figures and **bold** indicate tables in the text.

## M